Seventh Edition

EXERCISE PHYSIOLOGY

LABORATORY MANUAL

William C. Beam

California State University, Fullerton

Gene M. Adams

California State University, Fullerton

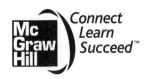

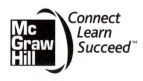

Published by McGraw-Hill, an imprint of The McGraw-Hill Companies, Inc., 1221 Avenue of the Americas, New York, NY 10020. Copyright © 2014. All rights reserved. No part of this publication may be reproduced or distributed in any form or by any means, or stored in a database or retrieval system, without the prior written consent of The McGraw-Hill Companies, Inc., including, but not limited to, in any network or other electronic storage or transmission, or broadcast for distance learning.

This book is printed on acid-free paper.

3 4 5 6 7 8 QVS/QVS 19 18 17 16 15

ISBN 978–0–07–802265–4
MHID 0–07–802265–7

Senior Vice President, Products & Markets: *Kurt L. Strand*
Vice President, General Manager, Products & Markets: *Michael Ryan*
Vice President, Content Production & Technology Services: *Kimberly Meriwether David*
Executive Director of Development: *Lisa Pinto*
Managing Director: *Gina Boedeker*
Brand Manager: *Bill Minick*
Managing Editor: *Sara Jaeger*
Marketing Specialist: *Alexandra Schultz*
Editorial Coordinator: *Adina Lonn*
Director, Content Production: *Terri Schiesl*
Senior Project Manager: *Joyce Watters*
Buyer: *Nichole Birkenholz*
Media Project Manager: *Sridevi Palani*
Cover Designer: *Studio Montage, St. Louis, MO*
Typeface: *10/12 Times Roman*
Compositor: *S4Carlisle Publishing Services*
Printer: *Quad/Graphics*

The Internet addresses listed in the text were accurate at the time of publication. The inclusion of a Web site does not indicate an endorsement by the authors or McGraw-Hill, and McGraw-Hill does not guarantee the accuracy of the information presented at these sites.

www.mhhe.com

CONTENTS

PREFACE

The seventh edition of *Exercise Physiology Laboratory Manual* is a comprehensive source of information for instructors and students interested in practical laboratory experiences related to the field of exercise physiology. The manual provides instruction on the measurement and evaluation of muscular strength, anaerobic fitness, aerobic fitness, cardiovascular function, respiratory function, flexibility, and body composition. Each chapter, written in a research format, provides the rationale underlying the test to be completed, includes detailed methods and up-to-date comparative data, and concludes with a discussion of the results based on published studies. *Homework* forms at the end of each chapter can be completed in preview of an upcoming lab or in review of a completed lab. *Lab Results* forms direct students on the collection of laboratory data and the calculation and evaluation of results. *Exercise Physiology Laboratory Manual* can be used as a stand-alone lab manual for a separate exercise physiology laboratory course. It can also serve, however, as a complement to any exercise physiology textbook to provide direction for laboratory experiences associated with an exercise physiology lecture course. And finally, it is an excellent reference source for a variety of other kinesiology courses, including those involved in measurement and evaluation, strength and conditioning, and exercise testing and prescription. The laboratory and field test experiences in this laboratory manual are designed to reinforce the basic principles learned in the lecture and laboratory course and to teach the fundamental skills of measurement and evaluation in the field of exercise physiology. Although specific equipment is described in the laboratory manual, the methods for each test are written as generically as possible, so that differing equipment and instrumentation can be used to conduct the tests. Much of the equipment used today in an exercise physiology laboratory is highly automated and provides instant results at the touch of a button. *Exercise Physiology Laboratory Manual* takes a more "old school" approach, assuming that more learning occurs when students are required to collect the raw data and conduct many of the calculations necessary to derive the final test results.

The Seventh Edition

The seventh edition of *Exercise Physiology Laboratory Manual* remains faithful to the roots established in the previous six editions over the last three decades. Readers of the manual will find that many hallmarks of the previous editions remain. Numerous changes have been made to the content in the seventh edition, however, and many up-to-date references have been added.

Features of the sixth edition remaining include:

- Written in a research format, the manual includes the rationale behind each laboratory test, detailed methods, comparative data, and a discussion of the results based on published studies.
- Accepted terminology and units of measure are used consistently throughout the manual.
- *Homework* forms are written to emphasize the content of the chapter. They can be completed prior to the lab as a preview of material, or can be done following the lab as a review of material.
- *Laboratory Results* forms are written to provide direction in the measurement and evaluation of laboratory data.
- *Accuracy Boxes* appear throughout the manual for those who want to examine the reliability, validity and objectivity of the tests performed.
- *Calibration Boxes* appear throughout the manual for those who want to go into further depth with the instruments.
- *Chapter Preview/Review boxes* in each chapter include questions to be answered by students either in preview of an upcoming lab or in review of a completed lab emphasize the chapter content and place more responsibility for learning on the students.

Significant changes made to the seventh edition include:

- Text changes made throughout the manual intended to make the manual more readable and understandable to students.
- Revised and new text in introduction, methods, and discussion sections throughout the manual to better describe the rationale of the tests, methodology of data collection, and significance of the results. Specific changes include new introductory material in Chapters 20, 21 and 23; changes to the methods sections of Chapters 8, 9, 13, 17 and 23; and newly written discussion sections in Chapters 8, 10, 11, 17, 20 and 23.
- Updated and newly added references to original research studies and other sources of information throughout the manual, especially in Chapters 1, 2, 3, 6, 8, 9, 13, 15, 19, 20, 23 and 24.
- Updated comparative data in numerous chapters, especially height and weight data in Chapter 3, comparative anaerobic fitness data in Chapter 10, comparative aerobic fitness data in Chapter 13, and additional lung function data in Chapter 20.
- Changes to numerous tables throughout the manual to make them more "user-friendly," especially tables in Chapters 3, 4, 6, 13, 14, 15 and 25.
- Changes to numerous *Chapter Preview/Review* boxes throughout the manual, especially in Chapters 4, 6, 7, 8, 9, 10, 22 and 24.
- Changes to *Homework* and *Lab Results* forms throughout the manual, especially in Chapters 10, 13, 14, 17 and 22.
- Other significant changes include the addition of alternate aerobic fitness tests in Chapters 13 and 14; changes in tables, figures and discussion in Chapter 17 related to rate-pressure product; addition of lung function comparative data for Asian-Americans in Chapter 20; addition of goniometry in Chapter 22; changes to methods and discussion in Chapter 23; and addition of waist-to-height ratio in Chapter 24.

Content and Organization

The material contained in *Exercise Physiology Laboratory Manual* is divided into eight parts, each of which describes a different type of physiological test or response. Part I, Orientation to Measurement in Exercise Physiology, includes chapters that introduce topics, terminology, variables (e.g., force, work, power), and units of measure (e.g., N, N·m, W) and describe the collection of basic data. Part II, Muscular Strength, includes chapters on the measurement of isotonic, isometric, and isokinetic strength. Emphasis is placed on testing and describing strength in both absolute and relative terms. Part III, Anaerobic Fitness, includes chapters on sprinting, jumping, and anaerobic cycling, stepping, and treadmill running. Numerous modes of testing are described so that the instructor or student can choose the most appropriate test to use based on the specific sport or activity of interest. Before administering any of these tests that require a high degree of physical effort, instructors should consider the health history of the participants (students). Participants (students) completing these tests should be free of disease (i.e., cardiovascular, pulmonary, metabolic); should have no signs or symptoms suggestive of disease (e.g., angina, shortness of breath, irregular heartbeat, dizziness, etc.); and should have few major risk factors for cardiovascular disease (i.e., cigarette smoking, hypertension, hyperlipidemia, diabetes, physical inactivity, obesity, and family history of disease). Appendix A and Appendix B include material that can be used to assess exercise risk.

Part IV, Aerobic Fitness, includes chapters on aerobic walking, jogging, running, stepping, and cycling and on the direct measurement of maximal oxygen consumption ($\dot{V}O_2$max). This part emphasizes the value of directly measuring $\dot{V}O_2$max and why $\dot{V}O_2$max is considered to be the one best laboratory test reflecting overall aerobic fitness. The health history of the participants should again be considered before performing any of these tests. Numerous modes of testing are described (e.g., walking, running, stepping), but the instructor may choose not to include all tests from every part.

Part V, Cardiovascular Function, includes chapters on resting and exercise blood pressure and on the resting and exercise electrocardiogram. Part VI, Respiratory Function, include chapters on resting lung volumes and exercise ventilation. Emphasis is placed on the measurement of lung function and identification of any restrictive or obstructive lung conditions the participant may possess at rest or during exercise. Part VII, Flexibility, includes a description and discussion of the measurement of lower body flexibility. Part VIII, Body Composition, includes chapters on assessing body composition by means of body mass index, girth, skinfolds, and hydrostatic weighing.

Homework and Lab Results Files on McGraw-Hill Online Learning Center Website

Files for every chapter in *Exercise Physiology Laboratory Manual, 7e,* are posted on the McGraw-Hill Online Learning Center website. The files are intended to assist in the instruction of a laboratory course. They can be projected for use during class and can be used by the instructor to grade homework forms and evaluate lab results.

The *Interactive Homework and Lab Results Files* include an Excel™ file for each chapter. Each file consists of 4 worksheets. Sheet 1 is the blank version of the *Homework* form for that chapter, formatted to fit a standard 8½" × 11" page when printed. Sheet 2 is the completed version with all calculations completed and fitness categories identified. The completed *Homework* form is convenient for grading student work. Sheet 3 is the blank version of the *Lab Results* form for that chapter. Sheet 4 is an "interactive" version of the form that can be used by the instructor to calculate results and identify fitness categories for any desired raw data. Simply insert any raw data into the highlighted areas and all calculations are performed automatically.

The *Instructional Files* include an Excel™ file for each chapter. The *Instructional Files* provide background information, rationale behind the use of the test in assessing fitness, and step-by-step instructions for completing the calculations. Each *Instructional File* consists of multiple worksheets. Sheet 1 is the blank *Homework* form for that chapter. The subsequent sheets provide step-by-step instructions regarding the calculations to help students understand the context of the calculations and results. The file can be projected during class to facilitate discussion of the fitness component being assessed. The final sheet is the completed *Homework* form.

The *Interactive Group Data Files* include an Excel™ file for each chapter. These files allow for collection and display of data collected on the entire class. Sheet 1 is a blank *Group Data* sheet that can be used to manually record data. Sheet 2 in an "interactive" version that can be used by the instructor to enter raw data for each student in the class. Simply enter new raw data over the values printed in blue and the file automatically calculates all results and identifies the corresponding fitness categories. The results can be projected for use during class and can be used by the instructor for grading student lab work. Sheet 3 is a sample data file that can be used for various purposes.

Philosophical Approach

Our philosophical approach to learning laboratory procedures is consistent with the following quote:

> A learner does not act without thinking and feeling, or think without acting and feeling, or feel without acting or thinking.[1]

To us, this means that teachers encourage students to be *active* during the laboratory session and not only administer the test but *feel* what it is like to be tested. Then teachers encourage students to *think* about their actions and feelings, so students can truly *know* the material.

Custom Version Available

To meet the needs of your specific course, you can create a customized version of *Exercise Physiology: Laboratory Manual* through McGraw-Hill Primis Custom Publishing. You can select the chapters you want, rearrange chapters, and personalize the manual by adding your own original content, including your own equipment list. Your customized content can be delivered to your students either electronically or as a print product. For more information, visit www.primisonline.com or contact your local McGraw-Hill sales representative.

---

[1] Barrow, H. M., & McGee, R. (1971). *A practical approach to measurement in physical education* (p. 145). Philadelphia: Lea & Febiger.

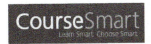

This text is available as an eTextbook from CourseSmart, a new way for faculty to find and review eTextbooks. It's also a great option for students who are interested in accessing their course materials digitally and saving money. CourseSmart offers thousands of the most commonly adopted textbooks across hundreds of courses from a wide variety of higher education publishers. It is the only place for faculty to review and compare the full text of a textbook online, providing immediate access without the environmental impact of requesting a print exam copy. At CourseSmart, students can save up to 50% off the cost of a print book, reduce their impact on the environment, and gain access to powerful web tools for learning, including full text search, notes and highlighting, and email tools for sharing notes between classmates. For further details contact your sales representative or go to www.coursesmart.com.

Acknowledgments

Every author must acknowledge that the knowledge, ability, motivation, and inspiration to write a work like this laboratory manual comes from many sources. It comes from former teachers, role models, colleagues, students, and family members. We are both especially appreciative of the students in our lab classes. We would like to acknowledge that the enthusiasm our students show in the lab inspires us to continue to teach and write.

From William Beam:

I am grateful to my parents for providing me the opportunity to begin my education at the College of Wooster, a small liberal arts college in my home state of Ohio. The basic science education I received in biology, chemistry, math, and physics prepared me well for graduate study. I took my first exercise physiology course from Dr. Edward Fox at The Ohio State University and it was during this course that I first got a sense of what I really wanted to do professionally. I am grateful also to my other graduate exercise physiology professors, including Dr. Robert Bartels and Dr. Timothy Kirby. I am especially grateful to my colleague of 23 years at Cal State Fullerton, Dr. Gene Adams. He provided me the opportunity to coauthor this manual, facilitated my involvement in the Southwest Chapter of the ACSM, and has simply been a wonderful colleague and friend. Thanks also go to my family including my wife, Terri, my son, Dan, and my daughter, Sara. I dedicate this book to each one of them and the love and support they have shown me over the course of these last 3 editions.

From Gene Adams:

My first teacher, Dr. Larry Morehouse, introduced me to exercise physiology and set the framework for my future knowledge in this field. My second teacher, Dr. Herbert deVries, contributed to my technical and research skills, while enhancing my knowledge and encouraging my involvement in the profession. My role model, Dr. Fred Kasch, showed me how to apply what I knew to the general public and to students. I am grateful to my colleagues from all parts of the country who contributed their encouragement and ideas. A big thank you goes to my wife, Janet, the illustrator for this manual, and to my son, Mannie, and my daughter, Shawn, who served as my wife's models.

Thanks also go to those who reviewed this manual:

Steven Devor, The Ohio State University
Cynthia Ferrara, University of Massachusetts Lowell
Marla Marie Graves, Arkansas State University
Jacalyn McComb, Texas Tech University
Susan Muller, Murray State University
Alexander Ng, Marquette University
Bulent Sokmen, Sonoma State University
Sean Walsh, Central Connecticut State University
Carena Winters, Slippery Rock University

INTRODUCTION AND TERMINOLOGY

Much of the terminology used to introduce and orient the beginning student to an exercise physiology course may be organized into the following categories: (1) components of fitness, (2) variables of interest, (3) statistical and evaluation terms, and (4) types of tests. Emphasis is placed on those fitness components, variables, terms, and tests that are included in this laboratory manual.

COMPONENTS OF FITNESS

Familiarization with fitness terms is essential for understanding the measurement of physical performance. Performance is often related to a person's fitness. One simple definition of physical fitness is "the ability to carry out physical activities satisfactorily."[16] Because the term *satisfactorily* has many interpretations, it behooves exercise physiologists to describe fitness more precisely in order to make the appropriate fitness measure. One perspective is to view fitness as having various components.[1] Some of the components of fitness include the following:

• Muscular strength and endurance
• Anaerobic fitness
• Aerobic fitness
• Flexibility
• Body composition

These purportedly independent fitness components are directed not only at exercise performance but also at diseases (e.g., cardiovascular) or functional disabilities (e.g., obesity, musculoskeletal pain) associated with hypokinetic (low activity) lifestyles.

Muscular Strength and Endurance

Muscular strength may be defined as the maximal force generated in one repetition at a given velocity of exercise. Strength is necessary for many functional tasks and activities of daily living across the life span. It is required for normal walking and running gait, climbing stairs, rising from a lying or seated position, and lifting and carrying objects. Strength is also an important contributor to higher intensity tasks associated with recreational and sporting events requiring sprinting, jumping, and throwing.

Strength tests included in this laboratory manual emphasize the measurement of one repetition maximum (1 RM), or the maximum amount of weight lifted or force

generated in a single repetition. The modes of measurement described involve various muscle actions, including isotonic, isometric, and isokinetic actions (Chapters 4 through 6).

Muscular endurance is a function of the muscle producing force over multiple consecutive contractions and can be assessed in time frames ranging from seconds, to minutes, to hours. Typical tests specifically geared to measure muscular endurance include timed push-ups and sit-ups; completing as many repetitions as possible of a specific load or weight (e.g., 15 lb dumbbell) or physical task (e.g., standing from a chair); or measuring the decline in peak torque over multiple repetitions with an isokinetic dynamometer. No specific tests of muscular endurance are included in this laboratory manual, but muscular endurance is a necessary fitness component for numerous tests, including tests of anaerobic fitness (Chapters 7 through 11) and aerobic fitness (Chapters 12 through 15).

Anaerobic Fitness

From a bioenergetic point of view, exercise and fitness may be categorized based upon the predominant metabolic pathways for producing adenosine triphosphate (ATP). The two anaerobic systems (the **phosphagen system** and the **glycolytic system**) produce ATP at high rates, but in relatively small amounts. Aerobic metabolism (or the aerobic system) produces ATP at a considerably lower rate but in essentially unlimited amounts.

The phosphagen system predominates for strength and power movements requiring anaerobic power and immediate maximal efforts of several seconds (< 15 s).[9] The force of these movements also depends upon the muscle mass and neuromuscular recruitment. The phosphagen system and glycolytic system together contribute substantially to activities requiring a combination of anaerobic power and anaerobic endurance that last approximately 15–30 s. The closer the exercise duration comes to 30 s, the greater the contribution from the glycolytic system.

The glycolytic system dominates for activities requiring anaerobic endurance that last approximately 30–60 s. The phosphagen system adds to the ATP being produced by the glycolytic system for maximally paced activities lasting just over 30 s, whereas the aerobic system contributes a meaningful amount of ATP for maximal effort activities lasting closer to 60 s.[21]

As exercise duration continues to increase, optimally sustained movements lasting between approximately 60 s (1 min) and 120 s (2 min) rely on substantial contributions from both the anaerobic and aerobic pathways. The ATP contribution from each pathway varies above and below 50 % of the total ATP, depending upon the duration. Shorter performances closer to 1 min will receive a greater (> 50 %) anaerobic contribution than longer all-out performances nearing 2 min, when > 50 % of the contribution comes from aerobic metabolism or the aerobic system. These types of activities result in high blood lactate levels indicating the significant involvement of the glycolytic system, along with elevated oxygen uptakes indicating the aerobic contribution to the exercise.

Aerobic Fitness

Aerobic metabolism, or the **aerobic system,** is the predominant pathway for ATP production in optimally paced exercise of duration longer than 3 min. Shorter duration activities from about 3 min to 60 min rely primarily on stored and dietary carbohydrates for ATP production. Longer duration activities, or prolonged exercise, lasting greater than 60 min, rely more on stored fats and dietary carbohydrate and also require more consideration of nutritional and hydration factors for successful performance than do shorter tasks.

Cardiorespiratory endurance depends on the level of **aerobic fitness** of the individual. In fact, the terms are sometimes used interchangeably. Cardiovascular function (including the control of heart rate, blood flow, and blood pressure) plays a fundamental role in the delivery of oxygen to working skeletal muscle. Respiratory function (including the control of breathing rate, tidal volume, and pulmonary ventilation) allows for the appropriate loading and unloading of oxygen and carbon dioxide from the circulating blood during exercise. The greater aerobic fitness an individual possesses, as indicated by the maximal oxygen uptake ($\dot{V}O_2$ max), the higher the cardiorespiratory endurance.

Many performance tests presented in this manual may be categorized based on their reliance on anaerobic or aerobic fitness (Table 1.1). Anaerobic fitness contributes greatly to 1 RM strength tests, sprint tests, vertical jump tests, and anaerobic cycling, stepping, and treadmill tests. And aerobic fitness contributes to numerous performance tests designed to measure cardiorespiratory endurance using walking, jogging, running, stepping, or cycling.

Flexibility

Flexibility is typically defined as the ability of a joint to move through its full, functional range of motion permitted by muscle and connective tissues. A lack of flexibility in single joints or in combinations of joints can reduce sport performance, physical function, and in some cases activities of daily living. Many people consider inflexibility a cause of certain athletic injuries (e.g., muscle strains) and a possible contributing factor in low-back pain. Excessive flexibility, however, may also be a problem because it potentially promotes joint laxity or hypermobility, which can lead to joint pathologies. Tests of flexibility are included in Chapter 22.

Body Composition

Body composition refers to the composition of the human body with regard to two primary components: fat tissue and fat-free or lean tissue. Most tests of body composition have as their objective an estimate of percent body fat. Once percent body fat is determined, other body composition variables can be calculated, including fat weight, lean weight, and estimated body weights at various desired percent body fats. Body composition can be assessed using numerous methodologies, including anthropometric measures of girths or skinfolds (Chapters 24 and 25), densitometry by underwater weighing (Chapter 26), bioelectrical impedance, volume displacement, absorptiometry (e.g., DXA), imaging techniques, and more.

There is significant interest in body composition among exercise physiologists and public health experts. Many sports benefit from athletes having low body fat (e.g., distance running, high jumping) or high lean weight (e.g., sprinting, football). Excess body fat and obesity play a role in determining the risk of chronic diseases, including metabolic syndrome, coronary heart disease, and diabetes mellitus.

Table 1.1	Fitness Component and Energy System Contributing to Performance Tests Based on Exercise Duration		
Exercise Duration	**Fitness Component**	**Energy System Contributing**	**Performance Test**
< 15 s	Anaerobic fitness	Phosphagen system	1 RM tests, Sprint tests, Vertical jump tests
15 to 30 s	Anaerobic fitness	Phosphagen system and Glycolytic system	Wingate test
30 to 60 s	Anaerobic fitness and Aerobic fitness	Glycolytic system and Aerobic system	Anaerobic treadmill test
1 to 3 min	Anaerobic fitness and Aerobic fitness	Glycolytic system and Aerobic system	Anaerobic step test
3 to 60 min	Aerobic fitness	Aerobic system (carbohydrate)	Rockport test, Cooper test, Forestry step test, Astrand cycle test, $\dot{V}O_2$max test
> 60 min	Aerobic fitness	Aerobic system (fat)	

VARIABLES OF INTEREST

When exercise physiologists measure fitness or exercise performance, they are typically interested in measuring quantities or variables such as mass, length, time, temperature, force, work, power, energy, speed, volume, pressure and more. Seven specific quantities are referred to in the metric system as **base quantities,** meaning they are assumed to be mutually exclusive, each of which is expressed in a **base unit** (included in parentheses). The base quantities used in this manual include length (meter, m), mass (kilogram, kg), time (second, s) and thermodynamic temperature (kelvin, K). The remaining SI base quantities, not used in this lab manual, include electric current (ampere, A), amount of substance (mole, mol), and luminous intensity (candela, cd). All of the other quantities or variables discussed in this lab manual (i.e., force, work, power, energy, volume, etc.) are **derived quantities,** derived from the base quantities through a system of equations, typically using multiplication or division.[32] For example, the base quantity *length* (m) can be used to derive *area* (m^2), *volume* (m^3), and in combination with *time* (s) the derived quantities *velocity* ($m \cdot s^{-1}$) and *acceleration* ($m \cdot s^{-2}$). A further discussion of base quantities, derived quantities, and the metric system of measurement is included in Chapter 2.

Mass and Weight

Mass is a base quantity defined as the quantity of matter in an object. Under the normal acceleration of gravity ($9.81 m \cdot s^{-2}$), mass is equivalent to **weight.** So generally, as long as we assume the effect of gravity is constant over the entire surface of the earth, we can assume that *mass* and *weight* are equal and the terms can be used interchangeably. However, should we travel to the moon (where the acceleration of gravity is 1/6 that of earth, or $1.62 m \cdot s^{-2}$), the weight of the object would be less. A person on earth with a body mass of 70.0 kg also has a body weight of 70.0 kg. On the moon, this same person still has a *body mass* of 70.0 kg, but has a *body weight* of only 11.6 kg, due to the reduced effect of gravity.

Length and Height

Length is the measure of how long an object is, most frequently from end to end. The length of an American football field from end to end is 100 yd; the length of a yardstick is 36 in. **Height** is also a measure of how long an object is, but is typically applied to the *vertical length* of an object from the ground. Typically, a person is described as having a height of 70 in. or 178 cm, instead of being 70 in. or 178 cm long. A mountain peak is described as being 4000 m high. It is interesting to note, however, in describing newborn babies, the term *length* is used instead of *height* because they cannot stand and therefore as traditionally viewed have no *vertical length,* or height.

Distance and Displacement

Distance and **displacement** are frequently interchanged and used to express the same variable. However, they are two distinct and separate terms expressing potentially different lengths. *Distance* is the total sum of the length of the path traveled by the exerciser. *Displacement,* on the other hand, is determined taking into account the starting and ending points of the exerciser. Displacement is literally the length of the straight-line path between the starting and ending points of the exerciser. As an example of the difference between distance and displacement consider a baseball player who hits an "inside-the-park home run." The *distance* run by the player is the sum of the length of the path traveled, or *360 ft* (knowing that each of the four bases is 90 ft apart). The *displacement* of the player, however, being the length of the straight-line path between the starting and ending points, is *0 ft* because the starting and ending points are the same point, home plate.

Force

Force is a derived quantity calculated as the product of mass and acceleration. It is defined as that which changes or tends to change the state of rest or motion in matter.[3] Thus, muscular activity generates force. Mass and force are two basic quantities that are similar under certain circumstances. For example, there are times when you will use your body weight (mass) as a measure of force in order to calculate your work load or work rate. A person applying a maximal force to a resistance or load, whether against gravity or a lever, is displaying the fitness component of strength. Most muscular activity, however, uses submaximal forces.

Work

Work is derived from the product of two basic quantities: force and length (distance or displacement). Mechanical work is the product of the force applied against an object and the distance the object moves in the direction of the force while the force is applied to the object. Mathematically, work is the product of the force (F) applied, the angle (θ) at which the force is applied on the object, and the distance (D) the object is moved. When the force is applied parallel to the line of displacement (or at an angle of 0°), the equation simplifies to Eq. 1.1. Often in exercise physiology, the amount of work done during a particular activity is of interest, such as stepping up and down on a bench, walking or running on a treadmill, or pedaling a cycle ergometer. In these cases, work is calculated based on body mass, step height and frequency, treadmill speed and grade, the cycle speed and resistance, and the total exercise time.

Work (W) = Force (F) * Distance (D)   Eq. 1.1

Power

Power is the variable that expresses the rate of work done. Mathematically, power is calculated as work divided by time, as in Eq. 1.2. A more powerful exercise is one in which there is either a larger amount of work done in a given time, or there is a given amount of work done in a shorter time. Power is a term often used when referring to the rate of transforming metabolic energy to physical performance, such as aerobic power and anaerobic power. However, instead of viewing these metabolic terms as power terms, as would a physicist, the exercise physiologist would typically view them as energy terms.

$$\text{Power (P)} = \text{Work (W)} / \text{Time } (t) \qquad \text{Eq. 1.2}$$

Energy

Energy is often simply defined as the ability to do work. Energy more specifically describes the amount of metabolic energy released due to the combination of mechanical work and the heat of the body itself. Energy expenditure during exercise can be measured using either direct or indirect calorimetry. Direct calorimetry is a complicated and expensive process of measuring metabolic rate by directly measuring heat production. Indirect calorimetry is based on measuring the exerciser's oxygen uptake, assuming that oxygen consumed is related to the amount of heat produced in the body during exercise. An oxygen uptake of 1 $L \cdot min^{-1}$ is assumed to have a caloric equivalent of approximately 5 $kcal \cdot L^{-1}$, or 22 $kJ \cdot L^{-1}$. This allows for the estimation of energy expenditure at rest and during exercise in kcal or kJ. By expressing oxygen uptake as a rate in $L \cdot min^{-1}$, a rate of energy expenditure in $kcal \cdot min^{-1}$ (Eq. 1.3a) or in $kJ \cdot min^{-1}$ (Eq. 1.3b), the preferred metric unit, can also be derived.

$$\text{Energy } (kcal \cdot min^{-1}) = \text{Oxygen uptake } (L \cdot min^{-1})$$
$$* 5 \, kcal \cdot L^{-1} \qquad \text{Eq. 1.3a}$$

$$\text{Energy } (kJ \cdot min^{-1}) = \text{Oxygen uptake } (L \cdot min^{-1})$$
$$* 22 \, kJ \cdot L^{-1} \qquad \text{Eq. 1.3b}$$

Speed and Velocity

Speed is the quotient of distance (D) divided by time (t), where distance represents the actual length covered (Eq. 1.4a). **Velocity** is calculated as displacement (d) divided by time (t), where displacement represents the straight-line distance between a specific starting point and ending point (Eq. 1.4b). In many instances, the term speed is substituted for velocity, but mechanically speaking, speed and velocity are different.[17] For example, a track athlete who runs 1 lap of a 400 m track in 50 s is running at a *speed* of 8 $m \cdot s^{-1}$ (400 m / 50 s). Technically, however, because the athlete starts and ends at the same point, the displacement is 0 m and therefore the *velocity* is 0 $m \cdot s^{-1}$ (0 m / 50 s).

$$\text{Speed} = \text{Distance (D)} / \text{Time } (t) \qquad \text{Eq. 1.4a}$$

$$\text{Velocity} = \text{Displacement (d)} / \text{Time } (t) \qquad \text{Eq. 1.4b}$$

Angular Velocity

The two variables just described, speed and velocity, are measured linearly (in a straight line). **Angular velocity** describes the velocity at which an object rotates or spins. It can be described in degrees per second ($deg \cdot s^{-1}$) as is frequently the case in isokinetic dynamometry (Chapter 6). The preferred SI unit, however, for expressing angular velocity is $radians \cdot second^{-1}$. There are 2π radians in a complete circle, so one radian is about 57.3.°

Torque and Peak Torque

Torque is a force or combination of forces that produces or tends to produce a rotating or twisting motion. Torque is used to describe muscular strength measurements taken with an isokinetic dynamometer (Chapter 6). It is mathematically the product of the linear force (F) applied to the device and the perpendicular length (D) of the lever arm at which that force is applied (Eq. 1.5). **Peak torque** is typically described as the greatest torque produced over several trials and is used as a measure of muscular strength.

$$\text{Torque } (\tau) = \text{Force (F)} * \text{Lever arm length (D)} \qquad \text{Eq. 1.5}$$

Volume

Several different measurements of **volume** are of interest in this manual with regard to the lungs, including static lung volumes (e.g., inspiratory reserve volume), lung function volumes (e.g., forced expiratory volume), and volumes and rates of exhaled air (e.g., pulmonary ventilation). Lung volumes, lung function, and exercise ventilation are discussed in Chapters 20 and 21. Each of these volumes is affected by changes in temperature and pressure, which vary between ambient (surrounding) conditions, body conditions, and standard conditions. *Body volume* is of interest due to its involvement in the determination of body density and percent body fat (Chapter 26). The measurement of *fluid volume* is also an important consideration in the exercise physiology lab.

Pressure

Pressure is exerted in different ways and expressed in a variety of units. Gases and liquids exert pressure on the walls of the containers in which they are held. *Blood pressure* is the pressure exerted by the circulating blood on the walls of the blood vessels, with most interest being in arterial blood pressure and its measurement at rest and during exercise (Chapters 16 and 17). *Barometric pressure* refers to the air pressure of the environment. Altitudes can be estimated from air pressures, and weather patterns can be dictated by changes in air pressures. Normal exercise responses occur at barometric pressures common near sea level (760 mm Hg). However, aerobic power is usually less at barometric pressures associated with altitudes above 1500 m (4920 ft).[10] Barometric pressures are used to correct respiratory ventilation volumes and metabolic volumes.

Temperature

Temperature is a measure of the hotness or coldness of any object and can be expressed on any one of three scales. Americans are familiar with the Fahrenheit scale, but the two most common scales for scientists are the Celsius scale and the scale using kelvin units. Usually, the Fahrenheit scale is not printed in scientific research journals, although sometimes it is presented in parentheses after the Celsius degree.

Celsius Scale

Celsius, formerly called the centigrade scale, is named for Anders Celsius, a Swedish mathematician. He created the centigrade scale by arbitrarily dividing the difference between the freezing point and boiling point of water into 100 equal degrees (0 °C and 100 °C, respectively). The appropriate term now in use for this scale is Celsius.[4]

Kelvin Scale

The basic thermal SI unit is the kelvin, named after 19th-century physicist William Kelvin. It has an absolute zero, meaning that the coldest possible temperature truly is zero kelvin (0 K), and there is no *minus* or *below zero* temperature for this scale. Because a kelvin unit is equal in size to a Celsius degree, absolute zero (0 K) corresponds to −273°C. Or conversely, 0 °C is equal to 273 K. To convert temperature between the two scales, one need only add or subtract 273. Notice that the *k* in kelvin is not capitalized, but the abbreviated symbol K is.

Fahrenheit Scale

Gabriel Fahrenheit, in developing the Fahrenheit scale, arbitrarily chose the number 32 to designate the melting point of ice and 96 as the temperature of human blood. Although this temperature scale accommodates most of earth's weather situations, it is not as convenient for calculations as the Celsius and kelvin scales. Thus, SI[30] does not recommend its use as a measurement scale.

STATISTICAL AND EVALUATION TERMS

The term *statistics* can have more than one meaning.[22] In a broad sense, it includes the method of organizing, describing, and analyzing quantitative (numerical) data, in addition to predicting outcomes or probabilities. The combined term *basic statistics* is sometimes used to describe group data with such statistics as the mean (*M*) and standard deviation (*SD*).

Independent and Dependent Variables

A **variable** is a characteristic. The characteristics, or variables, mentioned in this laboratory manual usually have quantitative values that vary among the members of a sample or population. Some of the measured variables discussed in this manual are strength, run/walk time, oxygen consumption, heart rate, blood pressure, and percent body fat. A variable is either independent or dependent.

An **independent variable** is manipulated, or changed, in order to determine its relationship to the dependent variable.[32] The independent variable's measuring unit is usually placed on the horizontal (X) axis of a graph. It is used to predict or estimate the dependent variable, as in using skinfold thickness (independent variable) to estimate percent body fat (dependent variable). The experimenter or technician controls the independent variable.[20]

A **dependent variable** is measured before and/or after manipulation of the independent variable. Its measuring unit is usually placed on the vertical (Y) axis of a graph. The dependent variable is predicted or estimated from the independent variable, as in estimating maximum oxygen uptake (dependent variable) from walking or running distance (independent variable) as seen in Figure 1.1.

Correlation and Prediction

Correlation analysis involves the observation of relationships between variables by plotting the data on a graph and calculating a correlation coefficient (*r* or *R*) The closer the points come to forming a straight line, the higher the correlation or the stronger the relationship between the two variables. The value of *r* can range from −1.00 to + 1.00, with the sign indicating the direction of the relationship (direct or inverse) and the value indicating the strength of the relationship. A positive *r* indicates a positive (direct) relationship between two variables, where an increase in one variable is associated with an increase in the other variable. A negative *r* indicates a negative (inverse) relationship between two variables, where an increase in one variable is associated with a decrease in the other variable. An *r* of 0.00 indicates no relationship between two variables; an *r* of 1.00 indicates a perfect, direct relationship between two variables; and an *r* of −1.00 indicates a perfect, inverse relationship. Figure 1.1 shows data from Chapter 14 demonstrating the strong, direct relationship (as indicated by the *r* of 0.91) between distance run/walked in 12 min and maximal oxygen uptake. An increase in distance run/walked is closely associated with an increase in maximal oxygen uptake.

Reliability, Validity, and Objectivity

A good test of body composition, aerobic fitness, or any other measure of physical performance should be reliable, valid, and objective. Each of these test characteristics can be described and assessed statistically using correlation analysis, as seen in Figure 1.2.

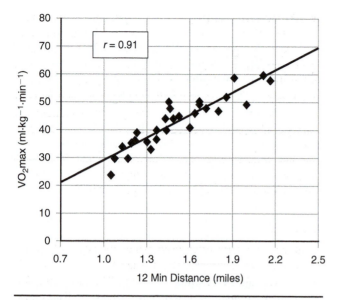

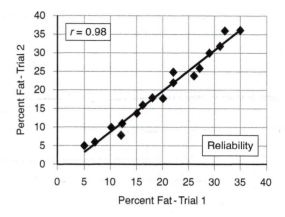

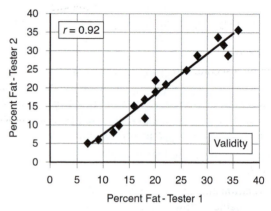

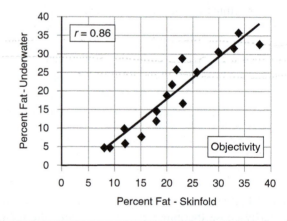

Figure 1.1 Data from Chapter 14 demonstrating the linear relationship between distance run/walked in 12 min and maximal oxygen uptake. The high, positive correlation coefficient ($r = 0.91$) indicates a strong, direct relationship between the two variables.

Figure 1.2 Demonstration of reliability (comparing 2 trials done by the same tester), objectivity (comparing 2 different testers using the same method), and validity (comparing 2 different methods) of measuring percent fat.

Reliability is an estimate of the reproducibility or consistency of a test. Reliabilities of tests should be based on a sample of at least 30 participants.[23] A reliable test generates a high intraclass correlation coefficient (R) and a high interclass correlation coefficient (r) when data from repeated trials of that test are compared. Based on input from other investigators,[8,18,21,26,29] the correlation coefficient criteria that may be used to qualitatively categorize reliability and validity ranging from poor to high are summarized in Table 1.2. The criterion for an acceptable correlation coefficient for reliability may vary with the opinions of various investigators; a recommended minimum test-retest correlation can be as low as .70[25,29] or, more stringently, as high as .85.[18]

The reliability of a test may be affected by the experimental and biological error (variability). Experimental variability is due to lab procedures, instrumentation, and environment; thus, it represents the technical error in a test. Biological variability or error is due to the natural periodicity (hourly, daily, weekly) or inherent biological fluctuations of the human participant.[19]

Validity is the ability of a test to measure what it claims to measure. A test with high validity has a good correlation (r) with the criterion measure (actual or true). For example, run-walk distances or times are often judged for concurrent validity by their correlation with scores on maximal oxygen uptake tests. The guidelines for qualifying meaningful criterion validity coefficients need not be as high as for those guidelines that qualify reliability coefficients (Table 1.2). For example, correlation coefficients

Table 1.2	Subjective Criteria for Assessing the Reliability and Validity of a Test		
Category for Test Reliability	**Correlation Coefficient**	**Category for Test Validity**	**Correlation Coefficient**
High reliability	.90–1.00	High validity	.80–1.00
Good reliability	.80–.89	Good validity	.70–.79
Fair reliability	.70–.79	Fair validity	.60–.69
Poor reliability	< .70	Poor validity	< .60

≥.80 can be interpreted as indicating high test validity; whereas correlation coefficients ≥.90 are required to indicate high test reliability.[29]

Two other types of validity are content validity and construct validity. Content validity relies on expert opinion or past research, and construct validity indicates the test's ability to discriminate among groups.[26] Most validity coefficients described in this laboratory manual are based on concurrent validity.

Objectivity, although similar to reliability, is distinct in that it represents the ability of a test to give similar results when administered by different administrators. It is sometimes referred to as *inter-observer reliability* or *inter-rater reliability*. Measuring skinfold thickness to estimate percent body fat, when done by one well-trained tester, typically is highly reliable and valid. If the same degree of reliability and validity is produced from measurements taken by a second tester, the objectivity of measuring skinfold thickness would also be considered high. The goal of any test is for it to be reliable (give the same results twice), valid (measure what it claims to measure), and objective (produce correct results regardless of the tester).

Prediction

The relationship between one variable and one or more other variables allows transformation into an equation to predict or estimate the dependent variable. The line of best fit of the graphic plot of one variable to another is termed a **regression line.** When it is transformed into an equation, it is called a **regression equation.** Sometimes regression equations are presented in the form of a **nomogram,** a series of two or more vertical or diagonal lines by which to predict one variable from one or more other variables without performing any calculations.

The statistical term that describes the predictive error of a regression equation is the **standard error of estimate (SEE).** This is a type of standard deviation around the predicted scores from the regression line. For example, if the predicted lean mass is 40 kg, and the *SEE* is 5 kg, then 68 % of the scores will be between 35 kg and 45 kg. Thus, the standard error of the estimate indicates the amount of error to be expected in a predictive score.[6] One researcher suggests an acceptable *SEE* criterion of less than 15 % for aerobic fitness estimation.[13]

Norms and Standards

Norms and standards enhance the interpretation of test scores. Although the two terms are often used interchangeably, they are different.

Norms

Norms are values that relate a person's score to those of the general population. Some authorities suggest that the minimum number of participants to establish norms be set at 100 for each category.[5] If the population sample number is less than 100, or if the samples within a population (e.g., specific age groups) are less than 100, it is probably more appropriate to refer to the data as *comparative scores*, rather than *norms*. The statistics derived from the norms are often used to develop descriptive categories such as poor, below average, average, above average, and excellent. For example, if a person is categorized as excellent in a certain fitness component on the Canadian Standardization Test and falls at the 85th percentile, then that person ranks better than 85 % of the population.[14] Table 1.3 shows three categorization scales based on percentiles.[14,15,27]

Standards

Standard is a term often used synonymously with norms. However, more appropriately, it is used to connote a desirable or recommended value or score.[2] The term *criterion-referenced standards (CRS)* is a professionally popular term.[12,18,24] It has an advantage over normative standards for fitness tests because CRS indicate the levels necessary for good health, regardless of the level of physical fitness of the reference group.[7,11,24,28] The CRS for fitness tests may be based upon professional expertise and scientific research, in addition to normative data.[11] Thus, CRS are standards that represent recommended levels of performance. Because the CRS are absolute standards, they do not consider the number of persons who meet the standard. The CRS levels allow easy recognition of the adequacy or inadequacy of a person on that particular fitness/health variable. Also, as long as a person meets the CRS criterion, he or she has the same merit as someone who scores extremely high on the variable.

Because the criterion standards are based partially on human judgment, and because of testing errors or participant motivation, the cutoff scores may cause false merit or false nonmerit. Also, the merit levels usually do not indicate fitness levels a person may need to be successful

Table 1.3	**Examples of Descriptive Categories Based on Percentiles**	
Test	**Percentiles**	**Category**
Canadian	81–100	Excellent
Standardization Test	61–80	Above average
	41–60	Average
	21–40	Below average
	1–20	Poor
Institute for Aerobics	90–100	Well above average
Research, YMCA	70–89	Above average
	50–69	Average
	30–49	Below average
	10–29	Well below average
Functional Fitness	76–100	Above average
Test	25–75	Average
	1–24	Below average

Sources: Based on Fitness and Amateur Sport Canada (1987)[14]; Institute for Aerobics Research, Dallas, TX; Golding, Myers, & Sinning (1989)[15]; Rikli & Jones (1999).[27]

Fitness Component	Examples of Laboratory Tests	Examples of Field Tests
Muscular strength and endurance	Peak torque (e.g., isokinetic dynamometry) Peak force (e.g., handgrip dynamometry)	1 Repetition max (RM) test Timed repetitions (e.g., sit-ups)
Anaerobic fitness	Peak power (e.g., Wingate test)	Sprint tests (e.g., 40, 50, 60 yd) Vertical jump and leg power tests
Aerobic fitness and cardiorespiratory endurance	Maximal oxygen uptake test	Walking test (e.g., Rockport test) Running test (e.g., Cooper test)
Flexibility	Range of motion (e.g., goniometry, electrogoniometry)	Flexibility (e.g., sit and reach) Height-weight measures
Body composition	Hydrostatic weighing, DXA, plethysmography	Skinfold and girth measures

in recreational or competitive sports; they are concerned mainly with health-related fitness. Thus, norms describe a person's position within a population, whereas standards describe the criteria suggested for appropriate health-related fitness of a population.

TYPES OF TESTS

The 30 or more tests described in this laboratory manual can be classified as laboratory tests or field tests based on the setting and equipment required, the degree of control maintained during the test, and the application of the results.

Laboratory Tests

A test is classified as a **laboratory test** when it can only be performed within the confines of the laboratory and requires the testing equipment found within the laboratory (e.g., metabolic measurement system, isokinetic dynamometer). An attempt is made during the test to maintain a high degree of control over many conditions involving the laboratory (e.g., temperature), the participant (e.g., diet, amount of rest, warm-up prior to the test), and the protocol (e.g., time intervals, specific treadmill speeds or cycle ergometer power levels). When the test results are to be used in research, it is common to use a laboratory test. To be useful, research requires test results that are highly reliable and valid, characteristics that should apply to well-conducted laboratory tests.

Field Tests

It is not always practical or possible to bring the population of interest into the laboratory to conduct the desired tests. Bringing participants into the laboratory frequently requires testing participants individually, providing transportation, arranging for entry into the laboratory (e.g., gaining access to a university campus), and sharing time in the laboratory and on the necessary laboratory equipment with other testers. Conducting the tests in the laboratory under controlled conditions also in some cases creates a contrived or artificial environment that differs from the more desired natural environment and can influence the results of the test. For

BOX 1.1   **Chapter Preview/Review**

What are the components of fitness?

What are the three energy systems?

How does exercise duration influence the contributions of the energy systems to physical performance?

What are some of the common variables measured in the exercise physiology laboratory?

What are the three scales that can be used to express temperature?

What is a correlation coefficient and what does it indicate about a relationship between variables?

What is meant by the reliability, validity, and objectivity of a test?

What is the difference between a laboratory test and a field test?

these and other reasons, testers have developed **field tests** that can be taken to the population of interest and conducted under more natural conditions.

Field tests are frequently used to assess a variety of fitness components, including muscular strength, muscular endurance, anaerobic fitness, aerobic fitness, flexibility, and body composition. Field tests in physical education were developed to test large groups of persons outside of a laboratory setting as accurately and economically as possible. Unless extrinsic variables (e.g., weather, terrain, motivation) are strictly controlled, field tests are not as appreciated in research as are the more controlled laboratory tests. This does not mean that field tests cannot be as valid as some laboratory tests. In addition to their use in physical education classes, field tests are popular as screening and maintenance tests for military and safety/ emergency personnel (e.g., firefighters, lifeguards, police, and rangers) and for college or professional sports recruiters. Table 1.4 gives examples of laboratory and field tests.

SUMMARY

Many of the basic terms used in exercise physiology are summarized in this chapter. As with learning any new language, the beginner should practice using these terms so that they become a natural part of the exercise physiology vocabulary. Students are encouraged to scan through the entire laboratory manual to get an idea of the scope of what is measured in the exercise physiology lab.

References

1. American College of Sports Medicine (2009). *ACSM's guidelines for exercise testing and prescription* (8th ed.). Philadelphia: Lippincott Williams & Wilkins.

2. American College of Sports Medicine (ACSM). (1988). ACSM opinion statement on physical fitness in children and youth. *Medicine and Science in Sports and Exercise 20,* 422–423.

3. American College of Sports Medicine (2012). Information for authors. In *Medicine and Science in Sports and Exercise,* (MSSE). Retrieved June 11, 2012 from https://www.editorialmanager.com/msse/.

4. American Psychological Association (2009). *Publication manual of the American Psychological Association* (6th ed.). Washington, DC: APA Publications.

5. Barrow, H. M., & McGee, R. (1971). *A practical approach to measurement in physical education.* Philadelphia: Lea and Febiger.

6. Baumgartner, T. A., & Jackson, A. S. (1987). *Measurement for evaluation in physical education and exercise science.* Dubuque, IA: Wm. C. Brown.

7. Blair, S. N., Falls, H. B., & Pate, R. R. (1983). A new physical fitness test. *The Physician and Sportsmedicine 11,* 87–91.

8. Blesh, T. E. (1974). *Measurement for evaluation in physical education.* New York: Ronald Press.

9. Brooks, G. A., Fahey, T. D., & Baldwin, K. M. (2005). *Exercise physiology: Human bioenergetics and its applications* (4th ed.). New York: McGraw-Hill.

10. Buskirk, E. R. (1969). Decrease in physical work capacity at high altitude. In A. H. Hegnauer (Ed.), *Biomedicine of high terrestrial elevations* (pp. 204–222). Natick, MA: U.S. Army Research Institute of Environmental Medicine.

11. Corbin, C. B., & Pangrazi, R. P. (1992). Are American children and youth fit? *Research Quarterly for Exercise and Sport, 63,* 96–106.

12. Cureton, K. J., & Warren, G. L. (1990). Criterion-referenced standards for youth health-related fitness tests: A tutorial. *Research Quarterly for Exercise and Sport, 61*(1), 7–19.

13. Davies, C. T. M. (1968). Limitations to the prediction of maximum oxygen intake from cardiac frequency measurements. *Journal of Applied Physiology, 24,* 700–706.

14. Fitness and Amateur Sport Canada. (1987). *Canadian Standardized Test of Fitness (CSTF) operations manual* (3rd ed.). Ottawa, Canada: Author.

15. Golding, L. A., Myers, C. R., & Sinning, W. E. (Eds.). (1989). *Y's way to physical fitness.* Champaign, IL: Human Kinetics.

16. Gutin, B., Manos, T., & Strong, W. (1992). Defining health and fitness: First step toward establishing children's fitness standards. *Research Quarterly for Exercise and Sport, 63,* 128–132.

17. Hay, J. G., & Reid, J. G. (1982). *The anatomical and mechanical bases of human motion.* Englewood Cliffs, NJ: Prentice-Hall.

18. Johnson, B. L., & Nelson, J. K. (1974). *Practical measurements for evaluation in physical education.* Minneapolis: Burgess.

19. Katch, V. L., Sady, S. S., & Freedson, P. (1982). Biological variability in maximum aerobic power. *Medicine and Science in Sports and Exercise, 14*(1), 21–25.

20. Kirk, R. E. (1968). *Experimental design: Procedures for the behavioral sciences.* Belmont, CA: Brooks/Cole.

21. Medbø, J. I., Mohn, A. C., Tabata, I., Bahr, R., Vaage, O., & Sejersted, O. (1988). Anaerobic capacity determined by maximal accumulated O_2 deficit. *Journal of Applied Physiology, 64,* 50–60.

22. Minium, E. W. (1970). *Statistical reasoning in psychology and education.* New York: John Wiley and Sons.

23. Morrow, J. R., & Jackson, A. W. (1993). How "significant" is your reliability? *Research Quarterly for Exercise and Science, 64,* 352–355.

24. Pate, R. (1983). *South Carolina physical fitness test manual.* Columbia: South Carolina Association for Health, Physical Education, Recreation and Dance.

25. Rarick, G. L., & Dobbins, D. A. (1975). Basic components in the motor performance of children six to nine years of age. *Medicine and Science in Sports and Exercise, 7,* 105–110.

26. Rikli, R. E., & Jones, C. J. (1999). Development and validation of a functional fitness test for community-residing older adults. *Journal of Aging and Physical Activity, 7,* 129–161.

27. Rikli, R. E., & Jones, C. J. (1999). Functional fitness normative scores for community-residing older adults, ages 60–94. *Journal of Aging and Physical Activity, 7,* 162–181.

28. Safritt, M. J. (1981). *Evaluation in physical education.* Englewood Cliffs, NJ: Prentice Hall.

29. Safritt, M. J. (1990). *Introduction to measurement in physical education and exercise science.* St. Louis: Times Mirror/Mosby.

30. Spencer, M. R., & Gastin, P. B. (2001). Energy system contribution during 200- to 1500-m running in highly trained athletes. *Medicine and Science in Sports and Exercise, 33,* 157–162.

31. Thompson, A., & Taylor, B. N. (2008). *NIST special publication 811, 2008 edition: Guide for the Use of the International System of Units (SI).* Gaithersburg, MD: United States Department of Commerce, National Institute of Standards and Technology.

32. Van Dalen, D. B. (1973). *Understanding educational research.* San Francisco: McGraw-Hill.

CHAPTER 2

UNITS OF MEASURE

Measuring units is the term given to describe the type of measure being made. For instance, in the United States we use *pounds* to describe weight and *feet* and *inches* to describe height. The units most commonly used in exercise physiology are those that measure variables associated with exercise, physiology, and meteorology. Some of these were introduced in Chapter 1. In accordance with the International System (SI) of nomenclature, numerous variables are described with such measuring units as kilogram, liter, meter, and kelvin. Many variables combine two or more measuring units to form such units as liters per minute and milliliters per kilogram per minute.

The quantification of exercise physiology requires that all variables have well-defined units of measure. Americans are most familiar with such units as inches, feet, and pounds, which they use in their daily lives. These units are sometimes referred to as *customary units*. However, the single measuring system that is officially approved worldwide by scientists is the International System of Units—abbreviated SI from its French name, "Système International."[2,5,7] SI is based upon the decimal and metric systems, thus simplifying the conversion of one unit to another.[3]

Only three countries in the world, at least according to current folklore,—the United States, Burma (also known as Myanmar), and Liberia—have not officially adopted, or are not fully committed to, the metric system.[6] Therefore, with apologies to Burma and Liberia, we can justify calling the nonmetric system the "American" system. However, American scientists, including exercise physiologists, have adopted SI metric units of measure. Although U.S. legislation has discouraged the use of the nonmetric system, the practice is dying slowly. Americans often overlook metric designations on such objects as engine sizes (e.g., cubic centimeters), food containers (e.g., grams), and liquid containers (e.g., liters). Metric markers in America are sometimes found on road mileage/ kilometer signs, auto tachometers, and speed-limit signs. Some U.S. buildings display temperature readings in Celsius. As more students become familiar with SI nomenclature—specifically, the metric system—perhaps the U.S. population will adopt, and use routinely, the worldwide metric system.

RECOGNIZING AND REPORTING SI (METRIC) UNITS

Students need to recognize SI units of measure when they see them and know how to report them after making measurements. As when learning any language, students must be concerned with the spelling, punctuation, and grammar of the SI "language." With respect to spelling, the SI guide published by the U.S. National Institute of Standards and Technology permits American scientists to spell *liter* and *meter* as such, whereas a Briton may spell them as litre and metre, respectively.[5] As noted in Chapter 1, although William Kelvin originated the kelvin temperature scale, the name is not capitalized when referring to the unit because the kelvin is adopted as one of the *base units* of the International System of units.[5] The same rationale applies when spelling out some of the derived units whose names are those of persons, such as newton, watt, joule, and pascal. When expressing the full name, not the abbreviation, of a two-component unit such as newton meter, use a space between the two words. Do not use a hyphen (e.g., not "newton-meter") and do not link terms into a single word (e.g., not "newtonmeter").

Obviously, symbols and abbreviations of measuring units avoid spelling problems and are convenient and space efficient. However, abbreviations (e.g., kg) and symbols (e.g., °) of measuring units should be used only when associated with the numeric value.[7] For example, *kilogram* should not be abbreviated as expressed in this sentence, but the abbreviation should be used if reporting that a person's body weight (mass) is 60 kg. Abbreviations are not capitalized unless associated with a person's name, such as N, W, C, and K, for Misters Newton, Watt, Celsius, and Kelvin, respectively.

Plural abbreviations are not acceptable in the SI. Thus, 60 kg or 175 cm is not reported as 60 kgs or 175 cms. Abbreviations are followed by a period only for the American abbreviation for inches (in.) or at the end of a sentence. A space is also required between the numeral and the unit; thus, the technician records "60 kg," not "60 kg," or records "10 %," not "10%." One exception to the rule regarding a space is when using the symbol for degrees as in "an angle of ninety degrees (90°)." When abbreviating a two-component unit, use a centered dot (·) to separate each component. Thus, you would abbreviate "newton meter" as "N·m." Unit abbreviations and unit names are not mixed; thus, do not use a mixed expression, such as "newton·m" or "N·meter." Similarly, do not mix numerals and names; thus, "the static force was 500 N," not ". . . 500 newtons," or ". . . five-hundred N."

The recommended style of expressing *per* in combined units, such as liters per minute, is to use the centered dot preceding the unit with its negative exponent. Thus, the unit would appear as L·min^{-1}, unless this is impractical for certain computers or typewriters. In that case, one slash (solidus; /) is acceptable (e.g., L/min). However, it is incorrect to use more than one solidus (accent on the first syllable *säl*) per expression, such as "ml/kg/min." The latter could be expressed with one solidus as ml/(kg·min) or as ml·kg^{-1}·min^{-1}.

The SI style also calls for scientists to record some numbers differently from what we are used to seeing. The general rule for numerical values with more than four digits is to insert a blank space to separate groups of three digits on either side of the decimal. For example, we are familiar with writing the number 10,500 with a comma, but we need to write it as 10 500 in accordance with SI recommendations (requirements). The one exception to this is when there are only four digits to the left or right of the decimal. For example, it is appropriate to record the number as 1500, or 1 500 for uniformity of numbers in a table, but not as 1,500. One reason for such rules is to avoid confusion where some countries use a comma instead of a decimal point.

VARIABLES AND UNITS OF MEASURE

Numerous variables were introduced and defined in Chapter 1. A main purpose of this chapter is to describe the units in which these quantities are typically measured and expressed. Emphasis is placed on SI (metric) units, but American or customary units are also discussed because of their frequent usage, at least in the United States.

Mass

Mass (M) is considered an SI base quantity and is represented by the SI base unit, the kilogram (kg). One of the most common measurements of mass in exercise physiology is body mass. Although the term *body mass* is the more appropriate term, *body weight* is still overwhelmingly used in the United States. For this reason, whenever the variable

mass refers to the mass of the human body, the term body weight will typically be used throughout this laboratory manual. Otherwise, the term mass will be used to refer to the mass of any other object. In some cases, where body weight is being described, it may be expressed in pounds (lb), again due to the popularity of the unit in the United States. But whenever body weight is described in pounds (mostly in tables or figures), it will also be expressed in kilograms.

Length and Distance

Length is also an SI base quantity described in the SI base unit, the meter (m). Longer lengths and distances are described in kilometers (km). For shorter lengths, a meter can be subdivided into 10 decimeters (dm), 100 centimeters (cm), or 1000 millimeters (mm). Table 2.1 lists common metric prefixes and the decimal and exponent they represent. The term height describes the "vertical length" of a person, which is expressed in meters or centimeters. It is actually more appropriate to refer not to a person's height, but to his or her *stature*. But again, because of the common usage of the term height, it will be used throughout the laboratory manual more so than the term stature.

Force

The recommended measuring unit for force is newton (N), named after mid-19th-century scientist Isaac Newton. The newton is a special name given to a derived SI unit, being mathematically derived from the three base quantities mass (kg), length (m), and time (s). Technically, the most appropriate unit in which to express force is kg·m·s^{-2}, due to its being the product of mass and acceleration. But the special term newton is more commonly used, to acknowledge the contributions made by this important scientist. Although the kilogram (kg) is a unit of mass, laboratories often use it as a measure of the force exerted to lift a weight, crank a cycle ergometer, or push against a dynamometer. Many grip strength dynamometers display force in both pounds and kilograms.

Table 2.1	Decimal and Exponent Expressions of SI (Metric) Prefixes				
Decimal	**Exponent**	**Prefix**	**Length (meter)**	**Mass (gram)**	**Volume (liter)**
1 000 000	10^6	mega	-	megagram (Mg)	-
1 000	10^3	kilo	kilometer (km)	kilogram (kg)	kiloliter (kl)
100	10^2	hecto	hectometer (hm)	hectogram (hg)	hectoliter (hl)
10	10^1	deka	dekameter (dam)	dekagram (dag)	dekaliter (dal)
1	10^0	-	meter (m)	gram (g)	liter (L)
0.1	10^{-1}	deci	decimeter (dm)	decigram (dm)	deciliter (dl)
0.01	10^{-2}	centi	centimeter (cm)	centigram (cm)	centiliter (cl)
0.001	10^{-3}	milli	millimeter (mm)	milligram (mg)	milliliter (ml)
0.000 001	10^{-6}	micro	micrometer (μm)	microgram (μg)	microliter (μl)

Work

The preferred unit for expressing work (w) is the joule (J) because it represents the "totality" of work rather than separating it into its two components—force and distance. Larger quantities of work can be expressed in kilojoules (kJ). When work is calculated as the product of the force unit (newton) and the distance unit (meter), another acceptable derived unit is produced—the newton meter (N·m). In the same way that force is still sometimes described in kg, work can still be described in kilogram meters (kg·m).

Power

The recommended unit for power (P) is the watt (W), a special name given in honor of Scottish inventor James Watt. Like the joule, the watt describes power in its totality. When power is broken down into its components, it is the product of the force (N) times the distance (m) that an object moves divided by the time (s) spent moving the object—or the derived unit, $N \cdot m \cdot s^{-1}$. Thus, 1 watt can be defined as either $1 \ N \cdot m \cdot s^{-1}$ or as $1 \ J \cdot s^{-1}$ since 1 N·m (derived unit) is equal to 1 J (special name for the derived unit). Although it is not an acceptable SI unit of power, you will still sometimes see power described in $kg \cdot m \cdot min^{-1}$, especially with reference to cycle ergometry.

Energy

The terms energy (E) and work are highly related to one another, in fact so much so that they use the same unit—the joule (J). The joule is named for James Joule, who proposed the law of the conservation of energy. The joule is the universally approved unit of measure for metabolic energy release, which is the result of energy done (work) and energy wasted (heat).[4] Energy is commonly expressed in kilocalories (kcal) in the United States, but this is not an SI unit of energy.

Energy expenditure at rest and during exercise can be estimated through indirect calorimetry using the measurement of oxygen uptake. It can be assumed that for every 1 liter of oxygen uptake, approximately 5 kcal or 21 kJ of energy is expended. These values are only approximations and are influenced slightly by exercise intensity with more energy expended per liter at higher intensity. (Data for more specific energy equivalents for 1 liter of oxygen, ranging from 4.69 to 5.05 $kcal \cdot L^{-1}$, can be found in Table 15.8.) Once the oxygen uptake and hence the oxygen cost is known, it is possible to estimate the *caloric expenditure* or *kilojoule expenditure* simply by multiplying the liters of oxygen consumed by 5 (Eq. 2.1a) or by 21 (Eq.2.1b), respectively.

Energy (caloric) expenditure (kcal)
   = Oxygen uptake ($L \cdot min^{-1}$) * 5   Eq. 2.1a

Energy (Kilojoule) expenditure (kJ)
   = Oxygen uptake ($L \cdot min^{-1}$) * 21   Eq. 2.1b

Speed and Velocity

Speed and velocity (v) are derived quantities based on distance and displacement, respectively, divided by time. The most appropriate unit in which to express speed and velocity is $m \cdot s^{-1}$, derived from the two base units meters and seconds. However, numerous other acceptable SI units can be derived from any unit of length (m, km, etc.) and time (s, min, h, etc.)—for example, $m \cdot min^{-1}$ and $km \cdot h^{-1}$. Speed limits in the United States are still posted in miles per hour ($mi \cdot h^{-1}$), although an attempt is being made to phase out this unit in favor of the SI unit of kilometers per hour ($km \cdot h^{-1}$).

Angular Velocity

Angular velocity (ω), instead of being linear, describes the velocity at which an object rotates. The preferred SI unit for expressing angular velocity is radians per second ($rad \cdot s^{-1}$). However, another unit that is frequently used, especially with regard to isokinetic dynamometry, is degrees per second ($deg \cdot s^{-1}$ or $° \cdot s^{-1}$). Because there are 2π radians in a complete circle, one radian is about 57.3 °, and therefore $1 \ rad \cdot s^{-1}$ is equivalent to 57.3 $° \cdot s^{-1}$ (or $deg \cdot s^{-1}$).

Torque

Torque (τ) is a derived quantity based on the "**moment of force**" created. The moment of force is the mathematical product of the length of the moment arm (measured from the center of rotation to the point where the force is applied) and the force applied at that moment arm length. The SI unit for torque is the newton meter (N·m), derived from the two base units of force (N) and length (m). In many earlier published studies involving isokinetic dynamometry, peak torque was described in foot pounds (ft·lb), but in general this unit is no longer used in scientific publications.

Volume

The SI unit of measure for volume (V) is the liter (L). Although logically *liter* would be abbreviated by a lowercase *l*, an uppercase *L* is acceptable and, in fact, is often used instead so that it is not confused with the numeral 1. Numerous volumes will be discussed in this laboratory manual related to lung volumes, pulmonary ventilation, cardiac output, and stroke volume, and the uppercase *L* will be used. For smaller volumes, a liter can be subdivided into 10 deciliters (dl), 100 centiliters (cl), or 1000 milliliters (ml); in these two-letter abbreviations, the lowercase *l* will be used.

METEOROLOGICAL UNITS

The primary meteorological concerns of the exercise physiologist are temperature, relative humidity, and barometric pressure. The units presented here for these terms are those accepted by the scientific community or adopted as the SI style.

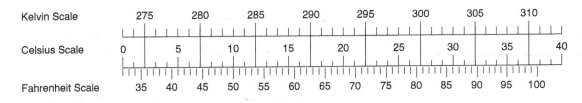

Figure 2.1 Conversion of temperature between different scales.

Temperature

The base unit of thermodynamic temperature (*T*) is the kelvin (K), named in honor of William Thomson Baron Kelvin. The Kelvin scale for describing temperature is based on an absolute zero (0 K), the lowest temperature possible in any macroscopic system. This absolute zero is equal to −273.15 °C (≈ −273 °C). For the purpose of this laboratory manual, converting temperature between kelvin units (K) and Celsius degrees (°C) will be done by adding or subtracting 273, as seen in Equation 2.2a and 2.2b. Although the kelvin is the base unit of temperature, most laboratory thermometers display in Celsius degrees, which are accepted SI units. Therefore, for selected calculations involving volume conversions, students need to be able to convert temperatures from Celsius degrees to kelvin units.

°C to K:	K = (°C + 273)	Eq. 2.2a
K to °C:	°C = (K − 273)	Eq. 2.2b

The Fahrenheit temperature scale and Fahrenheit degrees are not accepted by the International System, but they are described here because they are still so prevalent in the United States. The primary purpose of being able to convert °F to °C would be if the only thermometer or temperature available was in °F. For this conversion, it is necessary not only to change the "zero point" of the scale, designated by the freezing point of water (0 °C or 32 °F) but also to change the size of the degrees. Because there are 9 F degrees for every 5 C degrees, we multiply or divide by 9/5 (1.8). Converting temperatures between the Fahrenheit and Celsius scales is done using the formulas shown in Equation 2.3a and 2.3b. Figure 2.1 shows the conversion of temperatures between the three temperature scales.

°F to °C:	°C = (°F − 32) / 1.8	Eq. 2.3a
°C to °F:	°F = (°C ∗ 1.8) + 32	Eq. 2.3b

Relative Humidity

Relative humidity (RH) indicates the relative amount of water in the air. It is measured in the laboratory with an instrument called a hygrometer, which displays relative humidity in units of percent (e.g., 50 %). If the RH is 100 %, the air contains the most amount of water it can possibly hold at that air temperature. Air can hold more water at higher temperatures than it can at lower temperatures. Ideally, laboratories should also have instruments that display directly or indirectly the wet-bulb globe temperature index (WBGT index). This index considers the interaction of relative humidity with air temperature and radiant temperature and is important in identifying risk of heat illness.

Barometric Pressure

The pressure being exerted by the "weight" of the atmosphere is measured with an instrument called a barometer, so it is commonly referred to as *barometric pressure* (P_B). The derived unit for pressure is N·m² based on it being force (N) exerted per unit area (m²), which is specially named the pascal (Pa), in honor of 17th-century scientist Blaise Pascal. Because the unit is small, barometric pressure is commonly described in hectopascals (1 hPa = 100 Pa) or kilopascals (1 kPa = 1000 Pa). The standard barometric pressure at sea level is 1013 hPa. This same pressure (1013 hPa) can also be described as 1013 millibar (mbar) because the hPa and the mbar have the same numerical value. The millibar is a common unit used by meteorologists.

Barometric pressure, especially in the United States, is commonly described in other units not accepted as SI units. It is described in millimeters of mercury (mm Hg), or torr, and in inches of mercury (in. Hg). Standard barometric pressure, reported earlier as 1013 hPa, is also equivalent to 760 mm Hg (or torr) and 29.92 in. Hg. For much the same reason as was discussed with regard to temperature, it is useful to be able to convert between different units of pressure (Eq. 2.4a through 2.4d) if the only available measuring device does not measure in pascals or hPa.

mm Hg to hPa:	hPa = mm Hg ∗ 1.333	Eq. 2.4a
hPa to mm Hg:	mm Hg = hPa ∗ 0.75	Eq. 2.4b
in. Hg to hPa:	hPa = in. Hg ∗ 33.864	Eq. 2.4c
hPa to in. Hg:	in. Hg = hPa ∗ 0.0295	Eq. 2.4d

The American College of Sports Medicine (ACSM) permits exceptions to the SI units for physiological and gas pressures.[1] Thus, blood pressure units and lung pressures are reported in millimeters of mercury (mm Hg) in the journal *Medicine and Science in Sports and Exercise.*

Table 2.2 Conversions of SI (Metric) Units and American (Customary) Units

Mass and Weight (gram; g)

1 g = 1000 mg = 0.0022 lb = 0.0352 oz
1 oz = 28.3495 g
1 lb = 16 oz = 453.59 g = 0.4536 kg
1 kg = 1000 g = 2.2046 lb = 35.2736 oz
accel of gravity (g) = 9.81 $m \cdot s^{-2}$ = 32.2 $ft \cdot s^{-2}$

Length and Height (meter; m)

1 m = 1000 mm = 1.0936 yd = 3.281 ft = 39.37 in.
1 yd = 3 ft = 0.914 m = 91.4 cm
1 ft = 12 in. = 0.3048 m = 30.48 cm
1 in. = 25.4 mm = 2.54 cm = 0.0254 m
1 km = 1000 m = 0.6214 mile = 1093.6 yd
1 mile = 1.609 km = 1609.35 m

Force (newton; N)

1 N = 0.1020 kg = 0.2248 lb
1 kg = 1000 g = 2.2046 lb = 9.8067 N
1 lb = 0.4536 kg = 453.59 g

Work (joule; J)

1 J = 1 $N \cdot m$ = 0.1020 $kg \cdot m$ = 0.7375 $ft \cdot lb$
1 $kg \cdot m$ = 9.8067 J = 9.8067 $N \cdot m$ = 7.2307 $ft \cdot lb$
1 $ft \cdot lb$ = 1.3559 J = 1.3559 $N \cdot m$ = 0.1393 $kg \cdot m$

Power (watt; W)

1 W = 1 $J \cdot s^{-1}$ = 1 $N \cdot m \cdot s^{-1}$
1 W = 60 $J \cdot min^{-1}$ = 60 $N \cdot m \cdot min^{-1}$ = 6.1183 $kg \cdot m \cdot min^{-1}$
1 $N \cdot m \cdot min^{-1}$ = 0.0167 W = 0.1020 $kg \cdot m \cdot min^{-1}$
1 $kg \cdot m \cdot min^{-1}$ = 0.1634 W = 9.8067 $N \cdot m \cdot min^{-1}$
1 kW = 1000 W = 1.34 horsepower (hp)

Energy (kilojoule; kJ)

1 kJ = 1000 J = 0.239 kcal
1 kcal = 4.186 kJ = 4186 J
1 kcal = 426.85 $kg \cdot m$ (at 100 % efficiency)
1 L VO_2 ≈ 21 kJ ≈ 5 kcal (at R = 0.96)

Speed and Velocity (meter·second⁻¹; $m \cdot s^{-1}$)

1 $m \cdot s^{-1}$ = 2.2371 $mi \cdot h^{-1}$ (mph) = 3.281 $ft \cdot s^{-1}$
1 $m \cdot min^{-1}$ = 0.0373 mph = 3.281 $ft \cdot min^{-1}$
1 $km \cdot hr^{-1}$ = 1000 $m \cdot h^{-1}$ = 0.6215 mph
1 mph = 1.6093 $km \cdot h^{-1}$ = 26.822 $m \cdot min^{-1}$ = 0.447 $m \cdot s^{-1}$
= 1.4667 $ft \cdot s^{-1}$

Angular Velocity (radian·second⁻¹; $rad \cdot s^{-1}$)

2 π rad (~ 6.2832 rad) = 360° (1 full circle)
1 rad = 360° / 2π = 57.2958°
1 $rad \cdot s^{-1}$ = 57.2958° $\cdot s^{-1}$
1° $\cdot s^{-1}$ = 0.0175 $rad \cdot s^{-1}$

Torque (newton meter; $N \cdot m$)

1 $N \cdot m$ = 0.1020 $kg \cdot m$ = 0.7375 $ft \cdot lb$
1 $kg \cdot m$ = 9.8067 $N \cdot m$ = 7.2307 $ft \cdot lb$
1 $ft \cdot lb$ = 1.3559 $N \cdot m$ = 0.1393 $kg \cdot m$

Volume (liter; L)

1 L = 1000 ml = 1.0567 qt = 33.81 fluid ounce (fl oz)
1 qt = 32 fl oz = 0.9464 L = 946.4 ml
1 ml = 0.0338 fl oz
1 fl oz = 0.0313 qt = 0.0296 L = 29.574 ml

Pressure (pascal; Pa)

1 pascal (Pa) = 1 $N \cdot m^{-2}$ = 0.000145 $lb \cdot in.^{-2}$
1 hectopascal (hPa) = 100 Pa = 0.1 kilopascal (kPa)
1 hPa = 1 millibar (mbar) = 0.75 torr = 0.75 mm Hg
1 torr = 1 mm Hg = 1.333 hPa = 1.333 mbar
1 atmosphere (atm) = 1013 hPa = 1013 mbar
= 760 torr = 760 mm Hg = 29.92 in. Hg = 14.7 $lb \cdot in.^{-2}$

Temperature (kelvin; K)

°C to K: K = (°C + 273)
K to °C: °C = (K − 273)
°F to °C: °C = (°F − 32) / 1.8
°C to °F: °F = (°C * 1.8) + 32

METRIC CONVERSIONS

Metric units are simpler to use than the traditional or customary units of the American system. The metric system facilitates the conversion of base quantities (e.g., mass, length, time) expressed in base units (e.g., kilogram, meter, second) into derived quantities (e.g., force, power, speed, volume) expressed in derived units (e.g., $m \cdot kg \cdot s^2$, $m^2 \cdot kg \cdot s^{-3}$, $m \cdot s^{-1}$, m^3), respectively. The systematic nature of metric units is somewhat diminished, however, by the use of special names and symbols, such as expressing force in newtons (N) instead of $m \cdot kg \cdot s^{-2}$, or expressing pressure in pascals (Pa) instead of $m^{-1} \cdot kg \cdot s^{-2}$.

The metric system is also easier when it comes to measuring small or large quantities. For example, one meter (1m) can be systematically divided by 10 to create 10 decimeters (10 dm), or by 100 to create 100 centimeters (100 cm), or by 1000 to create 1000 millimeters (1000 mm). If long lengths or distances are being measured, 1 meter can be multiplied by 1000 (1000 m) to create one kilometer (1 km). This type of systematic approach does not apply to customary American units. The yard is the nonmetric equivalent of the meter. When a yard is divided into smaller units, it is divided into 3 feet and further into 36 inches. For measuring long distances, it is multiplied by 1760 (1760 yd) to create 1 mile (1 mi).

Table 2.2 provides a summary of conversion factors for converting between SI (metric) units and American (customary) units. It will be helpful to refer to this table frequently while reading the following discussion of metric conversions. These same conversion factors are also included in Appendix D for easy reference from any point throughout the manual.

Mass (Weight) Measures

Every exercise physiology student is expected to respond quickly and correctly in SI units to the question, "What is your body weight?" When expressing body weight (or mass), the correct response is to describe it in kilograms (kg). Components of body composition, including fat weight and lean weight (or lean body mass), are also expressed in kilograms. It is also appropriate to describe body weight in grams, but the more common measure is kilograms. If body weight is recorded on a measuring instrument that displays only pounds, it can be converted to kilograms by multiplying or dividing by the appropriate conversion factors (Eq. 2.5a and 2.5b). For smaller masses, the gram can be subdivided into 10 decigrams (dg), 100 centigrams (cg), and 1000 milligrams (mg).

Weight, X kg = **151 lb** * (0.4536 kg / 1 lb)
= **68.5 kg**   *ne = 86.18 kg*   Eq. 2.5a

Weight, X kg = **151 lb** * (1 kg / 2.2046 lb)
= **68.5 kg**   Eq. 2.5b

Instead of body weight being considered a mass, it can be thought of as a force, as in the force being exerted downward on a scale. When this is the case, body weight is expressed in newtons (N) and can be calculated by one of two conversion factors (Eq. 2.6a and 2.6b). A specific example of this can be found in Chapter 8, where body weight (or mass) in newtons (N) is used in conjunction with vertical distance to measure leg power.

Weight, X N = **151 lb** * (4.448N / 1 lb) = **672 N**   Eq. 2.6a

Weight, X N = **151 lb** * (1N / 0.2248 lb) = **672 N**   Eq. 2.6b

Length (Height) Measures

The next question would be, "What is your height?" Most devices for measuring height found in an exercise physiology laboratory should allow for the measurement of height directly in SI units. So measuring and expressing height (in centimeters) should be simple. When the measuring device displays inches instead of centimeters, however, it is necessary to convert them by multiplying or dividing the height in inches by one of two conversion factors (Eq. 2.7a and 2.7b). These two conversion factors are related mathematically in that they are reciprocals of one another.

Height, X cm = **70.5 in.** * (2.54 cm / 1 in.)
= **179 cm**   *ne = 190.5 cm*   Eq. 2.7a

Height, X cm = **70.5 in.** * (1 cm / 0.3937 in.)
= **179 cm**   Eq. 2.7b

Measurement Error and Significant Figures

No mention has been made to this point about **measurement error.** It is virtually impossible to measure any variable described in this laboratory manual (e.g., mass, length, force, power) without some degree of error. The error of any laboratory measurement is what determines the **precision** and **accuracy** with which that measurement can be made. The term *precision* refers to the *reliability* or reproducibility of a measurement or instrument. Precision is frequently characterized in terms of the variability of the measurement. A precise measure or instrument yields a low variability (standard deviation or standard error) and a high degree

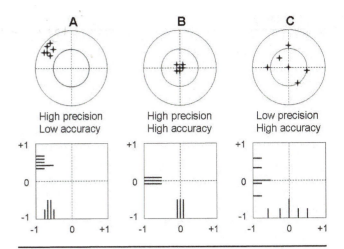

Figure 2.2 Demonstration of precision and accuracy. The upper portion of the figure shows six shots taken at each of three targets. The lower portion is the frequency with which each shot hit the target, with 0 in both directions (X and Y) being a "perfect" shot.

of reliability (high test-retest correlation coefficient). The term *accuracy* refers to the *validity* of the measurement, or how close a measurement is to the correct or "real" value (if it is known). The goal of every scientist and exercise physiology student should be to develop and use laboratory instruments and tests that are both precise and accurate.

A frequently used analogy to help demonstrate precision and accuracy is shooting at a target. Figure 2.2 shows three targets (A, B, and C) at which six shots each have been fired. Target B shows both high precision (the shots are tightly grouped with little variability or error) and high accuracy (the shots hit the correct or "real" target). Target A shows the same high precision (tightly grouped shots), but the accuracy is low because the shots do not hit the center of the target. Target C, even though it shows low precision (the shots are widespread with more variability or error), shows high accuracy because "on average" the shots are evenly arranged around the correct target. In the exercise physiology laboratory, a measuring device that is precise and accurate follows this same analogy, providing measurements that are tightly clustered around the "real" value.

It is important to be able to express the precision of a measurement or measuring device. Let's use a skinfold caliper as an example. Assume that a measuring device (e.g., ruler, scale, skinfold caliper) can be used to measure or "estimate" a quantity to one decimal place farther than the last decimal place on the scale of the device. So for the skinfold caliper, assuming it is marked in millimeters, a tester could measure a skinfold thickness to the closest millimeter (e.g., between 25 and 26 mm) and could still "estimate" the value between those two marks (e.g., 25.5 mm). So the *precision* of the skinfold caliper is considered 0.1 mm, and each of the figures in the estimated value (25.5 mm) is considered a **significant figure** (or significant digit). It would not be appropriate to express this value as 25.5000, because this is beyond the precision of the device.

Counting significant figures follows a general rule. Begin at the left end of the number and (ignoring any decimal point) count the number of digits until the precision of the measurement is reached. In the example above (25.5 mm), the skinfold thickness has three significant figures. Counting significant figures becomes difficult when the precision of the measuring device is uncertain. Assume in this chapter (for the purpose of unit conversions) that any values given are within the precision of the measuring device. An effort is made in each subsequent chapter to describe the precision and accuracy with which each measurement is made, so that the number of significant figures can be correctly determined.

Other Metric Measures and Conversions

The metric system facilitates the conversion from mass, length, and time measures to a variety of derived quantities, including force, work, power, energy, speed, torque, volume, pressure, and more. The emphasis in this laboratory manual is on the conversion of American or cus-tomary units (e.g., lb, ft·lb, mph, fl oz, lb·in.^{2}) into SI or metric units. This is most often necessary because a specific measuring device being used (especially an older one) does not display in metric units. Some examples of quantities being converted from American or customary units into metric units are shown in Equations 2.8a through 2.8h. Notice that each answer (or converted unit) is expressed in the *same number of significant figures* as the original quantity. This practice helps maintain the same level of precision before and after the conversion between units.

Force, X N = **71.5 kg** * (9. N / 1 kg)
    = **701 N**   Eq. 2.8a

Work, X J = **101 ft·lb** * (1.3559 J / ft·lb)
    = **137 J**   Eq. 2.8b

Power, X W = **515 kg·m·min^{-1}**
    * (1 W / 6.12 kg·m·min^{-1}) = **84.2 W**   Eq. 2.8c

Energy, X kJ = **125 kcal** * (4.186kJ / 1kcal)
    = **523 kJ**   Eq. 2.8d

Speed, X m·s^{-1} = **35 mph**
    * (1 m·s^{-1} / 2.2371 mph) = **16 m·s^{-1}**   Eq. 2.8e

Torque, X N·m = **63 ft·lb** * (1.3559 N·m / ft·lb)
    = **85 N·m**   Eq. 2.8f

Volume, X ml = **30.5 fl oz**
    * (29.574 ml / 1 fl oz) = **902 ml**   Eq. 2.8g

Pressure, hPa = **18.55 lb·in^2**
    * (1 hPa / 0.0145 lb·in^2) = **1279 hPa**   Eq. 2.8h

The Concept of Unit Analysis

In reviewing Equations 2.8a through 2.8h, notice that some quantities are multiplied by the metric conversion factor,

and others are divided. It is easy to get careless and multiply or divide by the incorrect factor and end up with the wrong answer. **Unit analysis** can increase the likelihood of getting the correct answer. It is a concept where special attention is given to the units, such that the problem is set up to yield the desired units before the calculation is performed.

As an example, look again at the conversion made in Equation 2.8g, where 30.5 fl oz is converted to 902 ml. Before performing the calculation, the problem is set up to insure that the correct units (ml) will result, as shown in Equation 2.9a. Once it is confirmed that the units are correct, the appropriate conversion factor can be chosen, in this case 29.574 ml = 1 fl oz. Furthermore, it should be clear that multiplying by the conversion factor will yield the correct units and therefore the correct answer. The problem could also be worked using the reciprocal correction factor, 1 ml = 0.0338 fl oz. In this case, based on an analysis of the units, the conversion factor should go in the denominator, again yielding the correct answer (Eq. 2.9b).

$$X \text{ ml} = 30.5 \ \cancel{\text{fl oz}} \ * \ \frac{29.574 \text{ ml}}{1 \ \cancel{\text{fl oz}}} = 902 \text{ ml} \qquad \text{Eq. 2.9a}$$

$$X \text{ ml} = 30.5 \ \cancel{\text{fl oz}} \ * \ \frac{1 \text{ ml}}{0.0338 \ \cancel{\text{fl oz}}} = 902 \text{ ml} \qquad \text{Eq. 2.9b}$$

Another example of unit analysis is to convert speed from miles per hour into meters per second. The conversion could be done in one step using one conversion factor (Eq. 2.10a). Instead, assume the conversion factor is not known, but what is known is that there are 1609.35 meters in 1 mile, 60 minutes in 1 hour, and 60 seconds in 1 minute. By setting up the problem with the units in the correct position (either in the numerator or denominator), so that the resultant units are meters per second, the calculation yields the same results, 55 mph equals 25 m·s^{-1} (Eq. 2.10b).

$$X \text{ m·s}^{-1} = 55 \ \cancel{\text{mph}} \ * \ \frac{0.447 \text{ m·s}^{-1}}{1 \ \cancel{\text{mph}}} = 25 \text{ m·s}^{-1} \quad \text{Eq. 2.10a}$$

$$X \text{ m·s}^{-1} = \frac{55 \ \cancel{\text{mi}}}{\cancel{\text{h}}} * \frac{1609.35 \text{ m}}{1 \ \cancel{\text{mi}}} * \frac{1 \ \cancel{\text{h}}}{60 \ \cancel{\text{min}}} * \frac{1 \ \cancel{\text{min}}}{60 \text{ s}}$$
$$= 25 \text{ m·s}^{-1} \qquad \text{Eq. 2.10a}$$

SUMMARY

The Système International (SI), or metric system, is the unit system of choice in the scientific community and is used by most people throughout the world. For this reason, the exercise physiology student must use and understand this system. The SI base quantities (e.g., length, mass, time, etc.) and SI base units (e.g., meter, kilogram, second, etc.) are used to derive all other quantities and units. Several derived units, such as newton, watt, and joule, have been named in honor of the scientists who have made significant contributions to various fields of science. Until the United States fully adopts

BOX 2.1	Chapter Preview/Review

What does the term *SI* mean?

When are abbreviations of units capitalized?

Who are some of the scientists who have had a metric unit named in their honor?

What is the relationship between meters, kilometers, and millimeters?

Which variables incorporate force?

What is the caloric equivalent of 1 L of oxygen uptake?

In what three scales may temperature be expressed?

In what units may pressure be expressed?

What do the terms *precision* and *accuracy* mean?

What is meant by the concept of unit analysis?

the SI system, wherever or whenever nonmetric units are used, students must understand how they can be converted. Remember also that nearly all measurements made in the exercise physiology lab are made with some degree of error. Therefore, the precision and accuracy of all measurement devices should be considered when possible, with the resultant measurements expressed in significant figures when the precision of the device is known.

At the conclusion of each chapter there are two forms: a **Homework** form and a **Lab Results** form. Form 2.1 (Homework) is a set of problems that the student may complete either as *preview* for an upcoming lab or as *review* of a completed lab, in whichever manner the instructor decides to use it. Form 2.2 (Lab Results) provides an opportunity for the student to collect laboratory data, and in this particular case to study the variables, instruments, and units discussed in Chapter 2. The data recorded on the Lab Results form in any chapter may also be used by the student to write a lab report or be used in any other project assigned by the instructor.

References

1. American College of Sports Medicine (2012). Information for authors in *Medicine and Science in Sports and Exercise* (MSSE). Retrieved June 11, 2012 from https://www.editorialmanager.com/msse/.

2. American Psychological Association (2009). *Publication Manual of the American Psychological Association* (6th ed.). Washington, DC: APA Publications.

3. Knuttgen, H. G. (1986). Quantifying exercise performance with SI units. *The Physician and Sportsmedicine, 14*(12): 157–161.

4. Knuttgen, H. G. (1995). Force, work, and power in athletic training. *Sports Science Exchange, 57*(4): 1–6.

5. Thompson, A., & Taylor, B. N. (2008). *NIST special publication 811, 2008 edition: Guide for the Use of the International System of Units (SI)*. Gaithersburg, MD: United States Department of Commerce, National Institute of Standards and Technology.

6. U.S. Metric Association (2009). Frequently asked questions about the metric system. Retrieved January 14, 2009, from http://www.metric.org.

7. Young, D. S. (1987). Implementation of SI units for clinical laboratory data. *Annals of Internal Medicine, 106*, 114–129.

Form 2.1
HOMEWORK

NAME Tyler Gilmore   DATE _____ SCORE _____

Units of Measure

Mass / Weight	X lb =	**78.5**	kg *	$78.5 kg \cdot \dfrac{2.2046 lbs}{1 kg}$	=	173.06 lb

Length / Height	X mile =	**5.2**	km *	$5.2 km \cdot \dfrac{0.6214 mi}{1 km}$	=	3.23 mi

Force	X lb =	**401**	N *	$401 N \cdot \dfrac{.2248}{1 N}$	=	90.14 lb

Work	X N·m =	**355**	ft·lb *	$355 ft lb \cdot \dfrac{1.3559 Nm}{1 ft lb}$	=	481.34 N·m

Power	X kg·m·min⁻¹ =	**305**	W *	$305 W \cdot \dfrac{6.1183 kg \cdot m \cdot min^{-1}}{1 W}$	=	1866.08 kg·m·min⁻¹

Energy	X kcal =	**1013**	J *	$1013 J \cdot \dfrac{.239 kcal}{1000 J}$	=	.24 kcal

Speed / Velocity	X mph =	**122**	km·h⁻¹ *	$122 km \cdot h^{-1} \cdot \dfrac{.6215 mph}{1 km \cdot h^{-1}}$	=	75.82 mph

Angular Velocity	X deg·s⁻¹ =	**1.5**	rad·s⁻¹ *	$1.5 rad \cdot s^{-1} \cdot \dfrac{57.2958°\cdot s^{-1}}{1 rad \cdot s^{-1}}$	=	85.94 deg·s⁻¹

Torque	X ft·lb =	**45**	N·m *	$45 N \cdot m \cdot \dfrac{.7375 ft lb}{1 N \cdot m}$	=	33.19 ft·lb

Volume	X ml =	**2.75**	cup *	$2.75 cup \cdot \dfrac{236.6 ml}{1 cup}$	=	650.65 ml

Pressure	X torr =	**999**	mbar *	$999 mbar \cdot \dfrac{.75 torr}{1 mbar}$	=	749.25 torr

Temperature	X K =	**212**	°F =	$(212°F - 32)1.8 = 100°C + 273$	=	373 K

Form 2.2
LAB RESULTS

NAME _Tyler Gilmore_   DATE _____   SCORE _____

Units of Measure

To gain an appreciation for variables and units of measure, take a <u>tour</u> of your exercise physiology lab and complete the following laboratory exercise *within the time available*.

<u>Observe</u> various laboratory instruments (e.g., scale, stadiometer, etc.). Attempt to <u>identify</u> an instrument in the lab that measures each of the variables listed below (e.g., weight, height, etc.) within the time available. Record the <u>units</u> in which the instrument measures (e.g., kg, cm, etc.). Record the <u>range</u> within which the instrument measures and the <u>precision</u> (or accuracy) with which it measures. *Some examples are provided.*

<u>Take one measurement</u> with the instrument in the units indicated (or alternatively <u>observe</u> the measurement scale on the instrument and record any value). <u>Convert</u> the measured or observed units into the units indicated below using the conversion factors in Appendix D. *Some examples are provided.*

Weight

Weight = **85.1** kg *   2.2046 lb / 1 kg   =   **188**   lb

   Scale   Units   kg, lb, N   Range   0–200 kg   Precision   0.1 kg

Height

Height = **175.0** cm *   0.3937 in. / 1 cm   =   **68.9**   in.

   Stadiometer   Units   cm, in. m   Range   0–200 cm   Precision   0.1 cm

Force

Force = _____ kg *   =   N

   Grip dynamometer   Units   Range   Precision

Power

Power = _____ W *   = $kg \cdot m \cdot min^{-1}$

   Cycle ergometer   Units   Range   Precision

Speed

Speed = _____ mph *   = $km \cdot h^{-1}$

   Treadmill   Units   Range   Precision

Volume

Volume = _____ L *   =   ml

   Spirometer   Units   Range   Precision

Pressure

Pressure = _____ mm Hg *   =   torr

   Sphygmomanometer   Units   mm Hg, torr   Range   0–300 mm Hg   Precision   1 mm Hg

Temperature

Temperature = _____ °F =   =   K

   Thermometer   Units   Range   Precision

CHAPTER

COLLECTION OF BASIC DATA

Nearly all test forms (data collection forms) include basic information or **basic data** about the participants and the conditions under which the data are collected. The information about the participants is typically referred to as either basic data or vital data, including such characteristics as name, gender/sex, age, height and weight. Sometimes more detailed vital data (e.g., heart rate, blood pressure, body temperature) are recorded. It is also common to record the conditions under which the data are collected, including test date, time of day, and in some cases the environmental conditions (e.g., temperature, barometric pressure, relative humidity). Form 3.2, at the end of this chapter, may be used to record basic data and assist in the evaluation of certain characteristics (especially height and weight) based on a review of comparative data.

RECORDING BASIC DATA

The art and technical skills of administering tests include the precise and thorough recording of all basic data. Some of the comments here may appear obvious, but there are numerous occasions when seemingly obvious items of basic data are omitted, much to the later chagrin of the investigators or the participants.

Name, Date, and Time

Name is typically written with the last name first, followed by a comma and then the first name. In potentially publishable research, an identification number (ID#) replaces the name for anonymity or confidentiality. Also, to resolve discrepancies or errors, especially if technicians have interobserver differences, it helps to include the technician's initials.

The test **date** is presented with the month in numerical form at the beginning; for example, September 4, 2006 would be recorded as 9/4/06 (or 09/04/06). Besides recording these on the data collection form (e.g., Form 3.2), name and date should be recorded on any type of chart paper, such as that from the electrocardiogram or isokinetic dynamometer.

It is important to record test **time** in addition to date on the data collection form because of the possible daily or monthly variations of many biological and performance variables (e.g., height, weight, strength, aerobic power, anaerobic power).

Age and Gender

Age is recorded to the closest year (y), except when it may be important to record to the closest one-tenth of a year. For example, if someone turned 32 y of age four months ago, the age might be recorded as 32.3 y.

Gender for a person is abbreviated as M (male) or F (female). For a group of adults (18 years old and above), the recommended group designation is M (men) and W (women).[1] But, if there are minors (under 18 y of age), the group designation is male or female, not men or women.

Height (Stature) and Body Weight (Mass)

In the field of anthropometry (defined as the measurement of humans), the term *stature,* derived from *statue,* is used to describe the standing height of a human (as if a statue). As noted earlier, although *stature* is the appropriate term to use in a scientific context when describing the anthropometric characteristics of the participants of a study, *height* is used throughout most of this laboratory manual because it is the more common term.

Mass, as noted in Chapter 2, is synonymous with weight when measured under the same acceleration of gravity. Because most measurements are assumed to be taken on earth, these two terms can be used interchangeably in most cases. The terms *mass, body mass,* and *lean body mass* are used in scientific publications, especially with reference to describing the body composition of the study participants. The terms *weight* and *body weight,* however, are also acceptable and again, because of their more common usage, are the terms of choice in this laboratory manual. The body mass and body weight of a person use the same unit of measure—the kilogram (kg). In Chapter 4, we will see that body weight can also be used as a measure of force, for the purpose of calculating work and power, in which case it is expressed in newtons (N).

Measurement Precision

The technician records height to the nearest tenth of a centimeter (0.1 cm; 1 mm) if the height scale (stadiometer; anthropometer) has such graduations (markings). If the measurement device is marked only in inches and the graduations are ¼ in. or ½ in., the technician records the inches to the closest ¼ in. or ½ in., respectively. Then the inch value is converted and recorded to the appropriately rounded centimeter or decimal centimeter.

The main considerations in rounding off numbers are conventionality, consistency of the significant digits, and precision of the measurement. The appropriate conventionality guide is that of the International System (SI).[16] SI recommends using the "5 rule" when reducing a certain number of digits. Fortunately, most Americans are familiar with this rule: "If the digits to be discarded begin with a digit less than 5, the digit preceding the 5 is not changed." For example, the number 7.44 changed to a two-digit number would become 7.4; changed to a one-digit number, it would become 7 (but not 7.0). Conversely, if the discarded digit or digits begin with a number greater than or equal to 5, then the digit preceding the 5 is increased by 1. For example, 167.66 cm becomes 167.7 cm as a four-digit number and becomes 168 as a three-digit number.

The degree of precision sought in a measure or mathematical calculation depends upon the purposes of the measurement and the precision of the instrument. In the United States the height of a person is often stated to the closest ½ in. (1.27 cm) or ¼ in. (0.64 cm), depending upon the accuracy of the stadiometer. Thus, when the mean (M) height is calculated from the heights of several persons, it should be rounded off either to the closest ½ in. or ¼ in., respectively. If converting the inches to centimeters, both the ½ in. (0.5 in.) and ¼ in. (0.25 in.) values should not be rounded to the closest tenth centimeter because the stadiometer does not justify such precision. The closest 0.5 cm would be a justifiably rounded number for the ¼ in. scale and to the closest centimeter for the ½ in. scale. Rounding off to the closest *tenth* centimeter provides unwarranted and false precision. However, if the purpose of the investigators is to detect the change in height in persons from morning to evening, then they should choose a more precise stadiometer. The use of a stadiometer with graduations in tenths of a centimeter allows measurement of height to the closest 0.1 cm (1 mm).

Environmental Conditions

Although environmental or meteorological conditions have no known effect on height or weight, they can affect other variables measured in the exercise physiology laboratory. It is recommended that the technician practice recording room temperature, barometric pressure and relative humidity. These laboratory or environmental conditions are most important when measuring air volumes (e.g. vital capacity, pulmonary ventilation, etc.). The conversion between ambient (ATPS), body (BTPS) and standard (STPD) conditions using these environmental data is discussed in Chapters 15, 20 and 21.

General Measurement Procedures

It is recommended that students test other students rather than a student testing him- or herself. Although this can

---

| BOX 3.1 | **Accuracy of Height and Body Weight Measures** |

Height

The test-retest reliability of height (stature) measurements is consistently high. A recent review article on anthropometric measurement error reported a mean reliability coefficient (*R*) for the measurement of height of .98 with a range of .93–.99.[17]

Height measurements may differ throughout the day due to compression of the spine.[17] Studies have shown height decreases of 6 mm to 8.8 mm later in the day.[3,8] Conversely, lying supine (for an average of 48 min) later in the day resulted in a 5 mm increase in height.[4]

Body Weight

The test-retest reliability of body weight (mass) measurements is also high. Range of reported reliability coefficients for the measurement of body weight is .95–1.00 with a mean of .98.[17]

Self-Reported Height and Weight

Generally speaking, the direct measurement of height and weight is preferred to the use of self-reported values when possible. Although highly correlated with actual height (*r* = .82–.91) and weight (*r* = .87–.94),[15] self-reported values differ significantly from the actual values. High school students[2] (n = 4619) overestimated height by 6.9 cm and underestimated weight by 1.6 kg. Adult males[13,14] overestimated height by 0.38–1.23 cm and underestimated weight by 1.40–1.85 kg, while adult females[13,14] overestimated height by 0.38–0.40 cm and underestimated weight by 0.54–0.85 kg.

Older Adults

The use of self-reported height and weight has limitations in older adults (over 60 years).[7] In research studies and clinical settings involving older adults, failure to directly measure height and weight can result in substantial error. Special consideration should also be given to diurnal variations in height in older adults if spinal osteoporosis is a concern.[4]

---

take more time, it mimics typical research procedures and gives students, who would be referred to as "technicians," or "testers," in this case, the chance to practice in their personal relationship with the participant. As an example, technicians (students) should call participants (other students) by their names and thank them for their cooperation and effort.

The methods sections in this manual usually include two major phases—preparations and procedures. Three items are usually included in the procedures phase—the technician's steps for administering the test, the calculations and conversions, and the recording of the data onto the forms. Box 3.1 discusses the accuracy of height and body weight measures.

METHODS

Height (Stature) Method

Height is a basic variable that is routinely measured in nearly all laboratories. Its accurate and standardized measurement should be given serious attention. The purposes for measuring height include (1) to familiarize students with standardized height measurements; (2) to characterize or describe the participant; (3) to relate the participant's height to norms or standards; (4) to relate body weight with height; (5) to relate height with growth or nutritional status; and (6) to relate height and body weight with risk of chronic diseases or conditions.

Height can be measured on a platform scale (sometimes also referred to as a physician's scale) equipped with a stadiometer (*stadio* = stature; *meter* = measure), as shown in Figure 3.1. The stadiometer includes a hinged lever that the technician can swing upward to a 90° angle and place on the crown of the participant's head to measure height. Stadiometers (especially newer ones) usually have both inch and centimeter graduations. Wall-mounted stadiometers, separate of a weight scale, are also available (e.g., Seca, Harpenden). These devices are often preferred to the stadiometer connected to the platform scale, because the mechanism allows for a smoother, more accurate measure of height. A stadiometer can also be improvised by attaching a measuring tape to a wall. The participant stands with the back against the wall, and any right-angled device is placed against the crown of the head and the measuring tape. It may be helpful to have a stool available for the technician to stand on to measure tall persons. The following procedures help to standardize and enhance the accuracy of height measurements.

Preparation by the Technician to Measure Height

1. If using the platform-beam scale, check its accuracy by confirming the distance from the platform base to the first graduated measure on the stadiometer.
2. Complete Form 3.2 with the prior basic data information (name, date, time, age, and gender).
3. Ask the participant to remove shoes; removing socks is also preferred, but thin socks may remain.
4. The hair should be worn down and low to the head. It may be necessary to ask the participant to remove accessories from the hair so that it may be worn down.

Procedures for Measuring Height

1. The participant steps onto the platform scale and turns away from the stadiometer. The technician asks the participant to lower the head in order to clear the swing of the hinged lever to a horizontal position. If using a wall-mounted stadiometer, the participant stands facing away from the wall, with heels, scapulae, and buttocks

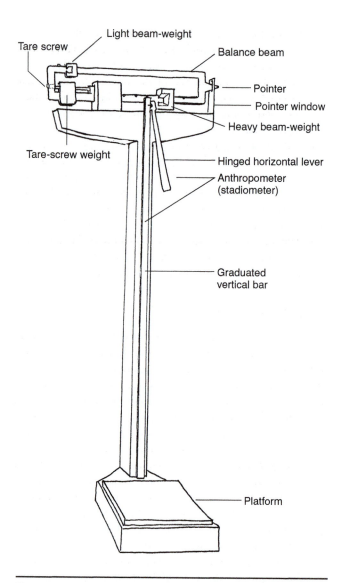

Figure 3.1 The platform scale is an instrument for body weight (mass) and height (stature). The anthropometer (stadiometer) with the sliding vertical bar and hinged horizontal head lever is the portion of the platform scale that measures height.

in contact with the wall. Some persons will not be able to maintain a natural stance if the posterior of the head is also touching the wall.[3]

2. The participant stands as tall as possible with heels together and feet evenly balanced at an angle of approximately 60°, using the medial borders (inside) of the feet and the wall as the reference lines. For example, a 90° angle would indicate that the feet were pointed directly forward.
3. The participant tucks the chin to bring the head into a position that horizontally aligns the lowest point of the orbit of the eye with the opening of the ear canal.
4. As the participant inhales deeply and maintains the designated position, the technician moves the hinged lever of the platform scale stadiometer into contact

with the crown of the head. It may be necessary to "compress" the participant's hair so that the lever contacts the head. If a stadiometer is not available, and height is being measured against a wall, the technician places one edge of the right-angled object against the wall and places the other edge on top of the participant's head.

5. The technician records height on Form 3.2 to the highest precision possible depending on the measurement device. If using a stadiometer, it should be possible to record height to the nearest tenth centimeter (0.1 cm). If using a less precise instrument, record height to the closest ½ in. or ¼ in., whichever is possible.

6. The technician (if necessary) converts the height from inches to centimeters and then records it on Form 3.2 to the appropriately rounded centimeter.

Body Weight (Mass) Method

Body mass is probably the most measured variable in exercise physiology laboratories. This basic variable is factored into many of the other variables described in this laboratory manual; hence, its importance cannot be overestimated. Body weight can fluctuate significantly based on the amount of food and water consumed throughout the course of a day. It is best, especially if tracking body weight longitudinally, that it is measured at the same time each day, preferably in the morning. Ideally, body weight would be measured nude in the morning following a 12-hour fast and following evacuation of all urine and feces from the body. This could be considered a "true" body weight. When longitudinal body weights are measured on the same person at different times of day they could vary by several kilograms just due to varying levels of food intake or hydration status.

Participants can be weighed in the attire that corresponds to the reference source. For example, if the reference source for comparison allowed 0.3 kg of clothing, such as underwear, shirt, and shorts, dress, or pants, then the person may be weighed in such attire. In some cases, especially when measuring body composition, nude weight is preferred. Because of the impracticality of obtaining nude weight, some researchers derive nude weight by weighing the clothes in which the participant is weighed and then subtracting the weight of the clothing from the clothed body weight. If a person wears only a nylon swimsuit or a disposable paper gown, it may be deemed as nude weight. The exercise-clothed weight should be used for the calculation of work or power when the participants are lifting their own body weight, such as in bench stepping, uphill walking, or uphill running. The following methods are helpful when measuring a participant's body weight.

Preparation by the Technician to Measure Weight

1. Calibrate the weighing scale, if it has not been calibrated within a month (Box 3.2).

BOX 3.2   Example of Calibration Procedures for the Platform Scale

Zero Calibration

1. Set both moveable beam-weights of the scale to the zero positions.
2. Observe the position of the pointer; it should come to rest in midair between the top and bottom of the pointer window.
3. If necessary, balance the pointer in this midair position by using a screwdriver to adjust the tare-screw weight of the platform scale. Turning the tare screw clockwise moves the tare-screw weight toward the screw's head, thus lifting the pointer higher in the pointer window.

High-Point Calibration

1. Set the beam-weights to the highest position for which you have calibration weights or to the position of the highest expected body weight of your participants. Typical platform scales cannot read body weights above 159 kg (350 lb). Ideally, if you have 350 lb of certified weights, place them on the scale. But, if you have only 100 kg (220.5 lb to closest 0.1 lb) certified weights, or weights that you have "certified" on a precision scale, set them on the scale and adjust the beam-weights accordingly. For example, set the heavy beam-weight to 200 lb and set the light beam-weight to 20.5 lb.
2. Observe the position of the pointer. If it is balanced in midposition in the pointer window, the scale is accurate at body weights near the high-point range.
3. If the pointer is above the balanced point, adjust the light beam-weight, if necessary, to the pointer's midair position.
4. Record any discrepancy between the original set position and the final balanced position.
5. If needed, derive a correction factor for the high-point readings. For example, if 120 kg of "certified" high-point weights showed 121 kg on the scale, subtract 1 kg from those persons' body weights that were between 110 kg and 130 kg (range chosen arbitrarily).

Midpoint Calibration

1. Estimate the average body weight of the participants.
2. Place "certified" weights on the scale that come close to the estimated participants' average weight. (A Cybex machine has certified weights.)
3. Balance the pointer to the midair position. If it is already balanced, the scale is accurate near the midpoint position of the pound or kilogram scale.
4. If the pointer is not in the midair position, adjust the light beam-weight to the balanced position.
5. Record any discrepancy between the original set position and the final midair position.
6. If needed, derive a correction factor for midpoint readings or readjust the tare-screw weight to the pointer's midair position. Unfortunately, this will change the zero point, thus distorting low-range body masses.

2. Insert the acquired basic data onto Form 3.2, including the participant's name, date, time, age, gender, and meteorological data.
3. Ask the participant to remove shoes, socks, jewelry, and accessories, empty all pockets, and remove as much clothing as feasible.
4. Weigh the person's "weigh-in clothing" and record onto Form 3.2 (optional).

Procedures for Measuring Body Weight

1. The participant stands on and faces the scale.
2. The technician places the heavy beam-weight (lower lever) to the estimated graduation mark first, followed by the light beam-weight (upper lever). The light beam-weight is moved slowly to balance the pointer in the midair position within the window of the scale. If the pointer cannot be balanced, the heavy beam-weight must be readjusted. If an electronic digital scale is being used, the technician simply reads the body weight on the indicator of the scale.
3. The technician records body weight on Form 3.2 to the highest precision possible depending on the measurement device. If using a platform scale, it should be possible to record body weight to the nearest ½ or ¼ lb. If using a more precise instrument, record body weight to the closest 0.02 kg (or to the maximum precision the instrument allows).
4. The technician (if necessary) converts the body weight from pounds to kilograms and then records it on Form 3.2 to the appropriately rounded kilogram.
5. The technician assists the participant off the scale, thanks the participant, and reminds the participant of any jewelry, accessories, or pocket contents that may have been removed.

Environmental Data

Environmental or meteorological data are frequently monitored using a simple electronic weather station. Such a device provides data for time of day, room temperature (typically in °C and °F), barometric pressure (typically in mm Hg and in. Hg), and relative humidity (%). Other laboratories are equipped with separate pieces of equipment including a thermometer for measuring temperature, a barometer (either mercurial or analog) for measuring barometric pressure, and a hygrometer (either digital or analog) for measuring relative humidity.

Procedures for Collecting Environmental Data

1. The technician records lab/room temperature (in °C) on Form 3.2 to the highest precision possible depending on the measurement device (weather station or thermometer).

2. The technician records barometric pressure (in mm Hg) on Form 3.2 to the highest precision possible depending on the measurement device (weather station or barometer).
3. The technician records relative humidity (in %) on Form 3.2 to the highest precision possible depending on the measurement device (weather station or hygrometer).

RESULTS AND DISCUSSION

The results section of a scientific report or study simply presents the findings in the text, tables, and figures. In the exercise physiology classroom, the results of the measurements are also recorded on the individual data collection form (e.g., Form 3.2). Frequently the results of an entire group are of interest. Group results typically include the mean *(M)*, standard deviation *(SD)*, and range of scores—that is, the lowest (minimum) to the highest (maximum) score.

The discussion section of a scientific report provides the reader with an interpretation of the results or measured values. An evaluation of the individual's height or body weight and the average of the group can be made by referring to the appropriate comparative data.

This particular discussion focuses on the effect of age, race/ethnicity, and time of day on height or body weight, and looks at how the height and body weight of the average American has changed over the years.

Effect of Age

The height and body weight of the average American is of interest with regard to growth, nutritional status, risk of chronic disease, the effect of aging, and other public health and research concerns. A recent publication[7] reviewed height and body weight data from national surveys conducted between 1999 and 2002. The mean or average height and body weight by gender and age group are seen in Table 3.1 and Table 3.2. The average American male has a height of 176.3 cm (69.4 in.) and a body weight of 88.3 kg (194.7 lb), with the average female having a height of 162.2 cm (63.8 in.) and body weight of 74.7 kg (164.7 lb). It can be seen in both genders that height reaches a peak by 49 years of age. Height then diminishes by about 1 cm per decade, resulting in a height loss of about 4–5 cm by the age of 79. Body weight appears to reach a peak at about the same age (40–49 y) in men and slightly later (50–59 y) in women, with a subsequent decline in the later years, especially after 70 years of age. Caution should always be used, however, in interpreting any trends in this way due to the fact that these are *cross-sectional* data and not *longitudinal* data. Cross-sectional data are collected at the *same time* on *different participants* in each category (in this case different age categories), whereas longitudinal data are collected on

Table 3.1	Average Height (cm; in.) by Gender and Age Group					
	Males	**Height (M ± SEM)**		**Females**	**Height (M ± SEM)**	
Age Group	N	cm	in.	N	cm	in.
6 years	176	120.6 ± 0.47	47.5 ± 0.19	193	119.0 ± 0.53	46.9 ± 0.21
10 years	171	142.3 ± 0.77	56.0 ± 0.30	189	144.2 ± 0.73	56.8 ± 0.29
14 years	260	168.7 ± 0.70	66.4 ± 0.28	270	160.5 ± 0.58	63.2 ± 0.23
18 years	284	176.8 ± 0.54	69.6 ± 0.21	304	163.0 ± 0.49	64.2 ± 0.10
20–29 years	808	177.6 ± 0.34	69.9 ± 0.13	1061	163.2 ± 0.31	64.3 ± 0.12
30–39 years	742	176.4 ± 0.33	69.4 ± 0.13	842	163.2 ± 0.32	64.3 ± 0.13
40–49 years	769	177.1 ± 0.28	69.7 ± 0.11	784	163.1 ± 0.29	64.2 ± 0.12
50–59 years	591	176.6 ± 0.38	69.5 ± 0.15	604	162.2 ± 0.34	63.9 ± 0.13
60–69 years	668	175.4 ± 0.28	69.0 ± 0.11	691	161.8 ± 0.33	63.7 ± 0.13
70–79 years	555	173.8 ± 0.41	68.4 ± 0.16	463	159.2 ± 0.34	62.7 ± 0.13
Total Mean	4 482	176.3 ± 0.17	69.4 ± 0.07	4 857	162.2 ± 0.16	63.8 ± 0.06

Source: McDowell, Fryar, Ogden & Flegal (2008).[11]

Table 3.2	Average Body Weight (kg; lb) by Gender and Age Group (United States, 2003–06)					
	Males	**Body Weight (M ± SEM)**		**Females**	**Body Weight (M ± SEM)**	
Age Group	N	kg	lb	N	kg	lb
6 years	176	24.2 ± 0.33	53.3 ± 0.72	193	23.4 ± 0.49	51.5 ± 1.08
10 years	172	40.1 ± 0.86	88.3 ± 1.89	189	42.4 ± 1.07	93.5 ± 2.35
14 years	260	63.1 ± 1.73	139.1 ± 3.81	269	58.8 ± 1.75	129.6 ± 3.85
18 years	283	77.2 ± 1.67	170.2 ± 3.68	272	67.6 ± 2.15	149.0 ± 4.75
20–29 years	811	85.4 ± 1.06	188.3 ± 2.33	706	70.7 ± 1.03	155.9 ± 2.27
30–39 years	741	88.1 ± 0.80	194.1 ± 1.77	663	74.7 ± 1.06	164.7 ± 2.34
40–49 years	769	91.8 ± 0.83	202.3 ± 1.83	787	77.7 ± 1.03	171.3 ± 2.27
50–59 years	591	90.2 ± 0.95	198.8 ± 2.10	593	78.0 ± 1.15	172.1 ± 2.53
60–69 years	669	90.0 ± 0.98	198.3 ± 2.16	728	77.3± 0.91	170.5 ± 2.02
70–79 years	555	85.0 ± 0.92	187.4 ± 2.03	486	70.6 ± 1.07	155.6 ± 2.35
Total Mean	4 489	88.3 ± 0.46	194.7 ± 1.02	4 330	74.7 ± 0.53	164.7 ± 1.17

Source: McDowell, Fryar, Ogden & Flegal (2008).[11]

the *same participants* over the *entire range* of interest (in this case that would mean measuring the same participants from age 6 through age 79).

For comparative purposes, Table 3.3 provides descriptive categories for body weight derived from percentiles. Body weight is described as well above average (> 95th percentile), above average (75th–95th percentile), average (25th–75th percentile), below average (5th–24th percentile), and well below average (< 5th percentile). Because of the effect of age on body weight, the categories are further subdivided by age group: 20–29 years, 30–39 years, and 40–49 years. This particular age range (20–49 years) is given special attention, as it was chosen to represent "young" adults, thinking that they would be the predominant users of this laboratory manual. However, data representing younger and older age groups are also included in numerous chapters throughout this laboratory manual whenever representative data sets were available in the research literature. No such table is provided for height in this case, as there are minimal differences in height throughout this particular age range (20–49 years).

Effect of Race/Ethnicity

A search for height and body weight data in the U.S. by race or ethnicity reveals good normative data for three groups: Caucasian-Americans (Whites), African-Americans (Blacks), and Mexican-Americans (Hispanics).[9] Large representative data sets for other racial and ethnic groups likely exist, but no sets with the same validity representing other ethnicities living in the U.S. could be found. Table 3.4 and Table 3.5 provide categories for height and body weight, respectively, for the three racial/ethnic groups living in the U.S.

The average heights for white men of 178 cm (69.6 in.) and black men of 177 cm (69.8 in.) both exceed the average height for Hispanic men of 170 cm (67.0 in.). The same trend holds true in women, where the average height of white women, 163 cm (64.2 in.), and the average height of black women, 163 cm (64.1 in.), both exceed the average height of Hispanic women of 158 cm (62.1 in.).[7] Data from citizens living in other countries show that Asians (living in Korea[5] and the Philippines[6]) are considerably shorter than all three U.S. ethnic groups previously described.

Table 3.3 — Category for Body Weight (kg; lb) by Gender and Age Group (United States, 2003–06)

Men Category	20–29 years kg	20–29 years lb	30–39 years kg	30–39 years lb	40–49 years kg	40–49 years lb
Well above ave (> 95th percentile)	> 122.6	> 270	> 120.8	> 266	> 124.7	> 275
Above ave (75th–95th percentile)	94.2–122.6	209–270	98.0–120.8	217–266	101.1–124.7	224–275
Average (25th–74th percentile)	71.5–94.3	158–208	74.2–98.1	165–216	79.2–101.2	176–223
Below ave (5th–24th percentile)	59.9–71.4	133–157	62.6–74.3	138–164	65.9–79.3	145–175
Well below ave (< 5th percentile)	< 59.9	< 132	< 62.6	< 138	< 65.9	< 145
Mean	85.4	188	88.1	194	91.8	202

Women Category	20–29 years kg	20–29 years lb	30–39 years kg	30–39 years lb	40–49 years kg	40–49 years lb
Well above ave (> 95th percentile)	> 110.7	> 244	> 114.2	> 252	> 116.9	> 258
Above ave (75th–95th percentile)	78.9–110.7	175–244	83.7–114.2	185–252	89.3–116.9	198–258
Average (25th–74th percentile)	56.4–78.8	125–174	59.9–83.6	133–184	62.9–89.2	139–197
Below ave (5th–24th percentile)	48.0–56.3	106–124	51.2–59.8	113–132	52.3–62.8	115–138
Well below ave (< 5th percentile)	< 48.0	< 106	< 51.2	< 113	< 52.3	< 115
Mean	70.7	156	74.7	165	77.7	171

Source: McDowell, Fryar, Ogden & Flegal (2008).[11]

Table 3.4 — Category for Height (cm; in.) by Gender and Race/Ethnicity (United States, 2003–06)

Men Category (Percentile)	Total cm	Total in.	White (Non-Hispanic) cm	White (Non-Hispanic) in.	Black (Non-Hispanic) cm	Black (Non-Hispanic) in.	Hispanic cm	Hispanic in.
Well above ave (> 95th)	> 189	> 74.3	> 189	> 74.5	> 190	> 74.6	> 182	> 71.6
Above ave (75th–95th)	183–189	71.6–74.3	183–189	71.7–74.5	181–190	71.7–74.6	176–182	68.9–71.6
Average (25th–74th)	172–182	67.5–71.5	174–182	67.9–71.8	172–182	67.9–71.6	166–175	65.1–68.8
Below ave (5th–24th)	164–171	64.4–67.4	166–173	65.0–68.0	165–172	65.1–67.8	159–165	62.5–65.0
Well below ave (< 5th)	< 164	< 64.4	< 166	< 65.4	< 165	< 65.1	< 159	< 62.5
Mean	176	69.4	178	69.9	177	69.8	170	67.0

Women Category (Percentile)	Total cm	Total in.	White (Non-Hispanic) cm	White (Non-Hispanic) in.	Black (Non-Hispanic) cm	Black (Non-Hispanic) in.	Hispanic cm	Hispanic in.
Well above ave (> 95th)	> 173	> 68.2	> 174	> 68.4	> 174	> 68.4	> 168	> 66.2
Above ave (75th–95th)	170–173	65.7–68.2	169–174	66.1–68.4	168–174	65.9–68.4	163–168	63.8–66.2
Average (25th–74th)	159–169	62.2–65.6	160–168	62.6–66.0	159–167	62.4–65.8	155–162	60.4–63.7
Below ave (5th–24th)	151–158	59.3–62.1	152–159	59.9–62.5	152–158	59.7–62.3	147–154	58.0–60.5
Well below ave (< 5th)	< 151	< 59.3	< 152	< 59.9	< 152	< 59.7	< 147	< 58.0
Mean	162	63.8	163	64.2	163	64.1	158	62.1

Source: McDowell, Fryar, Ogden & Flegal (2008).[11]

The average height for Asian men is about 162–165 cm, at least 5 cm shorter than Hispanic men in the U.S. The average height of Asian women is about 151–152 cm, at least 6 cm shorter than Hispanic women in the U.S.

The racial/ethnic trends in body weight are similar to height in men but not as much in women. White men and black men, with average body weights of 89.6 kg (197 lb) and 90.6 kg (200 lb), respectively, clearly outweigh Hispanic men, who average 81.9 kg (181 lb). However, black women, whose average body weight is 83.8 kg (185 lb), outweigh both white and Hispanic women with average body weights of 74.3 kg (164 lb) and 73.6 kg (162 lb), respectively.[9] The average body weight of two groups of Asian men is 60.1–69.8 kg,[5,6] at least 12 kg lighter than Hispanic men, and about 20 kg lighter than white and black men in the U.S. The average body weight of two groups of Asian women is 51.7–60.1 kg,[5,6] about 13 kg lighter than white and Hispanic women, and about 23 kg lighter than black women in the U.S.

Body Weight Ranges Derived from Height

What constitutes an ideal, appropriate, or normal body weight for the average adult is a subject for debate.

| Table 3.5 | Category for Body Weight (kg; lb) by Gender and Race/Ethnicity (United States, 2003–06) | | | | | | | | |

Men

Category (*Percentile*)	Total		White (*Non-Hispanic*)		Black (*Non-Hispanic*)		Hispanic	
	kg	lb	kg	lb	kg	lb	kg	lb
Well above ave (> *95th*)	> 122.6	> 270	> 122.7	> 271	> 137.2	> 303	> 112.9	> 249
Above ave (*75th–95th*)	98.5–122.6	218–270	99.3–122.7	220–271	100.6–137.2	223–303	90.1–112.9	199–249
Average (*25th–74th*)	75.3–98.4	167–217	76.9–99.2	170–219	75.1–100.5	166–222	70.6–90.0	157–198
Below ave (*5th–24th*)	62.2–75.2	137–166	64.2–76.8	142–169	62.3–75.0	137–165	60.0–70.5	132–156
Well below ave (< *5th*)	< 62.2	< 137	< 64.2	< 142	< 62.3	< 137	< 60.0	< 132
Mean	88.3	195	89.6	197	90.6	200	81.9	181

Women

Category (*Percentile*)	Total		White (*Non-Hispanic*)		Black (*Non-Hispanic*)		Hispanic	
	kg	lb	kg	lb	kg	lb	kg	lb
Well above ave (> *95th*)	> 113.6	> 250	> 111.6	> 246	> 125.2	> 276	> 103.9	> 229
Above ave (*75th–95th*)	84.4–113.6	187–250	83.5–111.6	185–246	95.2–125.2	211–276	83.2–103.9	184–229
Average (*25th–74th*)	60.3–84.3	134–186	60.4–83.4	134–184	68.7–95.1	152–210	60.8–83.1	135–183
Below ave (*5th–24th*)	50.5–60.2	111–133	50.9–60.3	112–133	53.0–68.6	117–151	50.5–60.7	111–134
Well below ave (< *5th*)	< 50.5	< 111	< 50.8	< 112	< 53.0	< 117	< 50.5	< 111
Mean	74.7	165	74.3	164	83.8	185	73.6	162

Source: McDowell, Fryar, Ogden & Flegal (2008).[11]

Numerous tables in books and magazines and on the Internet provide some form of "desirable" weight based on gender, age, height, race/ethnicity, frame size, or any combination of these variables. For the purpose of this laboratory manual, comparative body weight ranges are derived from height based on body mass index (BMI). BMI (discussed further in Chapter 23) is a measure of a person's degree of obesity and is calculated as the ratio of body weight divided by height squared. Values of BMI are used to classify a person's body weight into one of the following categories: "underweight" (BMI < 18.5), "normal weight" (BMI = 18.5−24.9), "overweight" (BMI = 25.0−29.9), "class I (mild) obesity" (BMI = 30.0−34.9), "class II (moderate) obesity" (BMI = 35.0−39.9), or "class III (extreme) obesity" (BMI > 40.0).[8] Table 3.6, using the "normal" BMI (18.5−24.9), demonstrates a "normal" body weight range for adults based on height, but regardless of gender or age.

Changes in Average Height and Body Weight over Years

The Department of Health and Human Services regularly administers surveys to collect anthropometric reference data for children and adults in the U.S. One long-running survey is known as the National Health and Nutrition Examination Survey (NHANES). A comparison of data from three cycles of the survey (1988–1994,[10] 1999–2002,[9] and 2003–2006[11]) is presented in Table 3.7. The comparison reveals a minimal increase in height in men of 0.7 cm and in women of 0.4 cm over the 12 years (from 1994 to 2006), with some minor differences based on race/ethnicity. The change in body weight over time is more dramatic with the average body weight in all U.S. men increasing 6.2 kg (7.6%) from 82.1 kg to 88.3 kg. The average body weight for women increased 5.5 kg (7.9%) from 69.2 kg to 74.7 kg.

| Table 3.6 | Body Weights Classified as "Normal" Derived from Height Using Body Mass Index (BMI) |

Height		"Normal Body Weight" (BMI = 18.5–24.9)	
cm	in	kg	lb
142	56.00	37–50	82–111
144	56.75	38–52	85–114
146	57.50	39–53	87–117
148	58.25	41–55	89–121
150	59.00	42–56	92–124
152	59.75	43–58	94–127
154	60.75	44–59	97–131
156	61.50	45–61	99–134
158	62.25	46–62	102–138
160	63.00	47–64	104–141
162	63.75	49–66	107–145
164	64.50	50–67	110–148
166	65.25	51–69	112–152
168	66.25	52–71	115–156
170	67.00	53–72	118–159
172	67.75	55–74	121–163
174	68.50	56–76	123–167
176	69.25	57–77	126–171
178	70.00	59–79	129–175
180	70.75	60–81	132–179
182	71.75	61–83	135–183
184	72.50	63–85	138–187
186	73.25	64–86	141–191
188	74.00	65–88	144–195
190	74.75	67–90	147–199
192	75.50	68–92	150–203
194	76.50	70–94	153–207
196	77.25	71–96	157–212
198	78.00	73–98	160–216

Note: "Normal" body weight is derived from a "normal" body mass index (BMI), which is 18.5–24.9.
Source: National Heart, Lung, and Blood Institute (1998).[12]

| Table 3.7 | Change in Mean Height and Body Weight by Survey Year, Gender, and Race/Ethnicity |

	Height			Height change from:		Body Weight			Weight change from:		
	1994[a]	2002[b]	2006[c]	94 to 02	02 to 06	1994[a]	2002[b]	2006[c]	94 to 02	02 to 06	94 to 06
Group	cm	cm	cm	cm (%)	cm (%)	kg	kg	kg	kg (%)	kg (%)	kg (%)
Men (Total)	175.6	176.0	176.3	0.4 (0.2%)	0.3 (0.2%)	82.1	86.3	88.3	4.2 (5.1%)	2.0 (2.3%)	6.2 (7.6%)
White	176.5	177.2	177.5	0.7 (0.4%)	0.3 (0.2%)	83.2	87.9	89.6	4.7 (5.6%)	1.7 (1.9%)	6.4 (7.7%)
Black	176.1	176.9	177.2	0.8 (0.5%)	0.3 (0.2%)	82.5	86.2	90.6	3.7 (4.5%)	4.4 (4.9%)	8.1 (9.8%)
Hispanic	169.7	169.6	170.3	−0.1 (−0.1%)	0.7 (0.4%)	77.5	80.0	81.9	2.5 (3.2%)	1.9 (2.3%)	4.4 (5.7%)
Women (Total)	161.8	162.1	162.2	0.3 (0.2%)	0.1 (0.1%)	69.2	74.1	74.7	4.9 (7.1%)	0.6 (0.8%)	5.5 (7.9%)
White	162.3	162.9	163.0	0.6 (0.4%)	0.1 (0.1%)	68.5	73.6	74.3	5.1 (7.4%)	0.7 (0.9%)	5.8 (8.5%)
Black	163.0	163.0	162.7	0.0 (0.0%)	−0.3 (−0.2%)	76.5	82.9	83.8	6.4 (8.4%)	0.9 (1.1%)	7.3 (9.5%)
Hispanic	156.7	157.4	157.8	0.7 (0.4%)	0.4 (0.3%)	68.9	71.2	73.6	2.3 (3.3%)	2.4 (3.3%)	4.7 (6.8%)

Source: [a]McDowell, Fryar & Ogden (2009)[10]; [b]McDowell, Fryar, Hirsch & Ogden (2005)[9]; [c]McDowell, Fryar, Ogden & Flegal (2008).[11]

The average body weight of African-American (Black) men increased 8.1 kg (9.8%), which means the *average* body weight of an African-American man in the United States as of 2006 was 90.6 kg (200 lb). The average body weights as of 2006 for all U.S. men and women are 88.3 kg (195 lb) and 74.7 kg (165 lb) respectively.

Effect of Time of Day

The time of day appears to have a small but significant effect on height. Based on measurements taken on one young male (age 13 y) in the morning (within 30 minutes of rising) and repeated before bed on 300 separate days, a 0.98 ± 0.2 cm decrease in height occurred during the course of the day.[6] Another study of 50 older women looked at diurnal changes in height. The results revealed a significant height decrease (> 6 mm) over the course of the day. Interestingly, it was also observed that height increased (> 5 mm) after lying supine for an average period of 49 minutes.[4] The observation of diurnal changes in height has practical consideration for the study of osteoporosis in particular. Because osteoporotic vertebral fractures result in loss of height, longitudinal measure of height in older adults may be useful in detecting the onset of osteoporosis and monitoring its progress. But these measurements should be taken at the same time of day to minimize any potential error due to normal daily variation in height.

It is also common to observe daily changes in body weight over the course of the day. Body weight can be influenced rapidly by food intake, fluid intake, salt intake, exercise, fluid loss, illness (vomiting and diarrhea), hormonal status (more so in women) and other factors. These daily changes in weight for the most part go unnoticed. However, some people, when trying to lose weight, choose to step on the scale frequently throughout the day. This can lead to confusing and frustrating results when they see 1–2 kg fluctuations in weight throughout the day. It might be recommended in this case that they weigh themselves only once per day, at the same time of day (typically in the morning),

---

after going to the bathroom, and before eating or drinking anything. This is the best way to get a "true" body weight, along with the use of an accurate scale.

References

1. American Psychological Association (2009). *Publication manual of the American Psychological Association* (6th ed.). Washington, DC: APA Publications.
2. Brener, N. D., Mcmanus, T., Galuska, D. A., Lowry, R., & Wechsler, H. (2003). Reliability and validity of self-reported height and weight among high school students. *Journal of Adolescent Health, 32,* 281–287.
3. Chumlea, W. C., & Roche, A. F. (1988). Stature, recumbent length, and weight. In T. G. Lohman, A. F. Roche, & R. Rartorell (Eds.), *Anthropometric standardization reference manual* (pp. 3–8). Champaign, IL: Human Kinetics.
4. Coles, R. J., Clements, D. G., & Evans, W. D. (1994). Measurement of height: practical considerations for the study of osteoporosis. *Osteoporosis International, 4,* 353–356.

5. Cui, L.-H., Choi, J.-S., Shin, M.-H., Kweon, S.-S., Park, K.-S., Lee, Y.-H., Nam, H.-S., Jeong, S.-K., & Im, J. S. (2008). Prevalence of osteoporosis and reference data for lumbar spine and hip bone mineral density in a Korean population. *Journal of Bone Mineral and Metabolism, 26,* 609–617.

6. Food and Nutrition Research Institute (2003). Philippine facts and figures 2003, Part II, Anthropometric facts and figures. Retrieved June 21, 2012, from http://www.fnri.dost.gov.ph/files/factsandfigures2003/anthropometric.pdf.

7. Kuczmarski, M. F., Kuczmarski, R. J., & Naijar, M. (2001). Effects of age on validity of self-reported height, weight, and body mass index: findings from the third National Health and Nutrition Examination Survey, 1988–1994. *Journal of the American Dietetic Association, 101,* 28–34.

8. Lampl, M. (1992). Further observations on diurnal variation in standing height. *Annals of Human Biology, 19,* 87–90.

9. McDowell, M. S., Fryar, C. D., Hirsch, R., & Ogden, C. L. (2005). *Anthropometric reference data for children and adults: U.S. population, 1999–2002. Advance data from vital and health statistics; no. 361.* Hyattsville, MD: National Center for Health Statistics.

10. McDowell, M. A., Fryar, C. D., & Ogden C. L. (2009). *Anthropometric reference data for children and adults: United States, 1988–1994. Vital and health statistics; series 11, no. 249.* Hyattsville, MD: National Center for Health Statistics.

11. McDowell, M. A., Fryar, C. D., Ogden, C. L., & Flegal, K. M. (2008). *Anthropometric reference data for children and adults: U.S. population, 2003–2006. National health statistics report; no. 10.* Hyattsville, MD: National Center for Health Statistics.

12. National Heart, Lung, and Blood Institute. (1998). *Clinical guidelines on the identification, evaluation, and treatment of overweight and obesity in adults. The evidence report.* (NIH Publication No. 98-4083). Washington, DC: U.S. Department of Health and Human Services.

13. Niedhammer, I., Bugel, I., Bonenfant, S., Goldberg, M., & Leclerc, A. (2000). Validity of self-reported weight and height in the French GAZEL cohort. *International Journal of Obesity and Related Metabolic Disorders, 24,* 1111–1118.

14. Spencer, E. A., Appleby, P. N., Davey, G. K., & Key, T. J. (2002). Validity of self-reported height and weight in 4808 EPIC-Oxford participants. *Public Health and Nutrition, 5,* 561–565.

15. Strauss, R. S. (1999). Comparison of measured and self-reported weight and height in a cross-sectional sample of young adolescents. *International Journal of Obesity and Related Metabolic Disorders, 23,* 904–908.

16. Thompson, A., & Taylor, B. N. (2008). *NIST special publication 811, 2008 edition: Guide for the Use of the International System of Units (SI).* Gaithersburg, MD: United States Department of Commerce, National Institute of Standards and Technology.

17. Ulijaszek, S. J., & Kerr, D. A. (1999). Anthropometric measurement error and the assessment of nutritional status. *British Journal of Nutrition, 82,* 165–177.

Form 3.1

NAME _____ DATE _____ SCORE _____

COLLECTION OF BASIC DATA

Homework

Laboratory / Meterological Data

Room termperature   **23**   °C   _____ K   _____ °F

Barometric pressure   **755**   mm Hg   _____ hPa   _____ in. Hg

Relative humidity   **40**   %

Male Participant   Participant initials   **AA**   Race/ethnicity* (W, B, H, O)   **W**

Age (y):   **22**   Height (in.):   **70.25**   Height (cm):   _____
                                   (closest 0.25 in.)   *(closest 0.1 cm)*

                    Weight (lb):   **165.75**   Weight (kg):   _____
                                     (closest 0.25 lb)   *(closest 0.1 kg)*

Weight category by age group   *(Table 3.3)*   _____

Height category by race/ethnicity   *(Table 3.4)*   _____

Weight category by race/ethnicity   *(Table 3.5)*   _____

"Normal" body weight   *(Table 3.6)*   _____ - _____ kg   _____ - _____ lb   Within range: _____

Female Participant   Participant initials   **BB**   Race/ethnicity* (W, B, H, O)   **B**

Age (y):   **21**   Height (in.):   **65.00**   Height (cm):   _____
                                     (closest 0.25 in.)   *(closest 0.1 cm)*

                    Weight (lb):   **158.25**   Weight (kg):   _____
                                       (closest 0.25 lb)   *(closest 0.1 kg)*

Weight category by age group   *(Table 3.3)*   _____

Height category by race/ethnicity   *(Table 3.4)*   _____

Weight category by race/ethnicity   *(Table 3.5)*   _____

"Normal" body weight   *(Table 3.6)*   _____ - _____ kg   _____ - _____ lb   Within range: _____

*Race/ethnicity: Caucasian, White (W); African-American, Black (B); Hispanic (H); Other/none (O)

Form 3.2

COLLECTION OF BASIC DATA

NAME _____ DATE _____ SCORE _____

Lab Results

Laboratory / Meterological Data

Date (mm/dd/yy) _____   Time of day _____

Room termperature _____ °C   _____ K   _____ °F

Barometric pressure _____ mm Hg   _____ hPa   _____ in. Hg

Relative humidity _____ %

Male Participant   Participant initials _____   Race/ethnicity* (W, B, H, O) _____

Age (y): _____   Height (in.): _____   Height (cm): _____
                              (closest 0.25 in.)   *(closest 0.1 cm)*

                              Weight (lb): _____   Weight (kg): _____
                              (closest 0.25 lb)   *(closest 0.1 kg)*

Female Participant   Participant initials _____   Race/ethnicity* (W, B, H, O) _____

Age (y): _____   Height (in.): _____   Height (cm): _____
                              (closest 0.25 in.)   *(closest 0.1 cm)*

                              Weight (lb): _____   Weight (kg): _____
                              (closest 0.25 lb)   *(closest 0.1 kg)*

Yourself   Race/ethnicity* (W, B, H, O) _____

Age (y): _____   Height (in.): _____   Height (cm): _____
                              (closest 0.25 in.)   *(closest 0.1 cm)*

Gender: _____   Weight (lb): _____   Weight (kg): _____
                              (closest 0.25 lb)   *(closest 0.1 kg)*

Weight category by age group *(Table 3.3)*   _____

Height category by race/ethnicity *(Table 3.4)*   _____

Weight category by race/ethnicity *(Table 3.5)*   _____

"Normal" body weight *(Table 3.6)*   _____ - _____ kg   _____ - _____ lb   Within range: _____

*Race/ethnicity: Caucasian, White (W); African-American, Black (B); Hispanic (H); Other/none (O)

Optional   Height *(closest 0.1 cm)*: Early in day _____   Late in day _____   Difference _____ cm

          Weight *(closest 0.1 kg)*: Early in day _____   Late in day _____   Difference _____ kg

          Nude weight *(closest 0.1 kg)*: Body wt _____   Clothes wt _____   Nude wt _____ kg

ISOTONIC (DYNAMIC) STRENGTH

Isotonic exercise is also referred to or defined as dynamic exercise. It is exercise that consists of muscle actions that are concentric or eccentric, depending on whether the muscles shorten or are lengthened. During isotonic or dynamic exercise, the speed of movement is variable throughout the movement, such as when lifting a barbell. Thus, the load being lifted changes speed, due to biomechanical, physiological, and anatomical factors of the lifter, but the absolute load itself (the mass of the load) does not change.[18]

Field tests of strength have existed since at least the time of the ancient Olympics, when contestants were required to lift a ball of iron in order to qualify for the games. In 1873, Dudley Sargent, a pioneer in early physical education, initiated strength testing at Harvard University. Currently, many strength trainees measure their strength in the weight room using free-weights and weight machines.

A popular free-weight exercise that is described as an isotonic or dynamic strength test in this chapter is the bench press. Depending on the controlled or standardized conditions, the free-weight test described here could be classified as a field or laboratory test.[11,36] This chapter includes a description of both direct and indirect (predicted; estimated) measures of dynamic strength for the muscle groups used in performing this free-weight exercise.

RATIONALE

One of the most operational (easily applied) definitions of dynamic strength states that it is expressed as a person's *one repetition maximum (1 RM)* for a specific movement, such as the bench press. This 1 RM is the maximum load or weight that a person can lift only one time. It can be directly measured from a maximal effort or it can be indirectly estimated from a submaximal effort.

Directly Measured 1 RM

A direct measure of strength is the maximal weight that a person can lift in the prescribed manner only one time. A brief preview of the traditional 1 RM test would show that it requires a person to exert maximally on a selected weight, chosen as close as possible to the person's expected 1 RM weight. If the person cannot lift it with correct form, then a lower weight is tried after a rest interval; if the person properly lifts the weight twice, then the participant stops. After a rest interval, a small additional

weight is added, and the person tries again. This process is repeated until only one repetition is possible.[24] Obtaining the 1 RM value for the first time in a person may be inaccurate and time consuming because of the number of attempts at achieving one, and only one, repetition at a given weight[21] and a lack of standardizing the lifting position or procedures. Direct 1 RM measurements also may be injurious for some persons, especially children[16] and the elderly.[33] The American Academy of Pediatrics[1] and the National Strength and Conditioning Association[31] endorse this sentiment in not recommending 1 RM performances by children.

Indirectly Estimated 1 RM

If for some reason directly measuring 1 RM is not possible or desirable, the 1 RM may be indirectly estimated by knowing the number of submaximal repetitions to fatigue (RTF) for any given weight lifted. The 1 RM may be estimated from equations based upon either a linear relationship[6,22,31] or a curvilinear (exponential) relationship[24,34] between the number of RTF and the percent of 1 RM (% 1 RM). An example of both of these relationships is seen in Figure 4.1. The 1 RM can be estimated from measuring the number of RTF at intensities between 75 % and 95 % 1 RM,[14,17,19] and possibly extended to intensities as low as 60 % 1 RM.[14,28] Generally, however, it is believed that estimations of 1 RM using such equations are best when using a load that results in no more than 10 repetitions to fatigue (~ 75 % of 1 RM).[6,26]

One indirect 1 RM method is based on a *linear* relationship between % 1 RM and the number of submaximal repetitions to fatigue.[31] If 4 repetitions to fatigue are completed, this would be considered the number of repetitions or 4 RM (4 reps to fatigue), 5 RM (5 reps to fatigue), etc. In general, the % 1 RM load decreases by about 2.5 % for each increase in the number of repetitions to fatigue, keeping in mind the assumption of a linear relationship. Thus, the 1 RM load represents 100 % 1 RM that can be lifted only once, whereas an 80 % 1 RM load could be lifted about 8 times. The % 1 RM can be estimated for a set of submaximal repetitions by assuming the 2.5 % decrease per RM, which can then be used to estimate the 1 RM. Another indirect 1 RM method is based on a *curvilinear* (or *exponential*) relationship between % 1 RM and the number of submaximal repetitions to fatigue.[24] This method is

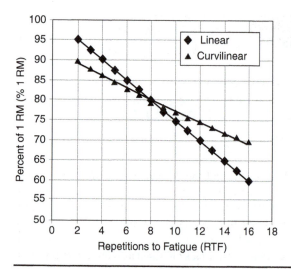

Figure 4.1 The linear and curvilinear (exponential) relationships between repetitions to fatigue (RTF) and percent of 1 repetition maximum (% 1 RM).

very similar to the linear method except that the estimated % of 1 RM is mathematically based on the exponent of the number of repetitions to fatigue. Because of this, the curvilinear method yields estimates of 1 RM that are slightly higher than the linear method when a low number of repetitions are completed (3–5 RM), but slightly lower estimates of 1 RM with higher numbers of repetitions to fatigue (10–12 RM).

Anatomical Rationale

Many major muscles in the upper body are involved in a bench press exercise. The primary muscles involved include those of the chest (pectoralis major), shoulders (anterior deltoid and coracobrachialis), and arms (triceps brachii). For this reason, the bench press was chosen to use in assessing 1 RM in this chapter.

Physiological Rationale

The biochemical pathway for maximal muscle actions—that is, strength—is the phosphagenic pathway. Even the longest of 1 RM movements is completed in less than 10 s; this includes the time spent holding the weight prior to the movement, raising the weight, holding it in the lifted position, and lowering the weight.[30] Thus, the actual time spent raising the weight is usually less than three seconds. Maximal exercise efforts of this duration are placed within the anaerobic fitness category.

TESTS OF STRENGTH (1 RM), WORK, AND POWER

Two tests of strength are described; one *directly measures* the most weight lifted one time (1 RM) and the

other *indirectly estimates* this value through the use of multiple submaximal lifts to fatigue (typically 3–12 repetitions). Strength testing serves purposes related to both performance and health. Before embarking on strength training programs, it is meaningful to evaluate participants in order to prescribe their programs and monitor their progress. For example, a trainee's exercise prescription may include performance of two or three sets of maximal repetitions at 80 % of the 1 RM load. Persons, especially women, who habitually exert forcefully against resistance may protect themselves from losing bone density.[2,4] It seems plausible that stronger persons are more likely to provide the necessary forces to prevent the advent of porous bones, associated with osteoporosis.

Additionally, directions are included for the quantification of work and power. This goes beyond the purpose of simply measuring strength. Because of the distinct terminology and measurement in exercise physiology, the purpose of this exercise is to familiarize the student with common exercise terms and measurement associated with work and power. Thus, in addition to learning how to administer the strength tests, students also learn how to measure positive (concentric) work, negative (eccentric) work, total work, and mean power.

METHODS

The Methods section of a research paper should enable the readers to replicate the researcher's study. This means that the equipment (instruments and materials), procedures, and calculations (analysis) are described in the Methods section. Box 4.1 provides a summary of the accuracy of 1 RM testing.

Equipment

Various instruments are available to measure muscle strength. Some of these are (a) free-weights (e.g., barbells), (b) dynamometers, (c) cable tensiometers, (d) load cells (electromechanical devices), and (e) isokinetic devices. The equipment for the isotonic strength and power tests includes the following: (1) weighing scale (e.g., platform scale or electronic scale); (2) bar; (3) assorted free-weights ranging from 1 kg (≈ 2.5 lb; 10 N) to 10 kg (≈ 25 lb; 100 N) each; (4) barbell collars (unless weights are welded onto the bar); (5) stopwatch capable of measuring to a tenth of a second; and (6) a metric tape or stick.

Weighing scales, used to measure the weight and force components, were discussed in Chapter 3. Most weight rooms have barbells and weights to measure the force component of work and power. A total weight of about 90 kg (200 lb) should accommodate most participants. One bench is needed for the strength exercise described here. Most exercise physiology laboratories have metric measurement tapes and stopwatches to measure

Executing the Bench Press Exercise

The accuracy of free-weight strength testing is enhanced if the execution of the lifts is standardized. The prescribed positions of the bench press are illustrated in Figure 4.2. These movements should be practiced a few times with only the bar. The technician ensures that the participant executes properly.

1. The participant lies supine on a wide bench with the knees bent and the soles of the feet on the floor. Alternately, the feet may be on the bench with novice lifters to prevent arching the back and risking injury.[10,23]
2. Two technicians, or spotters, at each side of the participant, or one spotter behind the participant, place the barbell in the participant's pronated hands (thumbs medial) spaced slightly wider (up to 20 cm) then shoulder width apart and at chest level.[41]
3. The participant raises the weight to a straightened-arms position directly above the chest.

the distance and time components of work and power, respectively. Students are encouraged to bring their own calculators and wristwatches (chronographs) to every laboratory session.

Safety is a concern for all fitness tests, especially those requiring intense or explosive movements and those leading to exhaustion. Box 4.2 provides a safety checklist for technicians and participants.

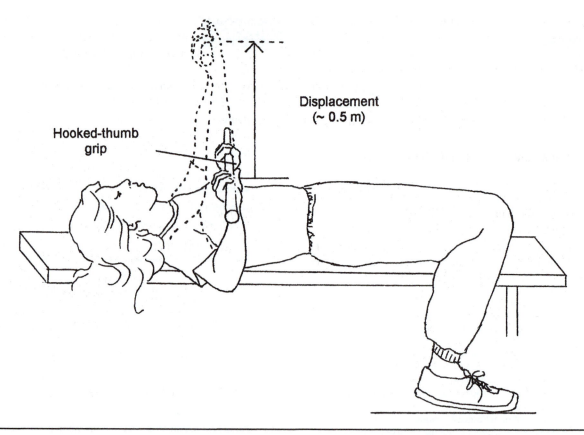

Hooked-thumb grip

Displacement (~ 0.5 m)

Figure 4.2 The beginning and end positions for the bench press. The arrow denotes the vertical displacement measurement needed for calculating work and power.

4. The participant returns the barbell to the preparatory position (in contact with the chest).
5. The participant stops at this position for about 1 s before initiating subsequent repetitions.

Preparation for 1 RM, Work, and Mean Power

As with all of the tests performed in this manual, the first step is to record the basic data. Thus, the name, date, age, gender, height, and weight are recorded on Form 4.2. An additional factor, specific for free-weight testing, might be the recording of the participant's experience in lifting free-weights. The body weight should be as close to the nude weight as possible and measured according to the procedures described in Chapter 3.

Another universal step is to calibrate the test equipment. The calibration of the platform scale was described in Box 3.2 of Chapter 3. It is not unusual for the poundage of commercial weights to be labeled inaccurately. For example, in one instance a sand-filled weight that was marked as 8.8 lb (4.0 kg) really weighed 10.4 lb (4.7 kg). Hence, the weights, barbells, and collars that are to be used for testing should be verified on an accurate scale prior to testing. The actual kilograms or pounds should be marked on the barbells or weights.

In some instances, weight (or mass) is considered equal to the force lifting the weight, such as when lifting a barbell against gravitational forces. The weight (free-weights), which in this case is the force, should be measured on a metric scale to the closest tenth kilogram or be converted to metrics after being weighed on a non-metric scale.

Before the subject performs the maximal repetitions for a given weight, displacement (d) measurements must be made in order to calculate the work (w = F * d) accomplished. The displacement[a] is measured to the closest centimeter with a metric tape. It is made with the participant using an unloaded bar at two points: the preparatory and end points of the movement. The criteria for measuring these lengths are illustrated in Figure 4.2.

After making the vertical displacement measures, the participant should be given 5–10 min of prior exercise, consisting of stretching and warming-up (weight lifting) exercises. These exercises should incorporate the muscles to be used in the strength test. Thus, the stretching exercises should stretch the upper body muscles and tendons. One

---

[a]The term *displacement* represents the straight-line length of the concentric phase of the exercise. The term *distance* includes the curved-line length (the arc) of concentric and eccentric phases of the exercise.

8 40-60
warm-up set of about eight repetitions should mimic the execution of the lift, but with weights that are about 40 %[37] to 60 %[18] of an estimated one repetition maximal. This can be followed by another set of three repetitions between 50 % and 70 % of estimated 1 RM or three to five reps at 60 % to 80 %. These preliminary estimates are rather exploratory for first-time participants (novices).

(margin handwritten: 3-5, 60-70)

Direct Measurement of Bench Press 1 RM

The direct method is the traditional trial-and-retrial method. The results may be compared with the results of the indirect method. Hence, the comparison can serve as a validation of the indirect method.

The procedures outlined here[20,32,44] combine those described by others. The procedural steps for the traditional direct measurement of 1 RM follow.

Technician Preparation

1. Calibrate the platform scale or electronic scale. (Refer to Box 3.2 in Chapter 3.)
2. Weigh and mark the barbells and assorted free-weights to the closest 0.1 kg.
3. Record basic data onto Form 4.2. Record height to the closest 1 cm and body weight (as close to nude weight as possible) to closest 0.1 kg.
4. Explain and demonstrate the proper execution of the bench press using only the bar. Provide as much detail as needed based on the previous weight lifting experience of the participant.
5. For novice lifters, load the bar with weight based on the body weight of the participant. For men, load the bar with about 50 % of body weight. For women, load the bar with about 30 % of body weight. For experienced lifters, load the bar with weight that approximates 50 % 1 RM.

Participant Preparation

1. Practice the bench press exercise with just the bar until performance is satisfactory to the technician.
2. Complete a warm-up set of 8–10 reps at the previously prescribed weight (50 % of body weight for novice men, 35 % of body weight for novice women, or 50 % 1 RM for more experienced lifters). The goal is a warm-up set of 8–10 reps at 40–60 % 1 RM. Rest for 1 minute with active recovery and stretching if desired.
3. Complete another warm-up set of 3–5 reps at a weight 5–10 kg (10–20 lb) higher than the first. The goal is another warm-up set of 3–5 reps at 60–80 % 1 RM. Rest for 1 minute with active recovery and stretching if desired.

Test Procedures

1. The technician loads the bar with an estimated near maximal weight (90–95 % 1 RM) by adding 5–10 kg

(10–20 lb) to the weight used for the second warm-up set. This weight is recorded as Trial 1 on Form 4.2.
2. The participant completes 2–3 reps at this weight (estimated to be 90–95 % 1 RM). The participant rests 1–2 min (or longer) with active recovery and stretching if desired.
3. The technician loads the bar with an additional 5–10 kg (10–20 lb) to estimate the 1 RM. The participant attempts one single rep at this weight.
   a. *If successful*, the technician records this weight as Trial 2 on Form 4.2. The participant rests 1–2 min (or more), then repeats Step 3 until the 1 RM is reached and recorded on Form 4.2.
   b. *If unsuccessful*, the technician unloads 5–10 kg (10–20 lb) from the bar. The participant rests 1–2 min (or more), then attempts another single rep at this reduced weight.
      i. *If successful*, the participant rests 1–2 min (or more), then repeats Step 3 until the 1 RM is reached.
      ii. *If unsuccessful*, the participant is done and Trial 1 is considered the 1 RM.
4. Ideally, the participant's 1 RM is reached within five trials. If more attempts are needed, the participant should be retested on another day.[44]

Indirect Estimate of Bench Press 1 RM

The prediction of 1 RM may be made based on either a linear relationship or a curvilinear relationship between % 1RM and # RM. The focus of the following is based on the more popular, but not necessarily more accurate, linear relationship. The ultimate step in predicting 1 RM is to determine the participant's maximal number of repetitions for a given weight (force). Repetitions maximal (# RM) is defined as the number of repetitions, without a rest interval, performed until no other properly executed repetition can be completed. In order to comply with the linearity rationale, it is best if the number of maximal repetitions does not exceed 20. If it is apparent that the participant is about to exceed 20 repetitions, stop the participant and wait for 5 min to 10 min before repeating the exercise at a heavier weight.

Technician Preparation

1. The technician completes Steps 1–5 as in the section "Direct Measurement of Bench Press 1 RM."

Participant Preparation

1. The participant completes Steps 1–2 as in the section "Direct Measurement of Bench Press 1 RM."

Test Procedures

1. The technician adds 5–10 kg (10–20 lb) to the bar over that weight used for the warm-up set. This weight is recorded as Trial 1 on Form 4.2.

Table 4.1

Table 4.1 Estimated Bench Press 1 RM from Number of Submaximal Repetitions (from 2 RM–12 RM) at Repetition Weight (kg or lb) Based on a Generalized Linear Prediction Model

Repetition Weight	2 RM 95.0%	3 RM 92.5%	4 RM 90.0%	5 RM 87.5%	6 RM 85.0%	7 RM 82.5%	8 RM 80.0%	9 RM 77.5%	10 RM 75.0%	11 RM 72.5%	12 RM 70.0%
30	32	32	33	34	35	36	38	39	40	41	43
35	37	38	39	40	41	42	44	45	47	48	50
40	42	43	44	46	47	48	50	52	53	55	57
45	47	49	50	51	53	55	56	58	60	62	64
50	53	54	56	57	59	61	62	65	67	69	71
60	63	65	67	69	71	73	75	77	80	83	86
70	74	76	78	80	82	85	87	90	93	97	100
80	84	86	89	91	94	97	100	103	107	110	114
90	95	97	100	103	106	109	113	116	120	124	129
100	105	108	111	114	118	121	125	129	133	138	143
110	116	119	122	126	129	133	138	142	147	152	157
120	126	130	133	137	141	145	150	155	160	166	171
130	137	141	144	149	153	158	163	168	173	179	186
140	147	151	156	160	165	170	175	181	187	193	200
150	158	162	167	171	176	182	188	194	200	207	214
160	168	173	178	183	188	194	200	206	213	221	229
170	179	184	189	194	200	206	213	219	227	234	243
180	189	195	200	206	212	218	225	232	240	248	257
190	200	205	211	217	224	230	238	245	253	262	271
200	211	216	222	229	235	242	250	258	267	276	286

Source: Data used to estimate percentages of 1 RM from National Strength and Conditioning Association (2000).[30] % 1 RM = 100 − (# RM * 2.5).

Note: Table can be used to estimate 1 RM in either kilograms (kg) or pounds (lb).

2. The participant lifts the weight as prescribed for the movement as many times as possible at a comfortable pace, but without a rest interval. Ideally, the goal of the test is to lift the weight about 3–12 times to fatigue (3–12 RM).

   a. If the participant fatigues in 3–12 reps, that is acceptable and the test is complete. The technician records the number of repetitions beside the weight lifted for Trial 1 on Form 4.2.

   b. If the weight can be lifted less than 3 times or more than 12 times, the test should be repeated after a 5–10 min rest. The technician increases or decreases the weight on the bar by 5–10 kg (10–20 lb) and the participant repeats the test until fatigue is reached in 3–12 reps.

3. The technician estimates the 1 RM of the participant using the number of repetitions to fatigue (# RM) and the amount of weight lifted (kg or lb).

   a. The estimation of 1 RM can be made using the mathematical method described previously based on the *linear relationship*[31] between % 1 RM and the number of reps to fatigue (# RM). The % 1 RM is estimated for a set of submaximal repetitions (Eq. 4.1a). The 1 RM is then estimated by factoring in the weight lifted (Eq. 4.1b). The 1 RM may also be estimated based on the data presented in Table 4.1.

$$\% \ 1 \ RM = 100 - (\#Reps * 2.5) \qquad \text{Eq. 4.1a}$$

$$1 \ RM = \text{Weight lifted} / (\% \ 1 \ RM / 100) \qquad \text{Eq. 4.1b}$$

For example, if a person completes 10 repetitions to fatigue of a particular weight, the % of 1 RM is estimated to be 75 % (Eq. 4.2a). If those 10 repetitions were completed with a load of 60 kg, then the 1 RM is estimated to be 80 kg (Eq. 4.2b). This same estimated 1 RM of 80 kg can be found in Table 4.1.

$$\% \ 1 \ RM = 100 - (\mathbf{10} * 2.5) = 75 \ \% \qquad \text{Eq. 4.2a}$$

$$1 \ RM = \mathbf{60} \ kg / (\mathbf{75} / 100) = \mathbf{80} \ kg \qquad \text{Eq. 4.2b}$$

   b. The 1 RM may alternately be estimated based on a *curvilinear (exponential) relationship*[24] between % 1 RM and the number of reps to fatigue and the weight lifted, as shown in Equations 4.3a and 4.3b. The symbol **e** in Eq. 4.3a represents the exponential function which is written e^x or often as exp(x) to avoid the use of the superscript. The calculation can be made on a scientific calculator using the e^x key or can be done in Excel® using the EXP function.

$$\% \ 1 \ RM = 52.5 + 41.9 \ e^{-0.055 * Reps} \qquad \text{Eq. 4.3a}$$

$$1 \ RM = \text{Weight lifted} / (\% 1 \ RM / 100) \qquad \text{Eq. 4.3b}$$

For example, using the same data as above, where the participant completed 10 repetitions of a 60 kg load, the estimated % 1 RM is slightly higher at 76.7 % (Eq. 4.4a), yielding a slightly lower estimated 1 RM of 78 kg (Eq. 4.4a). This same estimated 1 RM of 78 kg can be found in Table 4.2.

Table 4.2 Estimated Bench Press 1 RM from Number of Submaximal Repetitions (from 3 RM–12 RM) at Repetition Weight (kg or lb) Based on a Curvilinear (Exponential) Prediction Model

Repetition Weight	2 RM 90.0%	3 RM 88.0%	4 RM 86.1%	5 RM 84.3%	6 RM 82.6%	7 RM 81.0%	8 RM 79.5%	9 RM 78.0%	10 RM 76.7%	11 RM 75.4%	12 RM 74.2%
30	33	34	35	36	36	37	38	38	39	40	40
35	39	40	41	42	42	43	44	45	46	46	47
40	44	45	46	47	48	49	50	51	52	53	54
45	50	51	52	53	54	56	57	58	59	60	61
50	56	57	58	59	61	62	63	64	65	66	67
60	67	68	70	71	73	74	75	77	78	80	81
70	78	80	81	83	85	86	88	90	91	93	94
80	89	91	93	95	97	99	101	103	104	106	108
90	100	102	105	107	109	111	113	115	117	119	121
100	111	114	116	119	121	123	126	128	130	133	135
110	122	125	128	130	133	136	138	141	143	146	148
120	133	136	139	142	145	148	151	154	156	159	162
130	144	148	151	154	157	160	164	167	169	172	175
140	156	159	163	166	169	173	176	179	183	186	189
150	167	170	174	178	182	185	189	192	196	199	202
160	178	182	186	190	194	198	201	205	209	212	216
170	189	193	197	202	206	210	214	218	222	225	229
180	200	205	209	214	218	222	226	231	235	239	243
190	211	216	221	225	230	235	239	244	248	252	256
200	222	227	232	237	242	247	252	256	261	265	270

Source: Data used to estimate percentages of 1 RM from Mayhew, Ball, Arnold, & Bowen (1992).[24] % 1 RM = 52.2 + 41.9 e$^{-0.055 * \text{Reps}}$

Note: Table can be used to estimate 1 RM in either kilograms (kg) or pounds (lb).

$$\% \text{ RM} = 52.2 + 41.9\, e^{-0.055 * 10} = \mathbf{76.7} \% \qquad \text{Eq. 4.4a}$$

$$1 \text{ RM} = \mathbf{60}\text{ kg} / (\mathbf{76.7} \% / 100) = \mathbf{78}\text{ kg} \qquad \text{Eq. 4.4b}$$

Evaluation of Bench Press Measurements

1. The technician compares the directly measured 1 RM with the indirectly estimated 1 RMs and completes the related items on Form 4.2.
2. The technician selects a category from Table 4.3 to evaluate the absolute 1 RM bench press strength, selects a category from Table 4.4 to evaluate the relative 1 RM strength, and completes the related items on Form 4.2.

Estimation of Work and Mean Power

Timing the duration of the free-weight lift is necessary when calculating power because power is the rate of doing work. The timer should start the stopwatch at the participant's first movement of the bench press. The timer stops the watch when the participant returns the weight after the last complete or partial repetition. The timer records the time to the closest 0.1 s. The participant should execute the repetitions at a comfortable pace because the purpose of the power measurement is not to rank and compare the quality of the participant's mean power. If the latter were the goal, the participant would need to execute the maximal repetitions as fast as possible. No norms for this test could be found in the literature. The primary purpose of the mean power "test" is to become familiar with the concept of power and its calculation.[18]

The measurement of work and power can be completed in conjunction with the Indirect Estimate of 1 RM or independently. If it is to be completed in conjunction with this other test, the following preparation should be done prior to the Indirect Estimate of 1 RM.

Technician Preparation

1. The technician completes Steps 1–5 as in the section "Direct Measurement of Bench Press 1 RM."
2. Measure and record on Form 4.2 the vertical displacement of one concentric action of the participant's bench press (as indicated on Figure 4.2). This measurement allows for the calculation of work.
3. Have a stopwatch ready to measure the time elapsed during the complete exercise.

Participant Preparation

1. The participant completes Steps 1–2 as in the section "Direct Measurement of Bench Press 1 RM."

Table 4.3

Table 4.3 Category for 1 RM Bench Press Strength (kg) in Untrained Men and Women by Age Group

Category (percentile)	Men			Women		
	18–29 y	30–50 y	> 50 y	18–29 y	30–50 y	> 50 y
	(kg)	(kg)	(kg)	(kg)	(kg)	(kg)
Well above ave (> 95th %ile)	> 92.1	> 83.0	> 73.0	> 47.6	> 43.1	> 38.1
Above ave (75th–95th %ile)	76.9–92.1	69.4–83.0	61.0–73.0	42.2–47.6	38.3–43.1	33.8–38.1
Average (25th–74th %ile)	55.6–76.8	49.4–69.3	43.3–60.9	34.9–42.1	31.5–38.2	27.9–33.7
Below ave (5th–24th %ile)	40.4–55.5	35.8–49.3	31.3–43.2	29.5–34.8	26.8–31.4	23.6–27.8
Well below ave (< 5th %ile)	<40.4	<35.8	<31.3	<29.5	<26.8	<23.6
Mean	66.2	59.4	52.2	38.6	34.9	30.8

Source: Data from Hockey (1989).[13]

Test Procedures

1. The technician starts the stopwatch at the participant's first movement.
2. The participant lifts the weight as prescribed for the movement as many times as possible at a comfortable pace, but without a rest interval. Ideally, the goal of the test is to lift the weight about 6–10 times to fatigue (6–10 RM), but up to a maximum of 20 repetitions is allowed.
3. The technician counts and records on Form 4.2 the number of repetitions completed, including the fraction of a possible partial repetition on the last attempt. The weight lifted (kg) is converted into the force exerted (N), and recorded.
4. The technician stops the stopwatch at the end of the last attempt of a repetition and records the time to the closest 0.1 s onto Form 4.2.
5. If the participant exceeds 20 repetitions, the test should be repeated with a higher weight following a 5–10 min rest.
6. The technician completes the calculation of work and power as described below and completes the remaining items on Form 4.2.

Calculating Work and Power

only concentric work

Equation 4.5a is used to calculate the **positive work** (+w) from the weight lifted, expressed as force (F), the displacement (d) of a single concentric action, and the number of repetitions (# Reps). The latter will consist of more than one repetition (preferably 6 or more) and will include a somewhat subjective estimate of the fractional displacement of the final incomplete attempted repetition. For example, if the participant properly executes 9 complete repetitions of 50 kg (490 N) over 0.5 m, but attempts a 10th lift that only goes half the proper distance, then it is recorded as 9.5 reps and positive work is calculated as in Equation 4.5b. The result of the calculation ends up being in newton meters (N·m), which may also be expressed as joules (J), since 1 J is equal to 1 N·m.

$$+w \text{ (J)} = \text{Force (N)} * \text{Displacement (m / Rep)} * \text{\# Reps} \qquad \text{Eq. 4.5a}$$

$$+w \text{ (J)} = \textbf{490} \text{ N} * \textbf{0.5} \text{ m / Rep} * \textbf{9.5} \text{ Reps} = \textbf{2328} \text{ N·m} = \textbf{2328 J} \qquad \text{Eq. 4.5b}$$

Positive work, however, accounts only for the concentric muscle action lifting the weight vertically against gravity. To measure the total work of these dynamic exercises, the eccentric muscle action must be considered and the **negative work** (–w) calculated (Eq. 4.6a). Although the estimate of negative work is variable, for the purpose of expressing the total work accomplished during a bench press exercise, negative work is assumed here to be 1/3 the positive work, based on the relationship of the metabolic cost between concentric and eccentric work.[2] Thus, using the data from the example above, the negative work (–w) can be calculated as in Equation 4.6b and the total work accomplished during the exercise as in Equations 4.6c and 4.6d. Total work can also be calculated "collectively" in one step, as seen in Equations 4.6e and 4.6f.

$$-w \text{ (J)} = \text{Positive work (J)} * 0.33 \qquad \text{Eq. 4.6a}$$

$$-w \text{ (J)} = \textbf{2328} \text{ J} * 0.33 = \textbf{768 J} \qquad \text{Eq. 4.6b}$$

$$\text{Total work (J)} = +w \text{ (J)} + -w \text{ (J)} \qquad \text{Eq. 4.6c}$$

$$\text{Total work (J)} = \textbf{2328} \text{ J} + \textbf{768} \text{ J} = \textbf{3096 J} \qquad \text{Eq. 4.6d}$$

$$\text{Total work (J)} = \text{Force (N)} * \text{Displacement (m / Rep)} * \text{\# Reps} * 1.33 \qquad \text{Eq. 4.6e}$$

$$\text{Total work (J)} = \textbf{490} \text{ N} * \textbf{0.5} \text{ m / Rep} * \textbf{9.5} \text{ Reps} * 1.33 = \textbf{3096 J} \qquad \text{Eq. 4.6f}$$

Power, as described in Chapter 1, expresses the *rate* at which work is done. It is calculated as work divided by time. You have probably not thought much about how much work is done during a set of 8–10 bench press exercises or at what power the exercises are done. But knowing how much work is done and knowing the time in which it is done allows the calculation of mean power. Working with the example from above, we know that completing 9.5 reps of 50 kg (490 N) over 0.5 m resulted in 3096 J of work. If the work was completed in 30.5 s, the mean power of the bench press exercise can be determined as in Equations 4.7a and 4.7b. The units end up as joules per second ($J \cdot s^{-1}$), which can also be expressed in watts (W) since 1 W is equal to 1 $J \cdot s^{-1}$.

$$\text{Mean power (W)} = \text{Work (J) / Time (s)} \qquad \text{Eq. 4.7a}$$

$$\begin{aligned} \text{Mean power (W)} &= \textbf{3096 J / 30.5 s} = \textbf{102 } \mathbf{J \cdot s^{-1}} \\ &= \textbf{102 W} \end{aligned} \qquad \text{Eq. 4.7b.}$$

RESULTS AND DISCUSSION

Maximal bench press strength represents well the total upper body strength of a person. It is commonly measured by directly testing the maximal amount of weight that can be lifted in one repetition (1 RM) or estimating this value through multiple submaximal lifts. The accuracy of a submaximal, multiple repetition protocol to estimate 1 RM is improved by completing no more than about 10 repetitions to fatigue.[26] One source reports that the average free weight 1 RM bench press strength for young (18–29 y) men is 66.2 kg (146 lb) and for young women is 38.6 kg (85 lb).[13] Percentiles derived from this same source allow the creation of the descriptive categories seen in Table 4.3 for evaluating bench press strength. The bench press strength of women proved to be about 60 % that of men. With increasing age, it appears that maximal bench press strength decreases about 5 % per decade from age 30 to age 50 and beyond. Prior to the 1980s, strength was not emphasized as a fitness component for middle-aged and older adults. However, due to its effect on retaining muscle mass and preserving bone density, it has attained greater importance for persons of all ages.[2,4]

Strength up to this point has been described in *absolute* terms, regardless of an individual's body weight. A person's *absolute strength* is measured by the 1 RM, described in kilograms (e.g., 1 RM = 75 kg) or pounds. It is sometimes desirable to express strength on a *relative* basis, relative to body weight. A person with a 1 RM of 75 kg with a body weight of 75 kg could be described as having a *relative strength* of 1.00. This value can be expressed with units as 1.00 $kg \cdot kg^{-1}$, as a ratio of 1.00 (which is unitless), or as 100 % of body weight. The benefit of describing someone's relative strength might be made clearer with the following

example. Assume two people have the exact same absolute strength as defined by a 1 RM bench press of 75 kg. Further assume that one person weighs 75 kg but the other weighs 85 kg. This translates into two different relative strengths: 1.00 $kg \cdot kg^{-1}$ (75 kg / 75 kg) and 0.88 $kg \cdot kg^{-1}$ (75 kg / 85 kg). Depending on the situation, it is valuable to be able to express strength in either absolute or relative terms. Table 4.4 provides categories for evaluating relative bench press strength in untrained, college-aged men and women.[12]

Dynamic bench press strength is increased through training. Comparisons of untrained men and women with trained men and women show significant differences in absolute and relative strength, as seen in Table 4.5. Within trained participants, some groups show even greater bench press strength. Nearly every collegiate football program in the United States places great emphasis on bench press strength. Understandably, the strength developed by this particular group of athletes far exceeds the strength of the "average" person discussed throughout this chapter. The absolute 1 RM bench press strength of division II (DII) football players was nearly twice that of untrained men, and of division I (DI) players 2–3 times higher than untrained men. A more detailed description of absolute and relative bench press strength of DI college football players by position is shown in Table 4.6. Offensive and defensive linemen have the highest absolute strength, while running backs have the highest relative strength.

Although not described in this laboratory manual, a test that is sometimes used to estimate 1 RM bench press strength in college football players is the NFL-225 Test.[7,27,43] The test involves bench pressing 225 lb (102 kg) as many times as possible to fatigue. The number of repetitions to fatigue can then be used in a regression equation[26] to estimate 1 RM, as shown along with an example in Equations 4.7a and 4.7b. Strength tests such as these, using multiple repetitions to fatigue, instead of direct tests of 1 RM, are becoming popular with strength and conditioning specialists.[41] Essentially every lifting set to fatigue

Table 4.4	Relative Bench Press Strength in College-Age Men and Women	
	Men	**Women**
Category	**($kg \cdot kg^{-1}$)**	**($kg \cdot kg^{-1}$)**
Excellent	≥ 1.40	≥ 0.85
Good	1.20–1.39	0.70–0.85
Average	1.00–1.19	0.60–0.69
Fair	0.80–0.99	0.50–0.59
Poor	< 0.80	< 0.50

Source: Based on data adapted from Heyward (2000).[12]

Table 4.5	Absolute (Abs) and Relative (Rel) 1 RM for Bench Press in Various Groups		
	Wt	**Abs 1 RM**	**Rel 1 RM**
Group	**(kg)**	**(kg)**	**($kg \cdot kg^{-1}$)**
Untrained women[c]	61.6	28.7	0.47
Untrained women[b]	66.2	38.2	0.58
Trained women[a]	59.2	44.6	0.75
Untrained men[e]	73.1	62.8	0.85
Untrained men[b]	74.5	77.8	1.04
Trained men[g]	86.4	115.4	1.34
DII college football[f]	97.1	124.3	1.28
DI college football[d]	115.9	170.3	1.47

Source: Data from [a]Horvat, et al. (2003), [b]Mayhew, et al. (1992), [c]Mayhew, et al. (2008), [d]Secora, et al. (2004), [e]Shimano, et al. (2006), and [f]Ware, et al. (1995).

Table 4.6	Absolute (Abs) and Relative (Rel) 1 RM for Bench Press in College Football Players by Position		
Position	Body wt (kg)	Abs 1 RM (kg)	Rel 1 RM (kg·kg⁻¹)
Receivers	88.7	147 ± 25	1.50 ± 0.22
Quarterbacks	94.6	156 ± 24	1.59 ± 0.23
Tight ends	114.2	168 ± 21	1.31 ± 0.17
Running backs	96.9	170 ± 25	1.65 ± 0.25
Offensive line	134.3	176 ± 26	1.39 ± 0.20
Defensive line	122.3	180 ± 24	1.49 ± 0.19

Source: Data from Secora, Latin, Berg, & Noble (2004).[37]

(up to 10 RM) becomes an estimate of 1 RM and time is not wasted by performing frequent maximal 1 RM tests.

Assume: Reps@225 = **10**

$$1\ RM\ (lb) = (7.1 * Reps@225) + 226.7$$
$$r = .96, SEE = 14.1\ lb \qquad\qquad Eq.\ 4.7a$$

$$1\ RM\ (lb) = (7.1 * \mathbf{10}) + 226.7 = \mathbf{298}\ lb = \mathbf{135}\ kg \quad Eq.\ 4.7b$$

Norms for the tests of work and mean power described in this chapter are not available, so the results cannot be meaningfully evaluated. As was mentioned earlier, the tests were included primarily for demonstrating the concept of quantifying work and power during exercise. The mean power values derived from the bench press test reflect the relationship between the force (kg) generated during the lift, the distance (m) over which the force was applied, and the time (s) required to complete the lift. Interestingly, neither the highest forces nor the highest speeds necessarily produce the greatest powers. Moderate forces combined with moderate speeds most often produce the highest powers. Power during bench press exercise can be directly and accurately measured only through the use of special equipment that precisely measures force and time. When such measurements have been made, a peak power of 428 W

for "explosive" bench press exercise in men was reported using a load equal to 30 % of the measured 1 RM, which was 89 ± 30 kg. Peak power decreased with heavier loads until at 90 % of 1 RM it had dropped by half, to 214 W.[39] These power values, because they are "peak power" values measured during one "explosive" bench press trial, will be much higher than any "mean power" measurements you will record during multiple submaximal bench press trials.

References

1. American Academy of Pediatrics. (1983). Weight training and weight lifting: Information for the pediatrician. *The Physician and Sportsmedicine, 11*(3): 157–161.

2. American College of Sports Medicine. (2010). *ACSM'S guidelines for exercise testing and prescription* (8th ed.). Philadelphia: Lippincott Williams & Wilkins.

3. Berger, R. A., & Smith, K. J. (1991). Effects of the tonic neck reflex in the bench press. *Journal of Applied Sport Science Research, 5,* 188–191.

4. Block, J. E., Smith, R., Friedlander, G., & Genant, H. K. (1989). Preventing osteoporosis with exercise: A review with emphasis on methodology. *Medical Hypotheses, 30*(1): 9–19.

5. Braith, R. W., Graves, J. E., Leggett, S. H., & Pollock, M. L. (1993). Effect of training on the relationship between maximal and submaximal strength. *Medicine and Science in Sports and Exercise, 25*(1), 132–138.

6. Brzycki, M. (1993). Strength testing: prediction of one-rep max from reps-to-fatigue. *Journal of Health, Physical Education, Recreation and Dance, 64,* 88–90.

7. Chapman, P. P., Whitehead, J. R., & Brinkhert, R. H. (1996). Prediction of 1-RM bench press from the 225 lbs reps-to-fatigue test in college football players. *Medicine and Science in Sports and Exercise, 28,* Abstract #393, S66.

8. Claiborne, J. M., & Donolli, J. D. (1993). Number of repetitions at selected percentages of one repetition maximum in untrained college women. *Research Quarterly for Exercise and Sports, 64* (Suppl): (Abstract).

9. Clarke, D. H. (1975). *Exercise physiology.* Englewood Cliffs, NJ: Prentice-Hall.

10. Corbin, C. B., & Lindsey, R. (1996). *Physical fitness concepts.* Dubuque, IA: Brown & Benchmark.

11. Cronin, J. B., McNair, P. J., & Marshall, R. N. (2000). The role of maximal strength and load on initial power production. *Medicine and Science in Sports & Exercise, 32,* 1763–1769.

12. Heyward, V. H. (2000). Advanced fitness assessment and exercise prescription (4th ed., p. 121). Champaign, IL: Human Kinetics.

BOX 4.3	Chapter Preview/Review

How is isotonic or dynamic strength defined?

What does the abbreviation 1 RM mean?

How accurate is 1 RM testing?

How can 1 RM be estimated from submaximal repetitions to fatigue?

How do linear and curvilinear methods of estimating 1 RM differ?

What is the difference between absolute and relative strength?

How are work and power measured during weight lifting?

What is the NFL-225 test?

13. Hockey, R. V. (1989). *Physical fitness: The pathway to healthful living*. St. Louis: Times Mirror/Mosby.

14. Hoeger, W. K., Barette, S. L., Hale, D. F., & Hopkins, D. R. (1987). Relationship between repetitions and selected percentage of one repetition maximum. *Journal of Applied Sports Science Research, 1,* 11–13.

15. Horvat, M., Ramsey, V., Franklin, C., Gavin, C., Palumbo, T., Glass, L. A. (2003). A method for predicting maximal strength in collegiate women athletes. *Journal of Strength and Conditioning Research, 17,* 324–328.

16. Invergo, J. J., Ball, T. E., & Looney, M. (1991). Relationship of push-ups and absolute muscular endurance to bench press strength. *Journal of Applied Sport Science Research, 5,* 121–125.

17. Johnson, P. B., Updyke, W. F., Schaefer, M., & Stollberg, D. C. (1975). *Sport, exercise, and you*. San Francisco: Holt, Rinehart and Winston.

18. Knuttgen, H. G. (1995). Force, work, and power in athletic training. *Sports Science Exchange, 8*(4), 1–5.

19. Kraemer, R. R., Kilgore, J. L., Kraemer, G. R., & Castracane, V. D. (1992). Growth hormone, IGF-1, and testosterone responses to resistive exercise. *Medicine and Science in Sports and Exercise, 24,* 1346–1352.

20. Kramer, W. J., & Fry, A. C. (1995). Strength testing: Development and evaluation of methodology. In P. J. Maud & C. Foster (Eds.), *Physiological assessment of human fitness* (pp. 115–138). Champaign, IL: Human Kinetics.

21. Kuramoto, A. K., & Payne, V. G. (1995). Predicting muscular strength in women: A preliminary study. *Research Quarterly for Exercise and Sport, 66,* 168–172.

22. Lander, J. (1985). Maximum based on repetitions. *National Strength and Conditioning Association Journal, 6,* 60–61.

23. Liemohn, W. S., et al. (1998). Unresolved controversies in back management. *Journal of Orthopaedic and Sports Physical Therapy, 9,* 239–244.

24. Mayhew, J. L., Ball, T. E., Arnold, M. D., & Bowen, J. C. (1992). Relative muscular endurance performance as a predictor of bench press strength in college men and women. *Journal of Applied Sport Science Research, 6,* 200–206.

25. Mayhew, J. L., Johnson, B. D., LaMonte, M. J., Lauber, D., & Kemmler, W. (2008). Accuracy of prediction equations for determining one repetition maximum bench press in women before and after resistance training. *Journal of Strength and Conditioning Research, 22,* 1570–1577.

26. Mayhew, J. L., Prinster J. L., Wave, J. S., Zimmer, D. L., Arabas, J. R., & Bemben, M. G. (1995). Muscular endurance repetitions to predict bench press strength in men of different training levels. *Journal of Sports Medicine and Physical Fitness, 35,* 108–113.

27. Mayhew, J. L., Ware, J. S., Bemben, M. G., Wilt, B., Ward, T. E., Farris, B., Juraszek, J., & Slovak, J. P. (1999). The NFL-225 test as a measure of bench press strength in college football players. *Journal of Strength and Conditioning Research, 13,* 130–134.

28. McCarthy, J. J. (1991). *Effects of a wrestling periodization strength program on muscular strength, absolute endurance, and relative endurance*. Master's thesis, California State University, Fullerton.

29. McComas, A. J. (1994). Human neuromuscular adaptations that accompany changes in activity. *Medicine and Science in Sports and Exercise, 26,* 1498–1509.

30. Murray, J. A., & Karpovich, P. V. (1956). *Weight training in athletics*. Englewood Cliffs, NJ: Prentice-Hall.

31. National Strength and Conditioning Association. (2000). *Essentials of strength and conditioning,* (2nd ed. pp. 177, 407). T. R. Baechle, & R. W. Earle (Eds.). Champaign, IL: Human Kinetics.

32. *Penn State Sports Medicine Newsletter.* (1992). The RM prescription. *1*(2), 7.

33. Pollock, M. L., Graves, J. E., Leggett, S. H., Braith, R. W., & Hagberg, J. M. (1991). Injuries and adherence to aerobic and strength training exercise programs for the elderly. *Medicine and Science in Sports and Exercise, 23,* 1194–1200.

34. Reynolds, J. M., Gordon, T. J., & Robergs, R. A. (2004). Prediction of one repetition maximum strength from multiple repetition maximum testing and anthropometry. *Journal of Strength and Conditioning Research, 20,* 584–592.

35. Rikli, R. E., Jones, C. J., Beam, W. C., Duncan, S. J., & Lamar, B. (1996). Testing versus training effects on 1 RM strength assessment in older adults. *Medicine and Science in Sports and Exercise, 28* (5, Suppl.), Abstract #909, S153.

36. Sale, D. G. (1991). Testing strength and power. In J. D. MacDougal, H. A. Wenger, & H. J. Green (Eds.), *Physiological testing of the high-performance athlete* (pp. 21–106). Champaign, IL: Human Kinetics.

37. Secora, C. A., Latin, R. W., Berg, K. E., & Noble, J. M. (2004). Comparison of physical and performance characteristics of NCAA division I football players: 1987 and 2000. *Journal of Strength and Conditioning Research, 18,* 286–291.

38. Shimano, T., Kraemer, W. J., Spiering, B. A., Volck, J. S., Hatfield, D. L., (2006). Relationship between the number of repetitions and selected percentages of one repetition maximum in free weight exercises in trained and untrained men. *Journal of Strength and Conditioning Research, 20,* 819–823.

39. Siegel, J. A., Gilders, R. M., Staron, R. S., & Hagerman, F. C. (2002). Human muscle power output during upper- and lower-body exercises. *Journal of Strength and Conditioning Research, 16,* 173–178.
40. Wakim, K. G., Gersten, J. W., Elkins, E. C., & Martin, G. M. (1950). Objective recording of muscle strength. *Archives of Physical Medicine, 31,* 90–100.
41. Ware, J. S., Clemens, C. T., Mayhew, J. L., & Johnston, T. J. (1995). Muscular endurance repetitions to predict bench press and squat strength in college football players. *Journal of Strength and Conditioning Research, 9,* 99–103.
42. Weir, J. P., Wagner, L. L., & Housh, T. J. (1994). The effect of rest interval length on repeated maximal bench press. *Journal of Strength and Conditioning Research, 8,* 58–60.
43. Whisenant, M. J., Panton, L. B., East, W. B., & Broeder, C. E. (2003). Validation of submaximal prediction equations for the 1 repetition maximum bench press test on a group of collegiate football players. *Journal of Strength and Conditioning Research, 17,* 221–227.
44. Wilmore, J. H., & Costill, D. L. (1988). *Training for sport and activity.* Dubuque. IA: Wm. C. Brown.

Isotonic/Dynamic exercise = muscle lengthens/shortens, weight does not change
Dynamic strength is often measured through 1RM
 not recommended for children
Direct measurement: go until only do 1 rep
Indirect: submaximal then estimated using linear or curvilinear
Muscles used: pectoralis major, anterior deltoid, coracobrachialis, triceps brachii
Biochemical pathway is phosphogenic

Warm up sets of about 8, then 3-3
Direct uses trial+error method, hopefully in about 5 trials
Indirect uses #RM (repetitions maximal)... should be under 20 reps for given weight
 -ideally, fatigue/failure happens in 3-12 reps
Linear equation = %1RM = 100 - (#RM * 2.5)
$$1RM = \frac{Weight\ lifted}{(\%1RM/100)}$$

Can also calculate work (J) if measure displacement first
 can measure positive and negative work
 (concentric)   (eccentric)
 (against gravity) (with gravity)

Measured as absolute strength and relative strength
 - to calculate relative = $\frac{weight\ lifted}{body\ weight}$

normative values

	18-29	30-50	>50	
men	56-77	49-64	43-60	about -7 each group
women	35-42	32-38	28-34	about -4 each group

Form 4.1

ISOTONIC (DYNAMIC) STRENGTH

Homework

Gender: **F**   Initials: **AA**   Age (y): **22**   Height (cm): **158**   Weight (kg): **68.0**

Direct 1 RM	T1	T2	T3	T4	T5	Abs 1 RM	Rel 1 RM
Bench press (kg)	**47.5**	**50.0**	**52.5**	**55.0**		55 kg	55/68 = .8 kg·kg^{-1}

Strength Evaluation

Category for: Abs 1 RM *(Table 4.3)*   55   Rel 1 RM *(Table 4.4)*   .81 kg·kg^{-1}

Evaluation/comments: _____

_____

_____

Indirect 1 RM   Bench press: Weight lifted (kg) = **45.0** kg   # Reps (# RM) = **7**

Linear estimate of 1 RM   % 1 RM = 100 − (# Reps * 2.5) = _____ % 1 RM

Abs 1 RM (kg) = $\underset{\text{Weight lifted}}{\rule{2cm}{0.4pt}}$ / ($\underset{\text{\% 1 RM}}{\rule{1.5cm}{0.4pt}}$ / 100) = _____ kg   Abs 1 RM *(Table 4.1)* = _____ kg

Curvilinear estimate of 1 RM   % 1 RM = 52.5 + 41.9 e$^{-0.055 \, * \, \# \text{Reps}}$ = _____ % 1 RM

Abs 1 RM (kg) = $\underset{\text{Weight lifted}}{\rule{2cm}{0.4pt}}$ / ($\underset{\text{\% 1 RM}}{\rule{1.5cm}{0.4pt}}$ / 100) = _____ kg   Abs 1 RM *(Table 4.2)* = _____ kg

Comparison of direct/indirect 1 RM: _____

_____

Determination of Work and Mean Power *(Optional)*   *Note:* 1 kg = 9.8067 N

Work	Weight lifted (kg)	Force (N)	Displacement (m / Rep)	# RM
Bench press	**40**		**0.5**	**10**

Total work (J) = $\underset{\text{Force (N)}}{\rule{2cm}{0.4pt}}$ * $\underset{\text{Displacement}}{\rule{2cm}{0.4pt}}$ * $\underset{\text{\# Reps}}{\rule{1.5cm}{0.4pt}}$ * 1.33 = _____ J

Mean Power   Work (J) = _____ J   Time (s) = **33.5** s

Mean power (W) = $\underset{\text{Work}}{\rule{2cm}{0.4pt}}$ / $\underset{\text{Time}}{\rule{2cm}{0.4pt}}$ = _____ W

1RM = 160 lbs   Submax weight 135   100-(8·2.5) = 80 % 1RM   Absolute 1RM = 160 lbs = 72.58 kg
Direct   reps   8   135/(80/100) = 168.75 lbs   Relative 1RM = 168.75 lbs = 76.54 kg
                                                                                    Indirect

Form 4.2
ISOTONIC (DYNAMIC) STRENGTH

NAME Tyler Gilmore   DATE 2/11   SCORE _____

Lab Results

Gender: M   Initials: TG   Age (y): 21   Height (cm): 190.40   Weight (kg): 83.92

Direct 1 RM   T1   T2   T3   T4   T5   Abs 1 RM   Rel 1 RM

Bench press (kg) ___ ___ ___ ___ ___   72.58 kg   76.54 kg·kg⁻¹

Strength Evaluation

Category for: Abs 1 RM *(Table 4.3)* 72.58 kg   Rel 1 RM *(Table 4.4)* .86 = 86% of mass

Evaluation/comments: In absolute terms, my one repetition max fell at the upper end of average and I likely ended near the 70th percentile. As for relative strength, I fell into the fair category.

Indirect 1 RM   Bench press: Weight lifted (kg) = 61.24 kg   # Reps (# RM) = 8

Linear estimate of 1 RM   % 1 RM = 100 − (# Reps * 2.5) = 80 % 1 RM

Abs 1 RM (kg) = 61.24 / (80 / 100) = 76.54 kg   Abs 1 RM *(Table 4.1)* = 76.54 kg
$\underbrace{}_{\text{Weight lifted}}$ $\underbrace{}_{\text{\% 1 RM}}$

Curvilinear estimate of 1 RM   % 1 RM = $52.5 + 41.9 e^{-0.055 * \text{\# Reps}}$ = ____ % 1 RM

Abs 1 RM (kg) = ____ / (____ / 100) = ____ kg   Abs 1 RM *(Table 4.2)* = ____ kg
 Weight lifted   % 1 RM

Comparison of direct/indirect 1 RM: _____

Determination of Work and Mean Power *(Optional)*   Note: 1 kg = 9.8067 N

Work	Weight lifted (kg)	Force (N)	Displacement (m / Rep)	# RM
Bench press	___	___	___	___
Total work (J) =	___ *	___ *	___ * 1.33 =	___ J
	Force (N)	Displacement	# Reps	

Mean Power   Work (J) = ____ J   Time (s) = ____ s

Mean power (W) = ____ / ____ = ____ W
 Work   Time

ISOMETRIC (STATIC) STRENGTH

The importance of handgrip strength is not just to have an impressive handshake. Good handgrip strength may prevent people from dropping various objects, such as jars, bottles, and cans, in addition to allowing them to open the lid of a jar. Especially for older persons, good handgrip strength may prevent a fall down stairs or in bathtubs by enabling them to grasp a rail; it may also permit them to squeeze the gas pump at the service station. Grip strength also has been used in the occupational setting as a pre-employment device, as a periodic monitoring device, and as a return-to-work rehabilitation device.[18] In summary, handgrip strength is important for successful performance in activities of daily living and occupational activities.

The monitoring of handgrip strength is meaningful in the diagnosis and prognosis of neck and, of course, hand injuries. Thus, the measurement of handgrip strength has implications for people's safety, convenience, and neuromuscular assessment.

RATIONALE

The rationale for the measurement of strength may be categorized into two areas: anatomical and physiological. The measurement of handgrip strength is one example of an isometric muscle action or static exercise. The muscles do not change in length, except that caused by the elasticity of the muscles and connective tissues. It is the only isometric or static test described in this laboratory manual, but measurements can also be made isometrically of the strength of other muscles and functions of the hand and back. The further use of a cable tensiometer would allow the isometric testing of virtually any joint motion and muscle group in the body.

Anatomical Rationale

Grip strength is related ($r = .60$) to muscle mass.[22] Handgrip strength is mainly a function of the muscles in the forearm, in addition to those in the hand. Eight muscles serve as the prime movers and stabilizers for handgrip strength; 11 other muscles within the hand itself assist in the contraction.[6]

Physiological Rationale

Some participants can reach their peak force of a static handgrip test of strength in 0.3 s,[5,32] whereas others may take 2.7 s.[3] Similar times to peak force occur in larger muscle groups, such as elbow flexors.[32] Men reach peak force faster than women,[5] possibly because women's more elastic connective tissues require more time to reach the end point of stretch. Some people may be able to hold the peak force for only 1 s,[21] whereas others might hold it for a few seconds.[32]

Based upon this rapid onset and decay of peak force, it should be obvious that the energy pathway predominantly involved in maximal muscle actions (strength) is the phosphagen system. Thus, the primary biochemical reaction for strength, or any muscle action, is

$$\text{Adenosine triphosphate(ATP)} \xrightarrow{\text{ATPase}} \text{ADP} + \text{P} + \text{Energy}$$

Because the need for large amounts of ATP is so urgent, the ATP and its quick rejuvenator, creatine phosphate (CP), must be immediately available for the interacting muscle filaments—actin and myosin. However, the stores of ATP and CP are very limited. Because they cannot be resupplied adequately by the slower glycolytic and oxidative systems, the actin and myosin filaments cannot interact in order to continue contracting forcefully. Consequently, a rapid decay occurs in the peak force despite the physical and mental efforts to sustain it.

METHODS

The methods for testing grip strength are simple. The procedures of handgrip dynamometry can be learned quickly by watching a brief demonstration and then practicing for a few minutes. Box 5.1 summarizes the accuracy of handgrip strength testing.

Equipment for Handgrip Strength Testing

The word *dynamometer* (dī-na-móm-e-ter) comes from the Greek word meaning *power measure*. Because time is not measured in the strength tests described here, the more apt description of the handgrip dynamometer would be as a force-measuring device, rather than as a power-measuring one.

A common laboratory dynamometer, the Jamar™, uses a sealed hydraulic system to activate its force indicator during static muscle action. For example, the movement of the grip for the Jamar™ instrument (Figure 5.1) cannot be perceived; however, grip handles on spring dynamometers, such as the Lafayette™, (Lafayette Instruments, Lafayette, IN), may move more than 1.5 cm during a maximal handgrip contraction.

Strength is usually measured in units of force or torque. The force units for static dynamometry should

Accuracy of Handgrip Strength Testing

Muscular strength is highly affected by the central nervous system. Thus, emotional or mental factors play an important role in strength testing. If the motivation of the performer is consistent, strength variability should be minimized.

Reliability

One group of investigators reported no significant differences in reliability (Intraclass Correlation Coefficients; ICC) between (1) the maximal force of one trial, (2) the mean maximal force of two trials, (3) the mean maximal force of three trials, and the highest maximal force of three trials.[18] However, another group reported the highest reliability when the mean of three maximal trials was used.[18] Individual daily variations in strength range from 2 % to 12 % in women and 5 % to 9 % in men.[37] Reliability coefficients for strength testing are usually .90 or higher. The grip-handle setting at position #1 of the Jamar™ dynamometer is significantly less reliable than the other four handle positions.[26] The objectivity, or inter-rater reliability, is very high when two technicians follow standard procedures (r = .97).

Validity

For the average person, handgrip strength correlates moderately (r = .69) with the total strength of 22 other muscles of the body.[10] Static tests of strength are more valid for static muscle actions than they are for dynamic actions.

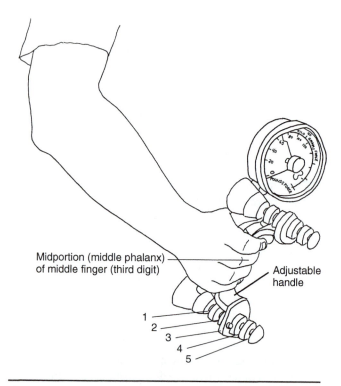

Midportion (middle phalanx) of middle finger (third digit)

Adjustable handle

1
2
3
4
5

Figure 5.1 The proper positioning of the body, upper arm, forearm, and hand during handgrip strength testing. Numbered slots indicate five different grip size positions of the Jamar™ dynamometer.

be expressed, preferably, in newtons (N). Although kilograms (kg) and pounds (lb) are commonly printed on the dials of most handgrip dynamometers, the scientific community encourages the use of newtons.[23] Most handgrip dynamometers provide scales that read up to 200–220 lb, or 90–100 kg. Most grip dynamometers have dual pointers, one pointer holding the maximal reading until it is reset and the other pointer returning to the zero position. Some have a single floating pointer that holds its position until reset.

Procedures for Handgrip Dynamometry

The procedures for handgrip strength testing are summarized as follows:

1. The participant should be in the standing position (Figure 5.2).
2. The participant's head should be in the midposition (facing straight ahead).
3. The grip size should be adjusted so that the middle finger's (third digit's) midportion (second phalanx) is approximately at a right angle.
   a. Grip adjustments of 1.3 cm (0.5 in) on the Jamar™ dynamometer (see Box 5.2 for calibration procedure) are made by slipping off the moveable handle and repositioning it into the five manufactured slots: #1 = the slot at the innermost position for the smallest grip size (see Figure 5.1).

   #5 = the slot at the outside position for the largest grip size.[a]
   b. Grip adjustments up to 4 cm for other dynamometers (e.g., Lafayette™) are possible.
4. The technician should record the grip setting (1 to 5 for Jamar™; 10 mm to 40 mm on inner scale for Lafayette™) on Form 5.2. Ideally, this same setting would be used for further tests on the same person.
5. The participant's forearm may be placed at any angle between 90° and 180° (right angle to straight) of the upper arm; the upper arm hangs in a vertical position.
6. The participant's wrist and forearm should be at the midprone position.
7. The participant should exert maximally and quickly after hearing the technician's following instructions:[28]
   a. "Are you ready?"
   b. "Squeeze as hard as you can." As the participant begins:
   c. "Harder! . . . Harder! . . . Relax."
8. The participant should make two[13,31,34] or three[35] trials alternately with each hand, with at least 30 s[26] or up to 1 min[35] between trials for the same hand.
9. The technician should record the force in kg, then convert the circled best score to approximate newtons by multiplying the kg value by 9.8067.
10. The technician resets the dynamometer's pointer to zero after each trial.

[a]Jamar™ position #2 spans ≈ 4.4 cm (≈ 1.75 in.).[11]

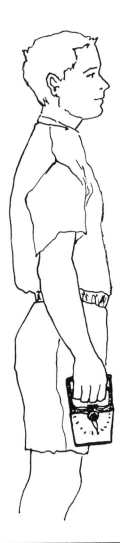

Figure 5.2 The participant squeezes the spring dynamometer maximally from a standing position and facing directly forward with the upper arm hanging straight down and the forearm at any position between 90° angle and 180° angle (straight down).

adjusting the grip-handle size, it appears that Jamar™ position #2[12] or #3[20] provides the highest force.

Although participants should make powerful exertions at the start of each trial, they should be careful to avoid jerking the dynamometer. No movement from the initial body position can take place during the trial, nor can the hand touch any other part of the body.

Consistent verbal instruction prior to and during the maximal effort enhances the reliability of the measures.[28] The participant should not gradually approach maximal; in fact, it is counterproductive to take more than five seconds to reach maximal contraction, especially in older persons.[24]

Based on the rapid recovery rate of the phosphagens, 30 s to 1 min should be sufficient as a rest interval between trials for the same hand, especially if each contraction is less than 5 s.

The score chosen to best represent the participant's strength has varied among investigators.[18,27,31,34,35] Most investigators have used the best of two or three[35] trials. Usually, the first trial of a three-trial protocol will be the highest.[11,33]

Comments on the Procedures

The standing position produces higher grip strengths than the sitting position.[1] The midposition of the head is recommended in order to avoid the bias of the tonic neck reflex.[4,16] Although this natural reflex may be diminished in adults, it causes the flexors of the opposite side (contralateral) of the body to be the most strong when the head is turned laterally away from the forearm being tested.[14,15] One group of investigators reported no difference in maximal forces of the dominant hand at 90° elbow flexion or full extension.[9] But other investigators found higher grip strengths with the elbow at full extension.[25,36]

Grip sizes do not make much difference except in participants with large hands who are tested at small grip settings, or persons with small hands who are tested at large settings.[30] However, when testing many persons without

RESULTS AND DISCUSSION

The measurement of handgrip strength is simple and widely used, especially in evaluating hand function in clinical and occupational applications.

The data in Table 5.1 provide categories for evaluating both the absolute and relative strength of the handgrip muscles. On an absolute basis, reflected by the maximum grip, the women are about 65 % as strong as the men. In comparing relative strength (i.e. ratio of combined sum to body weight), the women have an average ratio of 1.04, which is about 75 % as strong as the men, who have an average relative strength of 1.38 kg·kg⁻¹. Relative grip strength becomes important when evaluating the ability of a person to lift his or her own body weight or to assume and support certain body positions such as grasping a handrail or hanging from a chin-up bar.

Table 5.1	Category for Absolute Maximum Grip (kg; N) and Relative Combined Grip Sum (kg·kg⁻¹; N·kg⁻¹) for Young (18–25 y) Men and Women

| | Men (N = 312) | | | | Women (N = 601) | | | |
| | Absolute | | Relative | | Absolute | | Relative | |
Category	(kg)	(N)	(kg·kg⁻¹)	(N·kg⁻¹)	(kg)	(N)	(kg·kg⁻¹)	(N·kg⁻¹)
Well above ave (> 95th %ile)	> 67.7	> 664	> 1.80	> 17.7	> 41.7	> 409	> 1.40	> 13.7
Above ave (75th–95th %ile)	57.9–67.7	568–664	1.52–1.80	14.9–17.7	35.9–41.7	352–409	1.16–1.40	11.4–13.7
Average (25th–74th %ile)	48.1–57.8	472–567	1.24–1.51	12.2–14.8	30.1–35.8	295–351	0.92–1.15	9.0–11.3
Below ave (5th–24th %ile)	38.3–48.0	376–471	0.96–1.23	9.4–12.1	24.3–30.0	238–294	0.68–0.91	6.7–8.9
Well below ave (< 5th %ile)	< 38.3	< 376	< 0.96	< 9.4	< 24.3	< 238	< 0.68	< 6.7
Mean	53.0	520	1.38	13.5	33.0	324	1.04	10.2

Source: Data compiled by author, Beam (2003).[2]

Comparing grip strength between the two hands is interesting. In three studies of grip strength[7,19,27], 82–90 % of the participants were right-handed and 10–18 % were left-handed. When grip strength was reported in these studies as the average for right and left hands, the difference was 8–14 % for both men and women, with the right hand being stronger. When strength was expressed for dominant and non-dominant hands, the difference was 6–9 % for both men and women, with the dominant hand being stronger. It appears at first glance that the "dominant" hand (the right hand in right-handed persons and the left hand in left-handed persons) is stronger than the "non-dominant" hand. However, this appears to be true only in right-handed persons. The vast majority of right-handed persons (83 %) produced more force with their right hands, and on average were 7–8 % stronger in their right hand. However, a minority of left-handed persons (45 %) produced more force with their left hands than their right hands. In fact, in left-handed persons, the left hand (the "dominant" hand) is 1–2% weaker than the right hand.[7,19] Perhaps the similarity in right and left hand grip strength in left-handers is because they have more opportunity to use their right hand in mostly a "right-handed world" where tools and appliances are designed for right-handers.[7]

Mean grip strengths for males and females by age group from 6–7 y to 60–64 y are shown in Table 5.2. Grip strength is similar in boys and girls until puberty, at which time the strength of boys increases disproportionately.[32] Graphing these same data (Figure 5.3) more clearly demonstrates this trend and other trends observed across age groups. Young girls (6–11 y) are about 90 % as strong as their boy counterparts, but as they get older (14–19 y) they are only 65–75 % as strong as boys. Grip strength generally appears to peak in early adulthood (18–25 y) and for the most part remains unchanged through age 50 in both men and women.[17,29] After age 50, handgrip strength begins to decline. Men's grip strength after age 50 is reported to decline in a curvilinear fashion.[8]

It is important in testing isometric handgrip strength that as much as possible is standardized, including the type of grip dynamometer used; the position of the body, shoulder, and elbow; the protocol (e.g., number of repetitions);

Table 5.2	Average Right or Dominant Handgrip Strength (kg) by Gender

| | Males | | | | Females | | | |
Age Group	N	M	±	SD	N	M	±	SD
Right Handgrip (kg)								
6–7 y[a]	26	14.7	±	2.2	33	13.0	±	2.0
10–11 y[a]	43	24.4	±	4.4	40	22.5	±	3.7
14–15 y[a]	34	35.1	±	7.0	34	26.4	±	5.6
18–19 y[a]	33	49.0	±	11.2	30	32.5	±	5.6
Dominant Handgrip (kg)								
25–29 y[b]	103	53.1	±	10.4	90	33.1	±	6.4
30–34 y[b]	61	52.2	±	10.9	88	33.6	±	6.8
35–39 y[b]	60	53.5	±	10.4	75	33.6	±	7.3
40–44 y[b]	55	52.2	±	10.0	70	33.6	±	6.8
45–49 y[b]	51	54.9	±	11.3	72	33.1	±	7.7
50–54 y[b]	52	53.5	±	10.9	51	32.2	±	7.3
55–59 y[b]	48	43.1	±	9.1	58	29.0	±	6.4
60–64 y[b]	49	42.6	±	6.4	45	25.4	±	7.3

Sources: Data from [a]Mathiowetz, Wiemer, & Federman (1986)[29]; and [b]Hanten, et al. (1999).[19]

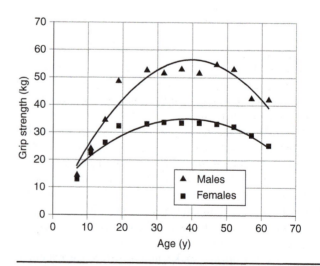

Figure 5.3 The relationship between age (y) and grip strength (kg) in males and females age 6–64 y.
Source: Data from Hanten, et al. (1999)[19]; and Mathiowetz, Wiemer & Federman (1986).[29]

How is isometric or static strength defined?

How well does handgrip strength correlate with total body strength?

In what units is grip strength (force) described?

Does grip strength differ when measured in the standing position versus the sitting position?

Does arm position (elbow angle) affect grip strength?

What is a sufficient rest interval between trials of grip strength measurement?

During which decade of life does handgrip strength appear to begin to decline?

Are bilateral differences in grip strength observed?

and the timing (e.g., time of day). If done well, grip strength testing can provide important information with regard to hand function and in a more general sense can reflect the overall strength of the body, within limitations.

References

1. Balogun, J. A., Akomolafe, C. T., & Amusa, L. O. (1991). Grip strength: Effects of testing posture and elbow position. *Archives of Physical Medicine and Rehabilitation, 72,* 280–283.

2. Beam, W. (2003). Unpublished data.

3. Bemben, M. G., Clasey, J. L., & Massey, B. H. (1990). The effect of the rate of muscle contraction on the force-time curve parameters of male and female subjects. *Research Quarterly for Exercise and Sport, 61*(1), 96–99.

4. Berntson, G. G., & Torello, M. W. (1977). Expression of Magnus tonic neck reflexes in distal muscles of prehension in normal adults. *Physiology and Behavior, 19,* 585–587.

5. Borsa, P. A., & Sauers, E. L. (2000). The importance of gender on myokinetic deficits before and after microinjury. *Medicine and Science in Sports and Exercise, 32,* 891–896.

6. Buck, J. A., Amundsen, L. R., & Nielsen, D. H. (1980). Systolic blood pressure responses during isometric contractions of large and small muscle groups. *Medicine and Science in Sports and Exercise, 12*(3), 145–147.

7. Crosby, C. A., & Wehbe, M. A. (1994). Hand strength: Normative values. *Journal of Hand Surgery, 19,* 665–670.

8. Desrosiers, J., Bravo, G., Hebert, R., & Dutil, E. (1995). Normative data for grip strength of elderly men and women. *American Journal of Occupational Therapy, 49,* 637–644.

9. Desrosiers, J., Bravo, G., Hebert, R., & Mercier, L. (1995). Impact of elbow position on grip strength of elderly men. *Journal of Hand Therapy, 8,* 27–30.

10. de Vries, H. A. (1980). *Physiology of exercise in physical education and athletics.* Dubuque, IA: Wm. C. Brown.

11. Fess, E. E. (1982). The effects of Jamar dynamometer handle position and test protocol on hand strength. *Journal of Hand Surgery, 1,* 308.

12. Firrell, J. C., & Crain, G. M. (1996). Which setting of the dynamometer provides maximal grip strength? *Journal of Hand Surgery, 21,* 397–401.

13. Fitness and Amateur Sport, Canada. (1987). *Canadian Standardized Test of Fitness (CSTF) operations manual* (3rd ed.). Ottawa, Canada: Author.

14. George, C. O. (1970). Effects of the asymmetrical tonic neck posture upon grip strength of normal children. *Research Quarterly, 41,* 361–364.

15. George, C. O. (1972). Facilitative and inhibitory effects of the tonic neck reflex upon grip strength of right- and left-handed children. *Research Quarterly, 43,* 157–166.

16. Gesell, A., & Ames, L. B. (1947). The development of handedness. *Journal of Genetic Psychology, 70,* 155–175.

17. Häger-Ross, C., & Rösblad, B. (2002). Norms for grip strength in children aged 4–16 years. *Acta Paediatrica, 91,* 617–625.

18. Hamilton, A., Balnave, R., & Adams, R. (1994). Grip strength testing reliability. *Journal of Hand Therapy, 7,* 163–170.

19. Hanten, W. P., Chen, W. Y., Austin, A. A., Brooks, R. E., Carter, H. C., Law, C. A., Morgan, M. K., (1999). Maximum grip strength in normal subjects from 20 to 64 years of age. *Journal of Hand Therapy, 12,* 193–200.

20. Harkonen, R., Piirtomaa, M., & Alaranta, H. (1993). Grip strength and hand position of the dynamometer in 204 Finnish adults. *Journal of Hand Surgery, 18,* 129–132.

21. Hislop, H. J. (1963). Quantitative changes in human muscular strength during isometric exercise. *Journal of the American Physical Therapy Association, 43,* 21–38.

22. Kallman, D. A., Plato, C. C., & Tobin, J. D. (1990). The role of muscle loss in the age-related decline of grip strength: Cross-sectional and longitudinal perspectives. *Journal of Gerontology: Medical Sciences, 45,* M82–88.

23. Knuttgen, H. G. (1986). Quantifying exercise performances with SI units. *The Physician and Sportsmedicine, 14*(12), 157–161.

24. Kroll, W., Clarkson, P. M., & Melchionda, A. M. (1981). Age, isometric strength, rate of tension development and fiber type composition. *Medicine and Science in Sports and Exercise, 13,* Abstract, 87.

25. Kuzala, E. A., & Vargo, M. C. (1992). The relationship between elbow position and grip strength. *American Journal of Occupational Therapy, 46,* 509–512.

26. Lind, A. R., & McNicol, G. W. (1967). Circulatory response to sustained handgrip contractions performed during other exercise, both rhythmic and static. *The American Journal of Cardiology, 38,* 46–51.

27. Mathiowetz, V., Kashman, N., Volland, G., Weber, K., Dowe, M., & Rogers, S. (1985). Grip and pinch strength: Normative data for adults. *Archives of Physical Medicine and Rehabilitation, 66,* 69–74.

28. Mathiowetz, V., Weber, K., Volland, G., & Kashman, N. (1984). Reliability and validity of hand strength evaluation. *Journal of Hand Surgery, 9A,* 222–226.

29. Mathiowetz, V., Wiemer, D. M., & Federman, S. M. (1986). Grip and pinch strength: Norms for 6- to 19-year-olds. *American Journal of Occupational Therapy, 40,* 705–711.

30. Montoye, H. J., & Faulkner, J. A. (1975). Determination of the optimum setting of an adjustable grip dynamometer. *The Research Quarterly, 35,* 30–36.

31. Montoye, H. J., & Lamphiear, D. E. (1977). Grip and arm strength in males and females, age 10 to 69. *Research Quarterly, 48,* 109–120.

32. Morris, A. F., Clarke, D. H., & Dainis, A. (1983). Time to maximal voluntary isometric contraction (MVC) for five different muscle groups in college adults. *Research Quarterly for Exercise and Sport, 54,* 163–168.

33. Patterson, R. P., & Baxter, T. (1988). A multiple muscle strength testing protocol. *Archives of Physical Medicine and Rehabilitation, 69,* 366–368.

34. Sale, D. G. (1991). Testing strength and power. In J. D. MacDougal, H. A. Wenger, & H. J. Green (Eds.), *Physiological testing of the high-performance athlete* (pp. 21–106). Champaign, IL: Human Kinetics.

35. Stoelting, C. H. (1970). *Smedley instruction manual.* Chicago: Author.

36. Su, C. Y., Lin, J. H., Chien, T. H., Chen, K. F., & Sung, Y. T. (1994). Grip strength in different positions of elbow and shoulder. *Archives of Physical Medicine and Rehabilitation, 75,* 812–815.

37. Wakim, K. G., Gersten, J. W., Elkins, E. C., & Martin, G. M. (1950). Objective recording of muscle strength. *Archives of Physical Medicine, 31,* 90–100.

Form 5.1

NAME _____ DATE _____ SCORE _____

ISOMETRIC (Static) STRENGTH

Homework

Gender: **M**   Initials: **AA**   Age (y): **20**   Weight (kg): **95.0**

Dominant hand (R or L): **R**   Dynamometer type: **Jamar**   Setting: **3**

Right grip (kg): T_1 **62.5** T_2 **63.0** T_3 **62.0** Highest of 3 = _____ kg = _____ N

Left grip (kg): T_1 **61.5** T_2 **61.0** T_3 **60.0** Highest of 3 = _____ kg = _____ N

Absolute strength (maximum grip) = _____ kg = _____ N

Combined sum = _____ + _____ = _____ kg = _____ N
              Right   Left

Relative strength = _____ / _____ = _____ kg·kg^{-1} = _____ N·kg^{-1}
        Combined sum   Weight

% Difference = ((_____ − _____) / _____) * 100 = _____ %
        Max   Min   Max

Category for absolute strength (Table 5.1) _____

Category for relative strength (Table 5.1) _____

Evaluation / comments: _____

Gender: **F**   Initials: **BB**   Age (y): **20**   Weight (kg): **75.0**

Dominant hand (R or L): **R**   Dynamometer type: **Jamar**   Setting: **2**

Right grip (kg): T_1 **42.5** T_2 **44.0** T_3 **42.0** Highest of 3 = _____ kg = _____ N

Left grip (kg): T_1 **41.5** T_2 **41.0** T_3 **40.0** Highest of 3 = _____ kg = _____ N

Absolute strength (maximum grip) = _____ kg = _____ N

Combined sum = _____ + _____ = _____ kg = _____ N
              Right   Left

Relative strength = _____ / _____ = _____ kg·kg^{-1} = _____ N·kg^{-1}
        Combined sum   Weight

% Difference = ((_____ − _____) / _____) * 100 = _____ %
        Max   Min   Max

Category for absolute strength (Table 5.1) _____

Category for relative strength (Table 5.1) _____

Evaluation / comments: _____

Form 5.2

ISOMETRIC (Static) STRENGTH

Lab Results

Gender: _____   Initials: _____   Age (y): _____   Weight (kg): _____

Dominant hand (R or L): ____   Dynamometer type: _____   Setting: _____

Right grip (kg): T_1 _____ T_2 _____ T_3 _____   Highest of 3 = _____ kg = _____ N

Left grip (kg): T_1 _____ T_2 _____ T_3 _____   Highest of 3 = _____ kg = _____ N

Absolute strength (maximum grip) = _____ kg = _____ N

Combined sum = _____ + _____ = _____ kg = _____ N
 Right Left

Relative strength = _____ / _____ = _____ kg·kg^{-1} = _____ N·kg^{-1}
 Combined sum Weight

% Difference = ((_____ − _____) / _____) ∗ 100 = _____ %
 Max Min Max

Category for absolute strength *(Table 5.1)* _____

Category for relative strength *(Table 5.1)* _____

Evaluation / comments: _____

Gender: _____   Initials: _____   Age (y): _____   Weight (kg): _____

Dominant hand (R or L): ____   Dynamometer type: _____   Setting: _____

Right grip (kg): T_1 _____ T_2 _____ T_3 _____   Highest of 3 = _____ kg = _____ N

Leftt grip (kg): T_1 _____ T_2 _____ T_3 _____   Highest of 3 = _____ kg = _____ N

Absolute strength (maximum grip) = _____ kg = _____ N

Combined sum = _____ + _____ = _____ kg = _____ N
 Right Left

Relative strength = _____ / _____ = _____ kg·kg^{-1} = _____ N·kg^{-1}
 Combined sum Weight

% Difference = ((_____ − _____) / _____) ∗ 100 = _____ %
 Max Min Max

Category for absolute strength *(Table 5.1)* _____

Category for relative strength *(Table 5.1)* _____

Evaluation / comments: _____

CHAPTER 6

ISOKINETIC STRENGTH

An isokinetic muscle action is defined by its performance at a constant speed or velocity. To contract at constant speed requires a specialized device called an isokinetic dynamometer. Despite the high cost of the isokinetic instrument, the description of how it is used to measure isokinetic strength has been included in this manual because of the prevalence of such machines in many exercise physiology labs and athletic training facilities on college campuses and in sophisticated physical therapy and rehabilitation clinics. As with many laboratory ergometers and dynamometers, isokinetic machines serve both as fitness testing devices and fitness training devices.

Leg strength diminishes faster than upper body strength as one ages past young adulthood.[32] Thus, leg strength training and periodic monitoring are important for middle-aged and older persons if they intend to keep functioning optimally in activities of daily living.

In addition to determining the state of training of the legs, testing leg strength may provide insight into the risk of injury. The **bilateral** (or contralateral) comparison of strength between two limbs, and the **ipsilateral** comparison of strength between opposing or reciprocal muscles in the same limb is of interest. **Bilateral strength imbalance** can be described either as a ratio or as a percent difference or percent deficit between the two limbs. This chapter uses the term **percent deficit (% Def)**,[26] calculated as the percent difference between the higher and lower peak torque of the two limbs divided by the higher peak torque. For example, the % Def between right and left knee extension peak torques of 125 N·m and 110 N·m, respectively, is calculated as (125 − 110) / 125 * 100, which is equal to 12 %. Muscle strength asymmetry may be a predisposing factor in muscle strains.[7,26,49] Sources typically consider bilateral differences of 10–15 % between limbs to be a significant strength imbalance.[18,32,53] However, other studies report no difference in knee injury rate with bilateral strength imbalances in excess of 10 %.[69]

Similarly, an **ipsilateral imbalance** between the strength of the antagonist (hamstrings) and agonist (quadriceps) within the same leg could lead to a higher risk of leg injury.[36,50] Weak hamstring strength in comparison to quadricep strength potentially increases the risk of hamstring strain and anterior cruciate ligament (ACL) sprain. The rationale supporting the risk of injury to the ACL is based on the co-contraction of the less forceful hamstring and the more forceful quadriceps during forceful leg extensions. Stronger co-contraction of the hamstrings reduces the anteriorly directed shear of the tibia relative to the femur due to the high quadriceps force. This, in turn, reduces the strain (pull) on the ACL.[17,62] As with bilateral imbalance, uncertainty exists over the meaning of ipsilateral imbalance and its validity as an injury predictor. The term used in this chapter to make the ipsilateral or reciprocal comparison within the same limb between flexion strength (antagonist muscles) and extension strength (agonist muscles) is the flexion/extension (Fl/Ex) ratio. Criteria ratios for Fl/Ex range from 0.50 (50 %)[36] to 0.75 (75 %).[27,38] The wide range is attributed not only to differences of opinion but to the isokinetic velocities of the test, whereby the slower velocities elicit lower ratios than the higher velocities at least without gravity correction. Not all investigators report a relationship between imbalanced strength and injury susceptibility.[30] Confirmation of optimal Fl/Ex ratios still awaits evidence from controlled studies of injury incidence in persons having undergone isokinetic balance testing before their injury.[38]

Use of the isokinetic dynamometer also allows the study of various characteristics of skeletal muscle. Skeletal muscle consists of slow-twitch (ST) and fast-twitch (FT) cells. The speed of contraction of skeletal muscle cells is determined by differences in protein type (or myosin isoform) along with differences in the development of the sarcoplasmic reticulum.[11,60] The metabolic characteristics of the cells are based on the level of enzymes, mitochondria, capillaries and fuels stored within the cells. ST cells have a high aerobic capacity and power due to elevated blood supply, mitochondrial density, aerobic enzyme content, and stored intramuscular lipids. FT cells have greater anaerobic capacity and power due to a higher concentration of stored glycogen and anaerobic enzymes.[28] FT cells are also larger, with a greater cross-sectional area, allowing for more force production than ST cells.[11] A person with a higher distribution of ST cells (> 50% ST) in the quadriceps is likely to fatigue less when performing repeated knee extension exercises. Researchers have used isokinetic dynamometry to estimate fiber composition based on the fatigability of the quadriceps. In comparing the force generated in the first 3 repetitions versus the last 3 repetitions in a 50-repetition isokinetic protocol, the decline in force (or the fatigability of the muscle) was correlated with the fiber composition as measured by needle muscle biopsy.[74] By measuring force production at different speeds (60, 180 and 300 deg·sec^{-1}), the force-velocity characteristics of muscle can be studied. It is well known that the ability of skeletal muscle to generate force diminishes with increasing speed or velocity which creates a characteristic force-velocity curve. The shape of this curve is influenced by fiber composition.[31,73,75]

RATIONALE FOR ISOKINETIC TESTING

The rationale for isokinetic testing of leg strength may be categorized into mechanical and anatomical rationales.

Mechanical Rationale for Isokinetic Testing

In 1967, researchers first introduced isokinetics as a type of dynamic muscle action at a constant velocity; thus, no momentum was gained or lost throughout a truly isokinetic movement.[72] Once the participant reaches the set velocity, an increase in force causes the isokinetic device to counteract this force with an accommodating increase in resistance. Conversely, a decrease in the application of force results in a corresponding decrease in the resistance.[47] Thus, the movement does not change velocity significantly. The testing apparatus controls the angular velocity of the exercise, thus allowing the musculature to elicit maximal tension for each angle within the movement range. Isokinetic movements are rare in most daily, recreational, and sports activities.[38] One of those activities is when the arms pull through the water in swimming.

The laboratory measurement of isokinetic strength provides torque measurements throughout the active range of motion during this maximal effort. The unit of measure for isokinetic strength is a torque value, commonly referred to as newton meters (N·m) (see Chapter 1). Torque indicates the force rotating about an axis, such as the force produced by a wrench when tightening the nut on a bolt. Because isokinetic devices have lever arms connected to strain gauges, torque is produced and recorded from the angular motion. *Peak torque* is the term that indicates muscular strength.

Torque (τ) is a rotational force that is the mathematical product of the force (F) being exerted times the distance (D) from the axis of rotation at which that force is being exerted (Figure 6.1). The distance of the lever arm is measured from the axis of rotation to the point where the external force is applied (the line of action). This distance is often referred to as the moment arm. The torque shown in Figure 6.1 would be calculated in newton meters (Eq. 6.1a and 6.1b). Although not an acceptable SI unit, the foot pound (ft·lb) was used to express torque in many of the original isokinetic studies and as a result is still seen in the literature.

Torque (τ) = Force (F) * Distance (D) *from axis of rotation*   Eq. 6.1a

Torque (N·m) = 30 N * 0.5 m = 150 N·m   Eq. 6.1b

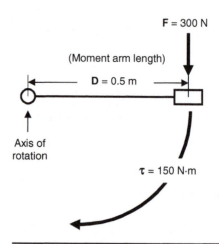

Figure 6.1 Production of rotational torque ($\tau = 150$ N·m) as a function of the external linear force (F = 300 N) applied at the distance (D = 0.5 m) from the axis of rotation, also referred to as the moment arm length.

Anatomical Rationale of Isokinetic Knee Extension and Flexion

Although isokinetic dynamometers are capable of measuring the torque of various joint movements (e.g., elbow extension and flexion, shoulder internal and external rotation, ankle inversion and eversion), this chapter will discuss only knee extension and flexion. Knee extension is represented by the strength of the quadriceps muscle group, which is made up of four muscles—the rectus femoris and the three vasti muscles, vastus medialis, lateralis, and intermedius. The rectus femoris crosses both the knee joint and hip joint, whereas the vasti muscles only cross the knee joint. The vasti contribute much more force ($\approx 85\%$) than the rectus femoris in a maximal knee extension.[46] Knee flexion is represented by the strength of the hamstring muscle group, which consists of three muscles—the biceps femoris, the semitendinosus, and the semimembranosus.

The seated knee extension and knee flexion during isokinetic leg strength testing is an open kinetic chain exercise (OKCE) utilizing single muscle groups, respectively. Also, OKCE are less functional than closed kinetic chain exercise (CKCE).[19,41] CKCE are multijoint exercises that are more functional because they are similar to running, jumping, squatting, and lunging. An example of OKCE is a leg press on a machine that causes your feet to move forward, but a CKCE leg press would cause your feet to remain stationary while your body moved away from your feet (in other words, the seat went backwards).

Fiber type plays an important role in determining the peak torque and duration of isokinetic contractions. For example, persons with higher percentages of fast-twitch fibers produce more torque (r = 0.69) at moderate (180°·s^{-1}) speeds, but have greater fatigability (r = 0.86), than persons with lower percentages.[74]

METHODS

The methods of testing isokinetic leg strength are much more elaborate than those for testing handgrip strength. Compared with handgrip dynamometers, the equipment for isokinetic testing is very expensive and complex. But no expensive machine can make up for any loss of accuracy by inappropriate procedures of the examiner (see Box 6.1).

Equipment

Numerous isokinetic dynamometers are in use today, including the Biodex™, Humac™, Cybex™, Kin-Com™, and Lido™. All of these dynamometers measure isometric (static) strength and concentric strength (where the muscle shortens during force production). The Biodex™, Humac™, and Kin-Com™ are also capable of measuring eccentric strength (where the muscle is lengthened while producing force). The typical position for testing leg strength is shown in Figure 6.2. Most of the information in this chapter, including the methods, refers specifically to the Cybex II+™ isokinetic dynamometer but can be applied to isokinetic strength measured with any brand of dynamometer.

Popular isokinetic velocities are 60°·s^{-1}, 180°·s^{-1}, and 300°·s^{-1}; these are often referred to as slow, medium, and fast speeds, respectively. However, the fast velocity may be

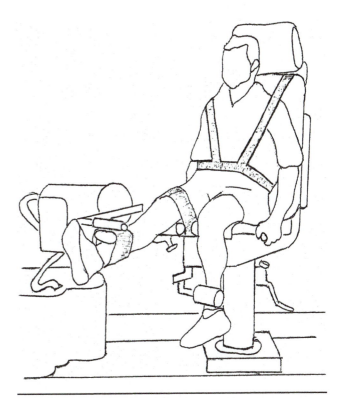

Figure 6.2 The position for isokinetic testing of leg strength places both the hip angle (trunk to upper leg) and knee angle (at full flexion) at approximately 90°.

construed as slow compared with the velocities required in many sports' movements, such as sprinting, throwing, striking, kicking, and jumping. Some models (e.g., Cybex II⁺™) provide increments of $15°·s^{-1}$ from $0°·s^{-1}$ to $300°·s^{-1}$ and may be controlled with an electronic remote device. When the velocity is set to $0°·s^{-1}$, static strength is measured.

Researchers sometimes express angular velocity in radians per second ($rad·s^{-1}$). A radian is an angle at the center of a circle described by an arc equal to the length of the radius of the circle.[33] There are 2π radians in a complete circle, so one radian is about $57.3°$. Thus, angular velocities in degrees per second can be converted to radians per second by dividing by 57.3 (Eq. 6.2a and 6.2b). It is important to understand radians in order to be able to interpret the unit used by some researchers and to use the unit of calculating work from the angular movement of isokinetic muscle actions.

$$X \, rad·s^{-1} = X°·s^{-1} / 57.3 \qquad \text{Eq. 6.2a}$$

$$X \, rad·s^{-1} = 300°·s^{-1} / 57.3 = 5.24 \, rad·s^{-1} \qquad \text{Eq. 6.2b}$$

Procedures

The procedures for testing the isokinetic strength of the legs include a description of the preparations in addition to the actual testing of the participant. They also include proper reading of the instrument and the graphic recording of torque. The procedures are specifically for the Cybex II⁺™ (Computer Sports Medicine, Inc., Stoughton, MA), but are also mostly applicable to the Biodex™ (Biodex Medical, Shirley, NY), Humac™ (CSMI, Stoughton, MA), Kin-Com™ (Chattecx, Chattanooga, TN), and other dynamometers. Some differences are noted with respect to the number of trials, rest interval, and activation force. As with most laboratory procedures, adequate preparations include those concerned with the equipment and the participant. See Box 6.2 for calibration procedures.

Instrument Preparation (for the Cybex II+™)

1. Procedures for periodic calibration are located in the calibration box (Box 6.2) or in the manufacturer's instruction manual.
2. The chart recorder is readied for testing by selecting a Damping setting of 2 (selected from a range of 1 to 4) on the Torque Channel. A Damping setting of 2 smoothes the torque curves somewhat without significantly reducing the peak torques.
3. The technician selects an appropriate Torque Scale on the chart recorder based on the estimated torque output of the performer. Four possible torque scales exist, including 30, 90, 180, and 360 ft·lb (which correspond to 41, 122, 244, and 488 N·m). Often the estimated torque is based on the joint and movement to be tested.

Joint / Movement	Torque Scale
Wrist extension/flexion	30 ft·lb (41 N·m)
Elbow extension/flexion	90 ft·lb (122 N·m)
Knee extension/flexion (female)	180 ft·lb (244 N·m)
Knee extension/flexion (male)	360 ft·lb (488 N·m)

4. The technician sets the Input Direction (on the Position Channel) to CW (clockwise) for the left limb and CCW (counterclockwise) for the right limb.
5. The Position Scale should be placed at the 150° scale (selected from 150° and 300°), representing the approximate range of motion (about 100°) for testing knee extension and flexion.

Participant Preparation

1. The participant removes shoes to minimize the effect of gravity on torque production. (Heavy shoes decrease knee extension torque and increase knee flexion torque.)
2. The participant sits in an upright position with the hips flexed at an angle of 90.°
3. The technician uses pelvic and thigh straps to stabilize the hips and thighs, respectively. If available, chest straps are used also.
4. The technician identifies the axis of rotation of the knee joint and visually aligns the input shaft of the dynamometer with this axis of rotation at the lateral epicondyle.
5. The technician adjusts the length of the lever arm so that the inferior rim of the tibia (shin) pad contacts the tibia just above the malleoli of the ankle; the technician secures the shin/ankle strap.
6. The participant flexes the knee at a minimum of 90° or as limited by the chair.
7. The participant grasps the sides of the chair throughout the warm-up and the test. Some protocols allow the participant to fold arms across the chest and maintain this position.

8. The technician explains and demonstrates the leg movements for the strength test. Aside from assuring that the participant understands that maximal efforts are made, no further encouragement during the test is advised so that uniformity in tester-participant interaction is maintained. Some protocols allow verbal encouragement.

9. The participant warms up by making 5 to 10 submaximal repetitions (about 50 % MVC), both during flexion and extension at each speed setting ($60°·s^{-1}$, $180°·s^{-1}$, and $300°·s^{-1}$).

10. The participant then rests for 2 min before the initial test, while the technician sets the velocity to $60°·s^{-1}$ and sets the paper recording speed to 5 mm·s^{-1} or 25 mm·s^{-1}.

Testing Peak Torque

1. The technician records the participant's name, the date of the test, the joint and joint motion being tested (i.e., knee extension and flexion), the limb being tested (right or left), the torque scale selected, and the test velocity on the chart recorder paper. (If the Biodex™ or Humac™ is used, this same basic information is entered into the computer program prior to testing.)

2. If desired (and available with regard to the specific dynamometer in use), a gravity correction maneuver may be done. This typically calls for the participant to relax the leg, at which time the leg is weighed and this weight is used to increase the extension torque and decrease the flexion torque to "correct" for the effects of gravity. Gravity correction is not included in this testing protocol.

3. With the chart recorder on the higher paper speed (25 mm·s^{-1}), the participant completes 3–5 maximal repetitions at $60°·s^{-1}$. Typically, the higher paper speed is used only for the first testing speed. This provides a wide, detailed printout of the torque curves, which is useful in qualitatively assessing the shape of the torque curves. Verbal encouragement may be provided by the technician throughout the test, but the most "standardized" condition would be to give no encouragement.

4. After a 30–60 s rest, the participant completes 3–5 maximal repetitions at $180°·s^{-1}$.

5. After another 30–60 s rest, the participant completes 3–5 maximal repetitions at $300°·s^{-1}$.

6. The technician rearranges the apparatus for testing the opposite leg and repeats the steps.

7. The technician determines the peak torque (N·m), the highest of the 3–5 trials, for knee extension and knee flexion of each leg at each of the three speeds tested, and records on Form 6.2.

8. The technician calculates the relative torque (N·m·kg^{-1}), the ipsilateral comparative ratios of flexion to extension (Fl/Ex) strength, and the bilateral percent deficit (% Def), as shown in Equations 6.3a through 6.3f, and records on Form 6.2. (Note: The % Def value is preceded by an *R* if the right limb is weaker, an *L* if the left limb is weaker, or an *E* if the two limbs are equal.)

Assume: Right extension torque = **125** N·m; Body weight = **70** kg

$$\text{Relative torque (N·m·kg}^{-1}) = \text{Absolute torque (N·m) / Body weight (kg)} \qquad \text{Eq. 6.3a}$$

$$\text{Relative torque (N·m·kg}^{-1}) = \textbf{125} \text{ N·m / 70 kg} = \underline{\textbf{1.8}} \text{ N·m·kg}^{-1} \qquad \text{Eq. 6.3b}$$

Assume: Right extension torque = **125** N·m; Right flexion torque = **80** N·m

$$\text{Fl / Ex ratio} = \text{Absolute flexion torque (N·m) / Absolute extension torque (N·m)} \qquad \text{Eq. 6.3c}$$

$$\text{Fl / Ex ratio} = \textbf{80} \text{ Nm / } \textbf{125} \text{ Nm} = \underline{\textbf{0.64}} \qquad \text{Eq. 6.3d}$$

Assume: Right extension torque = **125** N·m; Left extension torque = **110** N·m

$$\text{\% Def} = [\text{Higher torque (N·m)} - \text{Lower torque (N·m)}] / \text{Higher torque (N·m)} *100 \qquad \text{Eq. 6.3e}$$

$$\text{\% Def} = [\textbf{125} - \textbf{110}] / \textbf{125} * 100 = \underline{\textbf{12}} \text{ \%.} \qquad \text{Eq. 6.3f}$$

Estimating Fiber Distribution *(Optional)*

1. The technician sets the speed to $180°·s^{-1}$ and the recorder to the slower paper speed of 5 mm/s.

2. The participant completes 50 to 55 maximal knee extension repetitions. The knee flexions between are completed as quickly as possible but typically not at a maximal effort. Verbal encouragement may be provided by the technician throughout the test, but the most standardized condition is to give no encouragement.

3. The technician determines and averages the peak torques for repetitions 1–3 and for repetitions 48–50 and records on Form 6.2. The percent decline from repetitions 1–3 to repetitions 48–50 is calculated and used to estimate fiber distribution[74] (Eq. 6.4a through 6.4e).

Assume: Ave torque (1–3) = **200** N·m; Ave torque (48–50) = **110** N·m

$$\text{\% Decline} = [(\text{Ave torque (1} - \text{3)} - \text{Ave torque (48} - \text{50)}) / \text{Ave torque (1} + \text{3)}] * 100 \qquad \text{Eq. 6.4a}$$

$$\text{FT \%} = (\text{\% Decline} - 5.2) / 0.90 \qquad \text{Eq. 6.4b}$$

$$\text{\% Decline} = [(\textbf{200} \text{ N·m} - \textbf{110} \text{ N·m}) / (\textbf{200} \text{ N·m})] *100 = \textbf{45.0} \text{ \% decline} \qquad \text{Eq. 6.4c}$$

$$\text{FT \%} = (\textbf{45.0} - 5.2) / 0.90 = \textbf{44} \text{ \% FT fiber} \qquad \text{Eq. 6.4d}$$

$$\text{ST \%} = 100 - \text{FT \%} = 100 \text{ \%} - \textbf{44} \text{ \%} = \textbf{56} \text{ \% ST fiber} \qquad \text{Eq. 6.4e}$$

Demonstrating the Force-Velocity Curve (Optional)

1. The technician uses the peak torque values previously recorded for knee extension at 60, 180 and 300°·s⁻¹ to demonstrate the force-velocity characteristics of skeletal muscle.
2. The technician divides each of the 3 peak torques by the highest of the 3 torques (the one recorded at 60°·s⁻¹) expressing each one relative to the maximum (highest) peak torque value (as seen in Eq. 6.5a and 6.5b) and records on Form 6.4.
3. The technician plots each of the 3 peak torques relative to the max torque at the given speeds on Form 6.4.

Assume: Peak torque = **160** N·m;
Highest peak torque (at 60°·s⁻¹) = **244** N·m

Relative to max = Peak torque /
Highest peak torque   Eq. 6.5a

Relative to max = **160** Nm / **244** Nm = **0.66**   Eq. 6.5b

Comments on Isokinetic Procedures

The most common procedure for measuring isokinetic leg strength is at a seated position (80–100° angle at hip) and over a range of motion starting at between 100° to 90° knee flexion angle and ending at 0° to 10° knee angle. The participant must maintain the original seated posture throughout all repetitions.

The sequence of the testing for knee extension and flexion at different speeds is usually from slowest to fastest (e.g., 30°·s⁻¹, 60°·s⁻¹, 180°·s⁻¹, 240°·s⁻¹, and 300°·s⁻¹). Athletes involved in power sports could be tested at the higher speeds. If a detailed analysis of the relationship between torque and angle is desired, then the tracing is usually recorded at a speed of 25 mm·s⁻¹; however, for routine testing the recording speed is usually 5 mm·s⁻¹. The dual tracings provide a recorded replay of the movement, one tracing showing the torque values and another showing the position (angle in degrees) of the lower leg, as seen in Figure 6.3.

In addition to the quantitative assessment of knee strength (i.e., absolute and relative peak torques, flexion/extension ratios, bilateral percent deficits), a qualitative assessment of knee extension and flexion strength can be important, especially with particular knee pathologies. Chondromalacia patellae is a patellofemoral condition sometimes seen in young female athletes resulting in a softening and degeneration of the cartilage underneath the patellae (kneecaps). The symptoms of the condition include knee tenderness, knee pain, and a grinding sensation when the knee is extended. Figure 6.4 is an isokinetic strength assessment of a young woman with chondromalacia patella of the right limb only (the affected limb). The torque curve of the affected limb is clearly not "normal" and can be explained in part by the symptoms and mechanics associated with the pathology.

RESULTS AND DISCUSSION

Differences in participants' strengths are affected by such factors as musculotendon architecture, musculoskeletal geometry, muscle fiber types, and voluntary neuromuscular excitation.[59] The greatest torque for *dynamic isokinetic* actions is generated at speeds of 30°·s⁻¹ for both knee extension and flexion. By its very nature, torque is indirectly related to the speed of the movement; that is, the slower

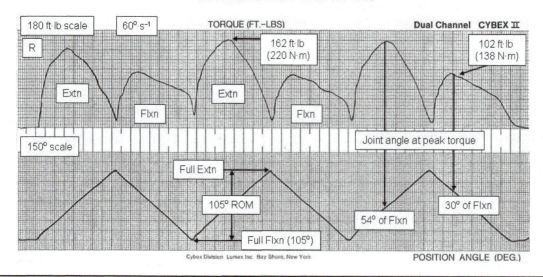

Figure 6.3   Recording of torque and position from the Cybex II+™ isokinetic dynamometer. Labeled components include torque scale (180 ft·lb), testing speed (60°·s⁻¹), peak torque for knee extension (162 ft·lb/220 N·m) and knee flexion (102 ft·lb/138 N·m), position scale (150°), range of motion (105°), and joint angle at peak knee extension (54° of flexion) and knee flexion (30° of flexion).

Knee Extension / Flexion Test

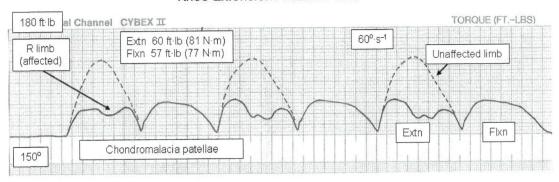

Figure 6.4 Recording of knee extension and flexion torque at $60°·s^{-1}$ for a female athlete with chondromalacia patellae. The knee extension peak torque in the affected limb is 81 N·m, compared to the nonaffected limb (superimposed) where it is 179 N·m, resulting in a bilateral deficit of 55 %.

the movement, the greater the torque. The flexion/extension (Fl/Ex) ratios are lowest at the highest torques, and the highest torques are at the lowest velocities.[50,72] The Fl/Ex ratio gets bigger as the velocity increases because the decrease in hamstring torque is typically less than the decrease in quadriceps torque.

Absolute and Relative Isokinetic Strength

Determining "normal" values for absolute and relative isokinetic strength is nearly impossible based on the number of variables that can potentially influence the results. All of the following factors add variability to the results: the specific dynamometer used (e.g., Biodex™, Cybex™); the sample selected (e.g., nonathletic, athletic, trained, elite); the testing protocol (e.g., testing velocity, velocity order, number of repetitions, recovery time, stabilization); the signal processing method; and the gravity correction method (if used). With this in mind, we will discuss the effect of gender, age, and sport participation on isokinetic strength based on a select number of studies, and within these stated limitations.

From the results presented in Table 6.1, it appears that knee extension and flexion peak torque measured at $60°·s^{-1}$ increases throughout adolescence (14–17 y) and probably peaks somewhere in young adulthood (18–35 y). A study of young male basketball players[25] showed a 39 % increase in mean absolute knee extension strength from 163 ± 42 N·m at age 14 to 227 ± 40 N·m at age 17, and a 12 % increase in relative knee extension strength from 2.44 ± 0.63 at age 14 to 2.73 ± 0.43 at age 17. A combination of three studies of adult nonathletes[4,24,78] revealed a 23 % decrease in absolute knee extension strength in men from 186 ± 30 N·m at age 25–34 y to 144 ± 30 N·m at age 65–78 y, and a 29 % decrease in women from 108 ± 19 N·m at age 25–34 y to 77 ± 14 N·m at age 65–78 y.

The absolute and relative strength of men and women in knee extension and flexion can be compared by calculating the ratio of female/male torque values. It appears that nonathletic and athletic women produce about 60 %

as much absolute torque (N·m) as their male counterparts, ranging from 55 % to 63 %. Women generally produce about 80 % as much relative torque (N·m·kg^{-1}) as men, ranging from 63 % to 82 %.[24,78]

Persons who train for and participate in sports, especially sports requiring power and sprinting (e.g., basketball, soccer), produce higher absolute and relative knee extension and flexion torque values than their nonathletic counterparts as seen in Table 6.2. It appears from a comparison of two studies[5,78] that athletes possess about 15–20 % more absolute strength and 5–10 % more relative strength than nonathletes. Those elite athletes who continue to compete beyond college on professional and national teams appear to continue to gain strength.[12,77]

Bilateral Comparison of Strength

Two different methods of bilateral strength comparison appear in the literature. One involves comparing the strength of a "dominant" limb to a "nondominant" limb. The dominant limb is sometimes defined as the "stronger" leg, but it is more common to see it defined *functionally* as that used by the participant to kick a ball, and the dominant arm as that used to throw a ball or handle a racquet. In this case, there is an assumption that the dominant limb should be stronger and hence produce a higher peak torque than the nondominant limb. This is typically the case in athletes who use one limb more than another (e.g., in tennis, baseball). However, in athletes and nonathletes who do not use one limb preferentially, there is no reason to expect a bilateral strength difference. Using dominant and nondominant limbs (identified by use) to make bilateral comparisons is probably better used in studying athletic performance and is not discussed further in this chapter.

The other method of bilateral strength comparison involves comparing the "weaker" limb to the "stronger" limb, regardless of right versus left or dominant versus nondominant (as previously defined). This approach assumes that the *weaker limb* produces a peak torque in "deficit" to

Table 6.1

Table 6.1 Concentric Absolute (N·m) and Relative (N·m·kg^{-1}) Peak Torque at 60 $^\circ$·s^{-1} by Gender and Age for Isokinetic Knee Extension and Flexion

Group	N	Weight (kg)	Knee Extension (N·m) M ± SD	Knee Extension (Nm·kg^{-1}) M ± SD	Knee Flexion (N·m) M ± SD	Knee Flexion (Nm·kg^{-1}) M ± SD
Men (Athletes)						
14 y [25]	30	66.8	163 ± 42	2.44 ± 0.63	114 ± 35	1.71 ± 0.52
15 y [25]	30	74.0	185 ± 27	2.50 ± 0.36	125 ± 22	1.69 ± 0.30
16 y [25]	30	77.9	212 ± 28	2.72 ± 0.36	140 ± 23	1.80 ± 0.30
17 y [25]	30	83.3	227 ± 40	2.73 ± 0.48	151 ± 23	1.81 ± 0.28
18-25 y [5]	168	81.8	242 ± 44	2.96 ± 0.54	151 ± 30	1.85 ± 0.37
Men (Non-Athletes)						
25-34 y [78]	50	77.6	186 ± 30	2.40 ± 0.39	133 ± 24	1.71 ± 0.31
45-54 y	24	80.8	180 ± 35	2.23 ± 0.43	100 ± 21	1.24 ± 0.26
55-64 y [24]	28	76.4	163 ± 30	2.13 ± 0.39	94 ± 20	1.23 ± 0.26
65-78 y	34	79.0	144 ± 30	1.82 ± 0.38	78 ± 19	0.99 ± 0.24
Women (Athletes)						
18-25 y	125	58.9	142 ± 27	2.41 ± 0.34	88 ± 18	1.51 ± 0.23
Women (Non-Athletes)						
25-34 y	50	58.0	108 ± 19	1.86 ± 0.33	79 ± 16	1.36 ± 0.28
45-54 y [24]	28	61.6	108 ± 22	1.75 ± 0.36	58 ± 14	0.94 ± 0.23
55-64 y	52	66.6	98 ± 20	1.47 ± 0.30	52 ± 10	0.78 ± 0.15
65-78 y [24]	34	63.3	89 ± 15	1.41 ± 0.24	49 ± 10	0.77 ± 0.16
75-83 y [4]	26	64.0	77 ± 14	1.20 ± 0.22	43 ± 9	0.67 ± 0.14

Based on data from Aquino et al. (1996)[4]; Beam et al. (1985)[5]; Frontera et al. (1991)[24]; Gerodimos et al. (2003)[25]; Wyatt & Edwards (1981).[78]

the *stronger limb*. The result is a percent difference or percent deficit (% Def) that is used in the clinical evaluation of an injury/surgery or to assess the potential risk for future injury.[26] A study of knee extension and flexion strength in 100 healthy nonathletes found on average a 10 % bilateral difference (ranging from 6 to 12 %) in men and an 11 % difference (ranging from 9 to 16 %) in women.[78] Another study of knee extension in 60 healthy college students found average bilateral differences of 15 % in men and 16 % in women.[29] A study of bilateral strength following knee surgery (arthroscopic meniscectomy) reported 25–40 % deficits in isokinetic knee extension strength and 17–23 % deficits in knee flexion at two weeks postsurgery.[45] When allowed to spontaneously recover (i.e., no supervised training), postsurgical strength deficits in the quadriceps return to about 15 % after 6 weeks, but further recovery does not appear possible without training, as the same deficit remains 12 weeks postsurgery. Another study showed a bilateral difference of 21 % in knee extensor peak torque following meniscectomy at 8 weeks postsurgery, even with a training program.[67] In general, a 10–15 % bilateral deficit between single muscle groups may be considered a significant difference,[18,26,78] and could be used as a criterion to hold an athlete out of practice or competition until the strength asymmetry is corrected.

Ipsilateral Comparison of Strength

The Fl/Ex ratios (or agonist/antagonist or hamstring/quadriceps ratios) described in this chapter are typically referred to as "conventional." They are defined by the comparison of *concentric flexion* (hamstrings) with *concentric extension* (quadriceps) strength within the same leg. Other references describe a "functional" or "mixed" ratio using a combination of *eccentric flexion* and *concentric extension,* thinking that this better reflects the actions that occur during running and jumping.[14,34] The conventional Fl/Ex ratios for the male athletes and nonathletes described in Table 6.2 range from 0.55–0.72 at 60°·s^{-1}, from 0.65–0.78 at 180°·s^{-1}, and from 0.78–0.83 at 300°·s^{-1}. Other studies[35,54,63,70,77] have reported conventional Fl/Ex ratios of 0.49–0.66, 0.58–0.85, and 0.75 at 60, 180, and 300°·s^{-1}, respectively. The variability in the ratios at each speed is likely due at least in part to the fact that some values are corrected for gravity,[54,63,70] whereas other values are not.[35,77] Gravity correction should be considered when interpreting the meaning of Fl/Ex ratios. A functional ratio between eccentric flexion and concentric extension of at least 1.00 is considered healthy,[1,34,43] and ratios as high as 1.40 have been reported.[14] Strength imbalance, as reflected by a decreased hamstring strength relative to quadriceps strength, provides a potential mechanism for lower extremity injuries.[22,23] It has been associated with hamstring muscle injury in some studies,[11,55,76] but other studies have shown no association between strength imbalance and injury.[7,77] Decreased hamstring strength has also been implicated in altering knee function with regard to anterior cruciate ligament (ACL) sprain or rupture, especially in women.[37,43,52]

Table 6.2

Table 6.2 Concentric Absolute (N·m) and Relative (N·m·kg^{-1}) Peak Torque by Group and Gender for Knee Extension and Flexion and Flexion/Extension (Fl / Ex) Ratio

Men Group	N	Weight (kg)		60°·s^{-1} (N·m)	60°·s^{-1} (N·m·kg^{-1})	180°·s^{-1} (N·m)	180°·s^{-1} (N·m·kg^{-1})	300°·s^{-1} (N·m)	300°·s^{-1} (N·m·kg^{-1})
Athletes [5]	168	81.8	Extension	242	2.96	159	1.95	110	1.35
(Collegiate)			Flexion	151	1.85	112	1.36	87	1.06
			Fl / Ex Ratio	0.62		0.70		0.79	
Soccer [12]	29	74.5	Extension	231	3.10	165	2.21	127	1.70
(Professional)			Flexion	152	2.04	123	1.65	99	1.33
			Fl / Ex Ratio	0.66		0.75		0.78	
Basketball [77]	61	88.2	Extension	274	3.11	164	1.86		
(National team)			Flexion	194	2.20	123	1.39		
			Fl / Ex Ratio	0.71		0.75			
Non-Athletes [78]	50	77.6	Extension	186	2.40	133	1.71	91	1.17
(Age 25–34 y)			Flexion	133	1.71	104	1.34	75	0.97
			Fl / Ex Ratio	0.72		0.78		0.82	

Women Group	N	Weight (kg)		60°·s^{-1} (N·m)	60°·s^{-1} (N·m·kg^{-1})	180°·s^{-1} (N·m)	180°·s^{-1} (N·m·kg^{-1})	300°·s^{-1} (N·m)	300°·s^{-1} (N·m·kg^{-1})
Athletes [5]	125	58.9	Extension	142	2.41	93	1.58	63	1.06
(Collegiate)			Flexion	88	1.51	65	1.11	50	0.86
			Fl / Ex Ratio	0.62		0.70		0.79	
Non-Athletes [78]	50	58.0	Extension	108	1.86	79	1.36	52	0.90
(Age 25–34 y)			Flexion	77	1.33	62	1.07	43	0.74
			Fl / Ex Ratio	0.71		0.78		0.83	
Non-Athletes [16]	103	61.0	Extension	137	2.25	88	1.44		
(Age 25–70 y)			Flexion	75	1.23	57	0.93		
			Fl / Ex Ratio	0.55		0.65			

Based on data from Beam et al. (1985)[5]; Cometti et al. (2001)[12]; DiBrezzo & Fort (1987)[16]; Wyatt & Edwards (1981)[78]; Zakas et al. (1995).[77]

Fiber Type

Table 6.3 summarizes various studies on fiber type distribution in men and women who are sedentary or participants in various sports. The large variations in percentages within each group testify to the influence of other factors besides fiber type in predicting success for each sport. The prediction of fiber type is enhanced by adding other influencing factors, such as fat-free thigh mass, to the equation.[68]

The fiber type test serves also as a fatigue index for muscular endurance (power endurance and mixed endurance). Some fatigue indexes use the number of repetitions until peak torque is 50 % of the initial peak torque[44] or the percentage derived from the last-third of work divided by the first-third of work derived from a Biodex™ isokinetic machine.[9]

Force-Velocity Characteristics

Successful sport and exercise performance depends not only on strength, but also on the speed of muscle contraction and on the development of power. The ability to generate force decreases with increasing speed of contraction. This relationship between the speed or velocity of movement and the amount of force or torque produced defines

Table 6.3 Fiber Type Distribution (% Fast Twitch) in Sedentary and Athletic Men and Women

Men Activity	% FT	Women Activity	% FT
Marathoners	19	800 m runners	39
Distance runners	30	X-country skiers	40
X-country skiers	36	Shot-putters	50
Race walkers	40	Distance cyclists	50
Distance cyclists	40	Sedentary	50
800 m runners	51	Long/high jump	52
Downhill skiers	51	Weight lifters	53
Sedentary	52	Sprints/jumpers	63
Shot-putters	62	Sprinters	73

Sources: Based on data from Burke et al. (1977)[10]; Costill et al. (1976)[13]; Gollnick et al. (1972)[28]; Thorstensson et al. (1977).[75]

the force-velocity or torque-velocity curve in human muscle. Figure 6.5 shows an "idealized" torque-velocity curve based on isokinetic strength measurements done at a range of velocities (from 60 to 300°·s^{-1}).[5,31] Maximum force production occurs at the lowest velocity (0°·s^{-1}), or isometrically, and diminishes with increasing speeds of contraction

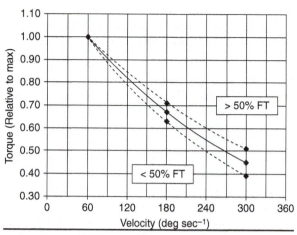

Figure 6.5 Idealized torque-velocity curve for isokinetic knee extension with lines indicating potential effect of fiber distribution.

BOX 6.3	**Chapter Preview/Review**

How is isokinetic strength defined?

What is meant by the terms *bilateral* and *ipsilateral*?

How is torque defined?

Is fiber type related to torque production?

What are some of the brands or models of isokinetic dynamometer?

How high is the test-retest reliability of peak torque?

What level of bilateral deficit is significant and used as a criterion for determining sport participation?

What isokinetic variable is related to risk of hamstring and ACL injury?

How is fiber type estimated from the results of isokinetic strength testing?

What is the force-velocity curve and how is it affected by fiber distribution?

---

until finally, at very high speed virtually no force can be generated. Think about lifting a very heavy weight. You typically do it slowly (at the low end of the force-velocity curve) so that you can apply more force. When pedaling a bike however, it is easier to pedal faster (at the high end of the force velocity curve) so that you are producing less force per pedal stroke. Fiber distribution (the percentage of slow and fast-twitch muscle) affects the force-velocity characteristics of muscle.[31,73,75] Athletes with a higher percentage of fast-twitch cells (> 50 % FT) can generate higher peak torques at the faster isokinetic velocities. The ability to produce higher forces at faster speeds makes an athlete more powerful, which is advantageous in sports requiring power like sprinting, football and basketball.

References

1. Aagaard, P., Simonson, E. B., Magnusson, S. P., Larsson, B., & Dyhre-Paulsen, P. (1998). A new concept for isokinetic hamstring:quadriceps muscle strength ratio. *American Journal of Sports Medicine, 26,* 231–237.

2. Abernethy, P. J., & Jurimae, J. (1996). Cross-sectional and longitudinal uses of isoinertial, isometric, and isokinetic dynamometry. *Medicine and Science in Sports and Exercise, 28,* 1180–1187.

3. Abler, P., Foster, C., Thompson, N. N., Crowe, M., Alt, K., Brophy, A., & Palin, W. D. (1986). Determinants of anaerobic muscular performance. *Medicine and Science in Sports and Exercise, 18,* (supplement), Abstract #3, S1.

4. Aquino, M. de A., Leme, L., Amatuzzi, M., Greve, J., Terreri, A., Andrusaitis, F., & Nardelli, J. (2002). Isokinetic assessment of knee flexor/extensor muscular strength in elderly women. *Revista do Hospital das Clinicas; Faculdade de Medicina da Universidade de Sao Paulo, 57,* 131–134.

5. Beam, W. C., Bartels, R. L., Ward, R. W., Clark, N., & Zuelzer, W. A. (1985). Multiple comparisons of isokinetic leg strength in male and female collegiate athletic teams. *Medicine and Science in Sports and Exercise, 17*(2), Abstract #20, 269.

6. Bemben, M. G., Grump, K. J., & Massey, B. H. (1988). Assessment of technical accuracy of the Cybex II isokinetic dynamometer and analog recording system. *Journal of Orthopaedic and Sports Physical Therapy, 19,* 12–17.

7. Bender, J. A. (1964). Factors affecting the occurrence of knee injuries. *Journal of Association of Physical and Mental Rehabilitation, 18,* 130–134.

8. Biodex Medical, Inc. (1994). *Biodex system 2 isokinetic dynamometer applications/operations manual.* Shirley, NY: Author.

9. Burke, E., Cerny, F., Costill, D., & Fink, W. (1977). Characteristics of skeletal muscle in competitive cyclists. *Medicine and Science in Sports and Exercise, 9,* 109–112.

10. Burkett, L. (1970). Causative factors in hamstring strains. *Medicine and Science in Sports, 2,* 39–42.

11. Close, R. (1967). Properties of motor units in fast and slow skeletal muscles of the rat. *Journal of Physiology (London), 193,* 45–55.

12. Cometti, G., Maffiuletti, N., Pousson, M., Chatard, J. C., & Maffulli, N. (2001). Isokinetic strength and anaerobic power of elite, subelite and amateur French soccer players. *International Journal of Sports Medicine, 22,* 45–51.

13. Costill, D., Fink, W., & Pollock, M. (1976). Muscle fiber composition and enzyme activities of elite distance runners. *Medicine and Science in Sports and Exercise, 8,* 96–100.

14. Croisier, J-L., Ganteaume, S., Binet, J., Gentry, M., & Ferret, J.-M. (2008). Strength imbalances and prevention of hamstring injury in professional soccer players. *American Journal of Sports Medicine, 36,* 1469–1475.

15. Cybex. 1983. *Isolated joint testing and exercise.* Ronkonoma, NY: Author.

16. DiBrezzo, R., & Fort, I. (1987). Strength norms for the knee in women 25 years and older. *Journal of Applied Sport Science Research, 1,* 45–47.

17. Draganich, L. F., & Vahey, J. W. (1990). An in vitro study of anterior cruciate ligament strain induced by quadriceps and hamstring forces. *Journal of Orthopedic Research, 8,* 57–63.

18. Ellenbecker, T., & Davies, G. (2000). The application of isokinetics in testing and rehabilitation of the shoulder complex. *Journal of Athletic Training, 35,* 338–350.

19. Escamilla, R. F., Fleisig, G. S., Zheng, N., Barrentine, S. W., Wilk, K. E., & Andrews, J. R. (1998). Biomechanics of the knee during closed kinetic chain and open kinetic chain exercises. *Medicine and Science in Sports and Exercise, 30,* 556–569.

20. Farrell, M., & Richards, J. G. (1986). Analysis of the reliability and validity of the kinetic communicator exercise device. *Medicine and Science in Sports and Exercise, 18,* 44–49.

21. Ford, W. J., Bailey, S. D., Babich, K., & Worrell, T. W. (1994). Effect of hip position on gravity effect torque. *Medicine and Science in Sports and Exercise, 26,* 230–234.

22. Ford, K. R., Myer, G. D., Schmitt, L. C., van den Bogert, A. J., & Hewett, T. E. (2008). Effect of drop height on lower extremity biomechanical measures in female athletes. *Medicine and Science in Sports and Exercise, 40,* S80.

23. Ford, K. R., van den Bogert, A. J., Myer, G. D., Shapiro, R., & Hewett, T. E. (2008). The effects of age and skill level on knee musculature co-contraction during functional activities: A systematic review. *British Journal of Sports Medicine, 42,* 561–566.

24. Frontera, W. R., Hughes, V. A., Lutz, K. J., & Evans, W. J. (1991). A cross-sectional study of muscle strength and mass in 45- to 78-yr-old men and women. *Journal of Applied Physiology, 71,* 644–650.

25. Gerodimos, V., Mandou, V., Zafeiridis, A., Ioakimidis, P., Stavropoulos, N., & Kellis, S. (2003). Isokinetic peak torque and hamstring/quadriceps ratios in young basketball players. Effects of age, velocity, and contraction mode. *Journal of Sports Medicine and Physical Fitness, 43,* 444–452.

26. Gleim, G. W., Nicholas, J. W., & Webb, J. N. (1978). Isokinetic evaluation following leg injuries. *The Physician and Sportsmedicine, 6*(8), 74–82.

27. Glick, J. M. (1980). Muscle strains: Prevention and treatment. *The Physician and Sportsmedicine, 8*(11), 74–82.

28. Gollnick, P., Armstrong, R., Saubert, C., Piehl, K., & Saltin, B. (1972). Enzyme activity and fiber composition in skeletal muscle of untrained and trained men. *Journal of Applied Physiology, 33,* 312–319.

29. Goslin, B. R., & Charteris, J. (1979). Isokinetic dynamometry: Normative data for clinical use in lower extremity (knee) cases. *Scandinavian Journal of Rehabilitation Medicine, 11,* 105–109.

30. Grace, T., Sweetser, E., Nelson, M., Ydens, L., & Skipper, B. (1984). Isokinetic muscle imbalance and knee-joint injuries. A prospective blind study. *Journal of Bone and Joint Surgery, 66,* 734–740.

31. Gregor, R. J., Edgerton, V. R., Perrine, J. J., Campion, D. S., & Debus, C. (1979). Torque-velocity relationships and muscle fiber composition in elite female athletes. *Journal of Applied Physiology, 47,* 388–392.

32. Grimby, G., & Saltin, B. (1983). The ageing muscle. *Clinical Physiology, 3,* 209–218.

33. Hamill, J., & Knutzen, K. M. (2009). *Biomechanical basis of human movement* (3rd ed.). Philadelphia: Wolters Kluwer.

34. Holcomb, W. R., Rubley, M. D., Lee, H. J., & Guadagnoli, M. A. (2007). Effect of hamstring-emphasized resistance training on hamstring: quadriceps strength ratios. *Journal of Strength and Conditioning Research, 21,* 41–47.

35. Housh, T., Johnson, G., Housh, D., Stout, J., Smith, D., & Ebersole, K. (1997). Isokinetic peak torque and estimated muscle cross-sectional area in high school wrestlers. *Journal of Strength and Conditioning Research, 11,* 45–49.

36. Housh, T. J., Johnson, G. O., Marty, L., Eischen, G., Eischen, C., & Housh, D. J. (1988). Isokinetic leg flexion and extension strength of university football players. *Journal of Orthopaedic and Sports Physical Therapy, 9,* 365–369.

37. Itoh, H., Ichihashi, N., Maruyama, T., Kurosaka, M., & Hirohata, K. (1992). Weakness of thigh muscles in individuals sustaining anterior cruciate ligament injury. *Kobe Journal of Medical Science, 38,* 93–107.

38. Kannus, P. (1994). Isokinetic evaluation of muscular performance: Implications for muscle testing and rehabilitation. *International Journal of Sports Medicine, 15* (Suppl 1), S11–S18.

39. Knapik, J. J., Wright, J. E., Mawdsley, R. H., & Braun, J. M. (1983). Isokinetic, isometric and isotonic strength relationships. *Archives of Physical Medicine and Rehabilitation, 64,* 77–80.

40. Kramer, J. F., Vaz, M. D., & Hakansson, D. (1991). Effect of activation force on knee extensor torques. *Medicine and Science in Sports and Exercise, 23,* 231–237.

41. Lansky, R. C. (1999). Open- versus closed-kinetic chain exercise: Point/counterpoint. *Strength and Conditioning Journal, 21,* 39.

42. Lesmes, G. R., Costill, D. L., Coyle, E. F., & Fink, W. J. (1978). Muscle strength and power changes during maximal isokinetic training. *Medicine and Science in Sports, 10,* 266–269.

43. Li, R., Maffulli, N., Hsu, Y., & Chan, K. (1996). Isokinetic strength of the quadriceps and hamstrings and functional ability of anterior cruciate deficient knees in recreational athletes. *British Journal of Sports Medicine, 30,* 161–164.

44. Lumex Inc. (1975). *Cybex II testing protocol.* Bay Shore, NY: Cybex Division of Lumex, Inc.

45. Matthews, P., & St-Pierre, D. (1996). Recovery of muscle strength following arthroscopic meniscectomy. *Journal of Orthopedic and Sports Physical Therapy, 23,* 18–26.

46. McNair, P. J., Marshall, R. N., & Matheson, J. A. (1991). Quadriceps strength deficit associated with rectus femoris rupture: A case report. *Clinical Biomechanics, 6,* 190–192.

47. Moffroid, M., Whipple, R., Hofkosh, J., Lowman, E., & Thistle, H. (1969). A study of isokinetic exercise. *Physical Therapy, 49,* 735–746.

48. Molczyk, L., Thigpen, L. K., Eickhoff, J., Goldgar, D., & Gallagher, J. C. (1991). Reliability of testing the knee extensors and flexors in healthy adult women using a Cybex II isokinetic dynamometer. *Journal of Orthopaedic and Sports Physical Therapy, 14,* 37–41.

49. Morris, A. F. (1974). Myotatic reflex on bilateral reciprocal leg strength. *American Corrective Therapy Journal, 28*(1) 24–29.

50. Morris, A. F., Lussier, L., Bell, G., & Dooley, J. (1983). Hamstring/quadriceps strength ratios in collegiate middle-distance and distance runners. *The Physician and Sportsmedicine, 11*(10), 71, 72, 75–77.

51. Murray, M. P., Gardner, G. M., Mollinger, L. A., & Sepic, S. B. (1980). Strength of isometric and isokinetic contractions: Knee muscles of men aged 20 to 86. *Physical Therapy, 60,* 412–419.

52. Myer, G. D., Ford, K. R., Barber Foss, K. D., Liu, C., Niek, T. G., & Hewett, T. E. (2009). The relationship of hamstrings and quadriceps strength to anterior cruciate ligament injury in female athletes. *Clinical Journal of Sports Medicine, 19,* 3–8.

53. Nicholas, J. A., Strizak, A. M., & Veras, G. (1976). A study of thigh muscle weakness in different pathological states of the lower extremity. *The American Journal of Sports Medicine, 4,* 241–248.

54. Oberg, B., Möller, M., Gillquist, J., & Ekstrand, J. (1986). Isokinetic torque levels for knee extensors and knee flexors in soccer players. *International Journal of Sports Medicine, 7,* 50–53.

55. Orchard, J., Marsden, J., Lord, S., & Garlick, D. (1997). Preseason hamstring muscle weakness associated with hamstring muscle injury in Australian footballers. *American Journal of Sports Medicine, 25,* 81–85.

56. Patterson, L. A., & Spivey, W. E. (1992). Validity and reliability of the LIDO active isokinetic system. *Journal of Orthopaedic and Sports Physical Therapy, 15,* 32–36.

57. Pavol, M. J., & Grabiner, M. D. (2000). Knee strength variability between individuals across ranges of motion and hip angles. *Medicine and Science in Sports and Exercise, 32,* 985–992.

58. Perrin, D. H. (1986). Reliability of isokinetic measures. *Athletic Training, 21,* 319–321.

59. Perrin, D. H. (1993). *Isokinetic exercise and assessment.* Champaign, IL: Human Kinetics.

60. Pette, D., & Staron, R. (1990). Cellular and molecular diversities of mammalian skeletal muscle fibers. *Review of Physiology, Biochemistry, and Pharmacology, 116,* 1–76.

61. Pincivero, D. M., Lephart, S. M., & Karunakara, R. A. (1997). Reliability and precision of isokinetic strength and muscular endurance for the quadriceps and hamstrings. *International Journal of Sports Medicine, 18,* 113–117.

62. Renström, P., Arms, S. W., Stanwyck, T. S., Johnson, R. J., & Pope, M. H. (1986). Strain within the anterior cruciate ligament during hamstring and quadriceps activity. *American Journal of Sports Medicine, 14,* 83–87.

63. Rosene, J., Fogarty, T., & Mahaffey, B. (2001). Isokinetic hamstrings: Quadriceps ratios in intercollegiate athletes. *Journal of Athletic Training, 36,* 378–383.

64. Salem, G. J., Wang, M.-Y., Young, J. T., Marion, M., & Greendale, G. A. (2000). Knee strength and lower- and higher-intensity functional performance in older adults. *Medicine and Science in Sports and Exercise, 32,* 1679–1684.

65. Stam, H., Binkhorst, R., Kuhlmann, P., & van Nieuwenhuyzen, J. (1992). Clinical progress and quadriceps torque ratios during training of meniscectomy patients. *International Journal of Sports Medicine, 13,* 183–188.

66. Suter, E., Herzog, W., Sokolosky, J., Wiley, J. P., Macintosh, B. R. (1993). Muscle fiber type distribution as estimated by Cybex testing and by muscle biopsy. *Medicine and Science in Sports and Exercise, 25,* 363–370.

67. Sweetser, E. R., Grace, T. G., Nelson, M. A., Ydens, L. R., & Skipper, B. J. (1983). Pre-season isokinetic muscle testing in high school athletes and relationship to knee injuries. *Medicine and Science in Sports and Exercise, 15,* Abstract, 154.

68. Theoharopoulos, A., Tsitskaris, G., Nikopoulou, M., & Tsaklis, P. (2000). Knee strength of professional basketball players. *Journal of Strength and Conditioning Research, 14,* 457–463.

69. Thistle, H. G., Hislop, H. J., Moffroid, M. T., & Lowman, E. (1967). Isokinetic contraction: A new concept of resistive exercise. *Archives of Physical Medicine and Rehabilitation, 48,* 279–282.

70. Thorstensson, A. (1976). Muscle strength, fibre type and enzyme activities in man. *Acta Physiologica Scandinavica, 98* (Suppl. 443), 1–45.

71. Thorstensson, A., Grimby, G., & Karlsson, J. (1976). Force-velocity relations and fiber composition in human knee extensor muscles. *Journal of Applied Physiology, 40,* 12–16.

72. Thorstensson, A., & Karlsson, J. (1976). Fatigability and fiber composition of human skeletal muscle. *Acta Physiologica Scandinavica, 98,* 318–322.

73. Thorstensson, A., Larsson, L., Tesch, P., & Karlsson, J. (1977). Muscle strength and fiber composition in athletes and sedentary men. *Medicine and Science in Sports and Exercise, 9,* 26–30.

74. Tornvall, G. (1963). Assessment of physical capabilities. *Acta Physiologica Scandinavica, 53* (Suppl. 210), 1–102.

75. Worrell, T., & Perrin, D. (1992). Hamstring muscle injury: the influence of strength, flexibility, warm-up and fatigue. *Journal of Orthopaedic and Sports Physical Therapy, 16,* 12–18.

76. Wyatt, M. P., & Edwards, A. M. (1981). Comparison of quadriceps and hamstring torque values during isokinetic exercise. *Journal of Orthopaedic and Sports Physical Therapy, 3,* 48–56.

77. Yamamoto, T. (1993). Relationship between hamstring strains and leg muscle strength. A follow-up study of collegiate track and field athletes. *Journal of Sports Medicine and Physical Fitness, 33,* 194–199.

78. Zakas, A., Mandroukas, K., Vamvakoudis, E., Christoulas, K., & Aggelopoulou, N. (1995). Peak torque of quadriceps and hamstring muscles in basketball and soccer players of different divisions. *Journal of Sports Medicine and Physical Fitness, 35,* 199–205.

Form 6.1
ISOKINETIC STRENGTH

NAME _____ DATE _____ SCORE _____

Homework

Gender: **M**   Initials: **AA**   Age (y): **22**   Weight (kg): **90.0**   Athlete (Y/N): **Y**

Peak torque (N·m)	60 deg·s⁻¹			180 deg·s⁻¹			300 deg·s⁻¹		
	R	L	% Def	R	L	% Def	R	L	% Def
Knee extension (Q)	**244**	**228**		**160**	**144**		**114**	**106**	
Knee flexion (H)	**138**	**138**		**100**	**92**		**76**	**68**	
Fl / Ex (H:Q) ratio			*			*			*
	Max	Max / kg	Est'd	Max	Max / kg	Est'd	Max	Max / kg	Est'd
Knee extension (Q)			*			*			*
Knee flexion (H)			*			*			*

* Estimated values from *Table 6.2* based on : _____

Bilateral Comparison (% Deficit) - Preferred that **% Def** < 10 % between two limbs

% Deficit = ((Higher t – Lower t) / Higher t) * 100   *e.g.*, % Def = ((244 - 228) / 244) * 100 = 7 %

Knee extn (quadricep) strength : _____

Knee flxn (hamstring) strength: _____

Ipsilateral Comparison (Fl / Ex ratio) - Preferred that **Fl / Ex** (H:Q) ratio exceeds estimated value*

Fl / Ex (H:Q) ratio = Knee flex / Knee extn   *e.g.* , Fl / Ex ratio = 138 / 244 = 0.57

Right knee flexion (hamstring) strength: _____

Left knee flexion (hamstring) strength: _____

Relative Strength Comparison (Max/kg) - Preferred that **Max/kg** exceeds estimated value*

Max/kg = Max value (N·m) of R vs L / Weight (kg)   e.g., Max/kg = 244 / 90.0 = 2.71 N·m/kg

Relative extn (quadricep) strength: _____

Relative flxn (hamstring) strength: _____

Evaluation / comments: _____

_____

_____

Form 6.2
ISOKINETIC STRENGTH

NAME _____ DATE _____ SCORE _____

Lab Results

Gender: _____ Initials: _____ Age (y): _____ Weight (kg): _____ Athlete (Y/N): _____

Peak torque (N·m)

	60 deg·s⁻¹			180 deg·s⁻¹			300 deg·s⁻¹		
	R	L	% Def	R	L	% Def	R	L	% Def
Knee extension (Q)	___	___	___	___	___	___	___	___	___
Knee flexion (H)	___	___	___	___	___	___	___	___	___
Fl / Ex (H:Q) ratio	___	___	*	___	___	*	___	___	*

	Max	Max / kg	Est'd	Max	Max / kg	Est'd	Max	Max / kg	Est'd
Knee extension (Q)	___	___	*	___	___	*	___	___	*
Knee flexion (H)	___	___	*	___	___	*	___	___	*

*Estimated values from *Table 6.2* based on : _____

Bilateral Comparison (% Deficit) - Preferred that **% Def** < 10 % between two limbs

% Deficit = ((Higher t – Lower t) / Higher t) * 100   *e.g.*, % Def = ((244 - 228) / 244) * 100 = 7 %

Knee extn (quadricep) strength : _____

Knee flxn (hamstring) strength: _____

Ipsilateral Comparison (Fl / Ex ratio) - Preferred that **Fl / Ex** (H:Q) ratio exceeds estimated value*

Fl / Ex (H:Q) ratio = Knee flex / Knee extn   *e.g.*, Fl / Ex ratio = 138 / 244 = 0.57

Right knee flexion (hamstring) strength: _____

Left knee flexion (hamstring) strength: _____

Relative Strength Comparison (Max/kg) - Preferred that **Max/kg** exceeds estimated value*

Max/kg = Max value (N·m) of R vs L / Weight (kg)   e.g., Max/kg = 244 / 90.0 = 2.71 N·m/kg

Relative extn (quadricep) strength: _____

Relative flxn (hamstring) strength: _____

Evaluation / comments: _____

_____

_____

Form 6.3

NAME _____ DATE _____ SCORE _____

ISOKINETIC STRENGTH (*OPTIONAL*)

Homework

Estimation of Fiber Distribution

Gender: **M**   Initials: **AA**   Age (y): **22**   Weight (kg): **90.0**

Torque (Reps 1–3): **160** N·m   Torque (Reps 48–50): **85** N·m

% Decline = ((_____ – _____) / _____) * 100 = _____ %

$\underset{\text{Reps 1–3}}{}$ $\underset{\text{Reps 48–50}}{}$ $\underset{\text{Reps 1–3}}{}$

% FT = (**46.9** % – 5.2) / 0.90 = _____ %   % ST = 100% – _____ = _____ %

$\underset{\text{% Decline}}{}$ $\underset{\text{% FT}}{}$

Demonstration of Force-Velocity Characteristics of Muscle

Gender: **M**   Initials: **A**   Age (y): **22**   Weight (kg): **90.0**

Knee Extension   60 deg·s⁻¹   180 deg·s⁻¹   300 deg·s⁻¹

	60 deg·s⁻¹	180 deg·s⁻¹	300 deg·s⁻¹
Peak Torque	**244** N·m	**160** N·m	**114** N·m
Relative to Max	___/___= ___	___/___= ___	___/___= ___
	Peak Max	Peak Max	Peak Max

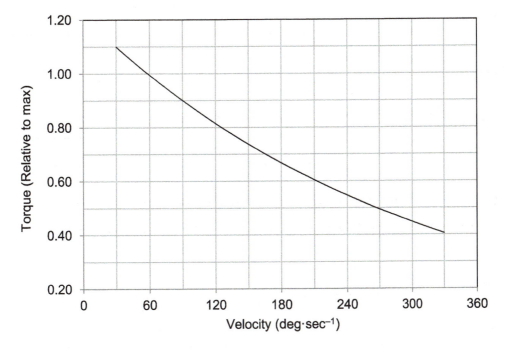

Evaluation / comments: _____

_____

_____

Form 6.4

NAME _____ DATE _____ SCORE _____

ISOKINETIC STRENGTH (*OPTIONAL*)

Lab Results

Estimation of Fiber Distribution

Gender: _____   Initials: _____   Age (y): _____   Weight (kg): _____

Torque (Reps 1–3): _____ N·m   Torque (Reps 48–50): _____ N·m

% Decline = ((_____ – _____) / _____) * 100 = _____ %
　　　　　　　　Reps 1–3　　Reps 48–50　　Reps 1–3

% FT = (_____ % – 5.2) / 0.90 = _____ %   % ST = 100% – _____ = _____ %
　　　　% Decline　　　　　　　　　　　　　　　　　　　　% FT

Demonstration of Force-Velocity Characteristics of Muscle

Gender: _____   Initials: _____   Age (y): _____   Weight (kg): _____

Knee Extension	60 deg·s^{-1}	180 deg·s^{-1}	300 deg·s^{-1}
Peak Torque	_____ N·m	_____ N·m	_____ N·m
Relative to Max	_____ / _____ = _____	_____ / _____ = _____	_____ / _____ = _____
	Peak　Max	Peak　Max	Peak　Max

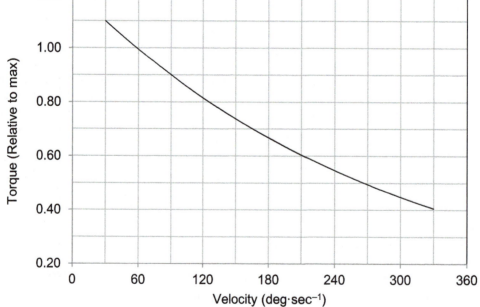

Evaluation / comments: _____

_____

SPRINTING—"HORIZONTAL POWER"

Contrary to aerobic exercise, anaerobic tasks do not rely predominantly upon the transport and extraction of oxygen by the cardiovascular and respiratory systems. Anaerobic fitness and its corresponding anaerobic activities are primarily dependent upon the energy sources already existing within the muscle fibers, those being adenosine triphosphate (ATP) and creatine phosphate (CP). As described in Chapter 1, high-intensity exercise relies on the two anaerobic energy systems, the phosphagen system and the glycolytic system. Exercise performed at a maximal pace for about 5–15 s, such as 50–100 m sprints in track, or intermittent sprinting during football, basketball, baseball, and soccer, rely more on phosphagen metabolism. Slightly longer maximal efforts ranging from a minimum of 15–30 s to a maximum of about 60 s rely predominantly on fast glycolysis to produce the needed energy.[3,10,17,23]

There is considerable interest among exercise physiologists and coaches in quantifying anaerobic fitness as it relates to physical performance and sports. Some of the more popular field tests for measuring "horizontal power" (as opposed to vertical power) include timed short sprints (ranging from 40 yd to 800 m), the standing long jump, and various shuttle runs. This chapter emphasizes the use of short, timed sprints (up to 60 m) as a test of anaerobic fitness. Ideally, only metric distances (i.e., 40 m, 50 m, 60 m) would be described. Comparative data can be found on these three metric distances.[13,22,31] However, the "40 yd dash" is so ingrained in high school, collegiate, and professional football in the United States that it must be included and discussed. The 40 yd sprint is used by football coaches because it theoretically represents the longest sprint football players are likely to make during long pass plays and punt and kickoff coverage. And in baseball, the 60 yd sprint is a popular distance because it corresponds to the distance a baseball player runs attempting to score from second base on a batter's single. Because of the popularity of football and baseball in America, and because of the frequent use of the 40 yd and 60 yd sprint, it is unlikely that these distances will be abandoned any time soon in favor of their metric equivalents.

ANATOMICAL RATIONALE

Two investigators suggested that faster sprinters have greater forward propulsion because they have more forceful and powerful hamstrings.[25] Along with the forceful action of the hip extensors and knee flexors during the ground phase, the ankle plantar flexors also contribute to sprint performance.[25] These investigators believe that the principal role of the arms is for balance, not cadence.

BIOMECHANICAL RATIONALE

Technically speaking, anaerobic power is not measured in these sprints. This is because of the lack of a true vertical distance component; only the horizontal distance[a] is known, but it cannot be used to calculate work as defined by a physicist ($w = F * D$). However, an estimate of "horizontal power"[b] may be made by multiplying the body mass (or force) of the participant by the sprint speed (Eq. 7.1). The unit produced by this multiplication is a $N \cdot m \cdot s^{-1}$, which is also equal to a watt.

"Horizontal power" (W) = Force (N)
$\quad$ * Speed ($m \cdot s^{-1}$) $\qquad$ Eq. 7.1

Tests for running speed are not exact estimates of anaerobic power because speed and power are not identical. The contribution of mass (weight) to power may be visualized by comparing the effect of dropping a table tennis ball versus a golf ball onto a pane of glass. Obviously, the golf ball will have a more powerful effect.

Also, the contribution of velocity may be visualized by comparing the power of two thrown baseballs—one going 50 mph and the other going 100 mph; although they both have the same mass, the faster one is more powerful. The concept of horizontal power is applicable to the collisions often encountered between competitors in such sports as football and ice hockey.

Sprint speed is not only dependent upon muscle power but also upon the elastic component (stiffness) of these muscles. Muscle power is important during the acceleration phase of the sprint and for maintaining maximal velocity, but high leg stiffness enhances rebound and also contributes to maximal velocity.[12,13,29]

PHYSIOLOGICAL RATIONALE

The duration of these sprints ranges from a minimum of about 4.3 s in the 40 yd sprint for a world-class runner to about 11 s in the 60 yd sprint for a slow college student.

---

[a]Distance and displacement are equal when assuming the runners go in a straight line from start to finish.
[b]Quotation marks emphasize the nontechnical term.

Thus, they are considered anaerobic power tests because they are usually performed in less than 15 s.

Biochemically, the tests are highly dependent upon the capacity and rate of splitting the phosphagens—adenosine triphosphate and creatine phosphate. One group of investigators reported the remaining percentage of creatine phosphate after 40 m and 60 m sprints as 37 % and 38 %, respectively, of the presprint concentrations.[22] A submaximal force, but high velocity, activity such as sprinting is probably more dependent upon the *rate* of myosin-actin interactions than upon the *number* of myosin-actin interactions.[18]

Fast-twitch skeletal muscle cells (Type IIa and IIx) predominate in fast, powerful anaerobic activities. They are good at rapidly generating high forces, but they fatigue much sooner than more aerobic slow-twitch cells (Type I).

METHODS

All three of the sprint tests may be administered simultaneously (see Figure 7.1). The facility can be any level terrain—marked-off football field, track, baseball diamond, gymnasium—that has an accurately measured sprint distance. For example, if you are using a baseball diamond, simply add 10, 20, and 30 yd to the distance between the bases in order to create 40, 50, and 60 yd, respectively. There should be a minimum of 25 yd beyond the 60 yd marker in order to provide the sprinter with ample space to slow down; this is called the **coasting**, or **deceleration, zone.** Box 7.1 discusses the accuracy of sprint tests.

Administrative Procedures

The procedures for administering the sprint tests (or any other high intensity anaerobic tests) should include adequate time for the participant to warm up prior to the sprint and cool down afterward. The participants need to know the proper starting procedures, and the technicians should be familiar with the timing of the events.

Warm-Up

It is common practice to warm up prior to anaerobic exercise through some combination of active warm-up, passive

warm-up (heating), and static and ballistic stretching. Whether there truly are benefits of any of these practices with regard to improving performance or reducing the risk of injury is not strongly supported by research. Of the evidence available, an active warm-up seems the most likely to positively affect anaerobic performance. The increased body temperature is believed to increase muscle and tendon compliance, increase nerve conduction velocity, and increase anaerobic energy contribution.[7] There may also be psychological benefits in that the participant senses an increased preparedness. A 15 min warm-up at 60–70 % VO_2max has been shown to improve anaerobic performance (treadmill running) by 10–13 %.[39] The active warm-up, however, if done at too high an intensity, can actually lead to fatigue and a reduction in performance,[8,9] especially in more untrained persons.[21] Passive warm-up, usually through the application of hot packs, has many of the same benefits of active warm-up but is typically not practical and therefore less frequently used.[7]

The use of static or ballistic stretching to improve anaerobic performance and reduce the risk of injury, although popular, is being seriously questioned. An acute

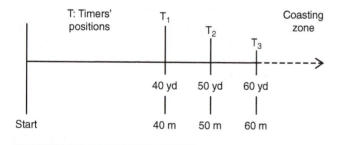

Figure 7.1 The sprint "layout" for measuring the times for the 40 yd, 50 yd, and 60 yd sprints (or 40 m, 50 m, and 60 m sprints).

bout of stretching has no positive effect on anaerobic performance,[35] or may even be detrimental.[6,33] And numerous studies that have systematically reviewed the literature can find no epidemiologic evidence that stretching before exercise reduces the risk of injury.[19,32,36,42]

Therefore, it is difficult to recommend a specific warm-up protocol. A 5 to 10 min warm-up at moderate intensity (60–70 % VO_2max) using the same exercise mode as the anaerobic fitness test (e.g., sprinting, cycling, etc.) will lead to an increased body temperature without undue fatigue. Short, intermittent bouts of higher intensity exercise (e.g., short runs, hops, jumps, or high speed spins) interspersed within the warm-up session may also be beneficial in fully warming up. Stretching immediately prior to anaerobic performance, however, is probably contraindicated due to a potential reduction in force production. Regular stretching to increase flexibility is still highly recommended, but it should not be done prior to performance.

Sprinter's Starting Technique

In order to reduce the effect of skill or past experience, participants should not use the specialized sprint-start technique of a track athlete. However, the starting position should assume a low center of gravity and a forward lean. Ideally, the participant should have shoes that will not slip upon starting. Starting blocks of any sort, such as using holes in the ground or by bracing against another person's feet, are not prescribed.

Timing of the Sprint

The three timers should use a stopwatch capable of measuring in hundredths of a second. After becoming familiar with the stopwatches, the timers should position themselves at the 40 yd, 50 yd, and 60 yd markers to allow an optimal view of the runner when starting and when breaking the plane of the finish line (see Figure 7.1). The timers should acknowledge a "Ready" signal of the runner. As soon as the runner makes the first movement to sprint, all timers start their watches. Thus, a "GO" signal is *not* given because the reaction time of the runner is not a consideration in this power test. As soon as the runner's trunk breaks the plane of the respective finish lines, technicians stop their watches. They record the times to the closest tenth of a second on Form 7.2. The mean time of the two or three trials is used as the sprinter's time for group statistical purposes.[14,29]

Number of Trials

Two trials of the sprint are typically performed. Three trials are recommended only if the difference in times between the first two trials is greater than 0.20 s. It is further recommended that no more than three trials are done to avoid the possible development of delayed-onset muscle soreness (DOMS). To avoid DOMS or injury and to allow restoration of the phosphagens, there should be a rest period between trials of at least 1–2 min if only sprinting 40 m,[2] and

3–8 min if performing 60 m sprints. Active recovery, such as fast walking or slow jogging, is superior to passive recovery, such as sitting or standing, during the relief interval for a supramaximal anaerobic activity, such as sprinting.[37]

Cool-Down

Unaccustomed anaerobic activity is conducive to delayed onset muscle soreness, whereby DOMS occurs as early as 6h, but usually 8–24 h post-exercise.[38] In addition to the warm-up prior to the exercise, and adhering to the three-trial maximum, the participant should also actively recover (cool down) at the same moderate intensity (60–70 % VO_2max) for about 5 min post-exercise. Static stretching of the sore muscles periodically over the next few days may have some benefit in relieving the DOMS, although this is not well proven.

Summary of Procedural Steps for Sprints

1. Sprint participants perform a warm-up routine.
2. The three timers stand at locations suitable for viewing the single sprinter's start and finish (review Figure 7.1). Thus, one timer is at the 40 yd (40 m) mark, another at the 50 yd (50 m) mark, and another at the 60 yd (60 m) mark.
3. The sprinter assumes the starting position by lowering the center of gravity and leaning slightly forward.
4. The sprinter and three timers acknowledge their readiness by (1) the sprinter's yelling, "Ready," and (2) the timers' yelling, "Ready," in return.
5. The timers start their watches at the first starting movement of the sprinter.
6. The sprinter runs as fast as possible through the 40 yd (40 m), 50 yd (50 m), or 60 yd (60 m) finish lines, depending upon the yardage comparisons desired by the sprinter or investigators.
7. The timers stop their watches when the sprinter breaks the plane of the respective finish lines; they record the time to the closest tenth of a second onto Form 7.2.
8. The sprinter repeats the trial after a recovery period consisting of a low-intensity activity, such as walking (40 m sprint only = 1–2 min recovery; 50 m = 2–5 min recovery; 60 m = 3–8 min recovery).
9. The sprinter performs a third trial if the difference between the first two trials is greater than 0.20 s.
10. The sprinter performs a proper cool-down by repeating a regimen similar to the first 5 min of the warm-up and by statically stretching the legs periodically during the next three days.

Calculation of "Horizontal Power"

As mentioned in the introduction to the chapter, it is not technically accurate to calculate or discuss "horizontal power." When exercise is performed "horizontally," as is the case in sprinting, no work is being done *against gravity*.

For this reason, there is no true work being done, so technically no measure of power can be calculated. The term horizontal power is used in this laboratory manual solely as a demonstration to students that the "instantaneous power" of an athlete is influenced by body mass (weight) and running speed. If two athletes possess the same body mass, but one is running at a faster speed, that athlete will generate more horizontal power upon impact in sports such as football and ice hockey. Similarly, if two athletes are running or skating at the same speed, but one athlete is heavier, that athlete will generate more power upon impact. Therefore, to demonstrate this point, horizontal power is calculated as the product of body mass (weight) and average running (or skating) speed as seen in the following example for a 40 m sprint (Eq. 7.2a through 7.2d). Either an increase in body mass at the same average speed, or an increase in speed at the same body mass would increase horizontal power.

$$\text{Average speed (m·s}^{-1}) = \text{Distance (m) / Time (s)} \quad \text{Eq. 7.2a}$$

$$\text{"Horizontal power" (W) = Body mass (N)} \\ * \text{Average speed (m·s}^{-1}) \quad \text{Eq. 7.2b}$$

Assume: Sprint time for **40 m = 4.75 s**
  (*or 40 yd = 5.20 s*); Body mass = **800 N**

$$\text{Average speed} = \textbf{40 m / 4.75 s = 8.4 (m·s}^{-1}) \quad \text{Eq. 7.2c}$$

$$\text{"Horizontal power"} = \textbf{800 N} * \textbf{8.4 m·s}^{-1} \\ = \textbf{6720 N·m·s}^{-1} = \textbf{6720 W} \quad \text{Eq. 7.2d}$$

RESULTS AND DISCUSSION

Sprint times are a measure of the ability to create horizontal power through the immediate breakdown of phosphagens within the skeletal muscle cells. Athletes involved in sports such as track and field, football, ice hockey, basketball, and baseball need a high degree of anaerobic power in order to run fast, skate fast, or jump far. The low creatine phosphate stores remaining after 5 s of sprinting may be responsible for the inability of sprinters to increase maximal speed after that time.[22] Sprint training can make any runner faster. Investigators appear to agree that sprint training does not convert Type I fibers into Type IIb (or IIx) fibers, although it may allow some Type IIa fibers to take on the characteristics of Type IIb (or IIx) fibers.[11]

Limited published data are available with which to compare sprint results. Table 7.1 provides normative data published by the American Alliance for Health, Physical Education, Recreation and Dance (AAHPERD) for 50 yd sprints in high school boys and girls. The median time for boys is 6.6 s, and the median time for girls is 7.9 s.[1] Compared with college men and women, high school boys and girls in general run about 90–95 % as fast over 50 yd.

Comparative times for various sprint distances in men and women are seen in Table 7.2. Published times for the 40yd sprint are most prevalent in the sport of football. A recent study of collegiate football players reported an average 40 yd sprint time of 4.74 s, with receivers recording the lowest times of 4.49 s when compared by position. The 40 yd sprint time of the receivers is 0.08 s faster than data

Table 7.1 50 yd Sprint Times for High School Boys and Girls

Category (percentile)	50 yd Time (s)	
	Boys	Girls
Well above ave (> 95th)	> 5.9	> 6.8
Above ave (75th–95th)	5.9 – 6.3	6.8 – 7.4
Average (25th–74th)	6.4 – 7.0	7.5 – 8.4
Below ave (5th–24th)	7.1 – 7.9	8.5 – 9.5
Well below ave (< 5th)	> 7.9	> 9.5

Source: Data from AAHPERD (1976).[1]

Table 7.2 Comparative Mean and World Record Times for Men and Women for Sprinting Distances of 40 yd / 40 m, 50 yd / 50 m, and 60 yd / 60 m

40 yd / 40 m	Time (s)	50 yd / 50 m	Time (s)	60 yd / 60 m	Time (s)
Men					
40 yd - College football mean[a]	4.78	50 yd - World best	5.15	60 yd - World best	5.99
Receivers mean[a]	4.49	50 m - World record[e]	5.56	60 m - World record[e]	6.39
Running backs mean[a]	4.55	50 m - College record[e]	5.67	60 m - College record[e]	6.45
Defensive line mean[a]	4.89	50 m - High school record[e]	5.69	60 m - High school record[e]	6.57
40 yd - NFL combine mean[b]	4.81	50 m - College athletes mean[f]	6.38	60 yd - Baseball "standard"[h]	6.8
40 yd - College students mean[c]	5.21	50 m - College students mean[g]	6.8	60 yd - Baseball "standard"[i]	7.0
Women					
40 yd - College athletes mean[d]	5.96	50 yd - World best	5.74	60 yd - World best	6.54
40 yd - College students mean[c]	6.12	50 m - World record[e]	5.96	60 m - World record[e]	6.92
		50 m - College record[e]	6.13	60 m - College record[e]	7.09
		50 m - High school record[e]	6.32	60 m - High school record[e]	7.22
		50 m - College students mean[g]	8.2		

Sources: Data from [a]Secora et al. (2004)[34]; [b]McGee & Burkett (2003)[28]; [c]Mayhew et al. (1994)[26]; [d]Moore et al. (2007)[30]; [e]Track & Field[41]; [f]Hanon, Bernard et al. (2012)[19]; [g]Johnson et al. (1975)[24].
Note: [h]Professional and [i]College baseball standard.

	College Male Students			College Female Students		
	Sprint Time	Sprint Time	"Horizontal"	Sprint Time	Sprint Time	"Horizontal"
Category	40-Yard (s)	40-Meter (s)	Power (W)	40-Yard (s)	40-Meter (s)	Power (W)
Well above ave (> 95th %ile)	< 4.72	< 4.31	> 8200	< 5.61	< 5.13	> 5113
Above ave (75th–95th %ile)	4.72–5.00	4.31–4.56	7395–8200	5.61–5.90	5.13–5.39	4742–5113
Average (25th–74th %ile)	5.01–5.40	4.57–4.93	6265–7394	5.91–6.32	5.40–5.78	4222–4741
Below ave (5th–24th %ile)	5.41–5.71	4.94–5.22	5459–6264	6.33–6.62	5.79–6.05	3850–4221
Well below ave (< 5th %ile)	> 5.71	> 5.22	< 5459	> 6.62	> 6.05	< 3850
Mean	5.21	4.76	6829	6.12	5.59	4481

Source: Data from Moore, Decker, Baarts, DuPont, Epema, Reuther, Houser & Mayhew.[30] Values for percentiles are estimated from reported means and standard deviations assuming the data are normally distributed. See text for definition of "horizontal" power, estimated from mean 40-yd sprint time (s) and mean body mass (N) of the study cited.

recorded on a similar group 13 years previously.[34] World record times are available in men and women for both 50 yd and 50 m distances. In setting these world records, men ran about 8.9–9.0 m·s^{-1} over this distance, while women ran 8.0–8.4 m·s^{-1}, which is about 90–93 % as fast as men. Sprint times for college men and women in one study averaged 6.8 s and 8.2 s for 50 m,[24] which is about 82 % and 73 % of world record pace, respectively. The 60 yd sprint is a popular distance in assessing speed and anaerobic fitness in baseball players because, as mentioned previously, it is the distance a player must run to score from second base on a single. A typical "criterion" time for the 60 yd sprint is 7.0 s in college baseball and 6.8 s in professional baseball. The 60 m distance is popular in indoor track and field because it is usually the longest straight sprint possible indoors.

No studies could be found in the literature to provide good normative data for sprint time or "horizontal power" derived from sprint time. Data are available from one recent study, however, that allow comparison values for college-aged male and female students (Table 7.3).[30] The mean 40-yd sprint time for non-athletes of 5.21 ± 0.24 s is considerably slower than that observed in college football players. The mean value for college men for "horizontal power" of 6829 ± 831 W is estimated based on their mean 40-yd sprint time and mean body weight (82.9 kg). It is also considerably lower than the estimated "horizontal power" for male football players of 9766 ± 522 W, which is extremely high based on the fact that football players are very fast (mean 40-yd sprint time of 4.78 s) and very big (mean body weight of 108.8 kg).[34]

The timed sprint measured over 40, 50, or 60 meters or yards is a good direct measure of running speed. It is also a measure of anaerobic fitness, as it reflects the participant's maximal ability to generate "horizontal power" by way of the phosphagen system. Because speed and anaerobic fitness are especially important in sports such as track and field, football, basketball, and baseball, measuring sprint times in these sports is likewise important.

BOX 7.2   Chapter Preview/Review

What muscles are involved in sprinting?
How do the energy systems contribute to sprinting?
What type of activity is best to perform in preparation for sprinting?
What two variables are used to determine the "horizontal power" associated with sprinting?
In what sports are the 40 yd, 60 yd, and 60 m sprints most popular?
According to AAHPERD, what are the median times for 50 yd sprints in high school boys and girls?
How does the "horizontal power" of football players compare with non-athletes?

References

1. AAHPERD. (1976). *AAHPERD youth fitness test manual.* Washington, DC: AAHPERD Publications.

2. Balsom, P. D., Seger, J. Y., Sjodin, B., & Ekblom, B. (1992). Maximal-intensity intermittent exercise: Effect of recovery duration. *International Journal of Sports Medicine, 13,* 528–533.

3. Bangsbo, J. (1998). Quantification of anaerobic energy production during intense exercise. *Medicine and Science in Sports and Exercise, 30,* 47–52.

4. Bar-Or, O., & Inbar, O. (1978). Relationships among anaerobic capacity, sprint and middle distance running of school children. In R.Shephard & H.Lavalle (Eds.), *Physical fitness assessment* (pp. 142–147). Springfield, IL: Charles C Thomas.

5. Baumgartner, T. A., & Jackson, A. S. (1987). *Measurement for evaluation in physical education and exercise science.* Dubuque, IA: Wm. C. Brown.

6. Behm, D., Bambury, A., Cahill, F., & Power, K. (2004). Effect of acute static stretching on force, balance, reaction time, and movement time. *Medicine and Science in Sports and Exercise, 36,* 1397–1402.

7. Bishop, D. (2003). Warm up I: Potential mechanisms and the effects of passive warm up on exercise performance. *Sports Medicine, 33,* 439–454.

8. Bishop, D. (2003). Warm up II: Performance changes following active warm up and how to structure the warm up. *Sports Medicine, 33,* 483–498.

9. Bishop, D., Bonetti, D., & Dawson, B. (2001). The effect of three different warm-up intensities on kayak ergometer performance. *Medicine and Science in Sports and Exercise, 33,* 1026–1032.

10. Boobis, L. H., Williams, C., & Wootton, S. A. (1982). Human muscle metabolism during brief maximal exercise. *Journal of Physiology, 338,* 21–22 P.

11. Cahill, B. R., Misner, J. E., & Boileau, R. A. (1997). The clinical importance of the anaerobic energy system and its assessment in human performance. *The American Journal of Sports Medicine, 25,* 863–872.

12. Cavagna, G. A., Komarek, L., & Mazzoleni, S. (1971). The mechanics of sprint running. *Journal of Physiology (London), 217,* 709–721.

13. Chelly, S. M., & Denis, C. (2001). Leg power and hopping stiffness: Relationship with sprint running performance. *Medicine & Science in Sports & Exercise, 33,* 326–333.

14. Costill, D. L., Miller, S. J., Myers, W. C., Kehoe, F. M., & Hoffman, W. M. (1968). Relationship among selected tests of explosive leg strength and power. *The Research Quarterly, 39*(3), 785–787.

15. Crews, T. R., & Meadors, W. J. (1978). Analysis of reaction time, speed, and body composition of college football players. *Journal of Sports Medicine and Physical Fitness, 18,* 169–174.

16. de Vries, H. A., & Housh, T. J. (1994). *Physiology of exercise for physical education, athletics, and exercise science.* Dubuque, IA: Brown & Benchmark.

17. Gaitanos, G. C., Williams, C., Boobis, L. H., & Brooks, S. (1993). Human muscle metabolism during intermittent maximal exercise. *Journal of Applied Physiology, 75,* 712–719.

18. Green, H. J. (1991). What do tests measure? In J. D. MacDougall, H. A. Wenger, & H. J. Green (Eds.), *Physiological testing of the high performance athlete* (pp. 7–19). Champaign, IL: Human Kinetics.

19. Hanon, C., Bernard, O., Rabate, M., & Claire, T. (2012). Effect of two different long-sprint training regimens on sprint performance and associated metabolic responses. *Journal of Strength and Conditioning Research, 26,* 1551–1557.

20. Hart, L. (2005). Effect of stretching on sport injury risk: a review. *Clinical Journal of Sports Medicine, 15,* 113.

21. Hawley, J., Williams, M., Hamling, G., & Walsh, R. (1989). Effects of a task-specific warm-up on anaerobic power. *British Journal of Sports Medicine, 23,* 233–236.

22. Hirvonen, J. S., Rehunen S., Rusko, H., & Härkönen, M. (1987). Breakdown of high-energy phosphate compounds and lactate accumulation during short supramaximal exercise. *European Journal of Applied Physiology, 56,* 253–259.

23. Jacobs, I., Bar-Or, O., Karlsson, J., Dotan, R., Tesch, P., Kaiser, P., & Inbar, O. (1982). Changes in muscle metabolites in females with 30-s exhaustive exercise. *Medicine and Science in Sports and Exercise, 14,* 457–460.

24. Johnson, P. B., Updyke, W. F., Schaefer, M., & Stolberg, D. C. (1975). *Sport, exercise, and you.* New York: Holt, Rinehart and Winston.

25. Mann, R., & Sprague, P. (1980). A kinetic analysis of the ground leg during sprint running. *Research Quarterly for Exercise and Sport, 51,* 334–348.

26. Mayhew, J. L., Bemben, M. G., Rohrs, D. M., & Bemben, D. A. (1994). Specificity among anaerobic power tests in college female athletes. *Journal of Strength and Conditioning Research, 8,* 43–47.

27. McArdle, W. D., Katch, F. I., & Katch, V. L. (1991). *Exercise physiology.* Philadelphia: Lea & Febiger.

28. McGee, K., & Burkett, L. (2003). The National Football League combine: a reliable predictor of draft status? *Journal of Strength and Conditioning Research, 17,* 6–11.

29. Mero, A., & Komi, P. V. (1986). Force-, EMG-, and elasticity-velocity relationships at submaximal, maximal and supramaximal running speeds in sprinters. *European Journal of Applied Physiology, 55,* 553–561.

30. Moore, A. N., Decker, A. J., Baarts, J. N., DuPont, A. M., Epema, J. S., Reuther, M. C., Houser, J. J., & Mayhew, J. L. (2007). Effect of competitiveness on forty-yard dash performance in college men and women. *Journal of Strength and Conditioning Research, 21,* 385–388.

31. Nesser, T. W., Latin, R. W., Berg, K., & Prentice, E. (1996). Physiological determinants of 40-meter sprint performance in young male athletes. *Journal of Strength and Conditioning Research, 10,* 263–267.

32. Pope, R., Herbert, R., Kirwan, J., & Graham, B. (2000). A randomized trial of pre-exercise stretching for prevention of lower-limb injury. *Medicine and Science in Sports and Exercise, 23,* 271–277.

33. Power, K., Behm, D., Cahill, F., Carroll, M., & Young, W. (2004). An acute bout of static stretching: effects on force and jumping performance. *Medicine and Science in Sports and Exercise, 36,* 1389–1396.

34. Secora, C., Latin, R., Berg, K., & Noble, J. (2004). Comparison of physical and performance characteristics of NCAA division I football players: 1987 and 2000. *Journal of Strength and Conditioning Research, 18,* 286–291.

35. Shrier, I. (2004). Does stretching improve performance?: A systematic and critical review of the literature. *Clinical Journal of Sports Medicine, 14,* 267–273.

36. Shrier, I. (1999). Stretching before exercise does not reduce the risk of local muscle injury: A critical review of the clinical and basic science literature. *Clinical Journal of Sports Medicine, 9,* 221–227.

37. Signorile, J. F., Ingalls, C., & Tremblay, L. M. (1993). The effects of active and passive recovery on short-term high intensity power output. *Canadian Journal of Applied Physiology, 18,* 31–42.

38. Smith, L. L., Brunetz, M. H., Chenier, T. C., McCammon, M. R., Houmard, J. A., Franklin, M. E., & Israel, R. G. (1993). The effects of static and ballistic stretching on delayed onset muscle soreness and creatine kinase. *Research Quarterly for Exercise and Sport, 64,* 103–107.

39. Stewart, I., & Sleivert, G. (1998). The effect of warm-up intensity on range of motion and anaerobic performance. *Journal of Orthopaedic and Sports Physical Therapy, 27,* 154–161.

40. Tharp, G. D., Newhouse, R. K., Uffelman, L., Thorland, W. G., & Johnson, G. O. (1985). Comparison of sprint and run times with performance on the Wingate anaerobic test. *Research Quarterly for Exercise and Sport, 56,* 73–76.

41. Track & Field News (2012). Website, *Archive.* Retrieved, June 24, 2012, from http://www .trackandfieldnews.com/.

42. Weldon, S., & Hill, R. (2003). The efficacy of stretching for prevention of exercise-related injury: A systematic review of the literature. *Manual Therapy, 8,* 141–150.

Form 7.1

NAME _____ DATE _____ SCORE _____

SPRINTING—"HORIZONTAL POWER"

Homework

Gender: **M**   Initials: **AA**   Age (y): **22**   Weight (kg): **85.0**   Body mass (N): _____

Sprint Times   *Record T_3 if T_1 and T_2 differ by > 0.20 s*   Distance (m or yd) :   **yd**

☐ 40 m / ■ 40 yd	T_1 **5.52**	T_2 **5.62**	T_3 _____	Mean _____	s (closest 0.01 s)
☐ 50 m / ■ 50 yd	T_1 **6.84**	T_2 **6.96**	T_3 _____	Mean _____	s (closest 0.01 s)
☐ 60 m / ☐ 60 yd	T_1 _____	T_2 _____	T_3 _____	Mean _____	s (closest 0.01 s)

Running Speeds   *Speed ($m \cdot s^{-1}$) = Distance (m) / Time (s)*   *1 m = 1.0936 yd ; 1 yd = 0.914 m*

☐ 40 m / ■ 40 yd	Speed = _____ m /	_____ s	= _____	$m \cdot s^{-1}$
☐ 50 m / ■ 50 yd	Speed = _____ m /	_____ s	= _____	$m \cdot s^{-1}$
☐ 60 m / ☐ 60 yd	Speed = _____ m /	_____ s	= _____	$m \cdot s^{-1}$

"Horizontal Power"   *Power (W) = Body mass (N) * Speed ($m \cdot s^{-1}$)*   *1 $N \cdot m \cdot s^{-1}$ = 1 W*

☐ 40 m / ■ 40 yd	Power = _____ N *	_____ $m \cdot s^{-1}$	= _____	W
☐ 50 m / ■ 50 yd	Power = _____ N *	_____ $m \cdot s^{-1}$	= _____	W
☐ 60 m / ☐ 60 yd	Power = _____ N *	_____ $m \cdot s^{-1}$	= _____	W

Category for: 40-yd/m time *(Table 7.3)* _____   "Power" *(Table 7.3)* _____

Evaluation/comments: _____

Gender: **F**   Initials: **BB**   Age (y): **21**   Weight (kg): **68.5**   Body mass (N): _____

Sprint Times   *Record T_3 if T_1 and T_2 differ by > 0.20 s*   Distance (m or yd) :   **yd**

☐ 40 m / ■ 40 yd	T_1 **5.95**	T_2 **6.18**	T_3 **6.13**	Mean _____	s (closest 0.01 s)
☐ 50 m / ■ 50 yd	T_1 **7.69**	T_2 **7.75**	T_3 **7.81**	Mean _____	s (closest 0.01 s)
☐ 60 m / ☐ 60 yd	T_1 _____	T_2 _____	T_3 _____	Mean _____	s (closest 0.01 s)

Running Speeds   *Speed ($m \cdot s^{-1}$) = Distance (m) / Time (s)*   *1 m = 1.0936 yd ; 1 yd = 0.914 m*

☐ 40 m / ■ 40 yd	Speed = _____ m /	_____ s	= _____	$m \cdot s^{-1}$
☐ 50 m / ■ 50 yd	Speed = _____ m /	_____ s	= _____	$m \cdot s^{-1}$
☐ 60 m / ☐ 60 yd	Speed = _____ m /	_____ s	= _____	$m \cdot s^{-1}$

"Horizontal Power"   *Power (W) = Body mass (N) * Speed ($m \cdot s^{-1}$)*   *1 $N \cdot m \cdot s^{-1}$ = 1 W*

☐ 40 m / ■ 40 yd	Power = _____ N *	_____ $m \cdot s^{-1}$	= _____	W
☐ 50 m / ■ 50 yd	Power = _____ N *	_____ $m \cdot s^{-1}$	= _____	W
☐ 60 m / ☐ 60 yd	Power = _____ N *	_____ $m \cdot s^{-1}$	= _____	W

Category for: 40-yd/m time *(Table 7.3)* _____   "Power" *(Table 7.3)* _____

Evaluation/comments: _____

Form 7.2

NAME _____ DATE _____ SCORE _____

SPRINTING—"HORIZONTAL POWER"

Lab Results

Gender: _____ Initials: _____ Age (y): _____ Weight (kg): _____ Body mass (N): _____

Sprint Times   *Record T_3 if T_1 and T_2 differ by > 0.20 s*   Distance (m or yd) : _____

☐ 40 m / ☐ 40 yd T_1 _____ T_2 _____ T_3 _____   Mean _____ *s (closest 0.01 s)*

☐ 50 m / ☐ 50 yd T_1 _____ T_2 _____ T_3 _____   Mean _____ *s (closest 0.01 s)*

☐ 60 m / ☐ 60 yd T_1 _____ T_2 _____ T_3 _____   Mean _____ *s (closest 0.01 s)*

Running Speeds   *Speed $(m \cdot s^{-1})$ = Distance (m) / Time (s)*   *1 m = 1.0936 yd ; 1 yd = 0.914 m*

☐ 40 m / ☐ 40 yd   Speed = _____ m / _____ s = _____ $m \cdot s^{-1}$

☐ 50 m / ☐ 50 yd   Speed = _____ m / _____ s = _____ $m \cdot s^{-1}$

☐ 60 m / ☐ 60 yd   Speed = _____ m / _____ s = _____ $m \cdot s^{-1}$

"Horizontal Power"   *Power (W) = Body mass (N) * Speed $(m \cdot s^{-1})$*   *$1 N \cdot m \cdot s^{-1} = 1 W$*

☐ 40 m / ☐ 40 yd   Power = _____ N * _____ $m \cdot s^{-1}$ = _____ W

☐ 50 m / ☐ 50 yd   Power = _____ N * _____ $m \cdot s^{-1}$ = _____ W

☐ 60 m / ☐ 60 yd   Power = _____ N * _____ $m \cdot s^{-1}$ = _____ W

Category for: 40-yd/m time *(Table 7.3)* _____   "Power" *(Table 7.3)* _____

Evaluation/comments: _____

Gender: _____ Initials: _____ Age (y): _____ Weight (kg): _____ Body mass (N): _____

Sprint Times   *Record T_3 if T_1 and T_2 differ by > 0.20 s*   Distance (m or yd) : _____

☐ 40 m / ☐ 40 yd T_1 _____ T_2 _____ T_3 _____   Mean _____ *s (closest 0.01 s)*

☐ 50 m / ☐ 50 yd T_1 _____ T_2 _____ T_3 _____   Mean _____ *s (closest 0.01 s)*

☐ 60 m / ☐ 60 yd T_1 _____ T_2 _____ T_3 _____   Mean _____ *s (closest 0.01 s)*

Running Speeds   *Speed $(m \cdot s^{-1})$ = Distance (m) / Time (s)*   *1 m = 1.0936 yd ; 1 yd = 0.914 m*

☐ 40 m / ☐ 40 yd   Speed = _____ m / _____ s = _____ $m \cdot s^{-1}$

☐ 50 m / ☐ 50 yd   Speed = _____ m / _____ s = _____ $m \cdot s^{-1}$

☐ 60 m / ☐ 60 yd   Speed = _____ m / _____ s = _____ $m \cdot s^{-1}$

"Horizontal Power"   *Power (W) = Body mass (N) * Speed $(m \cdot s^{-1})$*   *$1 N \cdot m \cdot s^{-1} = 1 W$*

☐ 40 m / ☐ 40 yd   Power = _____ N * _____ $m \cdot s^{-1}$ = _____ W

☐ 50 m / ☐ 50 yd   Power = _____ N * _____ $m \cdot s^{-1}$ = _____ W

☐ 60 m / ☐ 60 yd   Power = _____ N * _____ $m \cdot s^{-1}$ = _____ W

Category for: 40-yd/m time *(Table 7.3)* _____   "Power" *(Table 7.3)* _____

Evaluation/comments: _____

JUMPING—VERTICAL POWER

The vertical jump test, because of the vertical displacement of the body mass during the jump, provides a true measure of power. The test described in this manual is a modification of one developed by Dudley Sargent in the early 1900s—the Sargent Jump Test.[46] The original test was designed to measure only jumping height, by determining the distance between the standing-reach height and jumping-reach height. By also considering the body mass of the jumper, the current test allows a calculation of the power generated during the jump. It is logical to think that if two jumpers have the same vertical jump, but one jumper has a greater body mass, the heavier jumper needs to generate more power in order to lift the greater body mass the same vertical distance from the floor.

The power generated during the jump (W) depends on the force component, taken from the body mass (N), the vertical displacement (m) accomplished during the jump, and the time (s) in the air. The measurement or derivation of these three variables allows for the calculation of power in N·m·s⁻¹ (W). A force plate can be used to measure the forces and time involved during the jump.[12,38] The time in the air can also be measured using an electronic contact mat attached to a timer.[26,53] Or the time can also be estimated from the law of falling bodies or acceleration of gravity (g = 9.81 m·s⁻²) based upon the difference in the original height of the center of gravity and its height at the peak of the jump.[13,53]

$$W = \frac{Nm}{s}$$

PHYSIOLOGICAL AND BIOMECHANICAL RATIONALE

Power includes two basic components—dynamic strength and speed.[44] Although the vertical jump has been called an explosive strength test,[34] partly because the single jumping movement itself is accomplished in less than a second, it is not a true strength measure because a maximal muscle force is not elicited despite the maximal jump effort. Conceivably, repeated jumps within a 10 s period would have little decrement. Thus, the ability to perform well on this test may be related more to power than strength.

Correlations between strength and vertical jump have been quite variable. The ballistic act of vertical jumping correlated moderately high (r = 0.74; 0.81) with peak *relative* isokinetic torque[6] (N·m·kg⁻¹) and static force[22] of the leg extensors, respectively. However, others have reported insignificant[7,10,30] or low[11] (r < 0.2) or moderate[18,41] (r = 0.4

to 0.6) correlations between strength and jumping. Two reviewers[33] provide a rationale for this low strength vs. jump relationship, especially when the comparative strength measure is a slow static or slow muscle action. For example, the force applied in a 1 RM lift is longer than the force duration of a vertical jump in which the jumper's feet are in contact with the terrain for only about 350 ms (0.35 s). The reviewers conclude that the ability to generate the highest dynamic rate of force development is a very significant factor in such an explosive movement as the vertical jump. However, the contact time for vertical jump force is two to four times longer than the force in maximal sprinting.[40] Thus, it appears that anaerobic power is a fitness component that is too complex to be predicted by strength alone.

Disregarding biomechanical factors, jumping ability is dependent biochemically upon the individual's phosphagen system and the ability to use these phosphagen stores at a rapid rate. Although the percentage of fast-twitch fibers in the vastus lateralis—one of the four quadricep muscles—is significantly related (r = 0.48) to jump height as measured from a force platform, the correlation may not be high enough to have physiological relevance.[3]

Biomechanically, the jump test combines hip extension (glutei and hamstrings) and knee extension (vasti and rectus femoris) with ankle plantar flexion (gastrocnemius and soleus).[2,21,49] The jump movement has been compared to the snatch and clean Olympic events.[17] The type of vertical jump influences the ultimate vertical distance of the jump, although the same lower extremity muscles act in the jump. Two types of jumps often compared are the counter movement jump (CMJ) and the static squat jump. The CMJ is the natural way of jumping whereby the performer dips in the opposite direction of the goal prior to the start of the push-off phase. A static squat jump dispenses with the counter movement, meaning that the jumper assumes the push-off position, then delays and jumps from that position without dipping. Researchers agree that the CMJ results in higher jumps than the static squat jump.[2,3,4] One group of reviewers[2] provided five possible rationales for the CMJ advantage over the static squat jump: (1) accustomed skill; (2) added force from elastic recoil of tissues; (3) enhanced muscle fiber recruitment due to the stretch (myotatic) reflex; (4) altered properties of the contractile machinery; and (5) longer time available for force development. The reviewers' own findings favor the fifth rationale because the CMJ produces more work during the initial shortening distance. One must not dismiss the contribution of the arms during a vertical jump. Vertical jumps are enhanced when thrusting the arms upward.[3,4,49]

METHODS

The methods of conducting the vertical jump test consider (a) equipment, (b) procedures, (c) warm-up, (d) body positions and measurements, and (e) calculations. See Box 8.1 for a discussion on the accuracy of vertical jumps.

Equipment

The measurement of vertical jump and leg power can be accomplished using several different methods. Vertical jump can be measured directly by measuring the vertical difference between standing reach and maximal jumping reach with commercially available devices or with simple "homemade" devices. Vertical jump and leg power can also be measured with various electronic devices that measure the time and forces involved in the jump.

To directly measure the vertical jump height, a recommended commercially available device is the Vertec™ (Sports Imports, Hilliard, OH; Figure 8.1). This nonelectronic standing scale resembles a volleyball standard and has red, white, and blue vanes spaced 0.5 in. apart; the blue vanes mark the whole inches, the white vanes mark the half inches, and the red vanes indicate 6 in. intervals. The sweep of the jumper's hand causes the vanes to swivel and mark the highest point of the jump. If a Vertec™ is not affordable or available, a flat scale can be made on the wall for measuring jump height (Figure 8.2). A flat measuring scale about 1 ft wide and 4 ft long, with horizontal lines at 1 in. intervals, can be attached to a wall or post. If this flat scale is used, chalk or water should be applied to the jumper's fingers so that a visible mark is made at the highest point of the jump.

Various electronic systems can be used to analyze standing vertical jumps by measuring the time of the jump alone, or by measuring the time and forces involved in the jump. One such system is the Kistler™ 9281B multicomponent force measuring plate (Kistler Instrument Corporation, Amherst, MA). Kinetic and kinematic data recorded during the jump pertaining to body center of mass displacement, vertical takeoff velocity, and time in the air can be used to analyze vertical jump performance and leg power. The methodology for analyzing standing vertical jump using a force plate is not described in this manual, but can be found in other sources.[32,38]

Other pieces of equipment have been developed for field testing that are available to assess vertical jump employing different methodologies. The Just Jump® system (Probotics, Huntsville, AL) is a contact mat embedded with micro switches that time the interval between subject liftoff from the mat and landing. An attached computer records the flight time and uses it to determine the height of the jump. The Optojump® system (Microgate, Bolzano, Italy)

BOX 8.1 | Accuracy of the Vertical Jump

The measurement of vertical jump can be done utilizing different technologies, some requiring sophisticated laboratory equipment (motion analysis and/or force plate) while most, such as the "jump and reach" test, can be done in the field with inexpensive equipment. When measuring vertical jump with the Vertec®, investigators have expressed two concerns: (1) countermovement jump (CMJ) heights can only be measured in 1.27-cm increments, and (2) attaining a jump height on the Vertec® involves measuring standing reach and jumping reach, both of which contribute error. Although the Vertec® is considered a reliable and valid device, the sensitivity with which it can measure vertical jump is limited. Alternative approaches to measure vertical jump rely on: (1) measuring flight time using either a contact mat system (Just Jump®), or using an optical device with photoelectric cells (Optojump®), or (2) using an accelerometer which is worn during the jump that estimates jump height from vertical acceleration (Myotest®).

Reliability

When measuring jump height using the difference between standing reach and jumping reach, reports of test-retest reliability have been high, ranging from a correlation of 0.93 when using the technique described in this text[21,31] to 0.98 when using a more restrictive procedure.[22] Studies reported a correlation of 0.99 when testing university students[11], and correlations ranging from 0.90 to 0.97 in children.[36] A recent study of vertical jump height using a CMJ on a Vertec® device found a high degree of reliability in college students.[43] The study reported $ICC = 0.89–0.94$, $SEM = 2.1–2.7$ cm, and $CV = 5.5–6.9\%$. The investigators recommended that to maximize reliability when utilizing a CMJ and a Vertec®, the protocol should include extensive familiarization with the CMJ technique and a minimum of 3 trials or until performance plateaus. This same study reported that the contact mat system (Just Jump®) had an $ICC = 0.93$, $SEM = 1.6–2.3$ cm, and $CV = 4.2–4.4\%$; and the accelerometer system (Myotest®) had an $ICC = 0.91–0.95$, $SEM = 1.4–1.7$ cm, and $CV = 3.9–4.6\%$.[43] The reliability of the optical device (Optojump®) is also excellent with an $ICC = 0.98$; $SEM = 2.8$ cm; and $CV = 2.7\%$.[20]

Validity

The "gold standard" to which any measure of vertical jump is compared uses a motion analysis system to measure the displacement of the center of gravity from the standing position to its highest vertical displacement. Using such a standard, the validity of using the Vertec® has been reported as 0.906.[37] The validity of this type of "jump and reach" test is affected by the jumper's ability to contact the device while reaching maximal height which supports multiple attempts. The other methods do not have this limitation. Results from the Just Jump® system are highly correlated ($r = 0.967$) with results measured by motion analysis.[37] The Myotest[®9] and Optojump[®20] have both been reported to be valid tools for field-based evaluation. Peak power derived from measured vertical jump height is highly related to absolute ($r = 0.83$)[24] and relative ($r = 0.92$)[12] peak power measured directly on a force plate.

Vertical jump has been shown to be significantly related to 30-m sprint time in male basketball players ($r = -0.619$)[1] and to 30-m ($r = -0.79$) and 100-m sprint times ($r = -0.75$) in female sprinters.[28] Vertical jump is also related to power measured by the Wingate test in boys ($r = 0.70$)[52], and to a 20-s Wingate test in older adults ($r = 0.49$).[8]

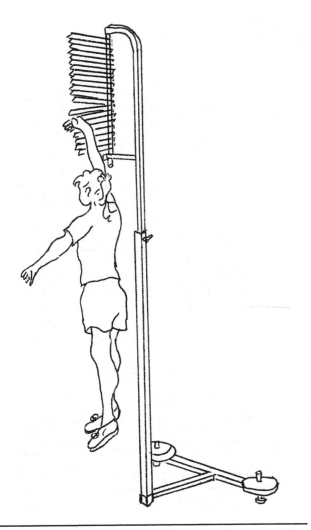

Figure 8.1 The Vertec™ is an example of a commercial vertical jump tester, showing the jumper displacing the vanes at the peak of the jump.

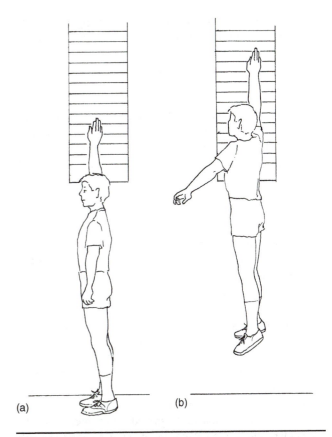

(a) (b)

Figure 8.2 The significant positions for the vertical jump: (a) the recorded standing-reach position and (b) the recorded jump position.

is an optical device with two rows of photoelectric cells (one row transmitting and the opposite row receiving) positioned at floor level that measure flight time from which vertical jump is determined. The Myotest® system (Myotest SA, Sion, Switzerland) is an accelerometer contained in a small case that is worn attached to the participant at the waist. It can estimate vertical jump height by measuring takeoff velocity or flight time.

Procedures for Vertical Jump

The emphasis in this manual is upon nonelectronic methods for measuring vertical jump. Regardless of the technical sophistication, a warm-up routine is recommended. The procedures should also include standardized body positions before and during the jump.

Warm-Up

This need not be quite so extensive as that typically recommended for sprint running. However, a warm-up appears

to enhance jumping performance.[14] About 5 min to 10 min of warming up, including a few vertical jumps at one-half to three-quarter effort, should be sufficient. The stretching exercises should include shoulder stretches because the arm reach requires a full range of motion.

Body Positions and Measurements

The jump distance is calculated from the two vertical measurements for the vertical jump test—the standing reach and the jump reach. These may be made in inches (in.) or centimeters (cm) to the closest 0.5 in. or 1 cm.

Standing Reach

The standing reach (Figure 8.2a) is measured as the jumper stands with the feet together and the dominant arm near the wall or standard of the commercial apparatus. The jumper then reaches as high as possible with the dominant arm so that the palm of the hand is against the measurement scale[39] or the wall. The highest point of the reach (usually tip of the middle finger) is observed and recorded onto Form 8.2.

Jumping Reach

After the standing reach is measured, the jumper moves the feet to a jumping position. The feet cannot change from this position prior to jumping, nor are any preparatory movements permitted other than one quick dip (countermovement) of the knees and one swing of the arms.

The participant makes the jump while touching or swatting the Vertec™ or measurement scale at the peak of the jump (Figure 8.2b). The jumping reach is indicated on the Vertec™ by the highest displaced vane. All of these vanes, below the jumping reach, may be moved out of the way before making subsequent jumps. The chalk or water mark on the wall scale is observed by a technician, who stands on a platform (e.g., a chair or a table) near eye level to the jump mark.

Three jump trials are usually given with the best trial used. If a jumper continues to improve on the third trial, then subsequent trials can be given until no further improvement is observed. Due to the rapid recovery of the relatively small volume of phosphagens used for performing one vertical jump, the time taken to observe and record the height of the jump and to prepare for the next trial (about 60 s) is adequate recovery time between trials.

Summary of Procedural Steps for Vertical Jumps

1. The participant executes a 5–10 min dynamic warm-up including several practice jumps. If using the Vertec, it is especially important to make several practice jumps to become familiarized with the equipment.
2. The technician explains and demonstrates the proper position for the standing reach. (It can be done with the dominant hand alone, or it can be done with the two hands held together.)
   a. Stand with feet together and dominant side near the Vertec or wall.
   b. Reach as high as possible with the dominant hand but keep both feet flat on the floor.
   c. Place the palm of the hand against the Vertec (and push the vanes forward slightly) or against the scale on the wall to make a mark.
3. The technician records the standing reach height (to the closest 0.5 in. if using the Vertec, or the closest 1 cm if using a wall-mounted scale) onto Form 8.2.
4. The technician explains and demonstrates the vertical jump and reach. (It can be done with or without a countermovement and with or without steps.)
   a. The participant lines up one large step back from the Vertec or scale (staying within 2 m).
   b. The participant takes one large, fast step toward the target, dips down into a semi-crouching position (the countermovement), then jumps maximally off both feet straight up from under the Vertec or scale while simultaneously swinging both arms forcefully upward. (Many protocols do not allow a step and some protocols do not allow an arm swing, but most allow a countermovement.)
   c. It is important to coordinate the jump so that the participant contacts the Vertec or wall-mounted scale at the peak height of the jump.
   d. The participant should land with the knees bent to help safely absorb the landing forces.
5. The participant completes at least 3 maximal trials (or continues until the jumping reach height plateaus) with about a 60-s rest between trials.
6. The technician records each trial or simply the highest jumping reach height (to the closest 0.5 in. if using the Vertec, or the closest 1 cm if using a wall-mounted scale) onto Form 8.2.

Calculation of Power for the Vertical Jump Test

Jump Distance (Difference)

The first step in calculating power, when using devices such as the Vertec™, is to determine the actual distance of the jump. The vertical jump distance, or difference (D), is calculated by subtracting the standing reach height from the best jumping reach height. For example, if a jumper's best jumping reach height is 110 in. (inches are used in this case because those are the units in which the Vertec™ measures), and the previously measured standing reach height is 90 in., then the vertical jump or difference is 20 in. (51 cm or 0.51 m).

Mean Power

Mean power, not peak or instantaneous power, can be estimated by knowing the work accomplished over a measured time period. Equation 8.1, also referred to as the Lewis equation,[15] calculates power by considering the duration of the ascending phase of the flight, not the total thrust (push-off) duration. In actuality, the flight time is not measured but is derived from a constant based upon the rate of falling bodies.

Mean power (W) = 2.21 * Body mass (N)

$$* \sqrt{\text{Vertical difference (m)}} \qquad \text{Eq. 8.1}$$

Where: $2.21 = \sqrt{4.9}$

$$2.21 \cdot \sqrt{22.75} \cdot \sqrt{.5} = 285.72$$

(Constant based on rate of falling bodies)

For example, if a person with a body mass of 657 N (67 kg or 148 lb) had a vertical difference between standing reach height and jumping reach height of 0.51 m (51 cm or 20 in), the following calculation (Eq. 8.2) would provide the mean power in watts.

Assume: Body mass = **657** N; Vertical difference = **0.51** m

Mean power (W) = 2.21 * **657** N * $\sqrt{\mathbf{0.51}\text{(m)}}$

$$= \mathbf{1037}\,\text{W} \qquad \text{Eq. 8.2}$$

The term *absolute mean power* is appropriate when the power unit is expressed only as watts (W). The term *relative mean power* is appropriate when absolute watts is divided by body weight (W·kg^{-1}), as in Equations 8.3a and 8.3b. There is a direct, linear relationship ($r = 0.99$)

between peak power output expressed as watts per kilogram body weight and the vertical distance of the center of gravity during the jump from a force platform.[18] The following calculation (Eq. 8.3a and 8.3b) produces the *relative mean power* for the person with an *absolute mean power* of 1037 W and a body weight of 67 kg.

Assume: Absolute mean power = **1037** W;
    Body weight = **67** kg

Relative mean power (W·kg^{-1}) = Absolute mean
    power (W) / Body weight (kg)   Eq. 8.3a

Relative mean power (W·kg^{-1}) = **1037** W
    / **65** kg = **15.5** W·kg^{-1} Eq. 8.3b

The Lewis equation (or Lewis nomogram) has been used to determine mean power since it was published in 1974.[15] The method is still valid today as a measure of average or mean power while jumping, but it is sometimes criticized due to the assumptions on which it is based and because it does not reflect the peak power generated during jumping.[16,24]

Peak Power

Recent studies analyzing force plate data collected during jumping directly measured peak power and formulated equations that can be used to accurately estimate peak power.[32,47] The peak leg power generated during vertical jumping may be more important with regard to predicting sport performance than is the mean power. One method for estimating peak power is known as the Sayers equation (Eq. 8.4a). This particular equation was formulated from a study of 108 participants who completed a counter movement jump (CMJ) on a force plate.[47] Through the use of statistical regression, absolute peak power was estimated from body mass (in kg) and from the height of the CMJ (in cm). In comparison with mean powers estimated from the Lewis equation, peak powers derived from the Sayers equation are about four times higher. Using the same data as were used in the example of mean power, the peak power value is calculated as seen in Equation 8.4b be estimated without calculations by using

Peak power (W) = [51.9 * CMJ height (cm)]
    + [48.9 * Body mass (kg)] − 2007   Eq. 8.4a

$(51.9 \cdot 50) + (48.9 \cdot 83.92) - 2007 = 4691.69 \text{ W}$

Assume: CMJ height = **51** cm; Body mass = **67** kg

Peak power = [51.9 * **51** cm] + [48.9 * **67** kg]
    − 2007 = **3916** W   Eq. 8.4b

The peak power calculated in this example is considered absolute peak power and is described in watts. A relative peak power can be calculated from the absolute peak power in the same way as before for mean power (Eq. 8.5a and 8.5b).

Assume: Absolute peak power = **3916** W;
    Body Weight = **67** kg

Relative peak power (W·kg^{-1}) = Absolute peak
    power (W) / Body weight (kg)   Eq.8.5a

Relative peak power W·kg^{-1} = **3916** W / **67** kg
    = **58.4** W·kg^{-1} Eq. 8.5b

RESULTS AND DISCUSSION

Vertical jump tests are often administered to track and field athletes and to basketball and volleyball players. Some of the high scores reported in the popular media were not produced under the same procedures as the vertical jump described in this manual. For example, some measures were made while the jumper took two or more preparatory steps. In various scientific studies, some low vertical jump scores are the result of using a *more* restrictive method than the one presented here. For example, the jumper's reaching arm may have been restricted to remain in the elevated position during the preparatory and jump phases,[22] or counter movements were disallowed.[23] Counter movements and arm swings combine to improve vertical jumps by more than 10%,[3,4] possibly due to the contributions of the stored elastic energy of the tendon-muscle complex and the neural facilitation of the stretch reflex, but more likely from the longer time available for force development, thus more work initially.[2] If timed optimally, the forward and upward thrusting of the arms enhances the momentum and, hence, the height of the jump.[49]

The results of numerous studies describing vertical jump and leg power are presented in Table 8.1 and Table 8.2. The values in Table 8.1 are representative of typical, active young people (age 21–25 y), with mean

Table 8.1 Norms for Vertical Jump (cm) and Mean Power (W) Derived from the Lewis Equation and Peak Power (W) Derived from the Sayers Equation

Category (percentile)	Vertical Jump (cm)		Mean Power (W)-Lewis		Peak Power (W)-Sayers	
	Men	Women	Men	Women	Men	Women
Well above ave (> 95th %ile)	>71.1	>48.3	>1446	>954	>5554	>3596
Above ave (75th–95th %ile)	62.2–71.1	39.4–48.3	1353–1446	861–954	5092–5554	3134–3596
Average (25th–74th %ile)	50.8–62.1	31.8–39.3	1223–1352	774–860	4500–5091	2740–3133
Below ave (5th–24th %ile)	41.9–50.7	25.4–31.7	1110–1222	692–773	4038–4499	2408–2739
Well below ave (<5th %ile)	<41.9	<25.4	<1110	<692	<4038	<2408
Mean	56.4	35.8	1309	833	4790	2948

Source: Data from Patterson & Peterson (2004)[45]. Based on young adult men (*N* = 312) and women (*N* = 182) from 21–25 y.

Table 8.2 Comparative Data for Mean Vertical Jump and Absolute and Relative Mean Power (Lewis Equation) and Peak Power (Sayers Equation) by Group

Group	Body Weight (kg)	Vertical Jump (cm)	(in)		Mean Power Absolute (W)	Mean Power Relative (W·kg⁻¹)	Peak Power Absolute (W)	Peak Power Relative (W·kg⁻¹)
Males								
Boys, age 10–12 y (N = 543)[a]	42.8	27.0	10.6	SJ	482	11.3	1523	35.6
Boys, age 13–15 y (N = 443)[a]	57.8	34.6	13.6	SJ	737	12.7	2664	46.1
Active college men (N = 52)[b]	77.3	53.0	20.9	CMJ	1220	15.8	4524	58.5
Active college men (N = 59)[c]	78.3	54.0	21.3	CMJ	1247	15.9	4624	59.1
Young men, 21–25 y (N = 312)[d]	78.9	56.4	22.2	CMJ	1284	16.3	4778	60.6
College athletes (N = 69)[e]	80.1	64.7	25.5	CMJ	1396	17.4	5268	65.8
Basketball (N = 58)[f]	91.5	68.4	26.9	CMJ	1640	17.9	6017	65.8
Volleyball (N = 16)[g]	84.0	70.5	27.8	CMJ	1529	18.2	5760	68.6
Females								
Girls, age 10–12 y (N = 544)[a]	44.2	27.1	10.7	SJ	499	11.3	1592	36.0
Girls, age 12–13 y (N = 315)[a]	54.9	34.6	13.6	SJ	700	12.7	2532	46.1
Young women, 21–25 y (N = 182)[d]	63.0	35.8	14.1	CMJ	817	13.0	2932	46.5
Active college women (N = 50)[b]	59.6	36.4	14.3	CMJ	779	13.1	2797	46.9
Active college women (N = 49)[c]	64.7	38.8	15.3	CMJ	873	13.5	3171	49.0
College athletes (N = 49)[e]	63.1	43.0	16.9	CMJ	897	14.2	3310	52.5
Basketball (N = 46)[h]	70.4	48.2	19.0	CMJ	1059	15.0	3937	55.9
Volleyball (N = 15)[i]	73.4	52.5	20.7	CMJ	1153	15.7	4307	58.7

Sources: Data from [a]Taylor et al. (2010)[51]; [b]Maud & Schultz (1986)[39]; [c]Sayers et al. (1999)[47]; [d]Patterson & Peterson (2004)[45]; [e]Johnson & Bahamonde[32]; [f]Hoffman et al. (1996)[29]; [g]Newton et al. (1999)[42]; [h]LaMonte et al. (1999)[35]; [i]Spence et al. (1980).[50]
Note: SJ Squat jump used; CMJ Countermovement jump used; Peak power calculated for boys and girls using "squat jump" Sayers equation[48]; Peak power calculated for men and women using "countermovement jump" Sayers equation.[47]

values of 56.4 cm (22.2 in.) in men and 35.8 cm (14.1 in.) in women.[45] The mean values for vertical jump in Table 8.2 show a steady progression from young boys and girls (10–15 y),[51] through young adults (21–25 y),[45] to trained athletes.[29,35,42,50] It is interesting to note that the increase in vertical jump observed in males with age and training (beyond 15 y of age), from 34.6 to 70.5 cm, is much greater than the increase observed in women, from 34.6 cm (equal to boys at this age) to 52.5 cm. In some athletes, evaluating vertical jump or maximal jumping reach is very important, as with basketball and volleyball. To rebound a basketball or to block a shot in volleyball requires an absolute jumping reach height, based on a combination of the athlete's height, arm length and vertical jump. Basketball and volleyball athletes[29,35,42,50] typically demonstrate high mean values for vertical jump (Table 8.2), which included with their high mean heights, provides the desired jumping reach heights.

Also shown in Table 8.2 are values for mean power and peak power, based on the combination of body mass and vertical jump. Mean power (derived using the Lewis equation) is estimated based on the force of gravity acting on the jumper's body throughout the entire flight time, as determined from the law of falling bodies.[15] Some researchers, however, question the accuracy of the Lewis

equation.[16,25] A more recent derivation, peak power (derived using the Sayers equation) is estimated from body mass and forces acting just during the push-off phase of the jump only.[47] These forces, which were originally measured directly on a force plate, are what allow the estimation of peak power. The leg power values for women are about 60–65% as high as men, which is similar to the comparisons observed in leg strength between men and women. In some sports, leg power is more important than actual vertical jump. Often, heavier persons or athletes, without the highest vertical jumps, can have the highest absolute leg power values. Football is a good example. Leg power, more than actual vertical jump, is an important characteristic of a successful football player. A study of high school football players, identified as "highly recruited" for college scholarships, reported 75 selected offensive linemen had a mean body weight of 131.1 kg and mean vertical jump of 65.1 cm.[19] While the vertical jump of 65.1 cm is not remarkable, the derived peak power of 7782 W far exceeds the peak powers observed in volleyball (5760 W)[42] and basketball (6017 W)[29] players. Leg power has also been determined during repeated jumps, done on a contact mat to measure the flight time of consecutive vertical jumps during a certain time period. Values for average relative power output (W·kg⁻¹) over 60 s of jumping (divided into

15-s intervals) in college-aged volleyball players have been reported as 26.7, 23.4, 21.2, and 16.7 W·kg^{-1} for 0–15 s, 15–30 s, 30–45 s, and 45–60 s, respectively.[5]

Leg power, in addition to being necessary for athletic performance, is also necessary for recreational activities and activities of daily living (ADL) in persons of all fitness levels and ages. Any person who hikes, surfs, snowboards or skis will benefit from additional leg power. Many researchers believe that leg power is more strongly related than strength to physical function and performance of activities of daily living in older adults.[27,47,48] This means that how fast muscles produce force may be more important to function than how much maximal force muscles produce. Sufficient leg power is required for older adults to rapidly cross a street before the light changes, or to move quickly and stabilize the body to prevent a fall. It is now being proposed that when the conditioning goal is to increase ADL ability, the focus of training should be on developing power, not just concentrating on increasing strength.[27]

> **BOX 8.2** **Chapter Preview/Review**
>
> The power generated during the vertical jump test depends on what three components of the jump?
>
> How do the static squat jump and the countermovement jump (CMJ) differ?
>
> What are some different methodologies (and equipment) used to measure vertical jump?
>
> What are five possible reasons that the CMJ results in a greater vertical jump than the static squat jump?
>
> How are vertical jump (or vertical difference) and body mass used to derive leg power?
>
> What is the Lewis equation and what is the Sayers equation?
>
> How much does vertical jump change comparing young children to highly trained adult athletes?
>
> Why is leg power important for older adults?

References

1. Alemdaroglu, U. (2012). The relationship between muscle strength, anaerobic performance, agility, sprint ability and vertical jump performance in professional basketball players. *Journal of Human Kinetics, 31,* 149–158.

2. Bobbert, M. F., Gerritsen, K. G. M., Litjens, M. C., & Van Soest, A. J. (1996). Why is countermovement jump height greater than squat jump height? *Medicine and Science in Sports and Exercise, 28,* 1402–1412.

3. Bosco, C., & Komi, P. V. (1979). Mechanical characteristics and fiber composition of human leg extensor muscles. *European Journal of Applied Physiology, 41,* 275–284.

4. Bosco, C., & Komi, P. V. (1980). Influence of aging on the mechanical behavior of leg extensor muscles. *European Journal of Applied Physiology, 45,* 209–219.

5. Bosco, C., Luhtanen, Pl, & Komi, P. V. (1983). A simple method for measurement of mechanical power in jumping. *European Journal of Applied Physiology, 50,* 273–282.

6. Bosco, C., Mognoni, P., & Luhtanen, P. (1983). Relationship between isokinetic performance and ballistic movement. *European Journal of Applied Physiology, 51,* 357–364.

7. Bosworth, J. M. (1964). *The effect of isometric training and rebound tumbling on performance in the vertical jump.* Master's thesis, Springfield College, MA.

8. Bowers, P., Coleman, A., & Oshiro, T. (1993). Measuring anaerobic power of aged men and women. *Sports Medicine, Training, and Rehabilitation, 4,* 304 (Abstract).

9. Casartelli, N., Muller, R., & Maffiuletti, N. A. (2010). Validity and reliability of the Myotest accelerometric system for the assessment of vertical jump height. *Journal of Strength and Conditioning Research, 24,* 3186–3193.

10. Clarke, H. H. (1957). Relationships of strength and anthropometric measures to physical performances involving the trunk and leg. *Research Quarterly, 28,* 223.

11. Considine, W. J., & Sullivan, W. J. (1973). Relationship of selected tests of leg strength and leg power on college men. *Research Quarterly, 44,* 404–416.

12. Davies, C. T. M., & Young, K. (1984). Effects of external loading on short term power output in children and young male adults. *European Journal of Applied Physiology, 52,* 351–354.

13. de Vries, H. A. (1971). *Laboratory experiments in physiology of exercise.* Dubuque, IA: Wm. C. Brown.

14. de Vries, H. A., & Housh, T. J. (1994). *Physiology of exercise for physical education, athletics, and exercise science.* Dubuque, IA: Brown & Benchmark.

15. Fox, E. L., & Mathews, D. K. (1974). *Interval training: conditioning for sports and general fitness.* Philadelphia: W.B. Saunders College.

16. Garhammer, J. (1993). A review of power output studies of Olympic and powerlifting: Methodology, performance prediction, and evaluation tests. *Journal of Strength and Conditioning Research, 7,* 76–89.

17. Garhammer, J., & Gregor, R. (1992). Propulsion forces as a function of intensity for weightlifting and vertical jumping. *Journal of Applied Sport Science Research, 6,* 129–134.

18. Genuario, S. E., & Dolgener, F. A. (1980). The relationship of isokinetic torque at two speeds to the vertical jump. *Research Quarterly for Exercise and Sport, 51,* 593–598.

19. Ghigiarelli, J. J. (2011). Combine performance descriptors and predictors of recruit ranking for the top high school football recruits from 2001 to 2009: Differences between position groups. *Journal of Strength and Conditioning Research, 25,* 1193–1203.

20. Glatthorn, J. F., Gouge, S., Nussbaumer, S., Stauffacher, S., Impellizzeri, F. M., & Maffiuletti, N. A. (2011). Validity and reliability of Optojump photoelectric cells for estimating vertical jump height. *Journal of Strength and Conditioning Research, 25,* 556–560.

21. Glencross, D. J. (1966). The nature of the vertical jump test and the standing broad jump. *Research Quarterly, 37,* 353–359.

22. Gray, R. K., Start, K. B., & Glencross, D. J. (1962). A test of leg power. *Research Quarterly, 33,* 44.

23. Harman, E. A., Rosenstein, M. T., Frykman, P. N., & Rosenstein, R. M. (1990). The effects of arms and countermovement on vertical jumping. *Medicine and Science in Sports and Exercise, 22,* 825–833.

24. Harman, E. A., Rosenstein, M. T., Frykman, P. N., Rosenstein, R. M., & Kraemer, W. J. (1989). Evaluation of the Lewis power output test. *Medicine and Science in Sports and Exercise, 21* (Suppl.), Abstract #305, S51.

25. Harman, E., Rosenstein, M., Frykman, P., Rosenstein, R., & Kraemer, W. (1991). Estimation of human power output from vertical jump. *Journal of Applied Sport Science Research, 3,* 116–120.

26. Harman, E. A., & Sharp, M. A. (1989). Prediction of power output during vertical jumps using body mass and flight time. *Medicine and Science in Sports and Exercise, 21* (Suppl. 2), Abstract #306, S51.

27. Hazell, T., Kenno, K., & Jakobi, J. (2007). Functional benefit of power training for older adults. *Journal of Aging and Physical Activity, 15,* 349–359.

28. Hennessy, L., & Kilty, J. (2001). Relationship of the stretch-shortening cycle to sprint performance in trained female athletes. *Journal of Strength & Conditioning Research, 15,* 326–331.

29. Hoffman, J. R., Tenenbaum, G., Maresh, C. M., & Kraemer, W. J. (1996). Relationship between athletic performance tests and playing time in elite college basketball players. *Journal of Strength and Conditioning, 10,* 67–71.

30. Hortobagyi, T., Houmard, J. A., Stevenson, J. R., Fraser, D. D., Johns, R. A., & Israel, R. G. (1993). The effects of detraining on power athletes. *Medicine and Science in Sports and Exercise, 25,* 929–935.

31. Johnson, B. L., & Nelson, J. K. (1974). *Practical measurements for evaluation in physical education.* Minneapolis: Burgess.

32. Johnson, D. L., & Bahamonde, R. (1996). Power output estimate in university athletes. *Journal of Strength and Conditioning Research, 10,* 161–166.

33. Kraemer, W. J., & Newton, R. U. (1994). Training for improved vertical jump. *Sports Science Exchange, 7* (6), 1–5.

34. Kujala, U. M., Viljanen, T., Taimela, S., & Viitasalo, J. T. (1994). Physical activity, VO$_2$ and jumping height in an urban population. *Medicine and Science in Sports and Exercise, 26,* 889–895.

35. LaMonte, M. J., McKinney, J. T., Quinn, S. M., Bainbridge, C. N., & Eisenman, P. A. (1999). Comparison of physical and physiological variables for female college basketball players. *Journal of Strength and Conditioning Research, 13,* 264–270.

36. Latchaw, M. (1954). Measuring selected motor skills in fourth, fifth, and sixth grades. *Research Quarterly, 25,* 439.

37. Leard, J. S., Cirillo, M. A., Katsnelson, E., Kimiatek, D. A., Miller, T. W., Trebincevic, K., & Garbalosa, J. S. (2007). Validity of two alternative systems for measuring vertical jump height. *Journal of Strength and Conditioning Research, 21,* 1296–1299.

38. Linthorne, N. P. (2001). Analysis of standing vertical jumps using a force platform. *American Journal of Physics, 69,* 1198–1204.

39. Maud, P. J., & Shultz, B. B. (1986). Gender comparisons in anaerobic power and anaerobic capacity tests. *British Journal of Sports Medicine, 20,* 51–54.

40. Mero, A., & Komi, P. V. (1986). Force-, EMG-, and elasticity-velocity relationships at submaximal, maximal and supramaximal running speeds in sprinters. *European Journal of Applied Physiology, 55,* 553–561.

41. Misner, J. E., Boileau, S. A., Plowman, S. A., Elmore, B. G., Gates, M. A., Gilbert, J. A., & Horswill, C. (1988). Leg power of female firefighter applicants. *Journal of Occupational Medicine, 30,* 433–437.

42. Newton, R. U., Kraemer, W. J., & Hakkinen, K. (1999). Effects of ballistic training on preseason preparation of elite volleyball players. *Medicine and Science in Sports and Exercise, 31,* 323–330.

43. Nuzzo, J., Anning, J., & Scharfenberg, J. (2011). The reliability of three devices used for measuring vertical jump height. *Journal of Strength and Conditioning Research, 25,* 2580–2590.

44. O'Shea, P. (1999). Toward an understanding of power. *Strength and Conditioning Journal, 21,* 34–35.

45. Patterson, D. D., & Peterson, D. F. (2004). Vertical jump and leg power norms for young adults. *Measurement in Physical Education and Exercise Science, 8,* 33–41.

46. Sargent, D. A. (1921). The physical test of a man. *American Physical Education Review, 26,* 188.

47. Sayers, S. P. (2007). High-speed power training: A novel approach to resistance training in older men and women. *Journal of Strength and Conditioning Research, 21,* 518–526.

48. Sayers, S. P., Harackiewicz, D. V., Harman, E. A., Frykman, P. N., & Rosenstein, M. T. (1999). Cross-validation of three jump power equations. *Medicine and Science in Sports and Exercise, 31,* 572–577.

49. Semenick, D. M., & Adams, K. O. (1987). The vertical jump: A kinesiological analysis with recommen-

dations for strength and conditioning programming. *National Strength and Conditioning Association Journal, 8*, 9–13.

50. Spence, D. W., Disch, J. G., Fred, H. L., & Coleman, A. E. (1980). Descriptive profiles of highly skilled women volleyball players. *Medicine and Science in Sports and Exercise, 12*, 299–302.

51. Taylor, M. J. D., Cohen, D., Voss, C. & Sandercock, G. R. H. (2010). Vertical jumping and leg power normative data for English school children aged 10–15 years. *Journal of Sports Sciences, 28*, 867–872.

52. Tharp, G. D., Newhouse, R. K., Uffleman, L., Thorland, W. G., & Johnson, G. O. (1985). Comparison of sprint and run times with performance on the Wingate anaerobic test. *Research Quarterly for Exercise and Sport, 56*, 73–76.

53. Viitasalo, J. T. (1988). Evaluation of explosive strength for young and adult athletes. *Research Quarterly, 59*, 9–13.

Vertical jump is used to measure power when also considering body mass

It's sport specific though, grandma wouldn't care

Force (W) = $\frac{Nm}{s} = \frac{J}{s}$

It's not a strength test because it's not a maximal effort from the muscle... more attempts wouldn't lead to performance decrement

CMJ = counter movement jump = higher than static jump because

1. accustomed skill
2. Added force from tissue recoil
3. enhanced muscle fiber recruitment from stretch reflex
4. altered properties of contractile machinery
5. longer time available for force development

Can use wall/chalk/meter stick, vertec, force plate (indirect measure)

Measure standing reach, jumping reach; measure difference (called vertical difference)

Calculate mean power

Absolute Mean power (W) = ~~[illegible]~~ 2.21 · Body weight (N) · √vertical difference (m)

Relative Mean power ($\frac{W}{kg}$) = absolute mean power (W) / Body mass (kg)

Calculate peak power

Peak power (W) = [51.9 · CMJ height (cm)] + [48.9 · Body mass (kg)] − 2007

Normative values

	Vert jump (cm)	absolute Mean Power (w)	Peak Power (w)	
men	51-62	1223-1352	4500-5091	) mean power ·4
women	32-39	774-860	2740-3133	to peak power
		relative mean power (w)	relative peak power ($\frac{W}{kg}$)	
men		16 W/kg	60 W/kg	
women		13 W/kg	46 W/kg	

Form 8.1

JUMPING—VERTICAL POWER

Homework

Gender: **M**   Initials: **AA**   Age (y): **20**   Weight (kg): **75.0**   Body mass (N): _____

Standing reach (in.)   **89.0**   *Measured with feet flat on floor using jumping hand*

Jumping reach (in.) T_1 **108.0** T_2 **109.0** T_3 **109.5** T_4 **109.5**   Best _____   *(closest 0.5 in.)*

Vertical jump = _____ in. = _____ cm =   Vertical difference (D) _____ m

Absolute mean power (W) =   2.21 * _____ * √ _____ = _____ W
Lewis equation   Body mass (N)   √ D (m)

Relative mean power (W·kg^{-1}) = _____ W / _____ kg = _____ W·kg^{-1}

Absolute peak power (W) =   [51.9 * _____] + [48.9 * _____] - 2007 = _____ W
Sayers CMJ equation   VJ (cm)   Wt (kg)

Relative peak power (W·kg^{-1}) = _____ W / _____ kg = _____ W·kg^{-1}

Category *(Table 8.1)* for: _____   _____   _____
                                            Vertical jump   Mean power   Peak power

Evaluation/comments: _____

_____

_____

Gender: **F**   Initials: **BB**   Age (y): **20**   Weight (kg): **60.0**   Body mass (N): _____

Standing reach (in.)   **83.0**   *Measured with feet flat on floor using jumping hand*

Jumping reach (in.) T_1 **101.5** T_2 **101.5** T_3 **102.5** T_4 _____   Best _____   *(closest 0.5 in.)*

Vertical jump = _____ in. = _____ cm =   Vertical difference (D) _____ m

Absolute mean power (W) =   2.21 * _____ * √ _____ = _____ W
Lewis equation   Body mass (N)   √ D (m)

Relative mean power (W·kg^{-1}) = _____ W / _____ kg = _____ W·kg^{-1}

Absolute peak power (W) =   [51.9 * _____] + [48.9 * _____] - 2007 = _____ W
Sayers CMJ equation   VJ (cm)   Wt (kg)

Relative peak power (W·kg^{-1}) = _____ W / _____ kg = _____ W·kg^{-1}

Category *(Table 8.1)* for: _____   _____   _____
                                            Vertical jump   Mean power   Peak power

Evaluation/comments: _____

_____

_____

jump distance = 50 cm = .5 m

mean absolute power (w) = 2.21 · 822.75 · √.5 = 1285.72 W

mean relative power (w/kg) = 1285.72 W/83.92 kg = 15.32 w/kg

peak absolute power = (51.9·50) + (47.9·83.92) - 2007
= 4691.69 W

peak relative power = 4691.69/83.92 = 55.91 w/kg

Form 8.2
JUMPING—VERTICAL POWER

NAME __Tyler Gilmore__   DATE __2/11__   SCORE _____

Lab Results

Gender: __M__   Initials: __TG__   Age (y): __21__   Weight (kg): __83.92__   Body mass (N): __822.75__

Mass *Weight*

Standing reach (in.) _____   *Measured with feet flat on floor using jumping hand*

Jumping reach (in.) T_1 ____ T_2 ____ T_3 ____ T_4 ____   Best ____   *(closest 0.5 in.)*

Vertical jump = ____ in. = ____ cm =   Vertical difference (D) ____ m

Absolute mean power (W) =   2.21 * ____ * √ ____ = ____ W
Lewis equation   Body mass (N)   √ D (m)

jump distance = .5 m
mean absolute power = 1285.72 W
mean relative power = 15.32 W/kg
peak absolute power = 4691.69 W
peak relative power = 55.91 w/kg

Relative mean power (W·kg⁻¹) = ____ W / ____ kg = ____ W·kg⁻¹

Absolute peak power (W) =   [51.9 * ____] + [48.9 * ____] - 2007 = ____ W
Sayers CMJ equation   VJ (cm)   Wt (kg)

Relative peak power (W·kg⁻¹) = ____ W / ____ kg = ____ W·kg⁻¹

Category (Table 8.1) for:
____ Vertical jump   ____ Mean power   ____ Peak power

Evaluation/comments: My vertical jump distance is near average for my demographic category. I also fell at average for mean absolute power, mean relative power and peak absolute power, while my peak relative power was slightly below average.

Gender: ____   Initials: ____   Age (y): ____   Weight (kg): ____   Body mass (N): ____

Standing reach (in.) _____   *Measured with feet flat on floor using jumping hand*

Jumping reach (in.) T_1 ____ T_2 ____ T_3 ____ T_4 ____   Best ____   *(closest 0.5 in.)*

Vertical jump = ____ in. = ____ cm =   Vertical difference (D) ____ m

Absolute mean power (W) =   2.21 * ____ * √ ____ = ____ W
Lewis equation   Body mass (N)   √ D (m)

Relative mean power (W·kg⁻¹) = ____ W / ____ kg = ____ W·kg⁻¹

Absolute peak power (W) =   [51.9 * ____] + [48.9 * ____] - 2007 = ____ W
Sayers CMJ equation   VJ (cm)   Wt (kg)

Relative peak power (W·kg⁻¹) = ____ W / ____ kg = ____ W·kg⁻¹

Category (Table 8.1) for:
____ Vertical jump   ____ Mean power   ____ Peak power

Evaluation/comments:
_____
_____
_____

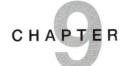

ANAEROBIC CYCLING

The most popular anaerobic cycling test is the Wingate Anaerobic Test (WAnT), named after a university in Israel. The original test[17] was designed for adolescents but became popular for adults in the late 1970s.[6] It fulfilled the need for a precisely measured anaerobic power test. It may be used to test either arm or leg power but is most commonly used to test the legs.

This anaerobic test can determine the participant's **peak anaerobic power, mean anaerobic power, total work,** and **fatigue index.** *Peak power* is based on the highest power level averaged usually over a 5 s period during the test, whereas *mean power* refers to the average power during the entire 30 s of the test. The *total work* represents the product of the number of pedal revolutions accomplished and the force or resistance during the 30 s test. The *fatigue index* measures the rate of power decrease from the point of peak anaerobic power to the finish of the test.

RATIONALE FOR THE WINGATE TEST

The Wingate Anaerobic Test is truly a supramaximal test when maximal oxygen consumption serves as the maximal reference point, because the WAnT usually requires a power level that, in turn, would require two to four times the participant's maximal oxygen consumption.[8] Thus, the physiological basis of the Wingate Test is best understood by focusing mainly on the contributions of the anaerobic pathways to the major components of the Wingate Test. One reviewer of anaerobic tests concluded that 30 s is an optimal duration for an all-out test of anaerobic work or mean anaerobic power.[24] The first several seconds of the WAnT rely predominantly on the phosphagen system. The total work during the 30 s WAnT requires energy production from both the phosphagen and lactic acid systems. Hence, participants in the WAnT test may receive from 60 %[42] or 66 %[11] up to 85 %[21] of their ATP from the powerful phosphagenic component and the enduring glycolytic component of the anaerobic pathways (see Figure 9.1).

Peak Anaerobic Power

We use *peak anaerobic power,* as opposed to *peak power,* to help identify the WAnT as a measure of anaerobic fitness. Cycle ergometry will also be used in a later chapter to measure peak aerobic power (determined by $\dot{V}O_2max$),

considered by many to be the best laboratory measure of aerobic fitness. Peak anaerobic power is usually reached within the first 2 s,[24] 5 s,[26,51,55] 8 s,[32] or 10 s[55] of supramaximal exercise. One group of investigators determined the ATP contribution of the phosphagenic pathway during the first 10 s of all-out cycling in recreational athletes by sampling biopsied muscle.[11] Discounting the ATP stores, they reported that the phosphagenic pathway contributed 43 % of the *anaerobic* energy supply. Contrary to earlier reports,[35,36] even in the first 10 s, the glycolytic pathway makes a significant contribution based on lactate values after 10 s that may be four times the resting value.[31]

Mean Anaerobic Power and Total Work

Mean anaerobic power has often been considered equivalent to anaerobic capacity,[24] but the promoter of the WAnT, Dr. Bar-Or,[8] prefers the term *mean anaerobic power* when watts is the unit of measure. Mean anaerobic power mainly reflects the ability to transform energy from the anaerobic glycolytic pathway. Whereas the phosphagenic pathway is the main contributor of ATP, the glycolytic pathway contributes most to a performer's mean anaerobic power and total work in the 30 s test. Based on vastus lateralis biopsies of recreational athletes who cycled all-out for 30 s, the phosphagen system contributed 21 %, the glycolytic system 45 %, and the aerobic system 34 % of the total required ATP production[11] as seen Figure 9.1. The 21 % from the phosphagen system agrees with earlier reports of 23 % in aerobically trained men.[51] Despite contributing as much as 45 %,[11] or 49 %[51] of all the ATP, and, therefore, being the main contributor during the Wingate Test, the glycolytic capacity is not fully utilized due to the short (30 s) duration of the test.[29] Thus, some investigators suggest that the term *anaerobic capacity* may be misleading,[30] despite the report[7] of its correlation with maximal accumulated oxygen debt (MAOD). The 30 s duration of the Wingate Test is certainly shorter than the 40 s[35] or 2 min[41] that may be required to exhaust the anaerobic capacity or maximize the lactate production volume. However, it is possible that the maximal *rate,* not total amount, of lactate production, which indicates anaerobic power,[40] may occur sometime during the Wingate Test. The anaerobic glycolytic production of ATP is evidenced by the moderate-to-high blood lactate values (ranging from 6 to 15 times the resting value) measured in Wingate Test participants.[30,53,56]

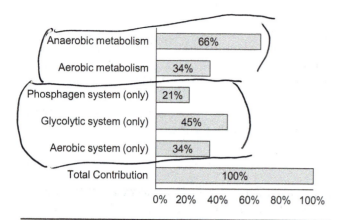

Figure 9.1 The percentage contribution of anaerobic and aerobic metabolism, and each energy system individually, to ATP production during 30 s of maximal exercise. Source: Bogdanis et al. (1996).[11]

The phosphagenic contribution to the entire 30 s of the test was substantiated by investigators[30] who found that female participants reduced their phosphagen levels to 70 % of their original adenosine triphosphate values

and 40 % of their original creatine phosphate values after performing the Wingate Test. Recreational men athletes reduced their creatine phosphate stores to 17 % of pre-exercise levels.[11]

It is appropriate to affix a higher role during the WAnT by Type II (fast-twitch) fibers than to Type I (slow-twitch) fibers because of the significant correlation between Type II fibers and mean anaerobic power.[20] Therefore, because the Wingate Test is a maximal-effort exercise bout for 30 s, it relies principally upon the two anaerobic pathways and secondarily upon the oxidative (aerobic) metabolic pathway to produce ATP.[28,51] Figure 9.1 illustrates the primary role of the anaerobic pathway during the WAnT.

METHODS

The methodology for the Wingate Test includes a brief description of the equipment, such as ergometer, counter, and timer; it also includes a description of the test procedures and calculations. For a discussion on the accuracy of the Wingate Test, see Box 9.1.

BOX 9.1   Accuracy of the Wingate Test (WAnT)

Reliability

It appears that the day-to-day variability of anaerobic power tests is similar to aerobic tests—that is, about 5 % to 6 %.[14,57] The variability of the Wingate Test is partly attributed to its reliability. Reliability coefficients (test-retest comparisons) for maximal anaerobic power/capacity are very high, usually ranging from 0.95 to 0.98.[21,28,31] The retesting reliability of the fatigue index can range from such low values as near 0.43 to moderate values near 0.73.[57] The intraclass correlation coefficient (ICC) for repeat WAnT within one week of each other was $r = 0.98$ for mean anaerobic power.[58]

Validity

There is no "gold standard" anaerobic performance test by which to compare the scores of the Wingate Test. It might be argued that for the Wingate Test to have physiological validity, the performers with the highest lactate values after the Wingate Test would be expected to have the highest glycolytic or anaerobic capacities. In a validation study,[53] only a moderate relationship ($r = 0.55$ and 0.60) was reported between mean anaerobic power (W and W·kg⁻¹) and blood lactates; the relationship between mean anaerobic power and maximal oxygen debt was slightly lower. These researchers concluded that the test's validity was tenuous. Another research group, using the accumulated oxygen deficit as a measure of anaerobic energy release, agrees that the WAnT "may not be a proper anaerobic capacity test" because it does not exhaust the anaerobic capacity.[42] However, because of the contributions of the phosphagenic and oxidative systems, the Wingate's validity should not be dependent upon its ability to incur maximal lactates or on its ability to exhaust anaerobic energy sources. For example, investigators supported the test's physiological validity by finding a significant relationship between both the peak anaerobic power and the total work versus the fast-twitch fiber area and percentage.[31]

Its performance validity was supported by the high relationship between peak power and the time for the 50 m run ($r = -0.91$),[31] and the vertical jump.[36] Low to moderate correlations have been reported between mean AnP and 50 m time ($r = -0.79$)[57] and 300 m cycling time ($r = -0.75$).[46] Low and moderate correlations also were reported between total work and the 300 m run ($r = -0.64$; -0.83).[10,46] Lean body mass and peak isokinetic torque are positively related to anaerobic mean power.[1] Further evidence of the test's validity is provided by the higher power outputs found in more elite cyclists than less elite cyclists.[54] It seems logical that the WAnT would relate more closely to anaerobic cycling events than to anaerobic running events.[22] However, the WAnT improves the predictability of run performance when power is divided by body mass (W·kg⁻¹).[55]

Finally, a brief comment on the mechanical validity of the WAnT is in order, though the details are beyond the scope of this laboratory manual. In the mid-1980s, it became apparent that corrections for acceleration and deceleration of the flywheel were necessary to produce valid power outputs.[16] The power outputs derived from WAnT on a mechanically braked (friction) cycle ergometer (e.g., Monark™ 324E), which provided much of the published data, included only the braking resistance (force) and flywheel velocity. Power outputs on such cycle ergometers are much lower than the corrected power outputs for peak power and slightly lower for mean power.[48] Fortunately, electrically braked ergometers reduce the inertial effects. Additionally, computer software makes corrections more practical. For more information, the reader is referred to detailed descriptions of the corrections.[15,48]

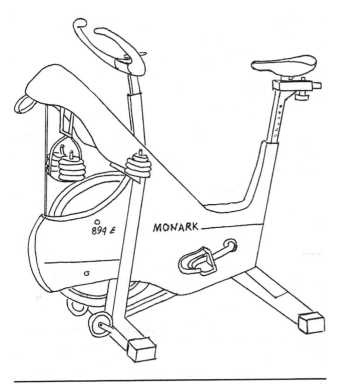

Figure 9.2 This model of Monark™ cycle ergometer is especially well suited for fast addition of force or resistance by loading weights on the basket, producing friction by way of the cord wrapped around the flywheel.

Equipment

The Wingate Anaerobic Test (WAnT) is most commonly done on a commercially available mechanically-braked cycle ergometer. Power during cycling is determined by the force or resistance (kg) and the cadence or speed (rpm) at which the cyclist pedals. By using a cycle ergometer set at a constant force, the cyclist can attempt to generate the most power possible by pedaling at the highest cadence possible. A popular ergometer in use is the Monark® 894E Peak Bike (Monark AB, Varberg, Sweden), shown in Figure 9.2. This particular "basket-style" of ergometer allows a pre-determined force to be loaded onto the ergometer, where it can be "suspended" during warm up, until it is "dropped" at the actual start of the test. This allows for an accurate force to be instantly applied to the ergometer at the very start of the WAnT. Other "pendulum-style" cycle ergometers can be used (similar to the Monark® 828E, etc.) that require turning a knob to adjust the force being exerted on the flywheel through a friction belt. Ergometers using this method of force application are not as accurate and take longer at the start of the test to set the desired force. They are still an appropriate piece of equipment and are frequently used. An isokinetic cycle ergometer, that controlled pedaling speed at 60 rpm, has also been used to measure exercise capacity during 30 s of cycling.[34]

Ideally, the cycle ergometer being used for the WAnT is interfaced with a computer, and through the use of special software, all required test data are automatically recorded. The Monark® 894E Peak Bike comes with such software (Monark Anaerobic Test Software) or other software is available (Sports Medicine Industries, Inc., St. Cloud, MN) which generates values for a variety of variables recorded in 5-s intervals over the 30-s test. When an automated system is not available, and the WAnT is being done manually, some type of timer is required. This can be a stopwatch, a digital watch (with a chronograph), or a laboratory clock. It is convenient, but not necessary, to have some hand-held "tally" counters that reset to zero to count the number of pedal revolutions. They are available at many office supply stores. An accurate platform-beam scale or electronic digital scale is also needed to measure the body weight of the participant.

Test Procedures

Teamwork among technicians is essential for the accurate administration of the WAnT; thus, the test procedures should be rehearsed prior to the actual test. Some of the factors to consider in the test procedures are (a) preparation, (b) Wingate Test protocol, and (c) the roles of timer, force setter, revolutions counter, and recorder.

Force Setting

The body weight is necessary not only to derive the relative power and work scores, but to prescribe the force setting on the ergometer. The force setting varies with such factors as the general anaerobic fitness of the performer, gender, age, and the type of ergometer.[9,23] Obtaining the optimal force for each person would require testing that person several times. Thus, for practical reasons, equations are presented that may approximate the optimal force setting for a person.

The original force settings for the WAnT were based on body weight, with a setting of 0.075 kg per kilogram of body weight for leg ergometry and 0.050 kg per kilogram for arm ergometry.[6,21,32,43] The force setting used for the WAnT is calculated as seen in Equations 9.1a and 9.1b. Because these force settings are both ratios with kg in the numerator and denominator, they may also be described as a percentage of body weight, as 7.5 % of body weight (kg) for leg ergometry and 5.0 % for arm ergometry. Other laboratories and researchers have chosen to use higher force settings for leg ergometry in more active participants (8.6–9.0 % of body weight)[8,12,19,57] and in anaerobically trained athletes (9–11 % of body weight).[13,45,52,54] One study reported that force settings greater than 10 % of body weight do not further increase WAnT scores.[18]

Leg ergometry: Force (kg) = Body weight (kg) * 0.075

Eq. 9.1a

Arm ergometry: Force (kg) = Body weight (kg) * 0.050

Eq. 9.1b

Table 9.1   Wingate Test Protocol

Period	Time Length	Activity
Warm-up period	5 min	Cycle at low to moderate intensity; intersperse with two to five sprints of 4–6 s at prescribed force (F).
Recovery interval	2–5 min	Rest or cycle slowly against minimal F.
Acceleration period	7–15 s	1st phase: Cycle for 5–10 s at one-third prescribed F at 60–70 rpm.
		2nd phase: Cycle 2–5 s against F; approaching prescribed F at near-maximal rpm.
Wingate Test	30 s	Cycle at highest rpm possible against prescribed F.
Cool-down period	2–3 min	Cycle at low to moderate aerobic power level (e.g., 25–100 W).

Wingate Test Protocol Components

The Wingate protocol (Table 9.1) has five distinct components or time periods: (1) warm-up, (2) recovery interval, (3) acceleration period, (4) Wingate Test, and (5) cool-down period.

As with the other anaerobic tests, warm-up is recommended for both safety (e.g., muscle injury and ischemic heart prevention)[4,5] and performance reasons.[39] The **warm-up** includes 5 min of low- to moderate-intensity pedaling at about 60–70 rpm, interspersed by two to five all-out sprints of 4–6 s duration; the sprints should progressively increase in resistance (force) so that by the fourth or fifth sprint approaches the prescribed resistance for the Wingate Test.[9,27]

The **recovery interval** between the end of the warm-up and the beginning of the Wingate Test should not be less than 2 min or more than 5 min after the warm-up period. The 2 min minimum provides adequate recovery time from any possible fatigue that the participant may have incurred during the warm-up. The 5 min maximum recovery still retains muscle temperature and blood flow to a significant extent. The activity during the recovery interval may consist of simply resting while seated on the bike or pedaling at a minimal resistance.

The **acceleration period** consists of two brief phases beginning immediately after the recovery interval. In the first phase, the participant pedals at about 60–70 rpm for about 5–10 s at a resistance that is about one-third of that prescribed from one of the chosen equations. In the second phase, the participant increases the rpm to a near-maximal rate while the technician loads the prescribed force (F) setting immediately, if using a basket-loaded ergometer, or within 2–5 s if using a pendulum-loaded ergometer. The total acceleration period, therefore, may last for as little as 7 s or as long as 15 s.

The actual **Wingate Test duration** of all-out cycling is 30 s. It begins at the end of the acceleration period and divides the 30 s into six continuous time intervals of 5 s each. The participant continuously tries to obtain the highest number of revolutions during each 5 s interval. For example, the participant does not pace the effort so that the last 5 s contains as many revolutions as the previous 5 s intervals. Thus, the test can be described as a rush to the peak power and a fading to the lowest power.

The **cool-down** period lasts 2–3 min[9] and consists of pedaling at a low to moderate power level (25–100 W) on the cycle ergometer immediately after the Wingate Test. If a repeat test on the same person and on the same day is necessary, then about 10 min of recovery is recommended.[2,25]

Technician Roles during Manually Administered Test

If the WAnT is being administered manually, a team of technicians is required all with specific roles, including a timer, force setter, counter and recorder. The *Timer* oversees the administration of the entire test. The timer directs the first two components of the protocol including the warm-up period and recovery interval prior to starting the acceleration period and the actual 30-s test. During the test, the timer loudly calls out the end of each 5-s period ("5!", "10!", etc.) until ending the test at the 30-s mark and initiating the cool-down period. The *Force Setter* calculates, applies and maintains the appropriate forces required during each component of the protocol. The *Counter (or Counters)* observes the pedaling of the participant and counts each full revolution, each time one pedal (i.e., the right) crosses a specific point in the 360° pedaling cycle. A piece of black tape placed horizontally on the ergometer at the level of the center of rotation of the pedals makes a good reference point. Thus, one revolution is when the pedal begins at the tape mark (which is at the 90° point in the rotation or the "3 o'clock" position) and finishes at the tape mark. The counter calls out the number of full revolutions completed in the 5-s interval ("15!", "12!", etc.) as prompted by the timer and begins counting the revolutions for the next 5-s interval. It can be difficult, because of the high initial pedal rates, for the counter to accurately "restart" counting each 5-s interval. For this reason, it is helpful to have 2 counters that can switch on and off between the alternating 5-s intervals. The *Recorder* is responsible for recording all data associated with the entire protocol. During the actual 30-s test, the recorder listens carefully for the counter to call out the number of revolutions completed in each 5-s interval and records them onto Form 9.2. Good teamwork among technicians is essential for administrating the WAnT. Therefore, the test procedures should be rehearsed prior to the actual test. The manually administered test, however, will still not be as accurate as the automated test using the interfaced computer.

Summary of Preparation and Procedural Steps

Preparation, Warm up, and Recovery Interval

1. Measure and record body weight (without shoes).
2. Determine the force (kg) to be used, ranging from 0.05 to 0.10 kg per kg of body weight.

3. Adjust the seat height on the ergometer so that the participant pedals with a slight knee bend at full down-stroke of the pedal. Using a goniometer to set knee angle to 25° at full down-stroke has been recommended.[47] Adjust the toe clips ("caged" pedals) if being used.

4. The participant begins pedaling for 5 min at 60–70 rpm at low force (1.0–1.5 kg) to warm up.

5. During the warm up, explain briefly all components of the protocol (Table 9.1) to the participant and further explain that it is very important to give an "all out effort" during the 30 s of the actual WAnT.

6. Interspersed during the warm up, the participant completes 2 to 3 short 5-s "high speed spins" at moderate force (2–4 kg) to become familiarized with the test.

7. A 2 to 5-min recovery interval follows the warm up, where the participant pedals at 60–70 rpm at very low force (0–1 kg).

Acceleration Period, WAnT, and Cool Down

1. The technicians prepare for the test, and the participant is told that it is time for the hard part of the test and to give an "all out effort" for the full 30 s, right from the start of the test.

2. The participant is instructed to accelerate over 3–5 s to a full sprint. During this time the technician (the timer) counts down, "3-2-1-Go!". If a pendulum-type ergometer is being used, the force is increased during this time to the desired level by the force setter.

3. At the command of "Go!", the weight is "dropped" (if using a basket-type ergometer) by the force setter and either the computerized system is activated, or if being done manually, the team goes to work.

4. At the end of each 5-s interval the timer calls out the time ("5", "10", etc.), the counter calls out the number of revolutions during that time interval ("15", "12", etc.), and the recorder records the number of revolutions on Form 9.2.

5. The technician (the force setter) verbally encourages the participant to give a maximal effort throughout the test ("Go!", "Don't stop!", "10 more seconds!"). If a pendulum-style ergometer is being used, the force setter monitors and adjusts the force if needed.

6. At the 30-s mark the test is concluded by the timer ("Stop!") and the final number of revolutions is recorded. If using the computerized system, the data collection is stopped.

7. The force is reduced to 0–1 kg and the participant completes a 2–3 min cool down by pedaling 60–70 rpm. (The technicians should be aware that the WAnT can frequently cause nausea and potentially vomiting in participants due to the high production of lactic acid.)

8. Calculations are performed to derive peak anaerobic power, total work, mean anaerobic power, and fatigue index.

Monark Test Report Monark Anaerobic Test
Created: 4.12.2012

Person Information

First Name:	Daniel	Height [cm]:	175
Last Name:	Scott	Weight [kg]:	80
Sex:	Male	Date of Birth:	10.23.1989

Test Information

Test Duration [s]:	30	Date:	4.12.2012
Brake Weight [kg]:	6.0	Supervisor:	
Person Weight [kg]:	80		

Analysis

Peak Power [W]:	707.94	Power Drop [W]:	353.65
Peak Power [W/kg]:	8.85	Power Drop [W/kg]:	4.42
		Power Drop [W/s]:	11.79
Avg. Power [W]:	531.25	Power Drop [W/s/kg]:	0.147
Avg. Power [W/kg]:	6.64	Power Drop [%]:	50.0
Min. Power [W]:	354.29		
Min. Power [W/kg]:	4.43		

Figure 9.3 Sample results from the Monark™ automated cycle ergometer power test.

Calculations

The data collected during the Wingate Test can be used to determine numerous related variables, including absolute peak and mean anaerobic power (W), relative peak and mean anaerobic power (W·kg^{-1}), absolute total work (kJ), relative total work (J·kg^{-1}), and fatigue index (%). Equations to calculate each of these variables are included. These same calculations can be performed by a computer interfaced with the appropriate hardware and software.[44] A sample of the results generated from a Wingate Test completed on a computerized Monark™ ergometer is included in Figure 9.3.

Peak Anaerobic Power

Peak anaerobic power (the highest power produced in any of the 5 s intervals; nearly always the *first* 5 s interval) is derived from the work done during the interval divided by the time. Work, being the mathematical product of force and distance, is calculated as the product of the force setting on the ergometer times the distance cycled during the 5s interval. To get the preferred units for power, which are watts (W), the force setting (kg) is converted to newtons (N) by multiplying by 9.8067 (Eq. 9.2a). The distance cycled is calculated for the specific ergometer used. Assuming a Monark™ cycle ergometer is used, completing 1 pedal revolution is equivalent to cycling 6 m (based on the size of the flywheel). So by knowing the number of pedal revolutions in any 5 s interval, the distance cycled during that interval is the product of the number of revolutions (# Rev) times 6 m per revolution (Eq. 9.2b). Once the force (N) and the distance cycled (m) are known, the work is calculated as the product of these two variables, which can then be divided by the time (5 s) to yield power, or the peak anaerobic power attained during the WAnT (Eq. 9.2c). The resultant unit for peak anaerobic power is a $N \cdot m \cdot s^{-1}$, which is equal to a watt (W). For example, if a participant completes 10 pedal revolutions (# Rev) against a force setting of 6.0kg (59 N) in 5 s, the calculated peak anaerobic power (Eq. 9.2d) is 708 W.

Force setting (N) = Force setting (kg) * 9.8067   Eq. 9.2a

Distance (m) = Number of revolutions
   * Distance per revolution (6 m)   Eq. 9.2b

Peak anaerobic power (W) = [Force (N)* #Rev
   * 6 m·rev^{-1}]/5 s   Eq. 9.2c

Assume: Force = **59** N(6.0 kg); #Rev = **10**; Time = **5** s

Peak anaerobic power = [**59** N* **10** rev
   * 6 m·rev^{-1}] / **5**s = **708** W   Eq. 9.2d

The value just described for peak anaerobic power is considered an "absolute" amount because it is expressed regardless of body weight. However, it is often desirable to express this value "relative" to a person's body weight so that persons of differing body weight can be more equally compared. Dividing the participant's peak anaerobic power by body weight yields relative peak anaerobic power (Eq. 9.3a). If we assume that the participant described above, who had a peak anaerobic power of 709 W, has a body weight of 80 kg, then the relative peak anaerobic power is determined to be 8.9 W·kg^{-1} (Eq. 9.3b).

Relative peak anaerobic power (W·kg^{-1})
   = Peak anaerobic power (W) / Body wt (kg)   Eq. 9.3a

Assume: Peak anaerobic power = **708** W; Body wt = **80** kg

Relative peak anaerobic power = **708** W / **80** kg
   = **8.9** W·kg^{-1} Eq. 9.3b

Total Work

Total work is based upon the total number of revolutions at the end of the 30 s test and the force setting against which the participant pedaled. If an automated counter set to zero at the start of the test is used, then the counter's display at the end of the 30 s test is the total number of revolutions. If the revolutions are counted by a technician's observation, then the total number of revolutions is the sum of the six 5 s revolutions. The calculation of total work (Eq. 9.4a) is similar to that described previously; it is the product of the force setting (N) times the total distance cycled (which is the number of revolutions cycled times 6 m per pedal revolution). The unit resulting from this calculation is a newton meter (N·m). This is an acceptable SI unit, but the preferred unit in which to express work is the joule (J) or kilojoule (kJ). The joule is equal to 1 N·m, and 1 kJ is equal to 1000 J. If a person completes 45 total revolutions

against a force of 59 N, the total work accomplished during this 30 s test is 15 930 N·m, which is equal to 15 900 J or 15.9 kJ.

Total work (kJ) = Force (N) * # Revolutions
   * 6 m·rev^{-1} / 1000   Eq. 9.4a

Assume: Force = **59** N (6.0 kg); **45** revolutions

Total work = **59** N * **45** rev * 6 m·rev^{-1} / 1000
   = **15.9** kJ   Eq. 9.4b

Total work may also be expressed relative to body weight by dividing the total work completed during the WAnT by the participant's body weight (Eq. 9.5a). This again allows for a more meaningful comparison of two persons who differ in body weight. If the participant described above, who completed 15 930 J of total work, has a body weight of 80 kg, the relative total work completed during the entire 30 s test would be 199 J·kg^{-1} (Eq. 9.5b).

Relative total work (J·kg^{-1}) = Total work (J)
   / Body wt (kg)   Eq. 9.5a

Assume: Total work = **15 930** J; Body weight = **80** kg

Relative total work = **15 930** J / **80** kg = **199** J·kg^{-1} Eq. 9.5b

Mean Anaerobic Power

The average or *mean* anaerobic power, in contrast to the *peak* anaerobic power, which was the highest power attained during one 5 s interval, is the power averaged over the entire 30 s test. Mean anaerobic power is a function of the total work completed during the test. Because power is work expressed per unit of time, power can be calculated by dividing the work performed by the time over which that work was completed. So in this case, mean anaerobic power can be calculated (Eq. 9.6a) as the total work done during the WAnT divided by the total time of the test (30 s). Going back to the previous example of total work, someone completing 15 930 J of work in 30 s would be working at a mean anaerobic power of 530 J·s^{-1} or 530 W (since 1 J·s^{-1} = 1 W) over the duration of the test (Eq. 9.6b). Furthermore, mean anaerobic power, just like many of the variables described previously pertaining to the Wingate Anaerobic Test, may also be expressed relative to body weight (Eq. 9.6c). The *relative* mean anaerobic power for a person with a mean anaerobic power of 531 W and a body weight of 80 kg works out to 6.6 W·kg^{-1} (Eq. 9.6d).

Mean anaerobic power (W) = Total work (J)
   / Time (s)   Eq. 9.6a

Assume: Total work = **15 930** J; Time = **30** s

Mean anaerobic power = 15930 J / 30 s = **531** W   Eq. 9.6b

Relative mean anaerobic power (W·kg^{-1})
   = Mean anaerobic power (W) / Body wt (kg)   Eq. 9.6c

Assume: Mean anaerobic power = **531** W; Body wt = **80** kg

Relative mean anaerobic power = **531** W / **80** kg
   = **6.6** W·kg^{-1} Eq. 9.6d

Table 9.2 **Category for Peak and Mean Anaerobic Power and Fatigue Index for Men and Women**

| Category | %ile | Peak Anaerobic Power | | | | Mean Anaerobic Power | | | | Fatigue Index | |
| | | Men (N = 52) | | Women (N = 50) | | Men | | Women | | Men | Women |
		Absolute (W)	Relative (W·kg⁻¹)	Absolute (W)	Relative (W·kg⁻¹)	Absolute (W)	Relative (W·kg⁻¹)	Absolute (W)	Relative (W·kg⁻¹)	(%)	(%)
Well above ave	95	867	11.1	602	9.3	677	8.6	483	7.5	21	20
Above average	90	822	10.9	560	9.0	662	8.2	470	7.3	23	25
	85	807	10.6	530	8.9	631	8.1	437	7.1	27	25
	75	768	10.4	518	8.6	604	8.0	414	6.9	30	28
Average	70	757	10.2	505	8.5	600	7.9	410	6.8	31	29
	50	689	9.2	449	7.6	565	7.4	381	6.4	38	35
	30	656	8.5	399	6.9	530	7.0	353	6.0	43	40
Below average	25	646	8.3	396	6.8	521	6.8	347	5.9	45	42
	15	594	7.4	362	6.4	485	6.4	320	5.6	47	44
	10	570	7.1	353	6.0	471	6.0	306	5.3	52	47
Well below ave	5	530	6.6	329	5.7	453	5.6	287	5.1	55	48
Mean		700	9.2	455	7.6	563	7.3	381	6.4	38	35
S.D.		95	1.4	81	1.2	67	0.9	56	0.7	10	8
Minimum		500	5.3	239	4.6	441	4.6	235	4.5	15	18
Maximum		927	11.9	623	10.6	711	9.1	529	8.1	58	49

Source: Data from Maud & Shultz (1989).[38]

Fatigue Index

The fatigue index reflects the degree of fatigue over the entire WAnT. Those individuals exhibiting a higher fatigue index do so because they are unable to maintain their power level over the duration of the test due to a greater level of neuromuscular fatigue. The fatigue index is calculated as the percent decrease in power (P) from the highest power (usually recorded during the first 5 s interval) to the lowest power (usually the last 5 s interval), as seen in Equation 9.7a. A participant starting with a power of 708 W (*highest power*) during the first 5 s interval and ending with a power of 354 W (*lowest power*) in the last 5 s would have a fatigue index of 50 %, as seen in Equation 9.7b.

$$\text{Fatigue index (\%)} = [\text{Highest P (W)} - \text{Lowest P (W)} / \text{Highest P(W)}] * 100 \qquad \text{Eq. 9.7a}$$

Assume: Highest P = **708** W; Lowest P = **354** W

$$\text{Fatigue index} = [(\textbf{708} \text{ W} - \textbf{354} \text{ W}) / \textbf{708} \text{ W}] * 100 = \textbf{50} \% \qquad \text{Eq. 9.7b}$$

RESULTS AND DISCUSSION

High scores on the WAnT indicate high anaerobic fitness. Some of those anaerobic factors reportedly[57] associated with higher scores are (1) greater capacity to produce lactic acid; (2) greater stores of the phosphagens; (3) greater buffering capacity; and (4) a combination of greater motivation and greater tolerance of discomfort. As mentioned in the introduction to this test, however, aerobic metabolism, thus aerobic fitness, plays a small but significant part in this all-out exercise bout that lasts for 30 s.

Although it would be impossible for persons to maintain their peak or mean Wingate anaerobic power for an entire minute, these anaerobic indices make for an interesting comparison with minute-based power levels that are frequently prescribed for aerobic cycle ergometry. For example, maintaining power levels aerobically of 150–200 W would be considered difficult for most untrained me, whereas mean anaerobic powers in similar subjects range from 450 W[27] to 563 W[38] for the 30-s WAnT.

The normative data and percentiles listed in Table 9.2 are based on men and women between the ages of 18 y and 28 y at a force setting of 7.5 % of body weight (0.075 kg·kg⁻¹). The average men's and women's peak anaerobic powers are 700 W and 455 W, respectively; their relative peak anaerobic powers are 9.2 W·kg⁻¹ and 7.6 W·kg⁻¹, respectively. The mean anaerobic powers are 563 W and 381 W, respectively; their relative mean anaerobic powers are 7.3 W·kg⁻¹ and 6.4 W·kg⁻¹, respectively. When comparing both peak and mean anaerobic powers between genders in absolute terms (W), women scored 65–68 % as high as men, but in relative terms (W·kg⁻¹), women scored 83–88 % as high as men. Expressing anaerobic power, or most any test of physical performance, relative to body weight, or lean body weight especially, minimizes the differences observed due to gender.[57]

The scores in Table 9.3 are for comparative purposes only. They should not be used as normative data because of the small sample sizes and varying forces and methodologies employed. The forces used vary from 0.075 kg per kg of body weight (7.5 % of body weight) to 0.110 kg·kg⁻¹. Using a higher force (resistance) during the WAnT results

Table 9.3 Comparative Data for the Wingate Anaerobic Test

Group	Peak Anaerobic Power Force* (kg·kg⁻¹)	Absolute (W)	Relative (W·kg⁻¹)	Mean Anaerobic Power Work (kJ)	Absolute (W)	Relative (W·kg⁻¹)	Fatigue Index
Men		M ± SD	M ± SD	M ± SD	M ± SD	M ± SD	M ± SD
Non-Athletes, 18–24y (N = 21)[a]	0.075	570	8.3	14.3	475	7.0	
Non-Athletes, 18–28y (N = 62)[b]	0.075	700 ± 95	9.2 ± 1.4	16.9 ± 2.0	563 ± 67	7.3 ± 0.9	38 ± 10
Trained athletes (N = 457)[c]	0.075	951 ± 141	11.7 ± 1.4	20.6 ± 2.7	686 ± 91	8.5 ± 0.9	47 ± 8
Trained cyclists (N = 30)[d]	0.095	963 ± 38	13.3 ± 0.3	23.5 ± 1.0	783 ± 32	10.8 ± 0.2	35 ± 1
Trained cyclists (N = 16)[e]	0.095	1350 ± 80	17.6 ± 0.4	22.0 ± 0.5	734 ± 17	9.5 ± 0.2	29 ± 1
Pro cyclists, endurance, (N = 5)[f]	0.110	1122 ± 65	17.0 ± 0.9	24.4 ± 0.7	813 ± 22	12.4 ± 0.3	32 ± 12
Pro cyclists, sprint (N = 5)[f]	0.110	1547 ± 128	20.6 ± 1.3	30.9 ± 1.6	1030 ± 52	13.8 ± 0.6	46 ± 12
Women		M ± SD	M ± SD	M ± SD	M ± SD	M ± SD	M ± SD
Non-Athletes, 18–28y (N = 68)[b]	0.075	455 ± 81	7.6 ± 1.2	11.4 ± 1.7	381 ± 56	6.4 ± 0.7	35 ± 8
Trained athletes (N = 64)[c]	0.075	598 ± 88	9.6 ± 1.0	13.4 ± 1.9	445 ± 64	7.2 ± 0.7	42 ± 8
Trained women (N = 107)[g]	0.085	673 ± 101	11.0 ± 1.0	13.7 ± 2.0	457 ± 66	7.5 ± 0.7	53 ± 6
Trained cyclists (N = 6)[d]	0.095	784 ± 50	12.2 ± 0.7	18.4 ± 0.9	615 ± 31	9.6 ± 0.5	38 ± 3
Trained cyclists (N = 13)[e]	0.095	1086 ± 28	16.8 ± 0.2	13.5 ± 0.4	450 ± 13	7.0 ± 0.2	27 ± 1

Sources: Data from [a]Inbar & Bar-Or (1986)[27]; [b]Maud & Shultz (1989)[38]; [c]Zupan et al. (2009)[59]; [d]Tanaka et al. (1993)[54]; [e]Richmond et al. (2011)[49]; and [f]Calbet et al. (2003)[13]; [g]Baker et al. (2011).[3]

* *Note:* Force is expressed as force (kg) per kg of body weight (kg·kg⁻¹).

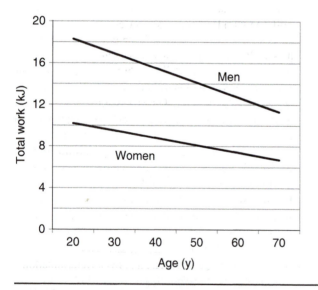

Figure 9.4 The relationship between age and total work (kJ) in males and females 15–70 y of age on an isokinetic cycle ergometer. Source: Modified from Makrides, Heigenhauser, McCartney, & Jones (1985).[34]

during the WAnT. Allowing the subject to "stand" (rise off of the saddle) during the WAnT results in peak powers 8.2 % higher and mean powers 10.0 % higher than when remaining in a seated position.[49] Greater powers with standing were attributed to: (1) greater muscle energy being transferred from the upper to lower body, (2) more weight being transferred to the pedals by removing the saddle forces, (3) an altered involvement of muscles due to different ranges of motion in the lower extremity joints, and (4) an altered body position while standing that allowed the cyclist to move forward or backward relative to the initial position by flexing or extending the trunk. It is important to consider all of these factors when making comparisons of the results of an anaerobic cycling test to previously published studies.

Anaerobic power and work values in a wide age range of adults are scarce in the literature. However, the values

in higher peak power, even within the same cyclists.[19,21,50] It appears that 0.075 kg·kg⁻¹ has been a frequently used resistive force,[27,38,59] but many studies have used higher forces up to a maximum observed load of 0.110 kg·kg⁻¹ to test trained and elite cyclists.[3,13,50,54] The use of toe stirrups ("caged" pedals) during the test, that allow "pulling" in addition to "pushing," has been shown to increase peak and mean power values by 5–12 %.[33] Many studies allow the cyclists to use their own pedals and cycling shoes

---

BOX 9.2 Chapter Preview/Review

What is the Wingate anaerobic test (WAnT)?
How do the energy systems contribute to the WAnT?
What are the typical force settings (kg per kg of body weight) used in the WAnT?
How do peak and mean anaerobic power differ?
What is the fatigue index and how is it calculated?
What is an average absolute and relative peak and mean anaerobic power for a man and woman?
What are four factors reportedly associated with higher scores on the Wingate test?
How does cycling experience affect WAnT scores?
What is the effect of aging on total work during cycling?

from one group of investigators[34] may be helpful despite their use of an isokinetic cycle ergometer, which makes comparisons with the traditional mechanically braked ergometer's scores less valid. Their participants, aged 15–70 y, pedaled with maximal effort for 30 s at a constant 60 rpm. The torque exerted on the pedals, which allowed the calculation of peak power, mean power, and total work, showed a 7–11 % decrease in these indices for each age decade. The values in this wider age group demonstrated that the women's anaerobic indices were 56–59 % of the men's values (see Figure 9.4).

References

1. Abler, P., Foster, C., Thompson, N. N., Crowe, M., Alt, K., Brophy, A., & Palin, W. D. (1986). Determinants of anaerobic muscular performance. *Medicine and Science in Sports and Exercise, 18,* Abstract #3, S1.

2. Ainsworth, B. E., Serfass, R. C., & Leon, A. S. (1993). Effects of recovery duration and blood lactate level on power output during cycling. *Canadian Journal of Applied Physiology, 18,*19–30.

3. Baker, U. C., Heath, E. M., Smith, D. R., & Oden, G. L. (2011). Development of Wingate anaerobic test norms for highly-trained women. *Journal of Exercise Physiology Online, 14,* 68–79.

4. Barnard, R. J. (1975). Warm-up is important for the heart. *Sports Medicine Bulletin, 10* (1), 6.

5. Barnard, R. J., Gardner, G. W., Diaco, N. V., MacAlpin, R. N., & Kattus, A. A. (1973). Cardiovascular responses to sudden strenuous exercise—Heart rate, blood pressure, and ECG. *Journal of Applied Physiology, 34,* 833–837.

6. Bar-Or, O. (1978). A new anaerobic capacity test: Characteristics applications. Proceedings of the 21st World Congress in Sports Medicine at Brasilia.

7. Bar-Or, O. (1981). Le test anaerobie de Wingate. *Symbiosis, 13,* 157–172.

8. Bar-Or, O. (1987). The Wingate Anaerobic Test: An update on methodology, reliability, and validity. *Sports Medicine, 4,* 381–394.

9. Bar-Or, O. (1994). *Testing of anaerobic performance by the Wingate Anaerobic Test.* Bloomington, IN: ERS Tech, Inc.

10. Bar-Or, O., & Inbar, O. (1978). Relationships among anaerobic capacity, sprint and middle distance running of school children. In R. J. Shephard & H. Lavallee (Eds.), *Physical fitness assessment—Principles, practice and application* (pp. 142–147). Springfield, IL: Charles C Thomas.

11. Bogdanis, G. C., Nevill, M. E., Boobis, L. H., & Lakomy, H. K. A. (1996). Contribution of phosphocreatine and aerobic metabolism to energy supply during repeated sprint exercise. *Journal of Applied Physiology, 80,* 876–884.

12. Bradley, A. L., & Ball, T. E. (1992). The Wingate Test: Effect of load on the power outputs of female athletes and nonathletes. *Journal of Applied Sport Science Research, 6,* 193–199.

13. Calbet, J. A. L., DePaz, J. A., Garatachea, N., DeVaca, S.C., & Chavarren, J. (2003). Anaerobic energy provision does not limit Wingate exercise performance in endurance-trained cyclists. *Journal of Applied Physiology, 94,* 668–676.

14. Coggan, A. R., & Costill, D. L. (1983). Day-to-day variability of three bicycle ergometer tests of anaerobic power. *Medicine and Science in Sports and Exercise, 15,* Abstract #1, 141.

15. Coleman, S. G. S., & Hale, T. (1998). The effect of different calculation methods of flywheel parameters on the Wingate Anaerobic Test. *Canadian Journal of Applied Physiology, 23,* 409–417.

16. Coleman, S. G. S., Hale, T., & Hamley, E. J. (1986). Correct power output in the Wingate Anaerobic Test. In *Kinanthropometry III* (pp. 308–309). London: E. & F. N. Spon.

17. Cumming, G. (1972). Correlation of athletic performance and aerobic power in 12- to 17-year-old children with bone age, calf muscle, total body potassium, heart volume and two indices of anaerobic power. *Proceedings of the Fourth International Symposium on Pediatric Work Physiology,* pp. 109–134.

18. Davy, K., Pizza, F., Guastella, P., McGuire, J., & Wygand, J. (1989). Optimal loading of Wingate power testing in conditioned athletes. *Medicine and Science in Sports and Exercise, 21* (Suppl., 2), Abstract #160, S27.

19. Dotan, R., & Bar-Or, O. (1983). Load optimization for the Wingate Anaerobic Test. *European Journal of Applied Physiology, 51,* 409–417.

20. Esbjornsson, M., Sylven, C., Holm, I., & Jansson, E. (1993). Fast-twitch fibers may predict anaerobic performance in both females and males. *International Journal of Sports Medicine, 14,* 257–263.

21. Evans, J. A., & Quinney, H. A. (1981). Determination of resistance settings for anaerobic power testing. *Canadian Journal of Applied Sport Science, 6,* 53–56.

22. Falk, B., Weinstein, Y., Dotan, R., Abramson, D. R., Mann-Segal, D., & Haffman, A. (1996). A treadmill test for sprint running. *Scandinavian Journal of Medicine and Science in Sports, 6,* 259–264.

23. Gledhill, N., & Jamnik, R. (1995). Determining power outputs for cycle ergometers with different sized flywheels. *Medicine and Science in Sports and Exercise, 27,* 134–135.

24. Green, S. (1995). Measurement of anaerobic work capacities in humans. *Sports Medicine, 19,* 32–42.

25. Hebestreit, H., Mimura, K., & Bar-Or, O. (1993). Recovery of anaerobic muscle power following 30 s supramaximal exercise: Comparison between boys and men. *Journal of Applied Physiology, 74,* 2875–2880.

26. Hill, D. W., & Smith, J. C. (1992). Calculation of aerobic contribution during high intensity exercise. *Research Quarterly for Exercise and Sport, 63,* 85–88.

27. Inbar, O., & Bar-Or, O. (1986). Anaerobic characteristics in male children and adolescents. *Medicine and Science in Sports and Exercise, 18,* 264–269.

28. Inbar, O., Dotan, R., & Bar-Or, O. (1976). Aerobic and anaerobic component of a thirty-second supramaximal cycling test. *Medicine and Science in Sports, 8,* 51.

29. Jacobs, I. (1980). The effects of thermal dehydration on performance of the Wingate Anaerobic Test. *International Journal of Sports Medicine, 1,* 21–24.

30. Jacobs, I., Bar-Or, O., Karlsson, J., Dotan, R., Tesch, P., Kaiser, P., & Inbar, O. (1982). Changes in muscle metabolites in females with 30-s exhaustive exercise. *Medicine and Science in Sports and Exercise, 14*(6), 457–460.

31. Jacobs, I., Tesch, P. A., Bar-Or, O., Karlsson, J., & Dotan, R. (1983). Lactate in human skeletal muscle after 10 and 30 s of supramaximal exercise. *Journal of Applied Physiology: Respiratory, Environmental, Exercise Physiology, 55,* 365–367.

32. Kaczkowski, W., Montgomery, D. L., Taylor, A. W., & Klissourous, V. (1982). The relationship between muscle fiber composition and maximal anaerobic power and capacity. *Journal of Sports Medicine and Physical Fitness, 22,* 407–413.

33. LaVoie, N. F., Dallaire, J., Brayne, S., & Barrett, D. (1984). Anaerobic testing using the Wingate and Evans-Quinney protocols with and without toe stirrups. *Canadian Journal of Applied Sport Sciences, 9,* 1–5.

34. Makrides, L., Heigenhauser, G. J. F., McCartney, N., & Jones, N. L. (1985). Maximal short term exercise capacity in healthy subjects aged 15–70 years. *Clinical Science, 69,* 197–205.

35. Margaria, R., Cerretelli, P., & Mangili, F. (1964). Balance and kinetics of anaerobic energy release during strenuous exercise in man. *Journal of Applied Physiology, 19,* 623–628.

36. Margaria, R., Oliva, D., DiPrampero, P. E., & Cerretelli, P. (1969). Energy utilization in intermittent exercise of supramaximal intensity. *Journal of Applied Physiology, 26,* 752–756.

37. Maud, P. J., & Shultz, B. B. (1986). Gender comparisons in anaerobic power and capacity tests. *British Journal of Sports Medicine, 20,* 51–54.

38. Maud, P. J., & Shultz, B. B. (1989). Norms for the Wingate Anaerobic Test with comparison to another similar test. *Research Quarterly for Exercise and Sport, 60*(2), 144–151.

39. McKenna, M. J., Green, R. A., Shaw, P. F., & Meyer, A. D. (1987). Tests of anaerobic power and capacity. *Australian Journal of Science and Medicine in Sport, 19,* 13–17.

40. Medbo, J. I., & Burgers, S. (1990). Effect of training on the anaerobic capacity. *Medicine and Science in Sports and Exercise, 22,* 501–507.

41. Medbo, J. I., Mohn, A. C., Tabata, I., Bahr, R., Vaage, O., & Sejersted, O. M. (1989). Anaerobic capacity determined by maximal accumulated O_2 deficit. *Journal of Applied Physiology, 64,* 50–60.

42. Medbo, J. I., & Tabata, I. (1993). Anaerobic energy release in working muscle during 30 s to 3 min of exhaustive bicycling. *Journal of Applied Physiology, 75,* 1654–1660.

43. Montgomery, D. L. (1982). The effect of added weight on ice hockey performance. *The Physician and Sportsmedicine, 10,* 91–95, 99.

44. Nicklin, R. C., O'Bryant, H. S., Zehnbauer, T. M., & Collins, M. A. (1990). A computerized method for assessing anaerobic power and work capacity using maximal cycle ergometry. *Journal of Applied Sports Science Research, 4,* 135–140.

45. Patton, J. F., Murphy, M. M., & Frederick, F. A. (1985). Maximal power outputs during the Wingate Anaerobic Test. *International Journal of Sports Medicine, 6,* 82–85.

46. Perez, H. R., Wygand, J. W., Kowalski, A., Smith, T. K., & Otto, R. M. (1986). A comparison of the Wingate Power Test to bicycle time trial performance. *Medicine and Science in Sports and Exercise, 18* (Suppl., 2), Abstract #1, S1.

47. Peveler, W. W., Pounders, J. D., & Bishop, P. A. (2007). Effects of saddle height on anaerobic power production in cycling. *Journal of Strength and Conditioning Research, 21,* 1023–1027.

48. Reiser, R. F., Broker, J. P., & Peterson, M. L. (2000). Inertial effects on mechanically braked Wingate power calculations. *Medicine and Science in Sports and Exercise, 32,* 1660–1664.

49. Reiser, R. F., Maines, J. M., Eisenmann, J. C., & Wilkinson, J. G. (2002). Standing and seated Wingate protocols in human cycling. A comparison of standard parameters. *European Journal of Applied Physiology, 88,* 152–157.

50. Richmond, S., Whitman, S., Acree, L., Olson, B., Carper, M., & Godard, M. P. (2011). Power output in trained male and female cyclists during the Wingate test with increasing flywheel resistance. *Journal of Exercise Physiology Online, 14*(5), 46–53.

51. Serresse, O., Lortie, G., Bouchard, C., & Boulay, M. R. (1988). Estimation of the contribution of the various energy systems during maximal work of short duration. *International Journal of Sports Medicine, 9,* 456–460.

52. Shaw, K., Davy, K., Coleman, C., & Kamimukai, C. (1988). Optimal resistance loading of the Wingate Power Test in female softball players. *Medicine and Science in Sports and Exercise, 20* (Suppl., 2), Abstract #105, S18.

53. Tamayo, M., Sucec, A., Phillips, W., Buono, M., Laubach, L., & Frey, M. (1984). The Wingate anaerobic power test, peak blood lactate, and maximal oxygen debt in elite volleyball players: A validation study. *Medicine and Science in Sports and Exercise, 16*(2), Abstract #10, 126.

54. Tanaka, H., Bassett, D. R., Swensen, T. C., & Sampredo, R. M. (1993). Aerobic and anaerobic power characteristics of competitive cyclists in the United States Cycling Federation. *International Journal of Sports Medicine, 14*, 334–338.

55. Tharp, G. D., Newhouse, R. K., Uffelman, L., Thorland, W. G., & Johnson, G. O. (1985). Comparison of sprint and run times with performance on the Wingate Anaerobic Test. *Research Quarterly for Exercise and Sport, 56*, 75–76.

56. Thompson, N. N., Foster, C., Crowe, M., Rogowski, B., & Kaplan, K. (1986). Serial responses of anaerobic muscular performance in competitive athletes. *Medicine and Science in Sports and Exercise, 18* (Suppl.), Abstract, S1.

57. Vandewalle, H., Peres, G., & Monod, H. (1987). Standard anaerobic exercise tests. *Sports Medicine, 4*, 268–289.

58. Weinstein, Y., Bediz, C., Dotan, R., & Falk, B. (1998). Reliability of peak-lactate, heart rate, and plasma volume following the Wingate Test. *Medicine and Science in Sports and Exercise, 30*, 1456–1460.

59. Zupan, M. F., Arata, A. W., Dawson, L. H., Wile, A. L., Payn, T. T., & Hannon, M. E. (2009). Wingate anaerobic test peak power and anaerobic capacity classifications for men and women intercollegiate athletes. *Journal of Strength and Conditioning Research, 23*, 2598–2604.

- Wingate is most popular anaerobic cycling test
    - can test arms or legs but most popularly legs
- measures peak anaerobic power, mean anaerobic power, total work, and fatigue index
    - (can also be relative measures)
    - peak power = highest ave over 5 sec. period
    - mean power = ave over 30 sec.
    - total work = Nm (revolutions (=6m) · force (resistance))
    - fatigue index = peak power to end of test
- it's a supramaximal test because it requires more O_2 than the Pp's maximal consumption rate
    - therefore it's best understood from perspective of metabolic pathways
- peak anaerobic power is usually reached within the first 2, 5, 8 or 10 seconds of supramaximal exercise
    - even in first 10 sec. Phosphagen supplies only 43% of ATP so glycolyte is major contributor
- mean anaerobic power reflects the ability to transform energy from the glycolyte pathway
    - however, the glycolyte pathway is not fully topped out so anaerobic capacity isn't the most accurate term
    - however however, maximal rate of lactate production (which indicates anaerobic power) may occur during the wingate test
- power is determined by product of force/resistance (kg) and cadence/speed (rpm)
- isokinetic cycle would hold rpm constant, not force... we held force constant per Pp and rpm was the varying variable
- force/resistance was determined by 0.075 kg per kg of body weight (or 7.5% of body weight (kg))
    - body weight (kg) · 0.075
- warm-up by pedaling at low/moderate intensity with interspersed 4-6s all out prints
- "recovery interval" is from end of warm up to beginning of test and should be 2-5 min
- immediately after the "recovery interval" there is an "acceleration period" where the Pp pedals as fast as possible without the resistance
- then the test begins and resistance is added, then pedal for 30s as fast as possible throughout
- cool-down should be 2-3 min at low intensity
- 3 Testing positions
    - Force setter
    - Counter
    - Timer
    - (Recorder of data)

- knee should be at 25° or 5-15°, depending on who you are, at down stroke of pedaling motion
- peak anaerobic power almost always happens in the first 5 seconds
- Power is in W, so force/resistance needs to be converted from (kg) to (N) by multiplying by 9.8067
- divide peak power by body weight to make it a relative measure
- total work (Nm, or J) is (# revolutions · force$^{(N)}$) · 6 m/revolution = x Nm
    - divide this by body weight to make it relative
- fatigue index

$$\left(\frac{\text{Highest Power} - \text{lowest power}}{\text{Highest power}} \right) \cdot 100$$

- relative values minimize gender differences
- standing out of saddle can result in 8.2-10% increase in power
- there's a 7-11% decrease per decade of aging

Values

	Peak Power	Relative Peak Power	Mean Power	Relative Mean Power	Fatigue index
men	700 - 900	8.3 - 11.7	475 - 686	7.0 - 8.5	38
women	455 - 600	7.6 - 11	380 - 450	6.8 - 7.5	38

(average - trained)

↑
better measure of
motivation than
fatigue

Form 9.1

NAME _____ DATE _____ SCORE _____

ANAEROBIC CYCLING (WINGATE)

Homework

Gender: **M** Initials: **AA** Age (y): **22** Weight (kg): **75.0** Force (kg·kg^{-1}): **0.075**

Leg force setting _____ kg = _____ N   *Force setting = Body wt (kg) * 0.075 (or 0.050-0.100)*

Interval (s) :	0-5	5-10	10-15	15-20	20-25	25-30	Rev Max	Rev Total
Pedal revolutions :	**12**	**9**	**8**	**7**	**7**	**6**		

Peak power = _____ * _____ * 6 m / 5 s = 723.6 W   Rel peak = _____ / _____ = 8.62 W·kg^{-1}
        F (N)   Rev$_{Max}$ Peak   Wt (kg)

Total work = _____ * _____ * 6 m / 1000 = 17,366 kJ   Rel work = _____ / _____ = 206.94 J·kg^{-1}
        F (N)   Rev$_{Tot}$ Work (J) Wt (kg)

Mean power = _____ * _____ * 6 m / 30 s = 578.87 W   Rel mean = _____ / _____ = 6.90 W·kg^{-1}
        F (N)   Rev$_{Tot}$ Mean   Wt (kg)

Category: _____   _____   _____   _____
      Abs Peak (Table 9.2)   Rel Peak (Table 9.2)   Abs Mean (Table 9.2)   Rel Mean (Table 9.2)

Fatigue index = (_____ - _____) / _____ * 100 = 40 %   Category: _____
         Highest P   Lowest P   Highest P

Evaluation: My peak power values, both absolute and relative, fell within the range of average values for men. The same is true for absolute mean power and relative mean power. My fatigue index also fell in the middle range for average for men

Gender: **F** Initials: **BB** Age (y): **20** Weight (kg): **65.0** Force (kg·kg^{-1}): **0.075**

Leg force setting _____ kg = _____ N   *Force setting = Body wt (kg) * 0.075 (or 0.050-0.100)*

Interval (s) :	0-5	5-10	10-15	15-20	20-25	25-30	Rev Max	Rev Total
Pedal revolutions :	**9**	**8**	**7**	**7**	**6**	**5**		

Peak power = _____ * _____ * 6 m / 5 s = _____ W   Rel peak = _____ / _____ = _____ W·kg^{-1}
        F (N)   Rev$_{Max}$ Peak   Wt (kg)

Total work = _____ * _____ * 6 m / 1000 = _____ kJ   Rel work = _____ / _____ = _____ J·kg^{-1}
        F (N)   Rev$_{Tot}$ Work (J) Wt (kg)

Mean power = _____ * _____ * 6 m / 30 s = _____ W   Rel mean = _____ / _____ = _____ W·kg^{-1}
        F (N)   Rev$_{Tot}$ Mean   Wt (kg)

Category: _____   _____   _____   _____
      Abs Peak (Table 9.2)   Rel Peak (Table 9.2)   Abs Mean (Table 9.2)   Rel Mean (Table 9.2)

Fatigue index = (_____ - _____) / _____ * 100 = _____ %   Category: _____
         Highest P   Lowest P   Highest P

Evaluation: _____

_____

Form 9.2

NAME _____ DATE _____ SCORE _____

ANAEROBIC CYCLING (WINGATE)

Lab Results

Gender: _____ Initials: _____ Age (y): _____ Weight (kg): _____ Force (kg·kg⁻¹): _____

Leg force setting _____ kg = _____ N   *Force setting = Body wt (kg) * 0.075 (or 0.050-0.100)*

Interval (s): 0-5   5-10   10-15   15-20   20-25   25-30   Rev $_{Max}$ Rev $_{Total}$

Pedal revolutions : _____ _____ _____ _____ _____ _____ _____ _____

Peak power = $\dfrac{\_\_\_\_}{F\ (N)}$ * $\dfrac{\_\_\_\_}{Rev_{Max}}$ * 6 m / 5 s = _____ W   Rel peak = $\dfrac{\_\_\_\_}{Peak}$ / $\dfrac{\_\_\_\_}{Wt\ (kg)}$ = _____ W·kg⁻¹

Total work = $\dfrac{\_\_\_\_}{F\ (N)}$ * $\dfrac{\_\_\_\_}{Rev_{Tot}}$ * 6 m / 1000 = _____ kJ   Rel work = $\dfrac{\_\_\_\_}{Work\ (J)}$ / $\dfrac{\_\_\_\_}{Wt\ (kg)}$ = _____ J·kg⁻¹

Mean power = $\dfrac{\_\_\_\_}{F\ (N)}$ * $\dfrac{\_\_\_\_}{Rev_{Tot}}$ * 6 m / 30 s = _____ W   Rel mean = $\dfrac{\_\_\_\_}{Mean}$ / $\dfrac{\_\_\_\_}{Wt\ (kg)}$ = _____ W·kg⁻¹

Category:
_____ Abs Peak (Table 9.2)   _____ Rel Peak (Table 9.2)   _____ Abs Mean (Table 9.2)   _____ Rel Mean (Table 9.2)

Fatigue index = ($\dfrac{\_\_\_\_}{Highest\ P}$ - $\dfrac{\_\_\_\_}{Lowest\ P}$) / $\dfrac{\_\_\_\_}{Highest\ P}$ * 100 = _____ %   Category: _____

Evaluation: _____

_____

_____

Gender: _____ Initials: _____ Age (y): _____ Weight (kg): _____ Force (kg·kg⁻¹): _____

Leg force setting _____ kg = _____ N   *Force setting = Body wt (kg) * 0.075 (or 0.050-0.100)*

Interval (s): 0-5   5-10   10-15   15-20   20-25   25-30   Rev $_{Max}$ Rev $_{Total}$

Pedal revolutions : _____ _____ _____ _____ _____ _____ _____ _____

Peak power = $\dfrac{\_\_\_\_}{F\ (N)}$ * $\dfrac{\_\_\_\_}{Rev_{Max}}$ * 6 m / 5 s = _____ W   Rel peak = $\dfrac{\_\_\_\_}{Peak}$ / $\dfrac{\_\_\_\_}{Wt\ (kg)}$ = _____ W·kg⁻¹

Total work = $\dfrac{\_\_\_\_}{F\ (N)}$ * $\dfrac{\_\_\_\_}{Rev_{Tot}}$ * 6 m / 1000 = _____ kJ   Rel work = $\dfrac{\_\_\_\_}{Work\ (J)}$ / $\dfrac{\_\_\_\_}{Wt\ (kg)}$ = _____ J·kg⁻¹

Mean power = $\dfrac{\_\_\_\_}{F\ (N)}$ * $\dfrac{\_\_\_\_}{Rev_{Tot}}$ * 6 m / 30 s = _____ W   Rel mean = $\dfrac{\_\_\_\_}{Mean}$ / $\dfrac{\_\_\_\_}{Wt\ (kg)}$ = _____ W·kg⁻¹

Category:
_____ Abs Peak (Table 9.2)   _____ Rel Peak (Table 9.2)   _____ Abs Mean (Table 9.2)   _____ Rel Mean (Table 9.2)

Fatigue index = ($\dfrac{\_\_\_\_}{Highest\ P}$ - $\dfrac{\_\_\_\_}{Lowest\ P}$) / $\dfrac{\_\_\_\_}{Highest\ P}$ * 100 = _____ %   Category: _____

Evaluation: _____

_____

_____

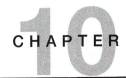

ANAEROBIC STEPPING

The performance of the Anaerobic Step Test is primarily dependent upon the glycolytic pathway (lactic acid system) of metabolism, but also receives ATP contributions from the phosphagen system and the aerobic system. It has been reported that maximal efforts involving large muscle groups of one-minute duration require metabolic contributions of about 30–35 % aerobic and 65–70 % anaerobic.[1] The highest lactate values observed occur in well-trained athletes at the end of competitive events of 1–2 minutes duration. Blood lactates in elite athletes engaging in all-out efforts of sustained power activities have been reported as high as 17 times (16.7 mmol·L^{-1}) the resting values.[5] Thus, the Anaerobic Step Test is expected to elicit moderately high lactate values because of its duration of 1 min.

However, because only one leg is used predominantly during the Anaerobic Step Test, the lactate values are less than maximal. Thus, despite presumably high lactate levels in the local muscle mass of the dominant leg, the lactate levels are diluted in the general circulation because of the smaller muscle mass compared with two-legged exercise. Indeed, the post–Anaerobic Step Test values of blood lactate were about six times greater (6 mmol·L^{-1}) than resting values (1 mmol·L^{-1}).[10]

METHODS

The Methods section in the description of most exercise physiology tests includes descriptions of equipment, preparations, procedures, and calculations. The accuracy of the Anaerobic Step Test is described in Box 10.1.

Equipment

The equipment for the Anaerobic Step Test is inexpensive. It requires only a bench (step), a laboratory clock or stopwatch, a calculator, and an accurate body weighing scale. The step height described for the Anaerobic Step Test in this chapter is lower than that used by the investigators in the original study.[3] A step height of 40 cm (15.75 in.) is currently used compared to the 18 in. (45.7 cm) step height used in the original study. This current step height (40 cm) was chosen because it corresponds to the same step height used for aerobic step tests, and steps or benches of this height would likely be more available in most laboratories.

BOX 10.1   Accuracy

Reliability

The test-retest reliability of the Anaerobic Step Test is high ($r > 0.90$) based upon two tests, each administered no more than one week apart to 30 university students.[10] However, significantly higher scores on the second trials indicate a likely learning effect.

Validity

The number of steps performed by ninth-grade girls in the earlier version of the Anaerobic Step Test was highly correlated ($r = -0.824$) with the time for the 600 yd run.[3] In the earlier test, however, they were allowed to change support legs during the test; this would lead, presumably, to higher anaerobic scores. Anaerobic Step Test power (W) for NCAA basketball players increased during their preseason training.[11] This shows that the Anaerobic Step Test is sensitive to the effects of heavy anaerobic training. There appears to be a strong relationship ($r = 0.87$) between the anaerobic power of the Anaerobic Step Test and lean body mass; there is a moderate relationship ($r = 0.61$) between the Anaerobic Step Test score and dominant-leg strength.[6] A report from a master's project indicated no relationship between the time in the 400 m run and mean anaerobic power ($r = -0.08$), but a significant relationship ($r = -0.79$) with the number of steps in 1 min.

Preparation

In preparation for the Anaerobic Step Test, the stepper should follow the basic plan of the warm-up regimen. The warm-up also familiarizes the stepper with the proper stepping technique. The participant should avoid becoming fatigued at any time during the warm-up.

- 0:00–2:00 min   Walk in place at a moderate rate; lift thighs to 90°.
- 2:00–3:00 min   Stretch: (1) groin; (2) quadriceps; (3) calf.
- 3:00–5:00 min   Step up and down on a step, stool, or bench using both legs in a traditional four-count cadence at a moderate pace (15–20 steps per minute).
- 5:00–7:00 min   Relief interval: Mild walking in place and/or stretching.

Procedures

The Anaerobic Step Test is a modification of three other step tests—the Forestry[7] and Skubic and Hodgkins[8] *aerobic* step tests and an earlier *anaerobic* step test.[3] There are four major differences between the Anaerobic Step Test and the aerobic step tests—one concerned with the position of the stepper, another concerned with cadence, another concerned with the primary leg, and, finally, another concerned with calculation of power or capacity. Also, the newer Anaerobic Step Test described here provides more information than the original because body mass is used to calculate anaerobic power.

Stepping Technique

The stepping technique is different from any of the common aerobic stepping techniques. The technique for the Anaerobic Step Test places a greater emphasis on one leg than the other. The initial position of the stepper is standing alongside the bench, not in front of it. The working leg (or preferred leg) rests on top of the step (bench) in preparation for the start of the test (Figure 10.1a). The other leg, called the free leg, does not touch the bench when the working leg lifts the body (Figure 10.1b).

During the test, each concentric muscle action of the working (preferred) leg raises the body to the top of the step. The free leg dangles in a straight position during the ascent, and its heel reaches the height of the bench. The foot of the free leg can push off when it contacts the floor. The foot on the step remains there for the duration of the test. The legs and the back must be straightened with each step. In fact, the back should start in a straight position and remain so throughout the test. The arms may be used for balance but cannot be pumped vigorously during the test. Ideally, the arms should be abducted to a "penguinlike" position at about 30° to 45° from the sides (Figurex 10.1b).

The cadence for the test is at a one-two count; "one" is up and "two" is down. This is different from the typical four-count cadence of aerobic step tests. An additional difference is that the participant goes as fast as possible at a pace designed to give a maximum number of steps during the one-minute time period. Thus, the stepper should barely be able to perform another step at the end of one minute.

Measurements

Measurements are made on only three items: (a) the body mass of the participant, (b) the participant's number of steps, and (c) the duration of the test.

Body Mass (BM)   The participant should be weighed to the closest tenth of a kilogram in the *same clothes and shoes* that are worn for the step test. The total mass is important because the stepper is lifting not only his or her body weight, but also the weight of the clothes and shoes.

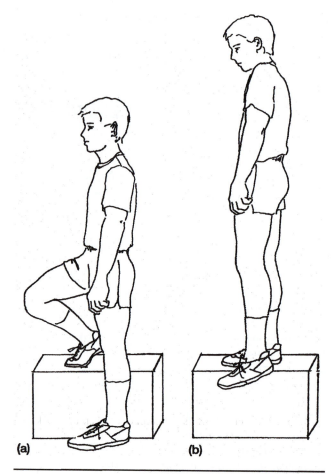

Figure 10.1 The positions for the Anaerobic Step Test including: (a) the starting ("down") position with the participant beside the box or bench, and (b) the "up" position with the working leg straight.

The measured body weight (kg) is then converted into body mass (N) for the calculation of anaerobic power.

Number of Steps   A step is counted for each time the stepper's working leg is straightened and then returned to the starting position. Steps are not counted if the working leg does not straighten or if the back is bent. Technicians count aloud in order to give immediate feedback to the participant. The counting should be as follows: "up-1, up-2, up-3, up-4, up-5," etc. Thus, a full step is considered to be a return to the starting position (down) after the ascent. The technician records the number of steps fully completed in 60 s onto Form 10.2. Optionally, the steps completed in the first 5 s (0–5 s) and the last 5 s of the test (55–60 s) can also be counted.

Duration   The duration of the test is 1 minute. The time begins with the first upward movement of the stepper. The technician should call out the time every 15 s or allow the timer to be visible for the stepper. The laboratory set-clock if used, can be set to buzz at the end of the test.

Recovery from the Anaerobic Step Test

The stepper's working or preferred leg is likely to be very weak at the end of this test, perhaps causing a few "buckled" walking steps. The quadriceps of the working leg and the calf of the free leg are the most likely muscle groups to become sore within about 12 h. In an effort to minimize delayed onset muscle soreness (DOMS), static stretching exercises should be repeated periodically after the test throughout the day. Based on the enhanced subsequent performance of 60 s events and lactate removal, active recovery, such as walking, mild jogging, or walking in place, is recommended immediately after the test.[12]

Summary of the Procedures

1. Weigh the participant in stepping attire to the closest 0.1 kg.
2. Convert the body mass to newtons and record on Form 10.2.
3. The stepper stands alongside the bench with the foot of the preferred (support) leg on the bench.
4. The time begins when the stepper starts.
5. The technician counts aloud the number of correct steps.
6. The technician reminds the stepper to keep the back straight and the arms in a "penguinlike" position.
7. The technician states the time every 15 s.
8. At the end of 1 min, the last repetition of a complete step is recorded.
9. The technician encourages the participant to actively recover immediately and to stretch the leg muscles periodically throughout the day.

Calculations

The Anaerobic Step Test is a measure of mean anaerobic power sustained over the full minute of exercise. In fact, the test may be said to measure "anaerobic capacity," as it relies heavily on the combination of the phosphagen and lactic acid systems. Participants are instructed to pace themselves over the duration of the test and try to complete the maximum number of steps possible in 1 minute. It is not an immediate all-out effort as in the Wingate Anaerobic Test (Chapter 9).

The determination of power is based first on the work accomplished during the concentric (against gravity) portion of stepping up onto the step. The positive work done during this phase is determined from the force exerted by the body weight (in this case expressed as body mass in newtons), the vertical distance the body mass raised (the step height), and the number of steps completed (or the number of times the body mass is raised the height of the step), as seen in Equation 10.1a. The negative work done during the eccentric (with gravity) portion of stepping down from the step is estimated to be one-third (33 %) of the concentric work. The total work (positive plus negative) done during the test, therefore, is equal to the positive work times 1.33 (Eq. 10.1b). The mean power sustained over the duration of the test is calculated as the total work divided by the time (Eq. 10.1c).

$$\text{Positive work (N·m)} = \text{Force (N)} * \text{Distance (m)} \quad \text{Eq. 10.1a}$$

Where: Force = Body mass (N); Distance = Step height (m·step^{-1}) * #Steps

$$\text{Total work (N·m)} = \text{Positive work} * 1.33 \quad \text{Eq. 10.1b}$$

$$\text{Mean power (W)} = \text{Total work (N·m)} / \text{Time (s)} \quad \text{Eq. 10.1c}$$

To mathematically calculate mean anaerobic power for the Anaerobic Step Test, the terms described in Equations 10.1a and 10.1b can be substituted into Equation 10.1c, with the result being Equation 10.2a. For example, if a person with a body weight of 70 kg (body mass or force = 686 N) steps up onto a 40 cm (0.40 m) step 50 times in 1 min (60 s), the resultant mean anaerobic power is 304 W (Eq.10.2b).

$$\text{Mean anaerobic power (W)} = [\text{Force (N)} * \text{Step ht (m)} * \text{\# Steps} * 1.33] / \text{Time (s)} \quad \text{Eq. 10.2a}$$

Assume: Force = **686** N; Step height = **0.40** m; # Steps = **50**; Time = **60** s

$$\text{Mean anaerobic power} = [\textbf{686} \text{ N} * \textbf{0.40} \text{ m} * \textbf{50} \text{ steps} * 1.33] / \textbf{60} \text{ s} = \textbf{304} \text{ W} \quad \text{Eq. 10.2b}$$

Optional Procedures and Calculations

The Anaerobic Step Test, although not specifically designed for it, can also provide a measure of "peak anaerobic power" and "fatigue index" in a manner similar to the Wingate anaerobic cycle test described in Chapter 9. As an option, students can count the number of steps taken within the first 5 s of the test (0–5 s), assumed to be the highest number of steps, and the last 5 s of the test (55–60s), assumed to be the lowest number of steps due to fatigue. Peak (highest) anaerobic power is calculated from the highest number of steps, assumed to be 0–5 s (Eq. 10.a); the lowest anaerobic power is calculated from the lowest number of steps, assumed to be 55–60 s (Eq. 10.b) 10.b; and fatigue index is calculated from these two powers (Eq. 10.c). The example provided results in a *peak anaerobic power* of 657 W (Eq. 10.d), which coupled with the *lowest anaerobic power* of 292 W (Eq. 10.e) results in a *fatigue index* of 57 % (Eq. 10.f). These calculated values can be used to investigate differences in peak anaerobic power and fatigue between students in the lab, no published data, however, are available with which to directly compare results. It may be expected, that the degree of fatigue, as indicated by the fatigue index, would be greater in the 1-min anaerobic step test compared to the 30-s Wingate anaerobic cycle test.

Peak (highest) anaerobic power (W) = [Force (N)

$\quad$ * Step ht (m) * # Steps * 1.33] / 5 s $\qquad$ Eq. 10.2a

Lowest anaerobic power (W) = [Force (N)

$\quad$ * Step ht (m) * # Steps * 1.33] / 5 s $\qquad$ Eq. 10.2b

Fatigue index (%) = [(Highest P (W) − Lowest P (W))

$\quad$ / Highest P (W)] * 100 $\qquad$ Eq. 10.2c

Assume: Force = **686** N; Step height = **0.40** m; # Steps

$\quad$ (0–5 s) = **9**; # Steps (55–60 s) = **4**

Peak anaerobic power (W) = [**686** N * **0.40** m

$\quad$ * **9** * 1.33] / 5 s = **657** W $\qquad$ Eq. 10.2d

Lowest anaerobic power (W) = [**686** N * **0.40** m

$\quad$ * **4** * 1.33] / 5 s = **292** W $\qquad$ Eq. 10.2e

Fatigue index (%) = [(657 W − 292 W) / 657 W]

$\quad$ * 100 = **56** % $\qquad$ Eq. 10.2f

RESULTS AND DISCUSSION

Mean values and percentiles for total number of steps taken in the 60-s Anaerobic Step Test and derived values for total work (or "anaerobic capacity"), and absolute and relative mean anaerobic power are included in Table 10.1. Because total steps are used to derive total work and absolute mean anaerobic power, the percentile categories for all three of these variables will be the same. A participant may fall into a different category, however, for relative mean anaerobic power, calculated per kg of body weight. The mean anaerobic powers for the Anaerobic Step Test of self-selected adults between the ages of 18 y and 30 y (M = 23 y) attending a fitness center were 460 ± 90 W for men and 307 ± 61 W for women.[6] These values are below those observed for mean anaerobic powers measured during the 30-s Wingate Anaerobic Test (WAnT), which were 563 ± 67 W for men and 381 ± 56 W for women.[4] The reduced values for mean anaerobic power in the 60-s step test are likely lower than the values for the 30-s cycling test because of the extended time of the test, resulting in a greater degree of fatigue. In both tests, comparing men and women, absolute values (W) of women are about 67–68 % those of men, but expressing values relative to body weight ($W \cdot kg^{-1}$) closes the gap, where women produce 88–91 % of the relative mean anaerobic power of men.[4,6]

Table 10.2 provides comparative scores for the anaerobic step test from various groups, such as high school athletes, college basketball players, active college students and adults, professional football players, and women college softball and volleyball players. Athletes trained in sports requiring significant anaerobic fitness (basketball, football, softball and volleyball), as expected, show anaerobic power scores greater than non-athletes. It should be noted that the high values for professional football players, the mean of 626 ± 108 W and the high score of 810 W, were measured with the participants facing the step bench and no restrictions were placed on arm movements.[9] Because of the mode used in the Anaerobic Step Test, stepping versus cycling, the step test could be considered a good alternative to the Wingate cycling test and more mode-specific in "non-cycling" sports. Further studies using the Anaerobic Step Tests could also generate normative data for using it to assess peak anaerobic power in the first 5 s of the test, minimal power in the last 5 s of the test, and a "fatigue index" similar to other anaerobic power tests.

| Table 10.1 | Categories for Total Number of Steps, Total Work (or "Anaerobic Capacity") and Absolute and Relative Mean Power Derived from the Anaerobic Step Test |

Category	%ile	Total Number of Steps		Total Work or "Anaerobic Capacity"		Absolute Mean Anaerobic Power		Relative Mean Anaerobic Power	
		Men (#)	Women (#)	Men (kJ)	Women (kJ)	Men (W)	Women (W)	Men ($W \cdot kg^{-1}$)	Women ($W \cdot kg^{-1}$)
Well above ave	95	87	81	36.5	24.4	608	407	7.6	7.0
Above average	90	84	78	35.0	23.5	584	391	7.3	6.7
	85	80	73	33.2	22.2	554	370	6.9	6.4
	80	77	71	32.2	21.5	536	358	6.7	6.2
	75	75	69	31.2	20.9	520	348	6.5	6.0
Average	70	73	67	30.4	20.3	507	339	6.3	5.8
	50	66	61	27.6	18.4	460	307	5.8	5.3
	30	59	55	24.8	16.5	413	275	5.2	4.7
Below average	25	58	53	24.0	16.0	400	266	5.0	4.6
	20	55	51	23.0	15.5	384	258	4.8	4.4
	15	53	48	22.0	14.6	366	244	4.6	4.2
	10	48	44	20.2	13.4	336	223	4.2	3.8
Well below ave	5	45	41	18.7	12.4	312	207	3.9	3.6
Mean		66	61	27.6	18.4	460	307	5.8	5.3
S.D.		13	12	5.4	3.7	90	61	1.1	1.1

Source: Data from Petersen (1989).[6] Based on active men (N = 130) and women (N = 70) between 18 y and 30 y of age.

Table 10.2 Comparative Data for Mean Power (W) for the Anaerobic Step Test

Group	Mean ± SD (W)	High (W)
Men		
High school athletes	405	
College students (N = 17)[a]	454	583
Active adults, 18–30y (N = 130)[b]	460 ± 90	
College basketball (N = 9)[c]	576 ± 53	
Pro football players (N = 15)[d]	626 ± 108	810
Women		
College students (N = 12)[a]	338	457
Active adults, 18–30y (N = 70)[b]	307 ± 61	
College softball players[e]	383 ± 60	
College volleyball players[e]	434 ± 58	

Sources: [a]Stojanovski (1989)[10]; [b]Petersen (1989)[6]; [c]Tavino et al. (1995)[11]; [d]Smith (1987)[9]; and [e]Covington et al. (1996).[2]

BOX 10.2 Chapter Preview/Review

How do the energy systems contribute to the Anaerobic Step Test?

What are the differences between the Anaerobic Step Test and aerobic step tests?

What is the mean anaerobic power (W) for a 76 kg person who completes 60 steps (40 cm step) in 60 s?

What is the average power (W) for the Anaerobic Step Test for active 18–30 year old men and women?

How does training for particular sports affect the Anaerobic Step Test?

References

1. Åstrand, P. O., & Rodahl, K. (1977). *Textbook of work physiology.* New York: McGraw-Hill.
2. Covington, N. K., Baylor, A. K., Kluka, D. A., Moltstad, S., Taylor, J., Cobb, T., & Cook, T. (1996). Body composition, flexibility, and selected anaerobic parameters of Division I female softball and volleyball athletes. *Research Quarterly for Exercise and Sports, 67* (Suppl.), A–31.
3. Manahan, J. E., & Gutin, B. (1971). The one-minute step test as a measure of 600-yard run performance. *Research Quarterly, 42,* 173–177.
4. Maud, P. J., & Shultz, B. B. (1989). Norms for the Wingate Anaerobic Test with comparison to another similar test. *Research Quarterly for Exercise and Sport, 60,* 144–151.
5. Parkhouse, W. S., & McKenzie, D. C. (1983). Anaerobic capacity assessment of elite athletes. *Medicine and Science in Sports and Exercise, 15* (Suppl. 2), Abstract, 142.
6. Petersen, M. (1989). "AnP norms and the relationship between anaerobic power versus leg strength and lean body mass." Master's thesis, California State University, Fullerton.
7. Sharkey, B. J. (1984). *Physiology of fitness.* Champaign, IL: Human Kinetics.
8. Skubic, V., & Hodgkins, J. (1963). Cardiovascular efficiency tests for girls and women. *Research Quarterly, 34,* 191–198.
9. Smith, C. D. (1987). "The effect of offseason training on anaerobic power training in pro football players." Master's project, California State University, Fullerton.
10. Stojanovski, J. (1989). "The reliability and validity of the AnP step test." Master's project, California State University, Fullerton.
11. Tavino, L. P., Bowers, C. J., & Archer, C. B. (1995). Effects of basketball on aerobic capacity, anaerobic capacity, and body composition of male college players. *Journal of Strength and Conditioning Research, 9,* 75–77.
12. Weltman, A., Stamford, B. A., Moffatt, R. J., & Katch, V. L. (1977). Exercise recovery, lactate removal, and repeated high-intensity exercise performance. *Research Quarterly, 48,* 786–796.

Form 10.1

ANAEROBIC STEPPING

NAME _____ DATE _____ SCORE _____

Homework

Gender: __**M**__   Initials: __**AA**__   Age (y): __**20**__   Height (cm): __**180**__   Weight (kg): __**85.0**__

Body mass = _____ * 9.8067 N·kg⁻¹ = _____ N   Step ht = __**40**__ cm / 100 = ____ m
                    Wt (kg)

Number of steps: 0-60 s __**64**__ steps   *Optional:*   0-5 s __**8**__ steps   55-60 s __**4**__ steps

Total work = [_____ * _____ * _____ * 1.33] = _____ J / 1000 = _____ kJ
                 Mass (N)   Step ht (m)   Steps 0-60 s

Abs power = _____ / 60 s = _____ W   Rel power = _____ / _____ = _____ W·kg⁻¹
              Work (J)   Abs power   Wt (kg)

Category for: Abs mean power _____   Rel mean power _____
                              (Table 10.1)   *(Table 10.1)*

Optional: Peak power = [_____ * _____ * 1.33 / 5] = _____ W
              (Highest)   Mass (N)   Step ht (m)   Steps 0-5 s

              Minimal power = [_____ * _____ * 1.33 / 5] = _____ W
              (Lowest)   Mass (N)   Step ht (m)   Steps 55-60 s

              Fatigue index = (_____ - _____) / _____ * 100 = _____ %
                                Highest   Lowest   Highest

Evaluation: _____

_____

_____

Gender: __**F**__   Initials: __**BB**__   Age (y): __**20**__   Height (cm): __**170**__   Weight (kg): __**65.0**__

Body mass = _____ * 9.8067 N·kg⁻¹ = _____ N   Step ht = __**40**__ cm / 100 = ____ m
                    Wt (kg)

Number of steps: 0-60 s __**55**__ steps   *Optional:*   0-5 s __**7**__ steps   55-60 s __**3**__ steps

Total work = [_____ * _____ * _____ * 1.33] = _____ J / 1000 = _____ kJ
                 Mass (N)   Step ht (m)   Steps 0-60 s

Abs power = _____ / 60 s = _____ W   Rel power = _____ / _____ = _____ W·kg⁻¹
              Work (J)   Abs power   Wt (kg)

Category for: Abs mean power _____   Rel mean power _____
                              (Table 10.1)   *(Table 10.1)*

Optional: Peak power = [_____ * _____ * 1.33 / 5] = _____ W
              (Highest)   Mass (N)   Step ht (m)   Steps 0-5 s

              Minimal power = [_____ * _____ * 1.33 / 5] = _____ W
              (Lowest)   Mass (N)   Step ht (m)   Steps 55-60 s

              Fatigue index = (_____ - _____) / _____ * 100 = _____ %
                                Highest   Lowest   Highest

Evaluation: _____

_____

_____

Form 10.2
ANAEROBIC STEPPING

NAME _____ DATE _____ SCORE _____

Lab Results

Gender: _____ Initials: _____ Age (y): _____ Height (cm): _____ Weight (kg): _____

Body mass = _____ * 9.8067 N·kg⁻¹ = _____ N   Step ht = _____ cm / 100 = _____ m
        Wt (kg)

Number of steps: 0-60 s _____ steps   *Optional:*   0-5 s _____ steps   55-60 s _____ steps

Total work = [_____ * _____ * _____ * 1.33] = _____ J / 1000 = _____ kJ
        Mass (N)   Step ht (m) Steps 0-60 s

Abs power = _____ / 60 s = _____ W   Rel power = _____ / _____ = _____ W·kg⁻¹
       Work (J)   Abs power Wt (kg)

Category for: Abs mean power _____   Rel mean power _____
                                    (Table 10.1)   *(Table 10.1)*

Optional: Peak power = [_____ * _____ * _____ * 1.33 / 5] = _____ W
        (Highest)   Mass (N)   Step ht (m)   Steps 0-5 s

            Minimal power = [_____ * _____ * _____ * 1.33 / 5] = _____ W
        (Lowest)   Mass (N)   Step ht (m)   Steps 55-60 s

            Fatigue index = (_____ - _____) / _____ * 100 = _____ %
                     Highest   Lowest   Highest

Evaluation: _____

_____

_____

Gender: _____ Initials: _____ Age (y): _____ Height (cm): _____ Weight (kg): _____

Body mass = _____ * 9.8067 N·kg⁻¹ = _____ N   Step ht = _____ cm / 100 = _____ m
        Wt (kg)

Number of steps: 0-60 s _____ steps   *Optional:*   0-5 s _____ steps   55-60 s _____ steps

Total work = [_____ * _____ * _____ * 1.33] = _____ J / 1000 = _____ kJ
        Mass (N)   Step ht (m) Steps 0-60 s

Abs power = _____ / 60 s = _____ W   Rel power = _____ / _____ = _____ W·kg⁻¹
       Work (J)   Abs power Wt (kg)

Category for: Abs mean power _____   Rel mean power _____
                                      (Table 10.1)   *(Table 10.1)*

Optional: Peak power = [_____ * _____ * _____ * 1.33 / 5] = _____ W
        (Highest)   Mass (N)   Step ht (m)   Steps 0-5 s

            Minimal power = [_____ * _____ * _____ * 1.33 / 5] = _____ W
        (Lowest)   Mass (N)   Step ht (m)   Steps 55-60 s

            Fatigue index = (_____ - _____) / _____ * 100 = _____ %
                     Highest   Lowest   Highest

Evaluation: _____

_____

_____

ANAEROBIC TREADMILL RUNNING

The treadmill running tests presented in this chapter are considered laboratory tests, not field tests, because of the need for a treadmill capable of moving a belt at 8 mph (3.58 m·s^{-1}) up a 20 % grade. Additionally, these treadmill tests do not lend themselves to the simultaneous measurement of multiple participants, as would be the case in other field tests. However, the protocol of these treadmill tests is as simple as most field tests. What is being measured is the total time a participant is able to run on a treadmill at a particular speed up a 20 % grade. Various versions of the Anaerobic Treadmill Test exist, including the Fast Test (run at 8 mph; 3.58 m·s^{-1}), the Moderate Test (run at 7mph; 3.13 m·s^{-1}), and the Slow Test (run at 6 mph; 2.67m·s^{-1}), all up a 20 % grade. A published review of Anaerobic Treadmill Tests concluded that the Fast Test was the most often used to measure anaerobic work capacity and anaerobic fitness.[7]

There is a problem in using the Fast Test exclusively, however, because many participants, especially women and untrained men, are not able to complete even 1 s of exercise because of the extremely high effort required of such an intense uphill run. The "goal" of an Anaerobic Treadmill Test is to provide an exercise intensity that results in fatigue in 15–60 s, to stress the production of ATP through a combination of the two anaerobic energy systems. When the time to fatigue is short (< 15 s), as is frequently the case in the Fast Test, there will be a much greater emphasis on the phosphagen system. If the participants are unable to complete the Fast Test (8 mph), or if the intention of the test is to truly measure sustained high-intensity exercise ($\sim$60 s), the Moderate Test (7 mph) may be used instead. The Slow Test (6 mph) provides a third option for those participants who are still unable to run at the speed required of the Moderate Test. Care should be taken in selecting a specific Anaerobic Treadmill Test based on the characteristics (e.g., gender, age) and anticipated anaerobic fitness (e.g., sport, training status) of the participants of interest.

PHYSIOLOGICAL RATIONALE

These tests certainly are supramaximal tests when maximal oxygen consumption is used as the reference point. An all-out treadmill sprint that lasts from 54 s to 105 s represents about 125 % of a runner's aerobic capacity and produces a pH of about 6.88 in the gastrocnemius and vastus lateralis muscles.[4] Because performance in the Fast Test rarely exceeds 100 s, and performance in the Slow Test is often more than 100 s in men, it is clear that these two tests represent oxygen consumptions exceeding 125 % of maximal. The Slow Test, especially, would be expected to incur higher lactic acid values due to the longer time to accumulate lactic acid during glycolysis. The derived anaerobic contribution to an exhaustive treadmill run, at a steady pace of 12.9 mph (5.75 m·s^{-1}) to 14.4 mph (6.43 m·s^{-1}) for about 60 s at a 5 % slope, ranges from about 64 % to 72 %, with the higher value elicited by trained sprinters. The contribution of the glycolytic pathway for this 60 s run was greater than that of the phosphagenic portion of the anaerobic pathway.[16]

The Moderate Test produced lactate levels in college women basketball players that were about 10 times greater than resting levels.[13] Using heart rate as a familiar variable by which to substantiate the high intensity of such anaerobic power treadmill tests, males had peak heart rates that averaged 192 b·min^{-1} when running for about 93 s ($\pm$29 s) at 16 km·h^{-1} on an 8 % slope.[9]

METHODS

High-intensity efforts on a treadmill are often induced by increasing both the speed and slope of the treadmill. It is best to use a combination of these, because if only one is used, the participant may be limited by a singular contributing factor to anaerobic performance. For example, if only a fast speed at a level slope is used, slow runners with strong legs might find themselves trailing off the back of the treadmill; if only a steep slope at a slow speed is used, those with inferior leg strength or power may not have sufficient force to lift the body for long. Thus, these anaerobic tests for anaerobic fitness use a combination of slope and speed to accommodate the supramaximal efforts of many people. The accuracy of Anaerobic Treadmill Tests is discussed in Box 11.1.

Equipment

Treadmill

Obviously, a treadmill is the major piece of equipment for the Anaerobic Treadmill Test. Theoretically, it is possible to use a road if it has the slope prescribed in these tests. However, roads at 20 % grade are rarely found; for example, interstate highway regulators discourage the construction of roads with more than a 6 % grade. Good treadmills are very expensive, especially research-precision ones. Treadmills with front and side handrails are required for the Anaerobic Treadmill Test. A novel treadmill (Gymrol, France), combined with software, is capable of directly measuring peak and mean anaerobic power.[6] It utilizes a pivoting bar that measures vertical displacement of the runner's center of gravity and a strain gauge to measure horizontal force.

Timer

A stopwatch is best used to measure the duration of the performance to the closest 0.1 s.

Treadmill Protocol

The protocol for the treadmill tests should include a warm-up and familiarization period, along with a cool-down period (Table 11.1). The warm-up should consist of a regimen that mimics the movements of running and stretches the running muscles, respectively. The warm-up should not cause fatigue; some investigators[4,8] did not allow a warm-up for the treadmill runners in their research studies.

The Anaerobic Treadmill Tests are constant load tests because each one's speed and slope never change throughout the run. The Fast Test should be performed first if two tests are given within one hour. This is because recovery from this shorter test is quicker than the others. However, it is probably wiser to do the tests on separate days so that the Slow Test can be administered first. This gives the participants and technicians some input into the runner's capabilities for the more intimidating Fast Test. For example, if runners in the longer test cannot continue longer than 30 s, they may not be able to run without the use of the handrails at the least, and only a few seconds at the most, on the faster treadmill test. For these latter participants, the speed of the Fast Test might be reduced from 8 mph to the moderate test's 7 mph. One or two trials may be run for each participant, depending upon the fatigue of the participant and the administrative considerations of the lab director.

The cool-down period should be done off the treadmill (to allow testing subsequent participants) and begin with fast walking and gradually slower walking for a combined time of about 3 min to 5 min.

Procedures

As with all test procedures, technicians must be concerned with the safety and psychological well-being of the participants prior to and during the treadmill test. The key measurement for these tests is the total time that the participant can continue running at the given speed and slope.

Safety

These treadmill tests can induce more psychological distress than any other tests described in this manual. A fast-moving treadmill belt can be intimidating, even to experienced treadmill users. Thus, the technician's sensitivity to the participant's fears should include a sincere effort to familiarize

Table 11.1 | **Protocols for the Slow, Moderate, and Fast Anaerobic Treadmill Tests**

Period	Time (min)	Activity	
Warm-up and familiarization	0:00–10:00	(1) Jog in place; (2) slow jogging; (3) short bouts on level treadmill: (a) one walk bout at 3 mph and another bout at 4 mph for 10 s each; enter and exit the treadmill for each bout; (b) one jogging bout at 6 mph and another bout at 8 mph for 10 s each; enter and exit the treadmill for each bout; (4) short bouts on sloped treadmill: (a) one walk bout at 3 mph at 5 % grade and a walk/jog bout at 5 mph at 10 % grade for 10 s each; enter and exit the treadmill for each bout; (b) one jog/run at 6 mph and at 15 % grade and a run bout at 8 mph at 20 % grade for 5 s each (if doing the Fast Test); enter and exit the treadmill for each bout.	
Relief interval	10:00–11:00	Slow walking or walking in place	
Treadmill Test	**Time (min)**	**Grade (%)**	**Speed**
Slow test		20	6 mph (2.67 m·s^{-1})
Moderate test		20	7 mph (3.13 m·s^{-1})
Fast test		20	8 mph (3.58 m·s^{-1})
Cool-down	3:00–5:00		Gradually slower jogging and walking; stretching

him or her with the safe and proper technique of using the handrails to get on and off the fast-moving treadmill belt. Participants should be given time to practice this procedure. The key to the runners' mental security is their contact with the handrails. If a person is too fearful to let go of the handrail, then the test should be modified to a speed that the participant selects. The technician in control of the treadmill should be prepared to stop the treadmill as soon as the runner touches the handrails in preparation of exiting, while a spotter at the rear end of the treadmill should be prepared to support the runner if necessary. A hip-belt harness attached from the runner to the treadmill rails or the ceiling is ideal for maximizing safety and promoting uninhibited efforts.

Measurements

There is only one measurement—the time (to the closest 0.1 s) spent at the prescribed speed and slope of the treadmill. The timer starts the clock as soon as the participant, while running, releases the handrails. The timer stops the clock when the runner takes hold of the handrails in preparation for exiting from the treadmill belt. If two trials are given, the better time is used for statistical purposes. In summary, the checklist of procedures is as follows:

1. Record the participant's weight in running attire onto Form 11.2.
2. The runner follows an appropriate warm-up and familiarization regimen similar to the one presented in Table 11.1.
3. A technician places the treadmill at the prescribed speed for the selected test (slow = 6 mph or 2.67 m·s⁻¹; moderate = 7 mph or 3.13 m·s⁻¹; fast = 8 mph or 3.58 m·s⁻¹) and grade (20 %).
4. With hands on the rails, the participant either straddles the treadmill belt or stands with both feet on one side of the treadmill belt.
5. With hands still holding onto the rails, the participant steps onto the moving treadmill belt.
6. A technician (timer) starts the watch as soon as the runner's hands release the handrail.
7. The timer stops the watch as soon as the runner touches the handrails.
8. Also at this time, the technician stops the treadmill.
9. The time is recorded to the closest 0.1 s on Form 11.2.
10. The participant cools down (see Table 11.1).

Calculations

The calculation of anaerobic work may be made from the body weight (mass) of the runner, the slope and speed of the treadmill, and the time spent on the treadmill. The percent grade (or slope) of the treadmill is defined as the projected distance of the vertical rise per 100 units of travel. Running up a 20 % grade means that, for every 100 m traveled on the treadmill belt, there will be a vertical rise of 20 m (see Figure 11.1).

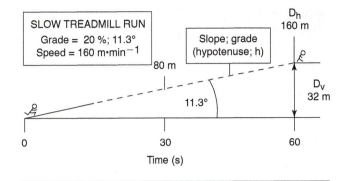

Figure 11.1 If a runner continues to run at a grade of 20 % and a speed of 160 m·min⁻¹ until exhaustion at the 60th s, the projected vertical distance (D_v) of the runner is 20 % of the covered distance of the treadmill belt/runner (hypotenuse; D_h = 160 m). Thus, the runner in this case would be projected vertically to a height of 32 m. If the runner stopped in 30 s, the hypotenuse distance would be 80 m and the vertical distance would be 20 % of 80 m, which is equal to 16 m.

Work can be calculated during treadmill running as the product of force (the runner's body mass in newtons) times distance (the vertical rise in m), as seen in Equation 11.1a. By substituting for force, vertical distance, and hypotenuse distance, work can be calculated through the use of Equation 11.1b. For example, a person with a body mass of 700 N, who runs for 60 s on the Slow Test at a speed of 6 mph (2.67 m·s⁻¹) up a 20 % grade, would complete 22.4 kJ of work (Eq. 11.1c).

Work (N·m) = Force (N) $*$ Vertical distance (m)   Eq. 11.1a

Where: Force = Body mass (N) = Body weight (kg) $*$ 9.8067

And where: Vertical distance = Hypotenuse distance $*$ % Slope / 100

And where: Hypotenuse distance = Speed (m·s⁻¹) $*$ Time (s)

By substitution:

Work (kJ) = Body mass (N) $*$ Speed (m·s⁻¹) $*$ Time (s) $*$ % Slope / 100   Eq. 11.1b

Assume: Force = **700** N; Speed = **2.67** m·s⁻¹;

    Time = **60** s; Slope = **20** % (0.20)

Work = **700** N $*$ **2.67** m·s⁻¹ $*$ **60** s $*$ **0.20** = **22 428** J
    = **22.4** kJ   Eq. 11.1c

RESULTS AND DISCUSSION

Norms, especially expressed in total work units, are needed for these treadmill tests. Table 11.2 presents unpublished percentiles from a master's project (2000) for time, total work and mean anaerobic power in men ages 18–25 y who performed the Fast Test.[3] The men (N = 105) averaged

Table 11.2	Norms for the Fast (8 mph) Anaerobic Treadmill Test for Active Men

Category	%ile	Time (s)	Work (kJ)	Power (W)
Well above ave	95	53.8	28.4	661
Above average	90	49.2	25.5	628
	85	46.3	24.0	605
	80	41.6	22.6	599
	75	40.7	21.7	587
Average	70	39.0	21.3	576
	50	33.3	18.8	541
	30	28.3	15.7	499
Below average	25	26.8	15.3	494
	20	22.8	15.1	454
	15	20.6	12.6	439
	10	19.2	11.0	421
Well below ave	5	17.9	10.2	401
Mean		33.6	18.8	535
S.D.		11.3	5.8	81
Minimum		5.9	7.3	377
Maximum		61.6	37.4	753

Source: Calmelat (2000).[3] Based on active men between the ages of 18 y and 25 y. Test results for Time (N = 105), Work (N = 71), and Power (N = 71).

Table 11.3	Comparative Data for Mean Exercise Time (s) for the Anaerobic Treadmill Test

Group	Mean ± SD (s)	Range (s)
Fast Test (8 mph; 3.58 m·s^{-1})		
College women (N = 14)[1]	14	8–22
College men (N = 38)[1]	33	18–66
College men (N = 105)[3]	34 ± 11	6–62
Trained men (N = 8)[5]	64 ± 13	44–90
Elite skiers, men (N = 20)[2]	77 ± 4	
Elite athletes, men (N = 6)[11]	82 ± 20	
Elite soccer, men (N = 16)[12]	93 ± 10	68–102
800 m runners, men (N = 6)[10]	114 ± 16	
Moderate Test (7 mph; 3.13 m·s^{-1})		
Basketball, women (N = 20)[13]	39 ± 2	
Slow Test (6 mph; 2.67 m·s^{-1})		
College women (N = 34)[1]	37	20–58
College men (N = 46)[1]	78	49–167

Sources: Adams (2000)[1]; Brown & Wilkinson (1983)[2]; Calmelat (2000)[3]; Cunningham & Faulkner (1969)[5]; McKenzie et al. (1982)[10]; Parkhouse & McKenzie (1983)[11]; Rhodes et al. (1986)[12]; Riezebos et al. (1983).[13]

33.6 ± 11.3 s for the 8 mph (3.58 m·s^{-1}) test, accomplished an average total work of 18.8 ± 5.8 kJ (N = 71), and a mean anaerobic power of 535 ± 81 N. Because work (kJ) and mean anaerobic power (W) are both derived from exercise time (s), the category will be the same for all 3 variables. The values presented in Table 11.3 are for the 3 different tests (the Fast, Moderate and Slow tests) and may be used for comparative purposes. The mean exercise time on the Fast Test goes from a low of 14 s in college women,[1] to 33–34 s for college men,[1,3] to 64 s for trained men,[5] up to 82–114 s for elite athletes.[10,11,12] The highest degree of anaerobic fitness observed was in 800 m runners, who's mean anaerobic power was 114 ±16 W.[10] Mean values on the Fast and Slow tests for men (33 s and 78 s respectively) were just over 2 times the values for women on the same tests (14 s and 37 s respectively).[1]

Running performance for such competitive distances as the 200 m, 300 m, and 400 m are predominantly anaerobic events. A pair of investigators used the accumulated maximal oxygen deficit (AMOD) to estimate the energy contribution by the aerobic pathway for treadmill simulated 200 m, 400 m, and 800 m run events in highly trained runners.[15] AMOD is calculated by subtracting the accumulated oxygen consumption from the accumulated oxygen demand for the duration of each run. For the 200 m run, the aerobic pathway contributed 29 % of the energy; hence, the anaerobic pathway contributed 71 %. The aerobic contribution for the 400 m run was 43 %—hence, 57 % by the anaerobic pathways. For the 800 m run, the aerobic pathway contributed 84 % of the energy; hence, the anaerobic pathways contributed only 16 % of the total energy. The treadmill tests described in this chapter often produce run times that presumably would require anaerobic contributions falling between the percentages of 16 % and 71 % reported for the 800 m and 200 m runs, respectively. The lower percentage (16 %), which was equivalent to a time of 113 s by the elite runners, was much lower than the 40 % contribution determined by another group of investigators.[14] One reviewer mentioned a maximum duration of 60 s as a criterion to qualify as a valid anaerobic test.[7] He suggested that times beyond 60 s would likely exceed 50 % energy contribution by the aerobic pathway. Thus, it appears that, if runners exceed 60 s on any of the Anaerobic Treadmill Tests, then the speed and/or the slope should be increased in order to get a true anaerobic fitness evaluation. However, times between 60 s and 120 s should still rely heavily on anaerobic metabolism.

BOX 11.2	Chapter Preview/Review

What are the three different versions of the Anaerobic Treadmill Test protocol?

How much work (kJ) would a 700 N person complete running for 60 s on the Slow Test at 6 mph (2.67 m.s^{-1}) up a 20% grade?

What is the average time (s) for the Slow Test for college men and women?

What is the average time (s) and work completed (kJ) for the Fast Test in active men (18–25y)?

References

1. Adams, G. (2000). Unpublished data.
2. Brown, S. L., & Wilkinson, J. G. (1983). Characteristics of national, divisional, and club male Alpine ski

racers. *Medicine and Science in Sports and Exercise, 15,* 491–495.

3. Calmelat, R. (2000). Unpublished master's project, California State University, Fullerton.

4. Costill, D. L., Barnett, A., Sharp, R., Fink, W. J., & Katz, A. (1983). Leg muscle pH following sprint running. *Medicine and Science in Sports and Exercise, 15,* 325–329.

5. Cunningham, D. A., & Faulkner, J. A. (1969). The effect of training on aerobic and anaerobic metabolism during a short exhaustive run. *Medicine and Science in Sports and Exercise, 1,* 65–69.

6. Falk, B., Weinstein, Y., Dotan, R., Abramson, D. A., Mann-Segal, D., & Hoffman, J. R. (1996). A treadmill test of sprint running. *Scandinavian Journal of Medicine and Science in Sports, 6,* 259–264.

7. Green, S. (1995). Measurement of anaerobic work capacities in humans. *Sports Medicine, 19,* 32–42.

8. Houston, M. E., & Green, H. J. (1976). Physiological and anthropometric characteristics of elite Canadian ice hockey players. *Journal of Sportsmedicine and Physical Fitness, 16,* 123–128.

9. Mackova, E. V., Melichna, J., Vondra, K., Jurimae, T., Tomas, P., & Novak, J. (1985). The relationship between anaerobic performance and muscle metabolic capacity and fibre distribution. *European Journal of Applied Physiology, 54,* 413–415.

10. McKenzie, D. C., Parkhouse, W. S., & Hearst, W. D. (1982). Anaerobic performance characteristics of elite Canadian 800 meter runners. *Canadian Journal of Applied Sport Sciences, 7,* 158–160.

11. Parkhouse, W. S., & McKenzie, D. C. (1983). Anaerobic capacity assessment of elite athletes. *Medicine and Science in Sports and Exercise, 15,* Abstract, 142.

12. Rhodes, E. C., Mosber, R. E., McKenzie, D. C., Franks, J. M., Potts, J. E., & Wenger, H. A. (1986). Physiological profiles of the Canadian Olympic Soccer Team. *Canadian Journal of Applied Sport Sciences, 11,* 31–36.

13. Riezebos, M. L., Paterson, D. H., Hall, C. R., & Yuhasz, S. (1983). Relationship of selected variables to performance in women's basketball. *Canadian Journal of Applied Sport Sciences, 8,* 34–40.

14. Scott, C. B., Roby, F. B., Lohman, T. G., & Bunt, J. C. (1991). The maximally accumulated oxygen deficit as an indicator of anaerobic capacity. *Medicine and Science in Sports and Exercise, 23,* 618–624.

15. Spencer, M. R., & Gastin, P. B. (2001). Energy system contribution during 200- to 1500-m running in highly trained athletes. *Medicine and Science in Sports and Exercise, 33,* 157–162.

16. Thomson, J. M., & Garvie, K. J. (1981). A laboratory method for determination of anaerobic energy expenditure during sprinting. *Canadian Journal of Applied Sport Sciences, 6,* 21–26.

Form 11.1

ANAEROBIC TREADMILL RUNNING

Homework

Gender: **M**   Initials: **AA**   Age (y): **20**   Height (cm): **180**   Weight (kg): **85.0**

Body mass = _____ * 9.8067 N·kg^{-1} = _____ N
⎯⎯⎯⎯ Wt (kg)

Test 1 : **Fast**   Speed (mph) = **8** = _____ m·s^{-1} Time (s) = **30.5**

Work (kJ) = [_____ N * _____ m·s^{-1} * _____ s * 0.20 / 1000] = _____ kJ
                Mass   Speed   Time   Grade

Evaluation for: Time (s) _____   Work (kJ) _____
                (Table 11.2 / 11.3)   *(Table 11.2 / 11.3)*

Test 2 : **Slow**   Speed (mph) = **6** = _____ m·s^{-1} Time (s) = **72.0**

Work (kJ) = [_____ N * _____ m·s^{-1} * _____ s * 0.20 / 1000] = _____ kJ
                Mass   Speed   Time   Grade

Evaluation for: Time (s) _____   Work (kJ) _____
                (Table 11.2 / 11.3)   *(Table 11.2 / 11.3)*

Evaluation / comments: _____

_____

Gender: **F**   Initials: **BB**   Age (y): **20**   Height (cm): **170**   Weight (kg): **75.0**

Body mass = _____ * 9.8067 N·kg^{-1} = _____ N
⎯⎯⎯⎯ Wt (kg)

Test 1 : **Fast**   Speed (mph) = **8** = _____ m·s^{-1} Time (s) = **17.3**

Work (kJ) = [_____ N * _____ m·s^{-1} * _____ s * 0.20 / 1000] = _____ kJ
                Mass   Speed   Time   Grade

Evaluation for: Time (s) _____   Work (kJ) _____
                (Table 11.2 / 11.3)   *(Table 11.2 / 11.3)*

Test 2 : **Slow**   Speed (mph) = **6** = _____ m·s^{-1} Time (s) = **38.5**

Work (kJ) = [_____ N * _____ m·s^{-1} * _____ s * 0.20 / 1000] = _____ kJ
                Mass   Speed   Time   Grade

Evaluation for: Time (s) _____   Work (kJ) _____
                (Table 11.2 / 11.3)   *(Table 11.2 / 11.3)*

Evaluation / comments: _____

_____

Form 11.2
ANAEROBIC TREADMILL RUNNING

NAME _____ DATE _____ SCORE _____

Lab Results

Gender: _____ Initials: _____ Age (y): _____ Height (cm): _____ Weight (kg): _____

Body mass = _____ * 9.8067 N·kg⁻¹ = _____ N
       Wt (kg)

Test 1 : _____ Speed (mph) = _____ = _____ m·s⁻¹ Time (s) = _____

Work (kJ) = [_____ N * _____ m·s⁻¹ * _____ s * 0.20 / 1000] = _____ kJ
       Mass   Speed   Time   Grade

Evaluation for: Time (s) _____ Work (kJ) _____
                    (Table 11.2 / 11.3)   *(Table 11.2 / 11.3)*

Test 2 : _____ Speed (mph) = _____ = _____ m·s⁻¹ Time (s) = _____

Work (kJ) = [_____ N * _____ m·s⁻¹ * _____ s * 0.20 / 1000] = _____ kJ
       Mass   Speed   Time   Grade

Evaluation for: Time (s) _____ Work (kJ) _____
                    (Table 11.2 / 11.3)   *(Table 11.2 / 11.3)*

Evaluation / comments: _____

_____

_____

Gender: _____ Initials: _____ Age (y): _____ Height (cm): _____ Weight (kg): _____

Body mass = _____ * 9.8067 N·kg⁻¹ = _____ N
       Wt (kg)

Test 1 : _____ Speed (mph) = _____ = _____ m·s⁻¹ Time (s) = _____

Work (kJ) = [_____ N * _____ m·s⁻¹ * _____ s * 0.20 / 1000] = _____ kJ
       Mass   Speed   Time   Grade

Evaluation for: Time (s) _____ Work (kJ) _____
                    (Table 11.2 / 11.3)   *(Table 11.2 / 11.3)*

Test 2 : _____ Speed (mph) = _____ = _____ m·s⁻¹ Time (s) = _____

Work (kJ) = [_____ N * _____ m·s⁻¹ * _____ s * 0.20 / 1000] = _____ kJ
       Mass   Speed   Time   Grade

Evaluation for: Time (s) _____ Work (kJ) _____
                    (Table 11.2 / 11.3)   *(Table 11.2 / 11.3)*

Evaluation / comments: _____

_____

_____

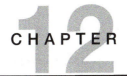
AEROBIC RUNNING, JOGGING, AND WALKING

This chapter discusses three popular field tests—the Cooper Run Test, the George Jog Test, and the Rockport Walk Test. These are good examples of field tests due to the use of minimal equipment, their application to large groups, and their ease of administration. Aerobic run/jog/walk tests are the most common field tests of cardiorespiratory fitness.[26] Despite their value in measuring functional fitness, these field tests are not usually considered replacement tests for the direct measurement of oxygen consumption in research studies.

The Cooper Run Test, developed by Kenneth Cooper for use by the U.S. Air Force,[6] evolved from the original 15min run test described by Bruno Balke.[3] Cooper developed a 12 Minute Run version and a 1.5 Mile Run version of the test. Although originally intended for measuring changes in fitness with training, the Cooper Run Test is now commonly used solely to assess the aerobic fitness of the general public. It is expected that participants will give a maximal effort and run as far as possible in 12 minutes or run the 1.5 mile distance as fast as possible. For this reason, the test applies better to a younger, fitter population. It is generally not considered an appropriate test for sedentary persons or for older adults.

James George and colleagues developed an alternative to the maximal Cooper Run Test, creating a submaximal 1mile jogging test, referred to in this laboratory manual as the George Jog Test. This test is more appropriate for less fit individuals due to its submaximal nature, but may still not be appropriate for sedentary persons or for older adults. It is typically used for assessing the aerobic fitness of fairly fit college-age persons.[14,15,16] In addition to recording the 1 mile jogging time, which is recommended to be no faster than an 8 to 9 minute mile pace, other variables, including gender, body weight, and heart rate, are used to estimate maximal oxygen consumption.

The third aerobic fitness test described here is the Rockport Walk Test, developed by James Rippe and colleagues.[19] The Rockport Walk Test, like the George Jog Test, uses gender, body weight, walk time, and heart rate to estimate maximal oxygen uptake and also incorporates the participant's age. The Rockport Walk Test was developed on adults ranging in age from 30 to 69 y. It has subsequently been modified for use in persons age 18–29 y.[12,14] It has been further validated for use with elderly women.[27] Although participants are asked to walk as fast as possible, the test is still considered a submaximal test, and is one of the more appropriate tests that can be used in sedentary persons and older adults.

PHYSIOLOGICAL RATIONALE FOR THE AEROBIC RUN/JOG/WALK TESTS

Aerobic metabolism predominates for events that last for about two or more minutes. A pair of investigators estimated that highly trained runners performing the 1500 m ($\approx$ 100 m short of one mile) in 3 min 55 s received 84 % of their energy from the aerobic system.[26] Thus, the aerobic system would dominate in the times required for the 1 mile and 1.5 mile tests. Oxygen is transported first by the respiratory (pulmonary) system to the cardiovascular system, and from there to the contracting muscles. The muscles consume the oxygen in order to provide sufficient amounts of adenosine triphosphate (ATP) for the myosin filaments to pull the actin filaments; the pulling within the muscles causes muscle action. Without a sufficient amount of oxygen, there is not enough ATP produced to sustain muscular action beyond a couple of minutes. Thus, other factors being equal, the runner who can supply the highest rate of oxygen to the muscles will be able to perform aerobic exercise at a faster speed. The highest possible rate of oxygen consumption is called the maximal oxygen consumption ($\dot{V}O_2max$).

METHODS

The Methods section includes descriptions of the (1) facility, (2) equipment, and (3) procedures and calculations. Comments pertaining to the accuracy of run/jog/walk tests are in Box 12.1.

Facility

The facility requires a level terrain that has accurately measured distances. Most new track facilities are ovals of 400 m, which means that each lap on the metric track is 2.5 yd shorter than the older 440 yd American ovals (Figure 12.1). This means that if performing on a metric track, the runner or walker must go 9 m (10 yd) beyond four laps for the 1.0 Mile Test, and 14 m (15 yd) beyond six laps for the 1.5 Mile Test. The two straightaways and the turns of a quarter-mile (440 yd) track are usually 110 yds. Thus, any distance halfway between any one of the four intervals is

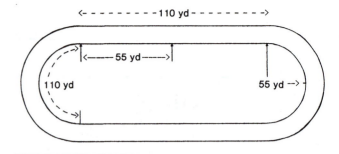

Figure 12.1   Layout of a quarter-mile (440 yd; 402.3 m) track. The straightaways and turns are 110 yd each; thus, the midpoints between these are 55 yd each (1 yd = 0.914 m; 1 m = 1.0936 yd).

for the George Jog Test and the Rockport Walk Test, electronic monitoring using miniature transmitters and receivers (e.g., Polar) are practical[21] and inexpensive. These monitors have a transmitting device and chest electrodes built into the chest strap. A receiver, which also serves other functions, digitally displays the heart rate. The runner or walker wears the strap and the "wristwatch" receiver, or the technician, within five feet of the participant, can hold the receiver.

    Large groups may be tested easily on these tests. At the "Go!" signal, all participants begin running, jogging, or walking, and the timer starts the clock. At the end of either the prescribed time or the prescribed distance, the timer yells out the times so that the participants or recorders can write down their times or distances.

Procedures and Calculations for the Aerobic Run/Jog/Walk Tests

The two versions of the Cooper Run Test described in this chapter, the Cooper 1.5 Mile Run Test and the Cooper 12 Minute Run Test, are based on a relationship between maximal oxygen consumption and running time or running distance. As seen in Figure 12.2, maximal oxygen consumption ($\dot{V}O_2$max) can be estimated based on the inverse relationship observed between 1.5 mi run time and $\dot{V}O_2$max, or the direct relationship observed between $\dot{V}O_2$max and running distance. The George Jog Test and Rockport Walk Test are both based on multiple regression models that estimate $\dot{V}O_2$max based on a number of independent variables, including age, gender, body weight, jogging or walking time required to cover 1 mile, and heart rate at the completion of the test or within the last lap (¼ mile).

The Cooper (1.5 mi) Run Test

1. The participant runs on level terrain (preferably a measured 440 yd or 400 m track) for the prescribed distance of 1.5 mi (2414 m).
2. The technician records the participant's time to the closest second onto Form 12.2. As an optional measure, the technician records the heart rate for 15 s immediately after the participant crosses the finish line.

55 yd. Also, keep in mind that the 400 m or 440 yd distance for one lap applies only to the inside lane (about 1 ft from the curb). A treadmill is optional when performing the Rockport Walk Test.[22]

Equipment

The only piece of equipment that is absolutely necessary to conduct the aerobic run/jog/walk tests is a watch with a seconds indicator. For greater accuracy in measuring heart rate

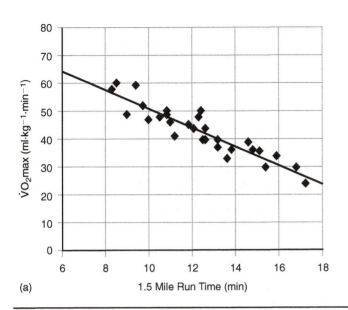

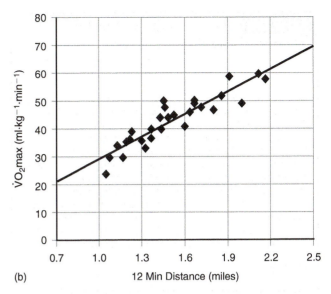

Figure 12.2 The inverse relationship observed between 1.5 mi running time and maximal oxygen consumption (a), and the direct relationship observed between 12 min distance run and maximal oxygen consumption (b). The longer the time required to run 1.5 mi or the shorter the distance run in 12 min, the lower the observed $\dot{V}O_2$max.

Table 12.1	Estimated Value (and Range) for Maximal Oxygen Consumption Based on 1.5 Mile Run Time

1.5 Mile Time (min:sec)	$\dot{V}O_2$max (ml·kg⁻¹·min⁻¹) Value	$\dot{V}O_2$max (ml·kg⁻¹·min⁻¹) (Range)	1.5 Mile Time (min:sec)	$\dot{V}O_2$max (ml·kg⁻¹·min⁻¹) Value	$\dot{V}O_2$max (ml·kg⁻¹·min⁻¹) (Range)	1.5 Mile Time (min:sec)	$\dot{V}O_2$max (ml·kg⁻¹·min⁻¹) Value	$\dot{V}O_2$max (ml·kg⁻¹·min⁻¹) (Range)
< 7:31	72.3	(> 72.3)	10:31–10:45	50.2	(49.5–50.9)	13:46–14:00	34.6	(34.2–35.0)
7:31–7:45	71.3	(70.3–72.3)	10:46–11:00	48.7	(48.0–49.4)	14:01–14:15	33.8	(33.4–34.1)
7:46–8:00	69.3	(68.3–70.2)	11:01–11:15	47.3	(46.7–47.9)	14:16–14:30	33.0	(32.6–33.3)
8:01–8:15	67.3	(66.4–68.2)	11:16–11:30	46.0	(45.3–46.6)	14:31–14:45	32.2	(31.8–32.5)
8:16–8:30	65.4	(64.5–66.3)	11:31–11:45	44.6	(44.0–45.2)	14:46–15:00	31.4	(31.1–31.7)
8:31–8:45	63.5	(62.6–64.4)	11:46–12:00	43.3	(42.7–43.9)	15:01–15:15	30.7	(30.4–31.0)
8:46–9:00	61.7	(60.8–62.5)	12:01–12:15	42.1	(41.5–42.6)	15:16–15:30	30.0	(29.7–30.3)
9:01–9:15	59.9	(59.1–60.7)	12:16–12:30	40.9	(40.3–41.4)	15:31–15:45	29.4	(29.1–29.6)
9:16–9:30	58.2	(57.4–59.0)	12:31–12:45	39.7	(39.2–40.2)	15:46–16:00	28.8	(28.6–29.0)
9:31–9:45	56.5	(55.7–57.3)	12:46–13:00	38.6	(38.1–39.1)	16:01–16:15	28.3	(28.1–28.5)
9:46–10:00	54.9	(54.1–55.6)	13:01–13:15	37.6	(37.1–38.0)	16:16–16:30	27.8	(27.6–28.0)
10:01–10:15	53.3	(52.5–54.0)	13:16–13:30	36.6	(36.1–37.0)	16:31–16:45	27.4	(27.2–27.5)
10:16–10:30	51.7	(51.0–52.4)	13:31–13:45	35.6	(35.1–36.0)	> 16:45	27.2	(< 27.2)

Source: Data for estimation of $\dot{V}O_2$max from Wilmore & Bergfeld (1979).[28]

3. The technician estimates $\dot{V}O_2$max from the 1.5 mi run time using Table 12.1. The fitness category is determined from the $\dot{V}O_2$max by using Table 12.3.

Example: If a 22-year-old man runs the 1.5 mi distance in 10:23, the maximal oxygen consumption can be estimated as 51.0–52.4 ml·kg⁻¹·min⁻¹ from Table 12.1. The corresponding fitness category is "excellent" from Table 12.3.

The Cooper (12 min) Run Test (*Optional*)

1. The participant runs on level terrain (preferably a measured 440 yd or 400 m track) as far as possible in 12 min.

2. The technician or participant estimates the distance covered to the closest 55 yd (or 50 m), which represents ⅛ of a lap on a 440 yd (400 m) track.

3. The technician estimates $\dot{V}O_2$max by using Table 12.2 or by inserting the distance covered in 12 min into Equation 12.1a (if in miles) or Equation 12.1b (if in kilometers) and records it on Form 12.2. The fitness category is determined from the $\dot{V}O_2$max by using Table 12.4.

$$\dot{V}O_2max \ (ml·kg^{-1}·min^{-1}) = (Distance \ (mi) - 0.3138) / 0.0278 \qquad Eq. \ 12.1a$$

$$\dot{V}O_2max \ (ml·kg^{-1}·min^{-1}) = (Distance \ (km) - 0.505) / 0.0447 \qquad Eq. \ 12.1b$$

Table 12.2 — Estimation of Maximal Oxygen Consumption Based on 12 Minute Performance

Distance (miles)	Number of Laps	Distance (miles and yards)		$\dot VO_2$max (ml·kg^{-1}·min^{-1})	Distance (miles)	Number of Laps	Distance (miles and yards)		$\dot VO_2$max (ml·kg^{-1}·min^{-1})
1.00	4.000	1 mile	0 yd	25.0	1.50	6.000	1 mile	880 yd	42.6
1.03	4.125	1 mile	55 yd	26.0	1.53	6.125	1 mile	935 yd	43.8
1.06	4.250	1 mile	110 yd	27.0	1.56	6.250	1 mile	990 yd	45.0
1.09	4.375	1 mile	165 yd	28.2	1.59	6.375	1 mile	1045 yd	46.0
1.13	4.500	1 mile	220 yd	29.0	1.63	6.500	1 mile	1100 yd	47.2
1.16	4.625	1 mile	275 yd	30.2	1.66	6.625	1 mile	1155 yd	48.0
1.19	4.750	1 mile	330 yd	31.6	1.69	6.750	1 mile	1210 yd	49.2
1.22	4.875	1 mile	385 yd	32.8	1.72	6.875	1 mile	1265 yd	50.2
1.25	5.000	1 mile	440 yd	33.8	1.75	7.000	1 mile	1320 yd	51.6
1.28	5.125	1 mile	495 yd	34.8	1.78	7.125	1 mile	1375 yd	52.6
1.31	5.250	1 mile	550 yd	36.2	1.81	7.250	1 mile	1430 yd	53.8
1.34	5.375	1 mile	605 yd	37.0	1.84	7.375	1 mile	1485 yd	54.8
1.38	5.500	1 mile	660 yd	38.2	1.88	7.500	1 mile	1540 yd	56.0
1.41	5.625	1 mile	715 yd	39.2	1.91	7.625	1 mile	1595 yd	57.0
1.44	5.750	1 mile	770 yd	40.4	1.94	7.750	1 mile	1650 yd	58.2
1.47	5.875	1 mile	825 yd	41.6	1.97	7.875	1 mile	1705 yd	59.2
					2.00	8.000	2 miles	0 yd	60.2

Sources: Data from Cooper (1968).[6]

Table 12.3 — Fitness Category and Estimated $\dot VO_2$max for 1.5 Mile Run Time by Gender and Age Group

Men	13–19 y		20–29 y		30–39 y		40–49 y	
Fitness Category	Time (min:sec)	$\dot VO_2$max (ml·kg^{-1}·min^{-1})	Time (min:sec)	$\dot VO_2$max (ml·kg^{-1}·min^{-1})	Time (min:sec)	$\dot VO_2$max (ml·kg^{-1}·min^{-1})	Time (min:sec)	$\dot VO_2$max (ml·kg^{-1}·min^{-1})
Superior	< 8:37	> 63.6	< 9:45	> 55.7	< 10:00	> 54.1	< 10:30	> 51.0
Excellent	8:37–9:40	56.2–63.6	9:45–10:45	49.5–55.7	10:00–11:00	48.0–54.1	10:30–11:30	45.3–51.0
Good	9:41–10:48	49.2–56.1	10:46–12:00	42.7–49.4	11:01–12:30	40.3–47.9	11:31–13:00	38.1–45.2
Fair	10:49–12:10	41.9–49.1	12:01–14:00	34.2–42.6	12:31–14:45	31.8–40.2	13:01–15:35	29.8–38.0
Poor	> 12:10	< 41.9	> 14:00	< 34.2	> 14:45	< 31.8	> 15:35	< 29.8

Women	13–19 y		20–29 y		30–39 y		40–49 y	
Fitness Category	Time (min:sec)	$\dot VO_2$max (ml·kg^{-1}·min^{-1})	Time (min:sec)	$\dot VO_2$max (ml·kg^{-1}·min^{-1})	Time (min:sec)	$\dot VO_2$max (ml·kg^{-1}·min^{-1})	Time (min:sec)	$\dot VO_2$max (ml·kg^{-1}·min^{-1})
Superior	< 11:50	> 43.6	< 12:30	> 40.3	< 13:00	> 38.0	< 13:45	> 35.1
Excellent	11:50–12:29	40.4–43.6	12:30–13:30	36.1–40.3	13:00–14:30	32.6–38.0	13:45–15:55	28.8–35.1
Good	12:30–14:30	32.6–40.3	13:31–15:54	28.8–36.0	14:31–16:30	27.6–32.5	15:56–17:30	26.2–28.7
Fair	14:31–16:54	27.0–32.5	15:55–18:30	25.6–28.7	16:31–19:00	25.5–27.5	17:31–19:30	25.5–26.1
Poor	> 16:54	< 27.0	> 18:30	< 25.6	> 19:00	< 25.5	> 19:30	< 25.5

Sources: Data for fitness category from Kusinitz & Fine (1991)[20]; data for estimation of $\dot VO_2$max from Wilmore & Bergfeld (1979).[28]

Table 12.4 — Fitness Category and Estimated $\dot VO_2$max for 12 Minute Performance Distance

Fitness Category	Distance (miles)	$\dot VO_2$max (ml·kg^{-1}·min^{-1})
Excellent	> 1.75	> 51.6
Good	1.50–1.74	51.6–42.6
Fair	1.25–1.49	42.5–33.8
Poor	1.00–1.24	33.7–25.0
Very Poor	< 1.00	< 25.0

Source: Data from Cooper (1968).[6]

Example: If the distance run in 12 min is 1 mi and 440 yd (1.25 mi), the maximal oxygen consumption can be determined as 33.8 ml·kg^{-1}·min^{-1} from Table 12.2, or it could be calculated as seen in Equation 12.2.

$$\dot VO_2\text{max (ml·kg}^{-1}\text{·min}^{-1}) = (\textbf{1.25 mi} - 0.3138)$$
$$/\ 0.0278 = \textbf{33.7 ml·kg}^{-1}\text{·min}^{-1} \qquad \text{Eq. 12.2}$$

The George Jog Test

1. The technician weighs the participant in running attire and records onto Form 12.2.
2. The participant jogs 1 mi at a slow to moderate steady pace (8 min per mi pace for men; 9 min per mi pace for women).

Table 12.5	Fitness Category for George Jog Test in College-Aged Men and Women (*N* = 106)	
Category	College Men	College Women
Well above ave	> 58.4	> 48.2
Above average	53.6–58.4	44.6–48.2
Average	47.0–53.5	39.6–44.5
Below average	42.2–46.9	36.0–39.5
Well below ave	< 42.2	< 36.0
Mean	50.3	42.1

Note: Values for percentiles are estimated using the reported means and standard deviations assuming the data are normally distributed.
Source: Data from George, et al. (1993).[16]

Table 12.6	Fitness Category for Rockport Walk Test in Men and Women 30–69 y (*N* = 343)	
Category	Men	Women
Well above ave	> 59.0	> 45.0
Above average	49.2–59.0	37.2–45.0
Average	35.4–49.2	26.4–37.1
Below average	25.5–35.3	18.6–26.3
Well below ave	< 25.5	< 18.6
Mean	42.3	31.8

Note: Values for percentiles are estimated using the reported means and standard deviations assuming the data are normally distributed.
Source: Data from Kline, et al. (1987).[19]

3. Heart rate (HR) is taken by the technician or by the participant immediately upon crossing the 1 mi mark or during the last quarter mile.
4. The technician records the participant's time to the closest second onto Form 12.2. The time is also converted into decimal form to the nearest hundredth minute and recorded. For example, a jogging time of 10:17 is converted by dividing 17 sec by 60 (0.28) and adding this to 10 min to yield 10.28 min.
5. The technician estimates $\dot{V}O_2max$ according to Equation 12.3 and determines a fitness category from Table 12.5.

$$\dot{V}O_2max\ (ml\cdot kg^{-1}\cdot min^{-1}) = 100 + (Gender * 8.344)$$
$$- (Weight\ (kg) * 0.1636 - (Jog\ time\ (min)$$
$$* 1.438) - (HR\ (bpm) * 0.1928) \qquad Eq.\ 12.3$$

Where: Gender = 1 (if male) or 0 (if female)

Example: If a 20-year-old man, who weighs 75 kg, jogs the 1.5 mi distance in 10:17 (10.28 min) with a heart rate of 150 bpm, the maximal oxygen consumption can be estimated as 52.9 ml·kg^{-1}·min^{-1} (Eq. 12.4).

$$\dot{V}O_2max\ (ml\cdot kg^{-1}\cdot min^{-1}) = 100.5 + (\mathbf{1} * 8.344)$$
$$- (\mathbf{75}\ kg * 0.1636 - (\mathbf{10.28}\ min * 1.438)$$
$$- (\mathbf{150}\ bpm * 0.1928) = \mathbf{52.9}\ ml\cdot kg^{-1}\cdot min^{-1} \quad Eq.\ 12.4$$

The Rockport Walk Test

1. The technician weighs the participant in running attire and records onto Form 12.2.
2. The participant walks on level terrain (preferably a measured 440 yd or 400 m track) 1 mi at the fastest pace possible.
3. Heart rate (HR) is taken by the technician or by the participant immediately upon crossing the 1 mi mark or during the last quarter mile.
4. The technician records the participant's time to the closest second onto Form 12.2. The time is also converted into decimal form to the nearest hundredth minute and recorded. For example, a walking time of 14:25 is converted by dividing 25 sec by 60 (0.42) and adding this to 14 min to yield 14.42 min.

Table 12.7	Fitness Category for Rockport Walk Test in Men and Women 18–29 y (*N* = 359)	
Category	Men	Women
Well above ave	> 57.8	> 45.4
Above average	51.0–57.8	40.7–45.4
Average	41.5–50.9	34.1–40.6
Below average	34.7–41.4	29.4–34.0
Well below ave	< 34.7	< 29.4
Mean	46.2	37.4

Note: Values for percentiles are estimated using the reported means and standard deviations assuming the data are normally distributed.
Sources: Dolgener, Hensley, Marsh, & Fjelstul (1994)[12]; George, et al. (1993).[16]

5. The technician estimates $\dot{V}O_2max$ according to Equation 12.5a (for adults)[18] or Equation 12.5b (for college-aged participants)[12,14] and determines a fitness category from Table 12.6 (for adults) or from Table 12.7 (for college-aged participants).

$$\dot{V}O_2max\ (ml\cdot kg^{-1}\cdot min^{-1}) = 132.853 + (Gender * 6.315)$$
$$- (Age\ (y) * 0.3877 - (Weight\ (kg)$$
$$* 0.1692) - (Walk\ time\ (min) * 3.2649)$$
$$- (HR\ (bpm) * 0.1565) \qquad Eq.\ 12.5a$$

$$\dot{V}O_2max\ (ml\cdot kg^{-1}\cdot min^{-1}) = 88.768 + (Gender * 8.892)$$
$$- (Weight\ (kg) * 0.2109 - (Walk\ time\ (min)$$
$$* 1.4537) - (HR\ (bpm) * 0.1194) \qquad Eq.\ 12.5b$$

Where: Gender = 1 (if male) or 0 (if female)

Example: If a college-aged participant (a 20-year-old woman), who weighs 60 kg, walks the 1 mi distance in 14:25 (14.42 min), with a heart rate of 150 bpm, the maximal oxygen consumption can be estimated as 37.2 ml·kg^{-1}·min^{-1} (Eq. 12.6).

$$\dot{V}O_2max\ (ml\cdot kg^{-1}\cdot min^{-1}) = 88.768 + (0 * 8.892)$$
$$- (60\ kg * 0.2109) - (14.42\ min * 1.4537)$$
$$- (150\ bpm * 0.1194) = \mathbf{37.2}\ ml\cdot kg^{-1}\cdot min^{-1} \quad Eq.\ 12.6$$

RESULTS AND DISCUSSION

The three run/jog/walk tests described in this chapter are presented as field tests of aerobic fitness. They are considered field tests because they use accessible facilities, minimal equipment, and simple procedures, and they may be administered to multiple persons simultaneously. They are aerobic fitness tests because they measure performance in large-muscle, rhythmic, continuous activities. They are physiologically meaningful because they allow the estimation of aerobic power in units of maximal oxygen consumption, an indicator of aerobic fitness and cardiorespiratory endurance. Norms and comparative data are available that allow participants to be categorized according to their fitness level. Before 1987, little information directly related aerobic fitness to health or disease.[9] But more recently the Surgeon General's Report on Physical Activity and Health indicates that inactivity as evidenced by low aerobic fitness is a serious health threat.[4,5,23,25]

The Cooper Run Test provides a very simple measure of aerobic fitness. The results of the test, however, can be influenced by many factors and differences between participants, including gender, age, body composition, running experience, running economy, fractional utilization of maximal oxygen consumption, and motivation. Because the test is typically performed outside, environmental factors (e.g., heat, altitude) can also lead to variable results. As of 1992, the Air Force ROTC standards for the Cooper (1.5 mi) Run Test for men and women between 17 and 29 y of age were 12:00 and 14:00, respectively. For ROTC personnel over 29 y of age, the standards for men and women were 12:30 and 14:52, respectively. The U.S. Navy requires its recruits to run 1.5 mi in 14 min or less. It has been recommended by Cooper[7,10] that a $\dot{V}O_2$max consistent with good health and functional capacity for daily living is 42 ml·kg^{-1}·min^{-1} for men and 35 ml·kg^{-1}·min^{-1} for women. These criteria were adopted in 1987 by the Institute for Aerobics Research for use in the FITNESSGRAM representing the mean aerobic fitness of young adults,[2,30] and are associated with a reduced risk of all-cause mortality.[4]

The maximal nature of the Cooper Run Test makes it less than conducive for all participants, especially older adults and those who are sedentary and deconditioned. Furthermore, maximal running tests have yielded a wide variety of correlation coefficients ($r = 0.13$ to $r = 0.90$) with directly measured $\dot{V}O_2$max,[16] and they potentially pose greater cardiovascular risk and risk of injury to the foot, ankle, and knee.[1] For these reasons, submaximal track tests involving jogging and walking have been developed. The George Jog Test[16] was developed using 149 college students, age 18–29 y, who performed a maximal treadmill test to directly determine $\dot{V}O_2$max, and then completed a 1 mi submaximal track jog at a self-selected, steady pace. The preferred jogging paces were no faster than an 8-min mile pace for men and a 9-min mile pace for women, so as not to exceed an exercise heart rate of 180 bpm. If too fast a pace is selected with an ending heart rate in excess

of 180 bpm, it is recommended that the test be repeated at a slower pace. Performing the test at an intensity above steady state has a tendency to overestimate $\dot{V}O_2$max because of a greater contribution from anaerobic energy sources. And sprinting at the end of the test weakens the relationship between exercise heart rate and $\dot{V}O_2$max. The specific variables utilized in the George Jog Test to estimate $\dot{V}O_2$max (e.g., gender, body weight, 1 mi jogging time, and heart rate) were selected based on their statistical and biological relationship to observed $\dot{V}O_2$max. Men typically demonstrate a higher observed $\dot{V}O_2$max than women, a lower body weight increases relative $\dot{V}O_2$max (expressed in ml·kg^{-1}·min^{-1}), and a lower submaximal exercise heart rate at a given elapsed jog time indicates a higher degree of aerobic fitness.

The Rockport Walk Test for the assessment of aerobic fitness, although not specifically developed for less fit and older participants, is more appropriate for these populations than either the Cooper Run Test or the George Jog Test. The developers of the Rockport Walk Test (also known as the Rockport Fitness Walking Test) questioned previous track tests on the basis of three main concerns: the accuracy and validity of the predictions, the ease and convenience of the tests, and the generalized application of the tests to broad populations.[19] In an attempt to create a better track test, they directly measured $\dot{V}O_2$max in 390 people ranging in age from 30 to 69 y, then had them complete a minimum of two 1 mile walks as fast as possible. Although 13 % of the participants appeared to show a learning effect due to faster walking times on the second trial, the researchers concluded that $\dot{V}O_2$max values predicted from walking times and heart rates during the first trial of the test compared favorably with the observed $\dot{V}O_2$max values. The correlation and *SEE* on the first trial were virtually identical to those obtained using subsequent trials, so for field use, data obtained from a single track walk appear sufficient to assess aerobic fitness in healthy adults 30–69 years of age. When the Rockport Walk Test was conducted in younger persons (< 30 y) and older persons (> 69 y), however, it was found to be less valid. It has since been modified for use in younger adults (18–29 y)[12,14] and in older women (67–85 y).[27] It is also possible to conduct the Rockport Walk Test on a treadmill if that is a better option.[22]

BOX 12.2 | **Chapter Preview/Review**

What are the three field tests of aerobic fitness described in this chapter?

What are the two versions of the Cooper Run Test?

What is the rationale behind each of the two versions of the Cooper Run Test?

How are weight, jog time, and heart rate related to $\dot{V}O_2$max in the George jog Test?

How are weight, walk time, and heart rate related to $\dot{V}O_2$max in the Rockport Walk Test?

Which of the three tests is best for assessing aerobic fitness in sedentary and older adults? Why?

References

1. American College of Sports Medicine. (1990). The recommended quantity and quality of exercise for developing and maintaining cardiorespiratory and muscular fitness in healthy adults. *Medicine and Science in Sports and Exercise, 22,* 265–274.

2. American Heart Association. (1972). *Exercise testing and training of apparently healthy individuals: A handbook for physicians.* New York: Author.

3. Balke, B. (1963). *A simple field test for the assessment of physical fitness.* (CARI Report 63-18). Oklahoma City: Civil Aeromedical Research Institute, Federal Aviation Agency.

4. Blair, S. N., Kohl, H. W., Paffenbarger, R. S., Clark, D. H., Cooper, K. H., & Gibbons, L. W. (1989). Physical fitness and all-cause mortality. A prospective study of healthy men and women. *Journal of the American Medical Association, 262,* 2395–2401.

5. Blair, S. N., & Morrow, M. S. (1997). Surgeon general's report on physical fitness: The inside story. *ACSM's Health and Fitness Journal, 1*(1), 14–18.

6. Cooper, K. H. (1968). A means of assessing maximal oxygen intake. *Journal of the American Medical Association, 203,* 135–138.

7. Cooper, K. H. (1968). *Aerobics.* New York: M. Evans & Bantam Books.

8. Cooper, K. H. (1968). Testing and developing cardiovascular fitness within the United States Air Force. *Journal of Occupational Medicine, 10,* 636–639.

9. Cureton, K. J. (1987). Commentary on children and fitness: A public health perspective. *Research Quarterly for Exercise and Sport, 58,* 315–320.

10. Cureton, K. J., & Warren, G. L. (1990). Criterion-referenced standards for youth health-related fitness tests: A tutorial. *Research Quarterly for Exercise and Sport, 61,* 7–19.

11. deVries, H. A., & Housh, T. J. (1994). *Physiology of exercise.* Dubuque, IA: Brown & Benchmark.

12. Dolgener, F. A., Hensley, L. D., Marsh, J. J., & Fjelstul, J. K. (1994). Validation of the Rockport Fitness Walking Test in college males and females. *Research Quarterly for Exercise and Sport, 65,* 152–158.

13. Fenstermaker, K. L., Plowman, S. A., & Looney, M. A. (1992). Validation of the Rockport Fitness Walking Test in females 65 years and older. *Research Quarterly for Exercise and Sport, 63,* 322–327.

14. George, J. D., Fellingham, G. W., & Fisher, A. G. (1998). A modified version of the Rockport Fitness Walking Test for college men and women. *Research Quarterly for Exercise and Sport, 69,* 205–209.

15. George, J. D., Fisher, A. G., & Vehrs, P. R. (1994). *Laboratory experiences in exercise science.* Boston: Jones and Bartlett.

16. George, J. D., Vehrs, P. R., Allsen, P. E., Fellingham, G. W., & Fisher, A. G. (1993). $\dot{V}O_2$max estimation from a submaximal 1-mile track jog for fit college-age individuals. *Medicine and Science in Sports and Exercise, 25,* 401–406.

17. Getchell, L. H., Kirkendall, D., & Robbins, G. (1977). Prediction of maximal oxygen uptake in young adult women joggers. *Research Quarterly, 48,* 61–67.

18. Kline, G. M., Porcari, J. P., Freedson, P. S., Ward, A., Ross, J., Wilke, S., & Rippe, J. (1987). Does aerobic capacity affect the validity of the one-mile walk $\dot{V}O_2$max prediction? *Medicine and Science in Sports and Exercise, 19,* Abstract #172, S29.

19. Kline, G. M., Porcari, J. P., Hintermeister, R., Freedson, P. S., Ward, A., McCarron, R. F., Ross, J., & Rippe, J. (1987). Estimation of $\dot{V}O_2$max from a one-mile track walk, gender, age, and body weight. *Medicine and Science in Sports and Exercise, 19,* 253–259.

20. Kusinitz, I., & Fine, M. (1991). *Your guide to getting fit.* Mountain View, CA: Mayfield.

21. Leger, L., & Thivierge, M. (1988). Heart rate monitors: Validity, stability, and functionality. *The Physician and Sportsmedicine, 16*(5), 143–151.

22. Nieman, D. C. (1995). *Fitness and sports medicine.* Palo Alto, CA: Bull.

23. Pate, R. R., Pratt, M., Blair, S. N., Haskell, W. L., Macera, C. A., Bouchard, C., Buchner, D., Ettinger, W., Heath, G. W., King, A. C., et al. (1995). Physical activity and public health: A recommendation from the Centers for Disease Control and Prevention and the American College of Sports Medicine. *Journal of the American Medical Association, 273,* 402–407.

24. Safrit, M. J., Hooper, L. M., Ehlert, S. A., Costa, M. G., & Patterson, P. (1988). The validity generalization of distance run tests. *Canadian Journal of Sport Science, 13,* 188–196.

25. Simons-Morton, B. G., O'Hara, N. M., Simons-Morton, D. G., & Parcel, G. S. (1987). Children and fitness: A public health perspective. *Research Quarterly for Exercise and Sport, 58,* 295–302.

26. Spencer, M. R., & Gastin, P. B. (2001). Energy system contribution during 200- to 1500-m running in highly trained athletes. *Medicine and Science in Sports and Exercise, 33,* 157–162.

27. Warren, B. J., Dotson, R. G., Nieman, D. C., & Butterworth, D. E. (1993). Validation of a 1-mile walk test in elderly women. *Journal of Aging and Physical Activity, 1,* 3–21.

28. Wilmore, J. H., & Bergfeld, J. A. (1979). A comparison of sports: Physiological and medical aspects. In R. H. Strauss (Ed.), *Sports medicine and physiology* (pp. 353–372). Philadelphia: W. B. Saunders.

29. Zingraf, S. A., & McClendon, T. (1986). An alternative index for cross-validating regression equations.

Abstract of Research Papers, 1986, AAHPERD Convention, Cincinnati, p. 28. Reston, VA: American Alliance for Health, Physical Education, Recreation and Dance. (Abstract)

30. Zuti, W. B., & Corbin, B. (1977). Physical fitness norms for college students. *Research Quarterly, 48,* 499–503.

31. Zwiren, L. D., Freedson, P. S., Ward, A., Wilke, S., & Rippe, J. M. (1991). Estimation of $\dot{V}O_2max$: A comparative analysis of five exercise tests. *Research Quarterly for Exercise and Sport, 62,* 73–78.

Form 12.1

NAME _____ DATE _____ SCORE _____

AEROBIC RUNNING, JOGGING, AND WALKING

Homework

Cooper (1.5-Mile) Run Test

Gender: **M**   Initials: **AA**   Age (y): **20**   Height (cm): **180**   Weight (kg): **85.0**

Run time (min:sec):   **11** : **57**   *Optional:*   Heart rate (bpm): **196**

Optional: Distance run in 12 min : _____ laps = _____ miles

VO_2max *(Table 12.1/12.2)* = _____ $ml \cdot kg^{-1} \cdot min^{-1}$ Fitness category *(Table 12.3/12.4)* _____

Evaluation / comments: _____

_____

_____

George (1-Mile) Jog Test

Gender: **F**   Initials: **BB**   Age (y): **20**   Height (cm): **160**   Weight (kg): **65.0**

Gender (M = 1, F = 0)   Jog time (min:sec) **10** : **45**   Jog time (min) _____   HR (bpm) **171**

VO_2max = 100.5 + (8.344 * _____) - (0.1636 * _____) - (1.438 * _____) - (0.1928 * _____)

          Gender   Body wt   Jog time   Heart rate

VO_2max $(ml \cdot kg^{-1} \cdot min^{-1})$ = _____   Fitness category *(Table 12.5)* _____

Evaluation / comments: _____

_____

_____

Rockport (1-Mile) Walk Test   *(Modified for 18-29 y)*

Gender: **F**   Initials: **CC**   Age (y): **20**   Height (cm): **165**   Weight (kg): **65.0**

Gender (M = 1, F = 0)   Walk time (min:sec) **16** : **14**   Walk time (min) _____   HR (bpm) **131**

VO_2max = 88.768 + (8.892 * _____) - (0.2109 * _____) - (1.4537 * _____) - (0.1194 * _____)

          Gender   Body wt   Walk time   Heart rate

VO_2max $(ml \cdot kg^{-1} \cdot min^{-1})$ = _____   Fitness category *(Table 12.7)* _____

Evaluation / comments: _____

_____

_____

Form 12.2

NAME _____ DATE _____ SCORE _____

AEROBIC RUNNING, JOGGING, AND WALKING

Lab Results

Cooper (1.5-Mile) Run Test

Gender: _____ Initials: _____ Age (y): _____ Height (cm): _____ Weight (kg): _____

Run time (min:sec): _____ : _____ *Optional:* Heart rate (bpm): _____

Optional: Distance run in 12 min : _____ laps = _____ miles

VO_2max *(Table 12.1/12.2)* = _____ $ml \cdot kg^{-1} \cdot min^{-1}$ Fitness category *(Table 12.3/12.4)* _____

Evaluation / comments: _____

_____

_____

George (1-Mile) Jog Test

Gender: _____ Initials: _____ Age (y): _____ Height (cm): _____ Weight (kg): _____

Gender (M = 1, F = 0) Jog time (min:sec) _____ : _____ Jog time (min) _____ HR (bpm) _____

VO_2max = 100.5 + (8.344 * _____) - (0.1636 * _____) - (1.438 * _____) - (0.1928 * _____)

Gender   Body wt   Jog time   Heart rate

VO_2max $(ml \cdot kg^{-1} \cdot min^{-1})$ = _____ Fitness category *(Table 12.5)* _____

Evaluation / comments: _____

_____

_____

Rockport (1-Mile) Walk Test *(Modified for 18-29 y)*

Gender: _____ Initials: _____ Age (y): _____ Height (cm): _____ Weight (kg): _____

Gender (M = 1, F = 0) Walk time (min:sec) _____ : _____ Walk time (min) _____ HR (bpm) _____

VO_2max = 88.768 + (8.892 * _____) - (0.2109 * _____) - (1.4537 * _____) - (0.1194 * _____)

Gender   Body wt   Walk time   Heart rate

VO_2max $(ml \cdot kg^{-1} \cdot min^{-1})$ = _____ Fitness category *(Table 12.7)* _____

Evaluation / comments: _____

_____

_____

AEROBIC STEPPING

*field =
predict*

*lab=
direct*

Aerobic step tests may be classified as field tests if they are designed to be submaximal tests that *predict* aerobic fitness; they may be categorized as laboratory tests if they are used as the exercise mode during the *direct* measurement of oxygen consumption or for clinical evaluation of a physiological system such as the cardiovascular (e.g., ECG) or respiratory systems. Lab tests usually require more stringent controls of the participant and environment than does the typical field test. Although step tests are simple, they lend themselves to the quantification of power and measure at least one physiological variable (e.g., heart rate). Their portability is demonstrated by the ease with which an appropriately dimensioned step box can be easily carried from one environmental site to another. Most step tests, including the time for heart rate measurement, can be completed in less than 6 min. In general, they are safe, convenient, inexpensive, and uncomplicated tests. The Forestry Step Test will be discussed as an example of the more than 30 step tests that have been used to measure aerobic fitness.

PURPOSES OF THE AEROBIC STEP TEST

The Forestry Step Test[14] is a modification of the original Harvard Test,[2] the modified Harvard Test,[11] and the Åstrand-Ryhming Step Test.[1,11] The purposes of the Forestry Step Test (FST) are to measure the aerobic fitness (cardiorespiratory endurance) of persons, to screen potential employees for their physical aptitude in an occupation, and to monitor changes in fitness associated with a physical training program. Because the final score derived from the FST is a maximal oxygen consumption value, the score may be used to determine an aerobic fitness category. The moderate exercise intensity required for the test enables its use in most younger and middle-aged adults, provided they can complete the prescribed duration of the test (5 min). However, the test is likely to be too strenuous for those persons with a very low fitness level or for older adults (> 60 y).

The Forestry Step Test was originally designed as a screening test for safety and emergency personnel (e.g., forestry firefighters, police, lifeguards).[14] The screening test prevents the employers for these physically demanding occupations from hiring unfit persons. At one time, many federal and state agencies adopted a maximal oxygen consumption standard for firefighters based on their performance on the FST. The U.S. Forestry Service adopted a maximal oxygen consumption of 45 ml·kg⁻¹·min⁻¹ as the minimum aerobic fitness required of forestry firefighters.[22] Such fitness tests allow fire and police departments to hire and fire persons based on the physical requirements of the job and alleviate the illegal practice of hiring or firing on the basis of gender or age. The Forestry Step Test may also be administered periodically to assess changes in aerobic fitness to ensure that fire, police, and safety personnel possess the required degree of aerobic fitness, or to assess the effectiveness of their physical training programs. The Queens College Step Test (QCST) is another version of an aerobic step test.[9] It was developed by researchers at Queens College, a part of the City University of New York (CUNY) system. The QCST evolved from earlier aerobic fitness tests including the Skubic and Hodgkins step test.[19] It was developed primarily to be used on multiple participants simultaneously, so that large groups of students could be measured quickly. Because the QCST was originally done on gymnasium bleachers that were 16¼ in. (41 cm) high, that is the step height currently in use. The QCST was initially used in the early 1970s as a measure of aerobic fitness in untrained young women in the United States, on whom there was limited data regarding maximal oxygen uptake and physical work capacity.[10] It was soon adapted, using a faster stepping rate, to also be used on college men.

Physiological Rationale

All tests in exercise physiology should be based upon a valid physiological rationale. The aerobic step test is based upon the relationships among oxygen consumption, heart rate, and power. Brian Sharkey, who developed the present version of the Forestry Step Test, wanted a simple test that would predict the success of wilderness firefighters. He determined that field measurements of wilderness firefighting tasks averaged 22.5 ml·kg⁻¹·min⁻¹.[14] Given the intermittent nature of firefighting tasks, Sharkey reasoned that a physically fit individual could sustain work rates not more than 50 % of capacity over an 8 h period. Therefore, he concluded that an aerobic capacity of at least 45 ml·kg⁻¹·min⁻¹ would be required for forestry firefighters. This criterion has been adopted by the U.S. Forest Service.[22]

As with oxygen consumption, most of the heart rate range is linearly related to exercise power. This also means that steady-state heart rate and oxygen consumption are related. Heart rates are not measured *during* the Forestry Step

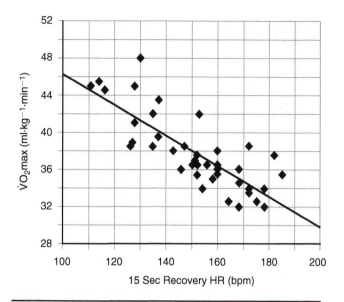

Figure 13.1 The inverse relationship observed between 15 sec recovery heart rate and maximal oxygen consumption. The higher the recovery HR, the lower the observed $\dot{V}O_2$max.

Test or the Queens College Step Test, but during *recovery* from the stepping exercise. Therefore, it is important that the recovery heart rate be relatively indicative of the exercise heart rate. There appears to be ample evidence to support a high relationship between exercise recovery heart rate and the actual exercise heart rate.[9,12,17]

The fitness of a person is related to both maximal oxygen consumption and submaximal exercise heart rate response. Low recovery heart rates reflect a low stress level by the participant, whereas high rates reflect a high stress level. This cardiovascular stress, as reflected by recovery heart rate, indicates the degree of aerobic fitness of the individual. Obviously, low stresses, or low heart rates, at any given exercise power equate with higher predicted maximal oxygen consumption values, which indicate a higher aerobic fitness level (Figure 13.1).

METHODS

The factors described for the aerobic step test are (a) equipment, (b) preparation, and (c) testing procedures. A discussion of the accuracy of the aerobic step test is presented in Box 13.1.

Equipment

The equipment necessary to complete the Forestry Step Test (FST) and the Queens College Step Test (QCST) are a step bench or box (of a specific height), a metronome to provide the stepping rate, a clock (preferably a lab clock) or stopwatch to monitor the duration of the test and to time the recovery pulse, and possibly a stethoscope if recovery pulse is to be determined by auscultation (listening to the heart). The

height of the step bench or box is chosen based on the gender of the participant. Men complete the FST using a step height of 40 cm (15¾ in.), while women use a step height of 33 cm (13 in.). All participants completing the QCST use a step height of 41 cm (16¼ in.). In some cases, existing benches or steps of the appropriate height can be found and used in the test. However, it is more typical that a step bench or step box is constructed specifically for conducting the aerobic step test. A long step bench (approximately 6–8 ft or 2 m in length) is convenient for testing two or three participants simultaneously. Accessory blocks may also be constructed that can adjust the height of the step bench to accommodate its use with different step tests. A step box, although it can be used to test only one person at a time, is smaller and therefore much more portable than a step bench. Because the stepping rate during the aerobic step test must be maintained at a specific rate, the use of a metronome is required. A good quality electronic metronome (that provides both auditory and visual signals of pace) is preferred. It is also possible to use a specially prepared audio recording that provides music or auditory cues ("up, up, down, down") at the specific rate necessary to complete the test. A timing device (e.g., clock, lab clock, stopwatch) is required to time the 3 or 5 min duration of the stepping portion of the test, and to time the 15 sec recovery pulse necessary to complete the test. A lab clock works especially well. The participants can watch the clock to monitor the stepping (exercise) time; then the remaining 20 to 30 s (the recovery time) is used to record the recovery pulse. In most cases, recovery pulse will be determined by the technician by palpating a carotid or radial pulse. However, if the technician prefers to determine recovery pulse by auscultation, a stethoscope is also an optional piece of equipment.

Preparation

Administration of any step test requires appropriate preparations on the part of both the participant and the technician. The preparation of the participant for this test applies to most field/lab tests.

Participant

1. The participant should be well rested and refrain from prior exercise the day of testing.[1]
2. The participant should not go more than 5–6 hours without food prior to the test, but should also not eat a large meal within 2–3 hours of the test. The participant should be normally hydrated and should refrain from consuming or taking any stimulants (e.g., caffeine, nicotine) or depressants (e.g., alcohol) that may have an effect on recovery pulse.
3. The participant should wear lightweight shoes and lightweight, loose clothing. (In some cases, however, where the objective of the stepping exercise is to determine the responses to specific occupational tasks, specific clothing such as firefighter turnout gear may be worn.)

Technician

The technician's preparations for the Forestry Step Test or the Queens College Step Test include four major factors: (1) preparation and calibration of the testing equipment, (2) measuring and recording basic data, (3) orienting the participant to the testing procedures, and (4) selecting the most appropriate method for determining recovery pulse.

The technician needs to prepare all equipment for the test. The height of the step bench or step box should be verified (see Box 13.2). The accuracy of the metronome should be checked by verifying the production of 90 audible and visible signals in 60 s. Basic data (e.g., age, height, body weight) are important in determining and interpreting the results. It is also useful to collect meteorological data during any laboratory testing. Although the meteorological data (e.g., temperature, barometric pressure, humidity) are not directly used in determining the results of the test, they may be useful in interpreting any unexpected test results.

BOX 13.2 Calibration for the Step Test

Calibration of some instruments does not have to be repeated on every test occasion. For example, after the initial verification of the step ergometer's height, it may never need to be measured again. The calibration of the platform weight scale was discussed in Chapter 3. The metronome should be checked for accuracy by counting the number of beats for 1 min at the prescribed test setting. For example, the setting for the Forestry Step Test is 90 beats.min[-1]. Thus, when starting a watch with a seconds hand simultaneously with a beat (sound) on the metronome and then counting the next beat as one, the 90th beat should occur at the end of 1 min.

Prior to the test, the technician orients the participant to the test by describing and demonstrating the proper testing procedures. The aerobic step test requires that the participant step at a constant rate in a four-count cadence (i.e., "up, up, down, down") in the following manner:

"Up"	The participant steps *up* onto the step bench/box with the *leading* foot.
"Up"	The participant steps *up fully* onto the bench/box with the *trailing* foot.
"Down"	The participant steps *down* from the bench/box with the *leading* foot.
"Down"	The participant steps *down fully* onto the floor with the *trailing foot*.

The technician emphasizes the importance of maintaining proper cadence and of straightening the back and legs at the top of the step (Figure 13.2). The four-count stepping cadence is maintained at the appropriate stepping rate in sequence with the metronome. If participants experience leg fatigue during the test, they may change the leading foot. This is done by taking two consecutive steps on the floor and then leading or stepping up onto the box with the opposite foot, which then becomes the leading foot.

At the conclusion of the 3 or 5 min of stepping exercise, it is necessary to measure and record the number of pulses within a 15 s period. This period, however, is not the immediate 15 s following the test. The technician and participant are given either 5 s (QCST) or 15 s (FST) immediately following the stepping exercise for the participant to be seated on the step bench or box and for the technician (and/or participant) to find the pulse. The pulse is then counted from 5:05 until 5:20 (QCST) or 5:15 until 5:30 (FST) by palpating the radial artery or carotid artery or by listening to the heart with a stethoscope. If palpating the pulse, the technician should palpate using the index and middle fingers, not the thumb. The thumb has a fairly strong pulse itself, so the technician could inadvertently feel and count the pulse in his or her own thumb instead of the participant's pulse. (If the participant is palpating his or her *own* pulse, he or she may use the thumb because it possesses the same pulse.) There is some concern over palpating the carotid artery. Because the carotid arteries

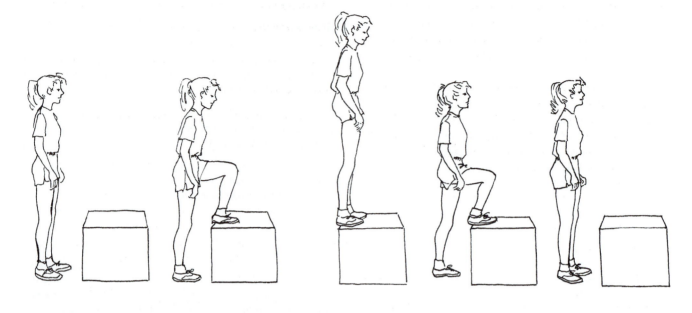

Figure 13.2 The four-count stepping technique for the step-test participant.

possess baroreceptors that are sensitive to arterial blood pressure, a bradycardic (slowing) effect on heart rate can occur when they are palpated or massaged. At least one study, however, has reported no significant difference between carotid and radial palpation of heart rate.[12] The recovery pulses may also be determined by listening to the heart with a stethoscope (as described in more detail in Chapter 14).

Testing Procedures

The testing procedures for various step tests are similar. The exercise protocol (Table 13.1) for the Forestry Step Test includes such factors as height of step, rate of stepping, duration of stepping, and time period of the recovery pulse count.

Timing the Recovery Pulse Count

The laboratory clock should continue to run after the fifth min; the time for counting pulses begins at 5:15 and ends at 5:30. The metronome is stopped at the fifth minute, however, because it may be disconcerting while trying to count heartbeats. The technician's and participant's 15 s pulse counts should not differ by more than two beats. (It is quite likely that only the participant will count the pulse under field conditions.) If the difference is greater than two beats, repeat the test after both palpators are confident that they are palpating correctly. It is very important to get accurate pulse counts. They will be used for estimating the individual's maximal oxygen consumption.

Cool-Down

The participant should walk for about three minutes immediately following the test. After mild walking, the participant should stretch the calves (e.g., wall-lean exercise) and

Table 13.1	Protocol for Forestry Step Test
Step bench height	
For men	40 cm (15.75 in.)
For women	33 cm (13 in.)
Stepping rate	22.5 steps·min^{-1}
Metronome rate	90 beats·min^{-1}
Stepping duration	5 min
Recovery pulse count	15 s (5:15–5:30)

quadriceps on three or four occasions for 3–60 s with 2 min relief intervals. The quadriceps stretch can be performed from the standing position by flexing the lower leg toward the buttocks, then grabbing the flexed leg's ankle with the opposite hand. You may need a wall, chair, or table to hold onto for balance.

Summary of Procedures for the Forestry Step Test

The procedures for administering the Forestry Step Test are summarized here. One technician can simultaneously test more than one participant.

1. The participant(s) stands facing the step bench or box (40 cm for men, 33 cm for women).
2. The technician starts the metronome that is set to 90 beats·min^{-1}.
3. The technician instructs the participant(s) to begin stepping by saying aloud, "Up, up, down, down" in time with the metronome.
4. The technician starts the timer and monitors the participant's cadence and form throughout the 5 min stepping exercise.
5. After 5 min, the technician stops the metronome and instructs the participant(s) to be seated. The technician

(and optionally the participant) finds the participant's pulse within the first 15 s of the recovery period. The 15-s recovery pulse is then counted from 5:15 until 5:30 (at which time the clock buzzes if using a lab clock).

6. The number of pulses palpated or auscultated during the designated 15 s period is recorded on Form 13.2.
7. The participant should cool down following the test by slowly walking or stepping in place for 2–3 min. Some static stretching of the quadriceps, hamstrings, and gastrocnemius may also be appropriate.
8. The technician estimates a non-adjusted $\dot{V}O_2$max from recovery pulse and body weight using Table 13.2,[12] adjusts the $\dot{V}O_2$max based on the participant's age using Table 13.3, and determines a fitness category from Table 13.4.

Example: If a 25-year-old man who weighs 82 kg counts 35 pulses in the 15 s recovery period (also equal to a recovery heart rate of 140 bpm) following the 5 min of stepping exercise, the non-adjusted maximal oxygen consumption is estimated to be 42 ml·kg⁻¹·min⁻¹ (from Table 13.2), the age-adjusted $\dot{V}O_2$max is 42 ml·kg⁻¹·min⁻¹ (from Table 13.3), and the fitness category is "good" (from Table 13.4).

Summary of Procedures for the Queens College Step Test

The procedures for the Queens College Step Test (QCST) are virtually identical to the Forestry Step Test (FST), with minor modifications in step height, stepping rate, exercise duration, and the timing of the 15-s recovery pulse noted below and described in Table 13.5.

1. The participant(s) stands facing the step bench or box (41 cm; 16¼ in.).
2. The technician starts the metronome that is set to 96 beats·min⁻¹ for men or 88 beats·min⁻¹ for women.
3. The technician instructs the participant(s) to begin stepping by saying aloud, "Up, up, down, down" in time with the metronome.
4. The technician starts the timer and monitors the participant's cadence and form throughout the 3 min stepping exercise.
5. After 3 min, the technician stops the metronome and instructs the participant(s) to be seated.
6. The 15-s recovery pulse is then counted from 3:05 until 3:20 and recorded on Form 13.2.
7. Follow the same cool down procedures as the Forestry Step Test.
8. The technician estimates $\dot{V}O_2$max and determines a fitness category from Table 13.6.

Table 13.2 Estimation of Non-Adjusted $\dot{V}O_2$max (ml·kg⁻¹·min⁻¹) from Recovery Pulse, Gender and Weight

Recovery Pulse 15 s (beats)	60 s (bpm)	(lb) (kg)	Men—Body Weight (lb or kg) 120 / 54	140 / 64	160 / 73	180 / 82	200 / 91	220 / 100	240 / 109	(lb) (kg)	Women—Body Weight (lb or kg) 80 / 36	100 / 45	120 / 54	140 / 64	160 / 73	180 / 82
45	180		34	34	33	33	32	32	32							30
44	176		35	34	34	33	33	33	33					32	32	31
43	172		35	35	34	34	34	34	33				33	32	32	32
42	168		36	35	35	35	34	34	34				33	33	33	32
41	164		36	36	35	35	35	35	35				33	33	33	33
40	160		37	37	36	36	36	36	36			34	34	34	34	34
39	156		38	38	37	37	37	37	37			35	34	35	35	35
38	152		39	39	38	38	38	38	38			35	35	36	36	36
37	148		40	40	39	39	39	39	39			36	36	37	37	37
36	144		41	41	40	40	40	41	40			37	37	38	38	39
35	140		42	42	41	42	42	42	41		39	38	38	39	40	40
34	136		44	43	43	43	43	43	43		39	39	40	41	41	41
33	132		45	45	44	44	44	44	44		40	41	41	42	42	43
32	128		47	46	46	46	46	45	45		41	42	43	44	44	44
31	124		48	48	47	47	47	47	46		42	44	45	45	46	46
30	120		50	50	49	49	49	48	48		43	46	47	47	47	47
29	116		52	51	51	50	50	50	49		45	48	49	49	49	49
28	112		54	53	53	52	52	51	51		47	50	51	51	51	51
27	108		56	55	55	54	53	53	52		49	53	53	54	53	
26	104		58	57	57	56	55	54	54		52	55	56	56	56	
25	100		60	59	59	58	57	56			54	58	59	58		
24	96		62	62	61	60	59	58			58	60	61	61		
23	92		65	64	63	62	61				61	63	64			
22	88		67	66	66	64	63				65	66	67			
21	84		70	69	68	66	65									

Note: The values for non-adjusted $\dot{V}O_2$max in this table assume the participant is 25 years old.
Source: Data adapted from Sharkey (1984).[15]

Table 13.3 — Determining Age-Adjusted $\dot{V}O_2$max from Non-Adjusted (Non-Adj) $\dot{V}O_2$max and Age (y)

Non-Adj $\dot{V}O_2$max		20–24	25–29	30–34	35–39	40–44	45–49	Non-Adj $\dot{V}O_2$max		20–24	25–29	30–34	35–39	40–44	45–49
				Age (y)								Age (y)			
30	-	31	30	29	28	26	25	50	-	52	50	48	46	44	42
31	-	32	31	30	29	27	26	51	-	53	51	49	47	45	43
32	-	33	32	31	29	28	27	52	-	54	52	50	48	46	44
33	-	34	33	32	30	29	28	53	-	55	53	51	49	47	45
34	-	35	34	33	31	30	29	54	-	56	54	52	50	48	45
35	-	36	35	34	32	31	29	55	-	57	55	53	51	48	46
36	-	37	36	35	33	32	30	56	-	58	56	54	52	49	47
37	-	38	37	36	34	33	31	57	-	59	57	55	52	50	48
38	-	40	38	36	35	33	32	58	-	60	58	56	53	51	49
39	-	41	39	37	36	34	33	59	-	61	59	57	54	52	50
40	-	42	40	38	37	35	34	60	-	62	60	58	55	53	50
41	-	43	41	39	38	36	34	61	-	63	61	59	56	54	51
42	-	44	42	40	39	37	35	62	-	64	62	60	57	55	52
43	-	45	43	41	40	38	36	63	-	66	63	60	58	55	53
44	-	46	44	42	40	39	37	64	-	67	64	61	59	56	54
45	-	47	45	43	41	40	38	65	-	68	65	62	60	57	55
46	-	48	46	44	42	40	39	66	-	69	66	63	61	58	55
47	-	49	47	45	43	41	39	67	-	70	67	64	62	59	56
48	-	50	48	46	44	42	40	68	-	71	68	65	63	60	57
49	-	51	49	47	45	43	41	69	-	72	69	66	63	61	58

Source: Data adapted from Sharkey (1984).[15] Age correction factor: 20–24y, 1.04; 25–29y, 1.00; 30–34y, 0.96; 35–39y, 0.92; 40–44y, 0.88; 45–49y, 0.84.

Table 13.4 — Fitness Category for Men and Women for the Forestry Step Test by Age Group

Category	Men—Age (y)				Women—Age (y)			
	18–29 y	30–39 y	40–49 y	≥ 50 y	18–29 y	30–39 y	40–49 y	≥ 50 y
Superior	≥ 55	≥ 53	≥ 51	≥ 49	≥ 52	≥ 50	≥ 48	≥ 46
Excellent	50–54	48–52	46–50	44–48	47–51	45–49	43–47	41–45
Very good	45–49	43–47	41–45	39–43	42–46	40–44	38–42	36–40
Good	40–44	38–42	36–40	34–38	37–41	35–39	33–37	31–35
Fair	35–39	33–37	31–35	29–33	32–36	30–34	28–32	26–30
Poor	30–34	28–32	26–30	24–28	27–31	25–29	23–27	21–25
Very poor	< 30	< 28	< 26	< 24	< 27	< 25	< 23	< 21

Source: Data adapted from Sharkey (1984).[15]

Table 13.5 — Protocol for Queens College Step Test

Step bench height	41 cm (16.25 in.)
Stepping rate	
For men	24 steps·min⁻¹ (beat = 96 bpm)
For women	22 steps·min⁻¹ (beat = 88 bpm)
Stepping duration	3 min
Recovery pulse count	15 s (3:05–3:20)

RESULTS AND DISCUSSION

The number of pulses (or the recovery heart rate) during the 15 s recovery period in combination with the body weight of the participant are used to estimate a non-adjusted maximal oxygen consumption when using the Forestry Step Test (Table 13.2). Getting accurate pulse counts is very important. In general, palpation or auscultation errors lead to a reduction in the number of pulses recorded because persons are more likely to *miss* pulses than add extra ones.[5] A lower recovery heart rate would lead to a higher $\dot{V}O_2$max value and an overestimation of the participant's aerobic fitness. It would typically be recommended that a trained technician count the number of pulses to get a true result. However, when multiple step tests are being administered simultaneously by one technician, it is necessary to rely on the participant to count his or her own pulse accurately. Notice also in Table 13.2 that $\dot{V}O_2$max varies little between participants of different body weights at the same recovery pulse. This is because the efficiency of stepping changes very little for given changes in body weight. The use of Table 13.2 to estimate non-adjusted $\dot{V}O_2$max is necessary because no regression equation for the Forestry Step Test is available.

The $\dot{V}O_2$max values shown in Table 13.2 are for young participants with an average age of 25 y. It is necessary to adjust these values for differences in age due to the natural decrease in maximal heart rate associated with aging. For younger participants, under the age of 25 y, $\dot{V}O_2$max is increased. For older participants, over the age of 25 y, $\dot{V}O_2$max is decreased. To find the *age-adjusted* $\dot{V}O_2$max, the first step is to find the participant's *non-adjusted* $\dot{V}O_2$max value in Table 13.3. For example, find the row corresponding to a non-adjusted $\dot{V}O_2$max of 45 ml·kg^{-1}·min^{-1}, remembering this value assumes an age of 25 y. Follow across the table horizontally to the age interval that includes the participant's age to see the age-adjusted $\dot{V}O_2$max value. The age-adjusted value for someone who is 20–24 y would be 47 ml·kg^{-1}·min^{-1}, and for someone 30–34 y, 35–39 y, 40–44 y, or 45–49 y, the value would be 43, 41, 40, or 38 ml·kg^{-1}·min^{-1}, respectively.

The interpretation of the maximal oxygen consumption value from the Forestry Step Test is made by consulting Table 13.4. The fitness categories distinguish between gender and age groups. For example, a 30-year-old man and woman whose age-adjusted $\dot{V}O_2$max is 40 ml·kg^{-1}·min^{-1} would be categorized as "good" and "very good," respectively. Neither of these persons, however, would meet the minimum criterion of 45 ml·kg^{-1}·min^{-1} that Sharkey determined to be necessary for a wilderness firefighter to safely and effectively execute the job.[15] The results of the Forestry Step Test can be used to assess aerobic fitness in the general population, or they can be used to assess whether a candidate is adequately fit to meet specific occupational demands. The results of the Queens College Step Test (QCST) were determined from Table 13.6 as described previously in the Methods section. Maximal oxygen uptake ($\dot{V}O_2$max) can also be estimated from the QCST by means of two regression equations, one for men (Eq. 13.1) and one for women (Eq. 13.2).[9] In this case, the 15-s recovery pulse (beats) counted following the test, has been multiplied by 4 to change it into a recovery pulse in beats·min^{-1} (bpm).

$$\dot{V}O_2\text{max (ml·kg}^{-1}\text{·min}^{-1}) = 111.33$$
$$- [0.42 * \text{Recovery pulse (bpm)}] \qquad \text{Eq. 13.1}$$

$$\dot{V}O_2\text{max (ml·kg}^{-1}\text{·min}^{-1}) = 65.81$$
$$- [0.1847 * \text{Recovery pulse (bpm)}] \qquad \text{Eq. 13.2}$$

The two step test protocols described, the Forestry Step Test and the Queens College Step Test, were developed and are used in healthy people, either firefighters or college students. The use of step tests in clinical populations is also sometimes considered. The Siconolfi Step Test, originally designed for epidemiological studies[18], was modified for use in a clinical population of patients with lupus[8], a systemic auto-immune disease. The step test was well tolerated and found to be a highly reliable and reasonably valid submaximal exercise test for assessing fitness in this clinical population. Some clinicians have questioned the safety of a "fixed-rate" step test in clinical populations, especially without physician supervision.[6] The concern is the intensity reached during the step test. In some cases, the step test becomes a vigorous, high-intensity exercise, increasing the risk for

Table 13.6	$\dot{V}O_2$max (ml·kg^{-1}·min^{-1}) Estimated from Recovery Pulse Using the Queens College Step Test

		Men		Women	
Category	%ile	Rec pulse	$\dot{V}O_2$max	Rec pulse	$\dot{V}O_2$max
Well above ave		30	60.9	33	41.4
		31	59.3	34	40.7
	95	32	57.6	35	40.0
Above average	90	33	55.9	36	39.2
	85	34	54.2	37	38.5
	80	35	52.5	38	37.7
	75	36	50.9	39	37.0
Average	70	37	49.2	40	36.3
	60	38	47.5	41	35.5
	50	39	45.8	42	34.8
	40	40	44.1	43	34.0
	30	41	42.5	44	33.3
Below average	25	42	40.8	45	32.6
	20	43	39.1	46	31.8
	15	44	37.4	47	31.1
	10	45	35.7	48	30.3
Well below ave	5	46	34.1	49	29.6
		47	32.4	50	28.9
		48	30.7	51	28.1

Note: $\dot{V}O_2$max (ml·kg^{-1}·min^{-1}) is estimated from recovery pulse (Rec pulse) counted for 15 s.
Source: Data adapted from McArdle, Katch & Katch (2007).[9]

myocardial ischemia, cardiac arrhythmias, and myocardial infarction in persons unaccustomed to exercise. When step tests are used with small, obese, and/or physically deconditioned subjects, it is recommended they be conducted with medical supervision.[6] An alternative step test, the Chester Step Test[20], alleviates some of the concern of overexertion. The test is done in 2-min stages on a 30 cm (< 12 in.) step at an initial stepping rate of 15 steps·min^{-1}, with stepping rate increased 5 steps·min^{-1} each 2-min stage. The participant completes as many stages necessary to reach 80 % of age-predicted max heart rate, up to a maximum of five 2-min stages (10 min). The submaximal test was shown to provide a valid estimate of aerobic fitness in rehabilitation settings.[20]

BOX 13.3	Chapter Preview/Review

Why was the Forestry Step Test developed and by whom was it developed?

Why is a $\dot{V}O_2$max of 45 ml·kg^{-1} min^{-1} required for wilderness firefighters?

What is the rationale behind the Aerobic Step Test?

What is the step cadence for the Forestry Step Test and Queens College Step Test and what are the step heights for men and women?

What is the effect of age on $\dot{V}O_2$max estimated from the Forestry Step Test?

References

1. Åstrand, P.-O., & Ryhming, I. (1954). A nomogram for calculation of aerobic capacity (physical fitness) from pulse rate during submaximal work. *Journal of Applied Physiology, 7,* 218–221.

2. Brouha, L. (1943). The Step Test: A simple method of measuring physical fitness for muscular work in young men. *Research Quarterly, 14,* 30–35.

3. Cicutti, N., Jette, M., & Sidney, K. (1991). Effect of leg length on bench stepping efficiency in children. *Canadian Journal of Sport Science, 16,* 58–63.

4. deVries, H. A. (1971). *Lab experiments in exercise physiology.* Dubuque, IA: Wm. C. Brown.

5. Greer, N. L., & Katch, F. I. (1982). Validity of palpation recovery pulse rate to estimate exercise heart rate following four intensities of bench step exercise. *Research Quarterly for Exercise and Sport, 53,* 340–343.

6. Hansen, D., Jacobs, N., Bex, S., D'Haene, G., Dendale, P., & Claes, N. (2011). Are fixed-rate step tests medically safe for assessing physical fitness? *European Journal of Applied Physiology, 111,* 2593–2599.

7. Johnson, J., & Siegel, D. (1981). The use of selected submaximal step tests in predicting change in the maximal oxygen intake of college women. *Journal of Sports Medicine and Physical Fitness, 21,* 259–264.

8. Marcora, S., Casanova, F., Fortes, M., & Maddison, P. (2007). Validity and reliability of the Siconolfi step test for assessment of physical fitness in patients with systemic lupus erythematosus. *Arthritis & Rheumatism, 57(6),* 1007–1011.

9. McArdle, W. D., Katch, F. I., & Katch, V. L. (2007). *Exercise physiology: Energy, nutrition and human performance, 6th ed.* Philadelphia, Lippincott Williams & Wilkins.

10. McArdle, W. D., Katch, F. I., Pechar, G. S., Jacobson, L., & Ruck, S. (1972). Reliability and interrelationships between maximal oxygen intake, physical work capacity and step-test scores in college women. *Medicine and Science in Sports, 4,* 182–186.

11. Ryhming, I. (1953). A modified Harvard step test for the evaluation of physical fitness. *Arbeitsphysiologie, 15,* 235–250.

12. Sedlock, D. A., Knowlton, R. G., Fitzgerald, P. I., Tahamont, M. V., & Schneider, D. A. (1983). Accuracy of subject-palpated carotid pulse after exercise. *The Physician and Sportsmedicine, 11*(4), 106–108, 113–116.

13. Shahnawaz, H. (1978). Influence of limb length on a stepping exercise. *Journal of Applied Physiology, 44,* 346–349.

14. Sharkey, B. J. (1977). *Fitness and work capacity.* (Report FS-315.) Washington, DC: U.S. Department of Agriculture.

15. Sharkey, B. J. (1984). *Physiology of fitness.* Champaign, IL: Human Kinetics.

16. Shephard, R. J. (1969). Learning, habituation, and training. *Internationale Z. Angew. Physiologi, 28,* 38–48.

17. Shephard, R. J. (1971). Standard test of aerobic power. In R. J. Shephard (Ed.), *Frontiers in fitness* (pp. 133–165). Springfield, IL: Charles C. Thomas.

18. Siconolfi, S. F., Garber, C. E., Lasater, T. M., & Carleton, R. A. (1985). A simple, valid step test for estimating maximal oxygen uptake in epidemiologic studies. *American Journal of Epidemiology, 121,* 382–90.

19. Skubic, V., & Hodgkins, J. (1963). Cardiovascular efficiency tests for girls and women. *Research Quarterly, 34,* 191–198.

20. Sykes, K., & Roberts, A. (2004). The Chester step test—a simple yet effective tool for the prediction of aerobic capacity. *Physiotherapy, 90,* 183–188.

21. Thomas, S. G., Miller, I. M. R., & Cox, M. H. (1993). Sources of variation in oxygen consumption during a stepping task. *Medicine and Science in Sports and Exercise, 25,* 139–144.

22. Washburn, R. A., & Safrit, M. J. (1982). Physical performance tests in job selection—A model for empirical validation. *Research Quarterly for Exercise and Sport, 53*(3), 267–270.

- Assesses aerobic fitness/cardio fitness via estimating VO₂ max (the max amount of O₂ that can be consumed for energy production per unit of time)
- Box height matters ≈ 40cm for men ≈ 32cm for women
- Pace matters 90 bpm
- wait 5 sec. then measure HR for 15 sec.
- non age adjusted score isn't relevant it's just a stepping store to age adjusted
- for the same submaximal load, a trained individual will have a lesser response
- developed w/ Forest Firefighters in mind
- straighten back and legs with each step

Graph: Heart rate (bpm) vs Exercise intensity / VO₂, showing "trained/untrained" lines and "estimated VO₂ max". Direct relationship between HR and VO₂ max

Form 13.1
AEROBIC STEPPING

NAME _____ DATE _____ SCORE _____

Homework

Gender: **M**   Initials: **AA**   Age (y): **20**   Height (cm): **180**   Weight (kg): **82.0**

Forestry Step Test

Participant maintained cadence and technique: ☐ always   ☒ usually   ☐ seldom

Recovery pulse (beats) =   **30**   beats

Non-adjusted $\dot{V}O_2$max =   54 $ml \cdot kg^{-1} \cdot min^{-1}$ Age-adjusted $\dot{V}O_2$max =   56 $ml \cdot kg^{-1} \cdot min^{-1}$
(Table 13.2)   (Table 13.3)

Fitness category _____   Qualified as firefighter :   ☐ yes   ☐ no
(Table 13.4)   ($\dot{V}O_2 max \geq 45\ ml \cdot kg^{-1} \cdot min^{-1}$)

Queen's College Step Test (Optional)

Recovery pulse =   **35**   beats $\dot{V}O_2$max = _____ $ml \cdot kg^{-1} \cdot min^{-1}$ Category _____
(Table 13.6)

Evaluation / comments: My age-adjusted VO_2 max was 56 ml·kg⁻¹·min⁻¹. This places me at the upper end of above average, and means that I can liberate approximately 0.056 Kcal of energy per minute

---

Gender: **F**   Initials: **BB**   Age (y): **20**   Height (cm): **170**   Weight (kg): **68.0**

Forestry Step Test

Participant maintained cadence and technique: ☐ always   ☒ usually   ☐ seldom

Recovery pulse (beats) =   **37**   beats

Non-adjusted $\dot{V}O_2$max = _____ $ml \cdot kg^{-1} \cdot min^{-1}$ Age-adjusted $\dot{V}O_2$max = _____ $ml \cdot kg^{-1} \cdot min^{-1}$
(Table 13.2)   (Table 13.3)

Fitness category _____   Qualified as firefighter :   ☐ yes   ☐ no
(Table 13.4)   ($\dot{V}O_2 max \geq 45\ ml \cdot kg^{-1} \cdot min^{-1}$)

Queen's College Step Test (Optional)

Recovery pulse =   **40**   beats $\dot{V}O_2$max = _____ $ml \cdot kg^{-1} \cdot min^{-1}$ Category _____
(Table 13.6)

Evaluation / comments: _____

Form 13.2
AEROBIC STEPPING

NAME _____ DATE _____ SCORE _____

Lab Results

Gender: _____ Initials: _____ Age (y): _____ Height (cm): _____ Weight (kg): _____

Forestry Step Test

Participant maintained cadence and technique: ☐ always ☐ usually ☐ seldom

Recovery pulse (beats) = _____ beats

Non-adjusted $\dot{V}O_2$max = _____ ml·kg^{-1}·min^{-1} Age-adjusted $\dot{V}O_2$max = _____ ml·kg^{-1}·min^{-1}
(Table 13.2)   *(Table 13.3)*

Fitness category _____   Qualified as firefighter : ☐ yes ☐ no
(Table 13.4)   ($\dot{V}O_2$ max ≥ 45 ml·kg^{-1}·min^{-1})

Queen's College Step Test *(Optional)*

Recovery pulse = _____ beats $\dot{V}O_2$max = _____ ml·kg^{-1}·min^{-1} Category _____
(Table 13.6)

Evaluation / comments: _____

_____

_____

_____

Gender: _____ Initials: _____ Age (y): _____ Height (cm): _____ Weight (kg): _____

Forestry Step Test

Participant maintained cadence and technique: ☐ always ☐ usually ☐ seldom

Recovery pulse (beats) = _____ beats

Non-adjusted $\dot{V}O_2$max = _____ ml·kg^{-1}·min^{-1} Age-adjusted $\dot{V}O_2$max = _____ ml·kg^{-1}·min^{-1}
(Table 13.2)   *(Table 13.3)*

Fitness category _____   Qualified as firefighter : ☐ yes ☐ no
(Table 13.4)   ($\dot{V}O_2$ max ≥ 45 ml·kg^{-1}·min^{-1})

Queen's College Step Test *(Optional)*

Recovery pulse = _____ beats $\dot{V}O_2$max = _____ ml·kg^{-1}·min^{-1} Category _____
(Table 13.6)

Evaluation / comments: _____

_____

_____

_____

AEROBIC CYCLING

Submaximal The Aerobic Cycle Test is one of the more popular submaximal exercise tests in exercise physiology laboratories and fitness clinics. It is a more sophisticated test than
the step test, partially due to its more complicated procedures and its more expensive and less portable ergometer.
Group testing is severely restricted due to the need for numerous cycle ergometers. It nearly qualifies as a laboratory
test because heart rate can be measured *during* exercise by
more sophisticated methods (e.g., ECG and auscultation)
than by palpation, such as in most step tests.

PURPOSE OF THE AEROBIC CYCLE TEST

The purpose of this submaximal exercise test is similar
to the run tests and the step tests—that is, to estimate a
person's aerobic fitness. Additionally, we have expanded
the designers'[2,3,5] original purposes to include educational
objectives, such as familiarization with cycle ergometry,
achievement of skill in auscultation of heartbeats, and
understanding of the rationale for the test.

PHYSIOLOGICAL RATIONALE

aerobic ↓ ATP

All submaximal cycle ergometer tests are designed to rely
predominantly upon the aerobic system to supply the majority of the ATP to the muscles. As is typical of exercise
meant to promote aerobic fitness, the muscles used in cycling are large. For example, the extension of the hip and
knee joints for the downstroke in cycling is accomplished
mainly by the gluteus maximus, rectus femoris, and the
vastus lateralis. Knee flexion is accomplished by the biceps
femoris and the gastrocnemius during the upstroke, while
hip flexion is accomplished by the rectus femoris during
the latter part of the upstroke.[10]

One particular aerobic cycle test, the Åstrand Cycle
Test, *predicts* maximal oxygen consumption ($\dot{V}O_2$max)
based upon the steady-state heart rate of a person exercising at a submaximal power level for 6 min. Thus,
the rationale is similar to that of step tests in that the
test depends upon the direct relationships among power
level, oxygen consumption, and heart rate. The positive
relationship between heart rate and oxygen consumption is most linear between 50 % and 90 % of maximal
heart rate.[9] Expressed in terms of the respective units
of measure, the physiological rationale for the Åstrand
Cycle Test can be stated as the following: A prediction of

maximal oxygen consumption ($L \cdot min^{-1}$) based upon the
participant's heart-rate response at a given power (W) or
submaximal oxygen consumption. Åstrand and Ryhming
observed that the heart rates for men and women at 50 %
$\dot{V}O_2$max were 128 bpm and 138 bpm, respectively. Thus,
if a man exercised at a power level that required an
oxygen consumption of 2.1 $L \cdot min^{-1}$ and his heart rate
was 128 bpm, then his predicted $\dot{V}O_2$max based on the
assumed linear relationship would be 4.2 $L \cdot min^{-1}$. Numerous alternative versions of aerobic cycling tests exist. The
YMCA Physical Working Capacity Test (PWCmax)[12]
utilizes the assumed linear relationship between power
on the cycle ergometer and submaximal exercise heart
rate. Cycling power is increased incrementally throughout
the test, resulting in an increase in submaximal exercise
heart rate. The test is typically discontinued at a submaximal heart rate (i.e, 150–170 bpm for young adults).
The submaximal values for heart rate and power are then
extrapolated to an age-predicted maximal heart rate which
allows for the estimation of a maximal cycling power,
had the participant continued to pedal to exhaustion. Further assuming that specific cycling powers require a given
oxygen uptake[1], the maximal power (Pmax) can be used
to estimate a maximal oxygen uptake ($\dot{V}O_2$max). Maximal
effort protocols also exist, one of which allows $\dot{V}O_2$max
to be estimated from the maximal cycling power attained
with cycling to fatigue.[29] There is reason to believe that a
maximal protocol may yield a better estimate of $\dot{V}O_2$max
than a submaximal protocol. Relying on a submaximal effort requires an estimation of maximal heart rate,
typically based only on the participant's age, which intro-
duces an added source of error or variability. By cycling
maximally to fatigue, the maximal cycling power is actually achieved and measured instead of being estimated by
extrapolation from the submaximal data.

METHODS

As with all field or laboratory tests, the methodology of
the Aerobic Cycle Test includes such factors as (a) equipment, (b) technician preparations, (c) test procedures, and
(d) calculations of $\dot{V}O_2$max Many of these methods apply
to numerous cycle ergometer tests that predict aerobic fitness, such as the YMCA Test.[11,12] The description of the
accuracy of the Aerobic Cycle Test is in Box 14.1, and the
calibration procedures are in Box 14.2.

BOX 14.1 Accuracy of the Aerobic Cycle Test

Reliability

The test-retest reliability coefficients were acceptable for older men (r = 0.835) and college women (r = 0.87)[35] who twice performed the Åstrand Cycle Test. When heart rates are taken daily on a person exercising at the same exercise power level, they vary by about ±5 bpm.[22]

Validity

All *predictive* tests should be interpreted with caution, especially if the original data from the test are from a different type of population. For example, both age and fitness may influence the interpretation of a test. With respect to age, low validity coefficients (approximately 0.60) were reported between the Åstrand Cycle Test and the directly measured maximal oxygen consumption of middle-aged men.[16] With respect to fitness, untrained persons are more likely to be underestimated by the Åstrand Cycle Test, whereas the highly trained are more likely to be overestimated in their maximal oxygen consumptions.[4]

The ability of the Åstrand Cycle Test to predict or estimate the actual measured maximal oxygen consumption varies considerably. The standard error of estimate *(SEE)* has ranged from as low as 6–10%[32] to as high as 15–20%.[16,21,24]

One investigator reported a validity coefficient of 0.74 between the Åstrand predicted values and the directly measured maximal oxygen consumption values.[8] In a review of 13 studies, validity coefficients ranged from as low as 0.34 to as high as 0.94, with the average being 0.64.[16] The rationale of the Åstrand Cycle Test assumes that the heart rate versus oxygen consumption relationship remains linear to maximal levels. This has been contested by some investigators[27,36] and is likely to contribute to the underestimation of $\dot{V}O_2$max in persons of average or low fitness. Although researchers report a linear increase in optimal pedaling rate with increased power output in cycle ergometry,[6] the 50 rpm prescribed for the Åstrand Cycle Test was the original rate in the development of the test's predictions and norms. Another group of investigators reported validity data for a maximal cycling test that increased 15 W·min^{-1} to the "limit of tolerance" in 115 men and 116 women aged 20–70 y. Direct measurement of oxygen uptake during the test allowed the determination of r and *SEE* values of 0.94 and 196 ml·min^{-1} for men and 0.93 and 134 ml·min^{-1} for women respectively. Equations reported in the study allowed the prediction of $\dot{V}O_2$max to within 10 % of its true value.

BOX 14.2 Calibration of the Cycle Ergometer

Mechanically Braked Ergometers

The mechanically braked (friction belt) ergometer (Figure 14.1) can be statically (no pedaling) calibrated based upon the movement of the pendulum to a given reading on the force scale (Figure 14.2), which corresponds to the amount of weight suspended from the friction belt.

Zero

1. Remove the belt from the spring-belt junction at the front of the ergometer.
2. Adjust the "winged-bolt" screw at the front rim of the force scale "quadrant" so that the zero point of the scale coincides with the red index mark on the pendulum weight.
3. Tighten the lock nut of the thumb screw.

Range

1. Hang a known weight from the spring or suspension hook where the friction belt attaches.
2. The pendulum weight should move to the corresponding marker on the Force scale (e.g., a 4 kg weight moves the pendulum to the 40 N or 4 kp [kilopond] marker). *Note:* kp is essentially the same as kg.
3. If not in agreement, adjust the weight pin inside the pendulum disk with the lock screw in the center of the back side of the disk.

Electronically Braked Constant-Power Cycle Ergometer

Although these cycle ergometers are calibrated by the manufacturer, they can lose their calibration with constant use. Advertisers of electronic calibrators claim that the typical accuracy of the power setting is 5–20 %. These cycles require either a technician's expertise in interfacing the cycle's electronic output to a volt/watt meter or the purchase of a special calibrating dynamometer (e.g., Quinton, model 805; Vacu·Med). The calibrators can measure the accuracy of powers up to 600 W from 40 rpm to 120 rpm. Some dynamometric calibrators can detect power variations of about 1 W. Manufacturers may perform the calibration periodically; however, this can be expensive. Rough checks of the accuracy can be made with a conventional torque wrench, following instructions from the manufacturer.

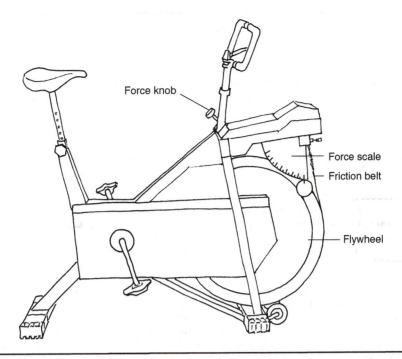

Figure 14.1 A mechanically braked cycle ergometer; the force (load) remains constant at its setting regardless of pedal revolutions.

Equipment

The equipment for administering the Aerobic Cycle Test varies according to the purposes of the investigator, technician, teacher, or student. For example, no equipment is necessary to palpate the pulse; however, if the goal of students is to develop auscultatory (listening) skills, then stethoscopes will be needed. Additionally, if assured accuracy is required, an investigator would use a heart-rate monitor or electrocardiogram to measure heart rate.

The equipment needed for the purposes presented in this manual are a cycle ergometer, a stopwatch, a metronome, a stethoscope, and a calculator.

Cycle Ergometer

Among the various types of cycle ergometers, most may be classified in two ways: according to their braking method or according to the constancy of the power level. There are usually two types of braking methods—mechanical or electrical; similarly, there are two types of power controls—one that is constant regardless of pedal speed and one that changes power according to pedal speed.

Mechanically braked cycle ergometers (e.g., Monark™, Tunturi™) used for testing in laboratories and fitness centers (Figure 14.1) control power by providing a *constant force,* or resistance. The resistance on the flywheel of a mechanically braked ergometer (sometimes called the braking force) is created by altering the tension on the friction belt (or brake belt) that contacts the flywheel. The

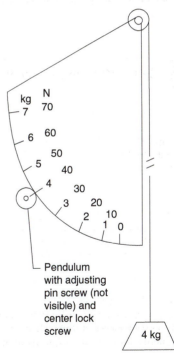

Figure 14.2 The force scale indicates by its pendulum the accuracy of a mass of 4 kg representing a force of 40 N on the friction belt of the mechanically braked cycle ergometer.

tighter the tension on the belt, the greater the resistance created by the friction between the belt and flywheel. A "pendulum type" Monark™ ergometer (e.g., 828E model) has a force scale (Figure 14.2) with gradations marked in kiloponds[a] (kp) ranging from 0 to 7 kp. In this manual, 1 kp is considered equivalent to 1 kg. The force scale is also marked in newtons (N). Although 1 kg technically is equal to 9.8067 N, it is sometimes assumed to be equivalent to or "rounded" to 10 N. This is the case on the force scale, because the newton values corresponding to the 7 kp values are given as 0 to 70 N in 10 N intervals.

When testing on the mechanically braked cycle, the power level (or the rate at which work is done) is determined based on three factors: the resistance or force setting (N), the pedaling rate (rev·min^{-1}), and the assumed distance traveled per pedal revolution (m·rev^{-1}). The circumference of the flywheel on a Monark™ ergometer (1.62 m) is such that one complete revolution of the pedals (resulting in 3.7 revolutions of the flywheel) results in a "constant" distance traveled of 6 m. The power can then be determined using Equation 14.1a. The resulting units are N·m·min^{-1}. The preferred unit for power in cycle ergometry, however, is the watt (W). Equations 14.1b through 14.1d show the derivation of determining power in watts. By dividing power by 60 s·min^{-1} (Eq. 14.1b), the units are converted from N·m·min^{-1} into N·m·s^{-1} (or also into watts because 1 Nm·s^{-1} is equal to 1 W). Furthermore, the constant distance traveled per pedal revolution (6 m) is substituted into Equation 14.1c. This all results in a simplified equation for calculating power on a Monark™ cycle ergometer from brake force and pedaling rate (Eq. 14.1d).

Power (N·m·min^{-1}) = Force (N) * Pedaling rate
(rev·min^{-1}) * (m·rev^{-1})　　　　　　　Eq. 14.1a

Power (N·m·s^{-1} or W) = Power (N·m·min^{-1})
/ 60 (s·min^{-1})　　　　　　　　　　　　　Eq. 14.1b

Power (W) = Force (N) * Pedaling rate
(rev·min^{-1}) * 6 (m) / 60 (s·min^{-1})　　Eq. 14.1c

Power (W) = Force (N) * Pedaling rate
(rev·min^{-1}) / 10　　　　　　　　　　　　Eq. 14.1d

For example, a person pedaling at a force of 30 N (or 3 kg) at a pedaling rate of 50 rpm (or rev·min^{-1}) is cycling at a power of 150 W, as seen in Equation 14.2a. Power is increased on a mechanically braked cycle by increasing either the brake force or the pedaling rate. An increase in brake force from 30 to 40 N at the same pedaling rate (50 rpm) results in an increase in power from 150 to 200 W (Eq. 14.2b). An increase in pedaling rate from 50 to 75 rpm at the same brake force (30 N) results in an increase in power from 150 to 225 W (Eq. 14.2c). Power is decreased by decreasing either brake force or pedaling rate. For this reason, it is important to maintain a constant pedaling rate

---

[a]One kilopond represents the force at normal acceleration of gravity that is dependent upon the global latitude. For example, a person's body mass is greater at the North Pole (90° latitude) than at the Equator (0° latitude) due to the greater pull of gravity at the pole. However, the difference between kilogram and kilopond has little practical significance for exercise laboratories.

| Table 14.1 | Calculation of Power (W) from Brake Force (N; kg) and Pedaling Rate (rpm) |

Force		Pedaling Rate (rpm)				
N	kg	50	65	75	85	100
5	0.5	25	33	38	43	50
10	1.0	50	65	75	85	100
15	1.5	75	98	113	128	150
20	2.0	100	130	150	170	200
25	2.5	125	163	188	213	250
30	3.0	150	195	225	255	300
35	3.5	175	228	263	298	350
40	4.0	200	260	300	340	400
45	4.5	225	293	338	383	450
50	5.0	250	325	375	425	500

Note: Power (W) = Force (N) * Pedaling rate (rpm) / 10.

to maintain a constant power. A sample of power levels based on various brake forces and pedaling rates is given in Table 14.1.

Power (W) = 30 N * 50 rpm / 10 = 150 W　　Eq. 14.2a

Power (W) = 40 N * 50 rpm / 10 = 200 W　　Eq. 14.2b

Power (W) = 30 N * 75 rpm / 10 = 220 W　　Eq. 14.2c

Electromagnetically braked cycle ergometers (e.g., Tectrix™, Biodex™, Cybex™) and computer-controlled ergometers (e.g., Monark™ 839E) actually provide a *constant power* during cycling by automatically altering the brake force or resistance in response to any changes in pedaling rate. That is to say, if the desired power is 150 W, and the person is pedaling at 50 rpm, the cycle ergometer will apply a force of 30 N (Power = 30 N * 50 rpm / 10 = 150 W). Should the person increase the pedaling rate to 75 rpm, the ergometer will automatically reduce the force to 20 N to maintain the 150 W power level (Power = 20 N * 75 rpm / 10 = 150 W). This means that maintaining a constant pedaling rate is not as important as it is on the mechanically braked ergometer.

Other Equipment

Most newer cycle ergometers are outfitted with an electronic display panel that displays time, pedaling rate (rpm), speed (km·h^{-1}; mi·h^{-1}), distance (km; mi), and other variables. And many have an integrated heart-rate receiver that allows the display of heart rate as well. When using an older cycle ergometer without an electronic display, it may be necessary to use a metronome to accurately maintain a specific pedaling rate. To maintain a pedaling rate of 50 rpm, it is common to set the metronome to 100 bpm and instruct the cyclist that each downstroke of the pedals should correspond to a beat on the metronome. For higher pedaling rates (80–100 rpm), it is common to set the metronome to the same rate (80–100 bpm) and instruct the cyclist to time the downstroke of one foot (right or left) to the beat of the metronome. If the ergometer does not display heart rate, it will be necessary to determine heart rate by palpation, stethoscope (auscultation), heart-rate monitor, or electrocardiograph.

Stethoscope

Heart rates can be determined by palpation, stethoscope, heart-rate monitors, or electrocardiograph. Auscultatory (by ear) heart rates are preferred over palpatory ones (by pulse or apical beat) for some tests when performed by experienced technicians.[12] The standard error between auscultation by stethoscope and recording by electrocardiograph for measuring heart rate was less than 2 bpm in one unpublished study. A stethoscope consists of a chestpiece that contacts the chest, and a sound tube that separates and becomes the binaurals (two tubes), ending in two earpieces. A wider, flatter chestpiece (or diaphragm) is often preferred. A double binaural stethoscope, also known as a "teaching" stethoscope, works especially well with students (Figure 14.3).

The basic purpose of the stethoscope—to bring the ear of the listener closer to the source of the sound—has not changed since a one-piece hollow tube was first used in 1819.[19] Typical stethoscopes do not amplify sounds, although some battery-powered ones may amplify by 100 times. The length of the tubing makes little, if any, practical difference in the sound intensity unless it exceeds three feet.[25] Heart-rate monitors are accurate as long as electrical interference from other heart-rate monitors or computerized equipment is avoided.[1,17]

Technician Preparation

Adequate preparation for the administration of the Aerobic Cycle Test consists of (1) periodic calibrations of equipment as described in Box 14.2, (2) orientation of the

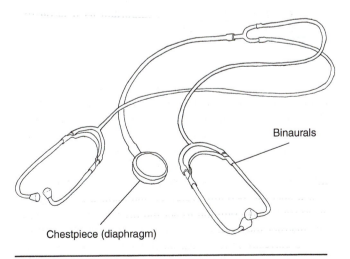

Binaurals

Chestpiece (diaphragm)

Figure 14.3 The "double binaural" or teaching stethoscope can be used by the instructor to teach students how to auscultate heart rate.

participant (3) development of the technician's auscultatory and timing skills, (4) adjustment of the ergometer's seat height, and (5) prescription of the participant's exercise protocol.

Orientation of the Participant

The participant should be in a condition that is standard for laboratory testing. This means that he or she is relaxed, drug free, euhydrated (normal hydration), appropriately attired, and is neither hungry nor full. The facility should be environmentally controlled so that the air temperature (T_a) is not higher than 23 °C ($\approx$ 74 °F).[1] Ideally, some investigators suggest an environmental temperature as low as 17 °C ($\approx$ 62 °F) for the best prediction of maximal oxygen consumption in trained persons.[27] The air's water vapor content should produce less than 60 % relative humidity (RH). Natural barometric pressures above 630 mm Hg (> 840 hPa)—equivalent to altitudes less than 1500 m or 5000 ft—will not affect the results of the exercise test.

The technician's explanations of the exercise task (e.g., intensity of the exercise) and the associated risks should satisfy most of the questions a participant might have regarding the Aerobic Cycle Test. For classroom purposes a verbal assent should be adequate, but for tests administered outside the classroom, a written consent should be obtained (see the Informed Consent information in Appendix C).

Auscultation of Heartbeats to Determine Heart Rate

Heart rate is most accurately determined by using an electrocardiogram or a heart-rate monitor (e.g., Polar™). It may also be determined by palpating or auscultating the participant's pulse. Palpation of pulse was described in Chapter 13. The following is a description of how to use a stethoscope to auscultate exercise pulse.

The vibrations of the heart valves and blood are responsible for the heart sounds. Their sounds are of low frequency and low decibel, making them difficult to hear for inexperienced technicians. The two distinct heart sounds heard under resting conditions are often referred to as *lub-dup*. The first sound, *lub*, is a systolic (ventricles contract) sound, and the second sound, *dup*, is the diastolic (ventricles relax) sound. The sound of systole is due primarily to the closing of the atrioventricular valves (mitral and tricuspid) and secondarily to the opening of the semilunar valves (aortic and pulmonic). *Lub* is heard best at the fourth to fifth intercostal space near the midclavicular line.[18,19] The *dup* sound of diastole is due mainly to the closing of the semilunar valves[20] and is heard best at the pulmonic area near the base of the heart, which is externally marked between the second and third intercostal space at a point about 2–3 cm left of the sternum.[7,18,19] Under exercise conditions, the duration between the *lub* and *dup* is usually too short to distinguish as two separate sounds. Thus, at exercise, each sound is equivalent to one heartbeat.

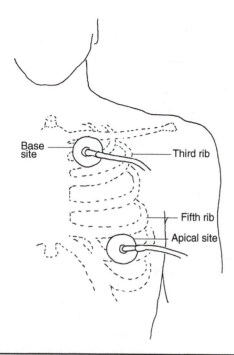

Figure 14.4 Two practical stethoscopic sites are at the base and apical regions of the heart.

Table 14.2		Calculation of Exercise Heart Rate (bpm) from the Time (s) for 30 Heart Beats			
Time (s)	HR (bpm)	Time (s)	HR (bpm)	Time (s)	HR (bpm)
18.0	100	13.8	130	11.3	160
17.6	102	13.6	132	11.1	162
17.3	104	13.4	134	11.0	164
17.0	106	13.2	136	10.8	166
16.7	108	13.0	138	10.7	168
16.4	110	12.9	140	10.6	170
16.1	112	12.7	142	10.5	172
15.8	114	12.5	144	10.3	174
15.5	116	12.3	146	10.2	176
15.3	118	12.2	148	10.1	178
15.0	120	12.0	150	10.0	180
14.8	122	11.8	152	9.9	182
14.5	124	11.7	154	9.8	184
14.3	126	11.5	156	9.7	186
14.1	128	11.4	158	9.6	188

Note: HR (bpm) = 1800 / Time (s) for 30 beats.

Stethoscopes, as mentioned, have binaurals, which sometimes curve near the ear tips; the direction of the binaurals should point toward the nose because the ear canals point in that direction. By tapping gently on the diaphragm, the listener can assure that the sound is being transmitted adequately. The diaphragm of a stethoscope should not be used over cloth and should be flush with the skin (i.e., no air spaces between it and the skin surface).

In general, the heartbeat is heard best at the apical region just below the pectoralis major muscle. Occasionally, it is more convenient to auscultate heartbeat at its base area just below and to the left of the manubrium (Figure 14.4).

The following procedures for timing the heartbeats and converting the number of beats to heart rate in the Åstrand Cycle Test are different from those commonly prescribed for run tests and step tests. By measuring the time elapsed during 30 heartbeats, the heart rate can be calculated by Equation 14.3. The heart rate may also be determined by using Table 14.2.

$$HR (bpm) = 1800 / Times (s) \qquad \text{Eq. 14.3}$$

1. Start the watch on a heartbeat while silently saying "zero."
2. Count 30 heartbeats.
3. Stop the watch on the 30th beat.
4. Record the time to closest 0.1 s for the 30 beats.
5. Determine heart rate (HR) by using Equation 14.3 or Table 14.2.

This 30-beat method of obtaining heart rate is considered more exact than the 15 s method prescribed for some field tests.[3] This is due to the elimination of partial intervals between beats at the start and finish of a timing period. Only whole intervals are in the 30-beat method, because the stopwatch is started and stopped on the respective beats, not on a go and stop signal or the movement of a seconds hand or display digit.

In cases where auscultation is difficult, it is helpful to get second opinions from more experienced technicians or to use a double-binaural stethoscope or an amplifying stethoscope. Also, heart-rate monitors have been perfected to provide accurate and practical measures.[18]

Seat Adjustment

The position of the cycle seat affects the efficiency of the rider.[28] Mechanical efficiency may vary by ± 6 % on the cycle ergometer even when appropriate seat adjustments are made.[4] With the ball of the cyclist's foot on the pedal, the leg should have a bend of only 5–15° at the bottom of the stroke (see Figure 14.5a). The leg should be nearly straight if the heel of the foot is on the pedal at the bottom of the stroke (Figure 14.5b). If the hips rock or if the heels slip off the pedals, the seat is too high. Most seat posts have numbers at intervals of about 2–3 cm. Once the proper seat height has been established, the seat setting can be recorded onto the individual's data collection form (Form 14.2).

Determining the Exercise Protocol

The original and most common pedaling rate is 50 rpm. However, any rate between 50 rpm and 80 rpm appears valid for predicting $\dot{V}O_2$max in a wide range of participants.[31] Experienced cyclists tend to be more economical at the higher end of this range (e.g., 70–80 rpm) at the high power levels.[6,13,30]

The goal of the Åstrand Cycle Test is to produce a steady-state heart rate of about 80–85 % of the participant's age-predicted maximal heart rate within 6 min of exercise.

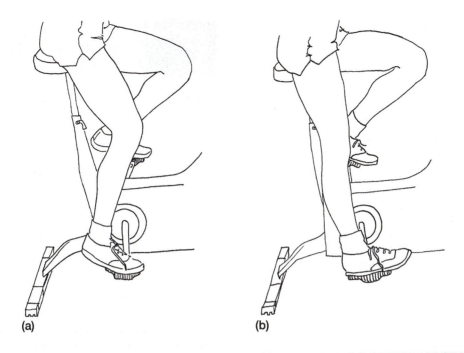

Figure 14.5 Adjusting the seat for the Åstrand Cycle Test: (a) slight bend in knee when the ball of the foot is on the pedal at the bottom of the pedal stroke; (b) straight leg when the heel is on the pedal. The cycling movement occurs with the ball of the foot on the pedal.

Table 14.3	**Target Heart Rate (HR) Zones and Initial Powers for the Åstrand Cycle Test**

		Power (W)	
Age (y)	Target HR (bpm)	Average Male	Average Female
< 30	150–160	150–175	125–150
30–39	145–155	125–150	100–125
40–49	140–150	100–125	75–100
50–59	135–145	100–125	75–100
60–69	130–140	75–100	50–75

Note: For the average person, a general guideline is to prescribe 1.65 W for each kg of body weight. Highly trained persons, especially of higher body weight, will require higher power levels.

For a person under 30 years of age this would be a steady-state or target heart rate of about 150–160 bpm. Approximate target heart-rate zones by age group are provided in Table 14.3. The initial power at which to begin the test is also an important consideration. General guidelines for initial power based on age and gender also appear in Table 14.3. It would be appropriate in young adults (< 30 y) to start the "average" man at 150–175 W and the "average" woman at 125–150 W. Two other factors to consider in selecting the initial power are fitness level and body weight. Higher initial powers would be selected for those who are more fit and for those of higher body weight. In fact, the initial power for sedentary persons may be estimated by using 1.65 W per kg of body weight. Using this formula, the initial power for a sedentary person who weighs 75 kg would be about 125 W (75 kg * 1.65 W·kg^{-1}). As mentioned previously, alternate submaximal and maximal protocols exist for aerobic cycling tests. These protocols consist of 1-min to 3-min stages where cycling power is incrementally increased typically by 10–15 W per 1-min stage or 25–50 W per 3-min stage. Two alternate aerobic cycling tests are described that can be completed in place of or in addition to the Åstrand Cycle Test. The first alternate test is a submaximal test that uses a "branching" protocol, where power is increased in 3-min stages in response to the participant's exercise heart rate (Form 14.3). The benefit of a branching protocol is that it allows participants of varying fitness levels to be tested in approximately the same amount of time, in about 9 to 12 min. The goal of the test in young adults is to raise the participant's HR to at least 150 bpm, but not to exceed 180 bpm by the end of the test, so as to keep the effort submaximal. The submaximal relationship between heart rate and cycling power is then extrapolated to age-predicted maximal HR to estimate maximal cycling power and $\dot{V}O_2$max. The second alternate test is a maximal effort test. Participants cycle at 0 W for 4 min then cycling power is increased at 15 W·min^{-1} until fatigue. $\dot{V}O_2$max is estimated from the maximal power achieved. The duration of the test may vary considerably based on the fitness level of the participants.

Summary of Technician's Preparatory Steps

1. Periodically calibrate the cycle ergometer (Box 14.2).
2. Orient the participant by explaining the purpose and protocol of the Aerobic Cycle Test.

3. Measure and record the participant's basic data (e.g., age, height, body weight) on Form 14.2.

4. Adjust the seat height so that the participant's leg is slightly bent (5–15°) with the ball of the foot on the pedal at the full down stroke (Figure 14.5).

5. If heart rate is to be determined by electrocardiography (ECG) or heart-rate monitor, prepare and attach the required equipment (e.g., ECG electrodes, heart-rate transmitter).

6. If heart rate is to be determined by palpation or auscultation, the technician should practice palpating at the radial and carotid sites, or should practice auscultating heartbeats (review Figure 14.4) with the participant seated comfortably on the ergometer.

7. Establish the desired pedaling rate (typically, 50–85 rpm) and power to be used to begin the test.

Test Procedures for the Åstrand Cycle Test

The normal duration of the Åstrand Cycle Test is six minutes. During this time the technician is responsible for monitoring the pedaling rate and power level of the participant, determining heart rate by any one of several methods described (e.g., heart-rate monitor, palpation, auscultation), and recording all data necessary to complete the test. The technician should also be aware of the participant's response to the exercise, watching for any signs or symptoms (e.g., chest pain, dizziness, nausea) that might warrant terminating the test. In some cases, adjustments may need to be made to the power at which the participant is cycling or to the length of the test so that the appropriate steady-state heart rate is achieved. A cool-down should be completed to allow for a gradual return of heart rate and blood pressure toward resting. Further description of these procedures and a detailed explanation of how to estimate and assess $\dot{V}O_2$max follow.

Power Adjustments During the Test

Adjusting the power during the test is often necessary because the initial power was set either too low or too high, resulting in an exercise heart rate outside the desired range. Table 14.4 provides guidelines for how much the technician should raise or lower the power based on the exercise heart rate of the participant after 3 min of exercise. Notice in Table 14.4 that no change in power would be necessary for a young adult (< 30 y) if the heart rate is in the desired range of 140–149 bpm. However, power level would be increased by 25 W if the heart rate is 130–139 bpm, by 50 W if heart rate is 110–129 bpm, and by 75 W if heart rate is far below desired (< 110 bpm). Conversely, if the heart rate is higher than the desired level, the power can be decreased by 25 or 50 W. If the difference between the heart rates during minutes 5 and 6 exceeds 10 beats (indicating HR is still rising), the participant should continue to exercise until the difference between the final two heart rates is 10 bpm or less.

| Table 14.4 | Power Adjustments for the Åstrand Test Based on Heart Rate After 3 Min and Age (y) |

Change in Power (W)	Heart Rate (bpm) After 3 Min		
	< 30 y	30–49 y	50–69 y
Raise 75 W	< 110	< 100	< 90
Raise 50 W	110–129	100–119	90–109
Raise 25 W	130–139	120–129	110–119
No change	140–149	130–139	120–129
Lower 25 W	150–159	140–149	130–139
Lower 50 W	> 160	> 150	> 140

Note: Adjust power up or down during the test if exercise heart rate after 3 min is outside the desired range. All exercise heart rates are decreased by about one-half beat per minute per year.

Time Adjustments During the Test

If the difference between the heart rates during minutes 5 and 6 exceeds 10 beats, the participant should continue to exercise until the difference between the final two heart rates is 10 bpm or less. One group of investigators suggested that if the difference between the final two heart rates is between 6 and 10 beats, then ignore the earlier minute's rate and use only the final minute's heart rate to make the calculation for predicting maximal oxygen consumption.[10]

Cool-Down

It is important that the cyclist be given a low-intensity exercise level after the regular test protocol. This will prevent the pooling of blood in the legs, which could lead to fainting if the participant were to stand still immediately after finishing the test. In general, the recovery exercise can be terminated when the heart rate is 100 bpm or less (18 s for 30 beats). Muscle soreness is unlikely in this aerobic submaximal test.

Estimation of Maximal Oxygen Consumption

The first step in estimating maximal oxygen consumption is to determine the steady-state or submaximal heart rate achieved at the end of the 6 min (or longer) exercise test. The final two heart rates (from minutes 5 and 6) are averaged to determine the submaximal heart rate. This averaged heart rate is then used in any one of three methods to estimate maximal oxygen consumption. It can be used to estimate $\dot{V}O_2$max by (1) using Equations 14.4a through 14.4c; (2) using Table 14.5; or (3) using the Åstrand—Ryhming nomogram.[2,3] By calculation, the oxygen consumption for submaximal exercise can be estimated (Eq. 14.4a). Then assuming age-predicted maximal heart rates ($HR_{max} = 220 - age$) and resting heart rates for men and women of 61 bpm and 72 bpm, respectively, the $\dot{V}O_2$max can be estimated for men (Eq. 14.4b) and women (Eq. 14.4c).

$$\text{Submaximal } \dot{V}O_2\text{max (L·min}^{-1}) = 0.012 * P\ (W) + 0.3 \qquad \text{Eq. 14.4a}$$

$$\dot{V}O_2\text{max (L·min}^{-1}) = \text{Submax } \dot{V}O_2\text{max (L·min}^{-1}) * (220 - \text{Age(y)} - 61)/(\text{Submax HR} - 61) \qquad \text{Eq. 14.4b}$$

Table 14.5	Estimation of Maximal Oxygen Consumption (L·min⁻¹) from Heart Rate and Power by Gender															

Submax HR (bpm)	Men Final Power Completed (W)									Submax HR (bpm)	Women Final Power Completed (W)				
	50	75	100	125	150	175	200	225	250		50	75	100	125	150
120	2.2	2.9	3.5	4.2	4.8					120	2.6	3.4	4.1	4.8	
125	2.0	2.7	3.3	3.9	4.4	5.2	5.9			125	2.3	3.0	3.7	4.4	
130	1.9	2.5	3.0	3.6	4.1	4.8	5.5			130	2.1	2.7	3.4	4.0	4.7
135	1.7	2.3	2.8	3.3	3.8	4.5	5.1			135	2.0	2.6	3.1	3.7	4.3
140	1.6	2.1	2.6	3.1	3.6	4.2	4.8	5.4	6.0	140	1.8	2.4	2.8	3.4	4.0
145			2.4	2.9	3.4	4.0	4.5	5.1	5.6	145	1.6	2.2	2.7	3.2	3.7
150			2.3	2.8	3.2	3.7	4.2	4.8	5.3	150		2.0	2.5	3.0	3.5
155			2.2	2.6	3.0	3.5	4.0	4.5	5.0	155		1.9	2.4	2.8	3.2
160			2.1	2.5	2.8	3.3	3.8	4.3	4.8	160		1.8	2.2	2.6	3.0
165			2.0	2.4	2.7	3.2	3.6	4.1	4.5	165		1.7	2.1	2.5	2.9
170			1.8	2.2	2.6	3.0	3.4	3.9	4.3	170		1.6	2.0	2.4	2.7

Source: Data from Åstrand (1988).[4]

$$\dot{V}O_2max \ (L·min^{-1}) = Submax \ \dot{V}O_2max \ (L·min^{-1})$$
$$* \ (220 - Age(y) - 72) \ / \ (Submax \ HR - 72) \quad \text{Eq. 14.4c}$$

For example, if a 35-year-old man's average heart rate during minutes 5 and 6 of the Åstrand Cycle Test is 155 bpm while cycling at 150 W, the calculations would be as shown in Equations 14.5a and 14.5b, yielding an estimated $\dot{V}O_2max$ of 2.77 L·min⁻¹.

$$\text{Submaximal } \dot{V}O_2max \ (L·min^{-1}) = 0.012 * \mathbf{150} \ W + 0.3$$
$$= \mathbf{2.10} \ L·min^{-1} \quad \text{Eq. 14.5a}$$

$$\dot{V}O_2max \ (L·min^{-1}) = \mathbf{2.10} \ L·min^{-1} * (220 - \mathbf{35} - 61) \ /$$
$$(\mathbf{155} - 61) = \mathbf{2.77} \ L·min^{-1} \quad \text{Eq. 14.5b}$$

Using the same data, but estimating $\dot{V}O_2max$ from Table 14.5, the estimated $\dot{V}O_2max$ is 3.0 L·min⁻¹. It should be noted, however, that the values in Table 14.5 assume an age of 25 y. If the participant is younger or older, it is necessary to correct the $\dot{V}O_2max$ using the correction factors in Table 14.6. Therefore, if the participant was 35 years old, the estimated $\dot{V}O_2max$ of 3.0 L·min⁻¹ would be corrected for age and yield a value of 2.61 L·min⁻¹ (Eq. 14.6).

$$\text{Age-adjusted } \dot{V}O_2max \ (L·min^{-1}) = \mathbf{3.00} \ L·min^{-1}$$
$$* \ \mathbf{0.88} = \mathbf{2.64} \ L·min^{-1} \quad \text{Eq. 14.6}$$

The $\dot{V}O_2max$ values derived in Equations 14.5b and 14.6 are considered the participant's *absolute* $\dot{V}O_2max$ and are expressed in liters·min⁻¹. More often, however, it is the *relative* $\dot{V}O_2max$ that is of interest. Relative $\dot{V}O_2max$ is the maximal oxygen consumption expressed relative to the participant's body weight in kilograms and is expressed in ml·kg⁻¹·min⁻¹ (Eq. 14.7a). For example, a person with an absolute $\dot{V}O_2max$ of 3.55 L·min⁻¹ who weighs 81.5 kg has a relative $\dot{V}O_2max$ of 43.6 ml·kg⁻¹·min⁻¹ (Eq. 14.7b).

$$\text{Relative } \dot{V}O_2 \ (ml·kg^{-1}·min^{-1}) = \text{Absolute } \dot{V}O_2$$
$$(L·min^{-1}) * 1000 \ / \ \text{Body wt (kg)} \quad \text{Eq. 14.7a}$$

$$\text{Relative } \dot{V}O_2 \ (ml·kg^{-1}·min^{-1}) = \mathbf{3.55} * 1000 \ / \ \mathbf{81.5}$$
$$= \mathbf{43.6} \ ml·kg^{-1}·min^{-1} \quad \text{Eq. 14.7b}$$

Table 14.6	Correction Factors (CF) for Adjusting Maximal Oxygen Consumption by Age (y)		

Age (y)	CF	Age (y)	CF
18	1.09	33	0.90
19	1.08	34	0.89
20	1.06	35	0.88
21	1.05	36	0.87
22	1.03	37	0.86
23	1.02	38	0.85
24	1.01	39	0.84
25	1.00	40	0.83
26	0.98	41	0.82
27	0.97	42	0.81
28	0.96	43	0.80
29	0.95	44	0.79
30	0.94	45	0.78
31	0.92	46	0.78
32	0.91	47	0.77

Note: Data adapted from Åstrand (1960).[2]

Summary of Test Procedures for the Åstrand Cycle Test

1. Measure and record the participant's basic data (i.e., age, height, weight, etc.) onto Form 14.2.
2. Adjust the seat height so that the cyclist's leg is slightly bent with the ball of the foot on the pedal at the full down stroke (Figure 14.5).
3. Instruct the participant to begin pedaling at the desired pedaling rate, typically 50–60 rpm during the Åstrand Cycle Test, although faster rates ranging up to 90 rpm can be used. If a metronome is to be used, it should be started at this point to help the participant maintain the desired pedaling rate.
4. Set the cycle ergometer to the desired initial power by adjusting either the braking force (on a *constant force* ergometer) or the power (on a *constant power* ergometer) and begin timing the test.

5. Determine heart rate (by any method) within the last 30 s of each minute and record on Form 14.2.

6. At the 3:00 mark, if the exercise heart rate is within the desired range (Table 14.4), maintain the same power on the cycle ergometer. If heart rate is *below* the desired range, *raise* the power 25–75 W. If heart rate is *above* the desired range, *lower* the power 25–50 W (Table 14.4).

7. At the 6:00 mark, if the difference in heart rates between min 5 and 6 was 10 bpm or less, end the test. If the difference was greater than 10 bpm, continue the test until the difference in heart rates between the final two minutes is 10 bpm or less.

8. Lower the power on the cycle ergometer to 25–50 W and instruct the participant to continue cycling (cool down) until the heart rate is less than 100 bpm.

9. Estimate *absolute* maximal oxygen consumption ($L \cdot min^{-1}$) from heart rate and cycle power using Table 14.5. Correct the $\dot{V}O_2max$ for age using Table 14.6. Calculate the *relative* $\dot{V}O_2max$ ($ml \cdot kg^{-1} \cdot min^{-1}$) and determine a fitness category from Table 14.7. Complete the rest of Form 14.2.

Test Procedures for the Alternate Cycle Tests

Summary of Submaximal Test Procedures

1. Measure and record the participant's basic data (i.e., age, weight, etc.) onto Form 14.4.

2. Adjust the seat height and instruct the participant on pedaling rate as described in the Åstrand Cycle Test.

3. Set the cycle ergometer to 25 W for women or 50 W for men and begin the test.

4. Determine heart rate (by any method) within the last 30 s of each 3-min stage and record power (W) and heart rate (bpm) on Form 14.4.

5. At the 3:00 mark, raise the power to the next desired level based on HR (see Form 14.4). In women, if HR < 110 bpm raise power to 75 W, or if HR ≥ 110 bpm raise only to 50 W. In men, if HR < 110 bpm raise power to 100 W, if HR ≥ 110 bpm raise only to 75 W. Record power and HR within 30 s of end of stage.

6. At the 6:00 mark, raise the power to the next desired level based on HR (see Form 14.4). Record power and HR within 30 s of end of stage.

7. At the 9:00 mark, if HR ≥ 150 bpm stop the test. If HR < 150 bpm, raise the power to the next desired level (see Form 14.4). Record power and HR within 30 s of end of stage.

8. Plot HR versus power, extrapolate to age-predicted HRmax, estimate maximal power (Pmax), estimate $\dot{V}O_2max$, and complete Form 14.4.

Summary of Maximal Test Procedures

1. Measure and record the participant's basic data (i.e., age, weight, etc.) onto Form 14.4.

2. Adjust the seat height and instruct the participant to pedal at 60 rpm.

3. Instruct the participant to pedal at 0 W for 4 min, then begin the test.

4. Increase the power in 15 $W \cdot min^{-1}$ increments until the participant fatigues or reaches what is described as his or her "limit of tolerance."

5. At the conclusion of the test, record the maximal power achieved (Pmax), estimate $\dot{V}O_2max$ using Equation 14.8a (men) or Equation 14.8b (women), and complete Form 14.4.

RESULTS AND DISCUSSION

Although the Åstrand Cycle Test originated in Sweden and was first used primarily on healthy Scandinavians, its popularity in other countries and its use in more clinical situations steadily grew. Throughout the world today, it is still used by researchers to test the aerobic fitness of a variety of people, including patients with back pain in Sweden,[26] cancer patients in Norway,[33] medical students in Thailand,[34] nurses in South Africa,[23] and soldiers in Israel.[15] The original data from the Åstrand Cycle Test, derived mainly from Swedish physical education students, resulted in norms higher than could be used in the United States. Different standards as shown in Table 14.7 were generated by testing 450 healthy Americans, nearly all of whom were tested on a cycle ergometer. A small fraction of the participants were tested using a treadmill. The mode of exercise affects the measurement of maximal oxygen consumption. Maximal oxygen consumptions elicited from treadmill tests can typically be 5 to 10 % greater than those elicited by cycle ergometry.[8,14]

Numerous other cycle ergometer tests exist for the estimation of maximal oxygen consumption. One test is the YMCA Maximum Physical Working Capacity Test (PWC_{max}).[12] This test assumes a linear relationship between power on the cycle ergometer and submaximal exercise heart rate. By extrapolating this submaximal relationship to the participant's age-predicted maximal heart rate ($HR_{max} = 220 - Age$), a maximal power associated with an assumed maximal cycling effort can be estimated. The example shown in Figure 14.6 is of a 40-year-old who at power levels of 50, 100, and 150 W had heart rates of 110, 138, and 164 bpm, respectively. Extrapolating the relationship between power and heart rate to the estimated HR_{max} of 180 bpm yields an estimated maximal power (P_{max}) of 175 W. It can be further assumed that each power level on a cycle ergometer (e.g., 50 W, 100 W, etc.) requires a specific oxygen consumption, and that this oxygen consumption is consistent between people. Oxygen uptakes for known power levels on the cycle ergometer can be estimated[1] as seen in Equation 14.8. The value of 10.8 in the equation is associated with the 10.8 ml increase in oxygen consumption required for each 1 W increase in power. The 7 represents the relative $\dot{V}O_2max$ ($ml \cdot kg^{-1} \cdot min^{-1}$) required when cycling against no resistive load. Therefore, the estimated maximal power (assuming the

Table 14.7	Aerobic Fitness Category for Men and Women for the Åstrand Cycle Test by Age Group

Maximal Oxygen Consumption (ml·kg⁻¹·min⁻¹)

	Men				Women			
Category	20–29 y	30–39 y	40–49 y	50–59 y	20–29 y	30–39 y	40–49 y	50–59 y
Very high	> 61	> 57	> 53	> 49	> 57	> 53	> 50	> 42
High	53–61	49–57	45–53	43–49	49–57	45–53	42–50	38–42
Good	43–52	39–48	36–44	34–42	38–48	34–44	31–41	28–37
Average	34–42	31–38	27–35	25–33	31–37	28–33	24–30	21–27
Fair	25–33	23–30	20–26	18–24	24–30	20–27	17–23	15–20
Low	< 25	< 23	< 20	< 18	< 24	< 20	< 17	< 15

Source: Data from Preventive Medicine Center, National Athletic Health Institute, Inglewood, CA.

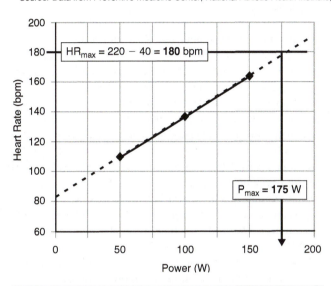

Figure 14.6 The assumed linear relationship between power (W) on the cycle ergometer and submaximal exercise heart rate (bpm) can be extrapolated to the estimated HR_{max} to estimate maximal cycle power (P_{max}). In this case, P_{max} is estimated to be 175 W based on a HR_{max} of 180 bpm.

participant could produce a maximal effort and heart rate) can be used to estimate a relative $\dot{V}O_2max$ (ml·kg⁻¹·min⁻¹) within a reasonable degree of error.

Estimated $\dot{V}O_2$ (ml·kg⁻¹·min⁻¹) = [Power (W)
  * 10.8/ Body wt (kg)] + 7   Eq. 14.8

Using an estimated maximal heart rate to estimate a person's maximal oxygen consumption adds to the variability and potential error of the test. To increase the accuracy of a cycle ergometer test to estimate $\dot{V}O_2max$, other researchers advocate employing a maximal test to directly measure the maximal power.[29] These same researchers further developed prediction equations to estimate $\dot{V}O_2max$ from the combination of gender, age, body weight, and the maximal power attained in a sample of 231 healthy males and females ranging in age from 20 to 70 years old. Participants cycled at 60 rpm for 4 min at 0 W (no load) then power was increased in increments of 15 W·min⁻¹ until fatigue, with heart rate and oxygen consumption measured directly throughout. $\dot{V}O_2max$ can be estimated in men and women from the resulting maximal power by using Equations 14.8a and 14.8b.[29] The high level of accuracy is such that it allows prediction of $\dot{V}O_2max$ to within 10 % of its true value in 95 out of every 100 persons.

Men: $\dot{V}O_2max$ (mL·min⁻¹) = 519.3 mL·min⁻¹
  + [10.51 * P_{max} (W)] + [6.35 * Body weight (kg)]
  − [10.49 * Age (y)]   Eq. 14.8a

Women: $\dot{V}O_2max$ (mL·min⁻¹) = 136.0 mL·min⁻¹
  + [9.39 * P_{max} (W)] + [7.71 * Body weight (kg)]
  − [5.88 * Age (y)]   Eq. 14.8b

Where: P_{max} = maximal power attained while increasing power in 15 W·min⁻¹ increments

Using cycle ergometry either to directly measure or indirectly estimate maximal oxygen consumption has several benefits. Because the participant is seated, cycle ergometry is very safe compared to treadmill running or other exercise modes. This seated position also allows for easier measurement of heart rate and blood pressure and results in less muscular artifact on the electrocardiogram, should these measurements be taken. The power on a cycle ergometer can be controlled at a constant level and is easy to quantify and use in the assessment of aerobic fitness. A possible disadvantage of cycle ergometry is that some persons who are unaccustomed to cycling may need to discontinue the test before the desired end point due to leg discomfort.

BOX 14.3	Chapter Preview/Review

What is the rationale behind the Åstrand Cycle Test?

How is power determined on a mechanically braked cycle ergometer?

What power is created on a Monark™ ergometer when pedaling 75 rpm against a 20 N (2 kg) resistance?

How can the time (s) for 30 heartbeats be converted into a heart rate (bpm)?

What is the target HR range and initial power for the Åstrand Cycle Test for a 40–49 year old?

What is the effect of age on $\dot{V}O_2max$ estimated from the Åstrand Cycle Test?

How can oxygen uptake (ml·kg⁻¹ min⁻¹) be estimated from power (W) on a cycle ergometer?

References

1. American College of Sports Medicine (2010). *ACSM's guidelines for exercise testing and prescription, 8th ed.* Philadelphia: Lippincott Williams & Wilkins.
2. Åstrand, I. (1960). Aerobic work capacity in men and women with special reference to age. *Acta Physiologica Scandinavica, 49* (Suppl. 169).
3. Åstrand, P.-O. (1988). *Work tests with the bicycle ergometer.* Varberg, Sweden: Monark Crescent AB.
4. Åstrand, P.-O., & Rodahl, K. (1977). *Textbook of work physiology.* San Francisco: McGraw-Hill.
5. Åstrand, P.-O., & Ryhming, I. (1954). A nomogram for calculation of aerobic capacity (physical fitness) from pulse rate during submaximal work. *Journal of Applied Physiology, 7,* 218–221.
6. Coast, J. R., & Welch, H. G. (1985). Linear increase in optimal pedalling rate with increased power output in cycle ergometry. *European Journal of Applied Physiology, 53,* 339–342.
7. DePasquale, N. P., Burch, G. E., & Philips, J. H. (1968). The second heart sound. *American Heart Journal, 76,* 419–431.
8. deVries, H. A. (1994). *Physiology of exercise.* Dubuque, IA: Brown & Benchmark.
9. Edington, D. W., & Cunningham, L. (1975). *Biological awareness.* Englewood Cliffs, NJ: Prentice-Hall.
10. Faria, I. E., & Cavanagh, P. R. (1978). *The physiology and biomechanics of cycling.* New York: John Wiley & Sons.
11. Golding, L. A. (2000). *YMCA fitness testing and assessment manual (4th ed.).* Champaign, IL: Human Kinetics.
12. Golding, L. A., Myers, C. R., & Sinning, W. E. (1989). *Y's way to fitness: The complete guide to fitness testing and instruction.* Champaign, IL: Human Kinetics.
13. Hagberg, J. M., Mullin, J. P., Giese, M. D., & Spitznagel, E. (1981). Effect of pedaling rate on submaximal exercise responses of competitive cyclists. *Journal of Applied Physiology, 51,* 447–451.
14. Hermansen, L., & Saltin, B. (1969). Oxygen uptake during maximal treadmill and bicycle exercise. *Journal of Applied Physiology, 26,* 31–37.
15. Huerta, M., Grotto, I., Shemla, S., Ashkenazi, I., Shpilbert, O., & Kark, J. (2004). Cycle ergometry estimation of physical fitness among Israeli soldiers. *Military Medicine, 169,* 217–220.
16. Kasch, F. W. (1984). The validity of the Åstrand and Sjostrand submaximal tests. *The Physician and Sportsmedicine, 12,* 47–51, 54.
17. Leger, L., & Thivierge, M. (1988). Heart rate monitors: Validity, stability, and functionality. *The Physician and Sportsmedicine, 16*(5), 143–151.
18. Lehmann, J. (1972). Auscultation of heart sounds. *American Journal of Nursing, 72,*1242–1246.
19. Littmann, D. (1972). Stethoscope and auscultation. *American Journal of Nursing, 72,*1238–1241.
20. Luisada, A. A., & Zalter, R. (1960). Phonocardiography. In American College of Chest Physicians (Eds.), *Clinical cardiopulmonary physiology* (pp. 75–83). New York: Grune and Stratton.
21. Mathews, D. K., & Fox, E. L. (1976). *The physiological basis of physical education and athletics.* Philadelphia: W. B. Saunders.
22. McArdle, W. D., Katch, F. I., & Katch, V. L. (2007). *Exercise physiology: Energy, nutrition and human performance, 6th ed.* Philadelphia, Lippincott Williams & Wilkins.
23. Naidoo, R., & Coopoo, Y. (2007). The health and fitness profiles of nurses in KwaZulu-Natal. *Curationis, 30,* 66–73.
24. Noble, B. J. (1986). *Physiology of exercise and sport.* St. Louis: Times Mirror/Mosby.
25. Rappaport, M. B., & Sprague, H. B. (1941). Physiologic and physical laws that govern auscultation, and their clinical application. *American Heart Journal, 21,* 257–318.
26. Rasmussen-Barr, E., Lundqvist, L., Nilsson-Wikmar, L, & Ljungquist, T. (2008). Aerobic fitness in patients at work despite recurrent low back pain: A cross-sectional study with healthy age- and gender-matched controls. *Journal of Rehabilitative Medicine, 40,* 359–365.
27. Rowell, L. B., Taylor, H. L., & Wang, Y. (1964). Limitations to prediction of maximal oxygen intake. *Journal of Applied Physiology, 19,* 919–927.
28. Shennum, P. L., & deVries, H. A. (1976). The effect of saddle height on oxygen consumption during bicycle ergometer work. *Medicine and Science in Sports, 8,*119–121.
29. Storer, T. W., Davis, J. A., & Caiozzo, V. J. (1990). Accurate prediction of $\dot{V}O_2$max in cycle ergometry. *Medicine and Science in Sports and Exercise, 22,* 704–712.
30. Swain, D. P., & Wilcox, J. P. (1992). Effect of cadence on the economy of uphill cycling. *Medicine and Science in Sports and Exercise, 24,* 1123–1127.
31. Swain, D. P., & Wright, R. L. (1997). Prediction of $\dot{V}O_2$max peak from submaximal cycle ergometry using 50 versus 80 rpm. *Medicine and Science in Sports and Exercise, 29,* 268–272.
32. Terry, J. W., Tolson, H., Johnson, D. J., & Jessup, G. T. (1977). A workload selection procedure for the Åstrand-Ryhming test. *Journal of Sports Medicine and Physical Fitness, 17,* 361.
33. Thorsen, L., Nystad, W., Stigum, H., Hjermstad, M., Oldervoll, L., Martinsen, W. W., Hornslien, K., Strømme, S. B., Dahl, A. A., & Fosså, S. D.

(2006). Cardiorespiratory fitness in relation to self-reported physical function in cancer patients after chemotherapy. *Journal of Sports Medicine and Physical Fitness, 46,* 122–127.

34. Tongprasert, S., & Wattanapan, P. (2007). Aerobic capacity of fifth-year medical students at Chiang Mai University. *Journal of the Medical Association of Thailand, 90,* 1411–1416.

35. Williams, L. (1975). Reliability of predicting maximal oxygen intake using the Åstrand-Ryhming nomogram. *Research Quarterly, 46,*12–16.

36. Wyndham, C. H., Strydom, N. B., Moritz, J. S., Morrison, J. F., Peter, J., & Potgieter, Z. U. (1959). Maximum oxygen intake and maximum heart rate during strenuous work. *Journal of Applied Physiology, 14,* 927–936.

Form 14.1

NAME _____ DATE _____ SCORE _____

AEROBIC CYCLING (ÅSTRAND TEST)

Homework

Gender: **M**   Initials: **AA**   Age (y): **22**   Height (cm): **180**   Weight (kg): **82.0**

Seat height: _____   Desired pedaling rate: **75** rpm   Maintained rate: ☐ always ☒ usually

Target HR zone *(from Table 14.3)* : _____ bpm   Initial power *(from Table 14.3)* : **150** W

HR at: Min 1 **118** bpm   Min 2 **124** bpm   Min 3 **132** bpm

After 3 min: ☐ raise power   ☐ no change   ☐ lower power   Power level for Min 4: _____ W

HR at: Min 4 **142** bpm   Min 5 **148** bpm   Min 6 **152** bpm   Submax HR _____ bpm

After 6 min: HR difference between Min 5 and Min 6:   ☐ 0-10 bpm (end test)   ☐ >10 bpm (continue test)

HR at: Min 7 _____ bpm   Min 8 _____ bpm   *(Only if necessary)*   Submax HR _____ bpm

Estimated $\dot{V}O_2$max *(from Table 14.5)* = _____ $L \cdot min^{-1}$

Age-adjusted $\dot{V}O_2$max = _____ * CF (_____) = _____ $L \cdot min^{-1}$
                                     VO₂max   Table 14.6

Relative $\dot{V}O_2$max = $\dot{V}O_2$max * 1000 / BW (kg) = _____ $ml \cdot kg^{-1} \cdot min^{-1}$

Fitness category *(from Table 14.7)*   _____

Evaluation / comments: _____

_____

Gender: **F**   Initials: **BB**   Age (y): **20**   Height (cm): **160**   Weight (kg): **62.0**

Seat height: _____   Desired pedaling rate: **75** rpm   Maintained rate: ☐ always ☒ usually

Target HR zone *(from Table 14.3)* : _____ bpm   Initial power *(from Table 14.3)* : **125** W

HR at: Min 1 **122** bpm   Min 2 **132** bpm   Min 3 **141** bpm

After 3 min: ☐ raise power   ☐ no change   ☐ lower power   Power level for Min 4: _____ W

HR at: Min 4 **145** bpm   Min 5 **148** bpm   Min 6 **152** bpm   Submax HR _____ bpm

After 6 min: HR difference between Min 5 and Min 6:   ☐ 0-10 bpm (end test)   ☐ >10 bpm (continue test)

HR at: Min 7 _____ bpm   Min 8 _____ bpm   *(Only if necessary)*   Submax HR _____ bpm

Estimated $\dot{V}O_2$max *(from Table 14.5)* = _____ $L \cdot min^{-1}$

Age-adjusted $\dot{V}O_2$max = _____ * CF (_____) = _____ $L \cdot min^{-1}$
                                     VO₂max   Table 14.6

Relative $\dot{V}O_2$max = $\dot{V}O_2$max * 1000 / BW (kg) = _____ $ml \cdot kg^{-1} \cdot min^{-1}$

Fitness category *(from Table 14.7)*   _____

Evaluation / comments: _____

_____

Form 14.2

AEROBIC CYCLING (ÅSTRAND TEST)

NAME _____ DATE _____ SCORE _____

Lab Results

Gender: _____ Initials: _____ Age (y): _____ Height (cm): _____ Weight (kg): _____

Seat height: _____ Desired pedaling rate: _____ rpm Maintained rate: ☐ always ☐ usually

Target HR zone *(from Table 14.3)*: _____ bpm Initial power *(from Table 14.3)*: _____ W

HR at: Min 1 _____ bpm Min 2 _____ bpm Min 3 _____ bpm

After 3 min: ☐ raise power ☐ no change ☐ lower power Power level for Min 4: _____ W

HR at: Min 4 _____ bpm Min 5 _____ bpm Min 6 _____ bpm Submax HR _____ bpm

After 6 min: HR difference between Min 5 and Min 6: ☐ 0-10 bpm (end test) ☐ >10 bpm (continue test)

HR at: Min 7 _____ bpm Min 8 _____ bpm *(Only if necessary)* Submax HR _____ bpm

Estimated $\dot{V}O_2$max *(from Table 14.5)* = _____ $L\cdot min^{-1}$

Age-adjusted $\dot{V}O_2$max = _____ * CF (_____) = _____ $L\cdot min^{-1}$
     VO₂max   Table 14.6

Relative $\dot{V}O_2$max = $\dot{V}O_2$max * 1000 / BW (kg) = _____ $ml\cdot kg^{-1}\cdot min^{-1}$

Fitness category *(from Table 14.7)* _____

Evaluation / comments: _____

_____

_____

Gender: _____ Initials: _____ Age (y): _____ Height (cm): _____ Weight (kg): _____

Seat height: _____ Desired pedaling rate: _____ rpm Maintained rate: ☐ always ☐ usually

Target HR zone *(from Table 14.3)*: _____ bpm Initial power *(from Table 14.3)*: _____ W

HR at: Min 1 _____ bpm Min 2 _____ bpm Min 3 _____ bpm

After 3 min: ☐ raise power ☐ no change ☐ lower power Power level for Min 4: _____ W

HR at: Min 4 _____ bpm Min 5 _____ bpm Min 6 _____ bpm Submax HR _____ bpm

After 6 min: HR difference between Min 5 and Min 6: ☐ 0-10 bpm (end test) ☐ >10 bpm (continue test)

HR at: Min 7 _____ bpm Min 8 _____ bpm *(Only if necessary)* Submax HR _____ bpm

Estimated $\dot{V}O_2$max *(from Table 14.5)* = _____ $L\cdot min^{-1}$

Age-adjusted $\dot{V}O_2$max = _____ * CF (_____) = _____ $L\cdot min^{-1}$
     VO₂max   Table 14.6

Relative $\dot{V}O_2$max = $\dot{V}O_2$max * 1000 / BW (kg) = _____ $ml\cdot kg^{-1}\cdot min^{-1}$

Fitness category *(from Table 14.7)* _____

Evaluation / comments: _____

_____

_____

Form 14.3

NAME _____ DATE _____ SCORE _____

AEROBIC CYCLING (ALTERNATIVE TESTS)

Home Work

Gender: **M**   Initials: **AA**   Age (y): **20**   HR max (bpm): _____   Weight (kg): **70.0**

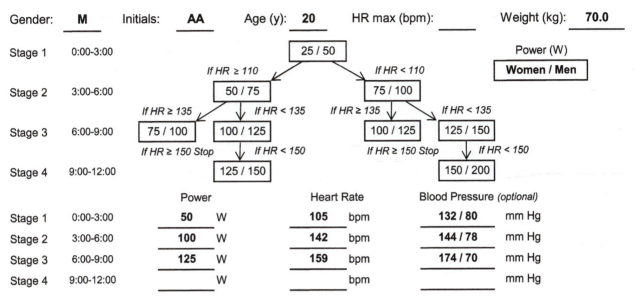

		Power		Heart Rate		Blood Pressure (optional)	
Stage 1	0:00-3:00	**50**	W	**105**	bpm	**132 / 80**	mm Hg
Stage 2	3:00-6:00	**100**	W	**142**	bpm	**144 / 78**	mm Hg
Stage 3	6:00-9:00	**125**	W	**159**	bpm	**174 / 70**	mm Hg
Stage 4	9:00-12:00		W		bpm		mm Hg

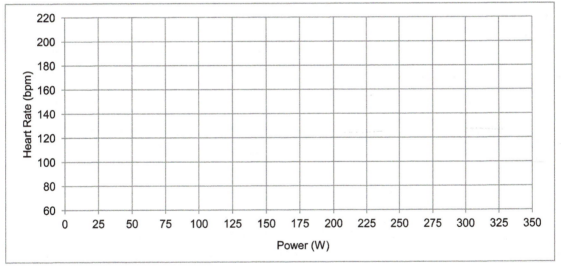

Pmax (W) = _____ $\dot{V}O_2$max (ml·kg^{-1}·min^{-1}) = [10.8 * Pmax / Body wt (kg)] + 7] = _____

Fitness category (from Table 14.7) _____

Evaluation / comments: _____

_____

Maximal Test   Gender: **M**   Pmax (W): **175**   BW (kg): **70.0**   Age (y): **20**

$\dot{V}O_2$max = _____ + (_____ * _____) + (_____ * _____) - (_____ * _____) = _____ ml·min^{-1}

                                     Pmax (W)   BW (kg)   Age (y)

$\dot{V}O_2$max = _____ ml·min^{-1} / _____ kg = _____ ml·kg^{-1}·min^{-1}

            $\dot{V}O_2$max   BW

Form 14.4

NAME _____ DATE _____ SCORE _____

AEROBIC CYCLING (ALTERNATIVE TESTS)

Lab Results

Gender: _____ Initials: _____ Age (y): _____ HR max (bpm): _____ Weight (kg): _____

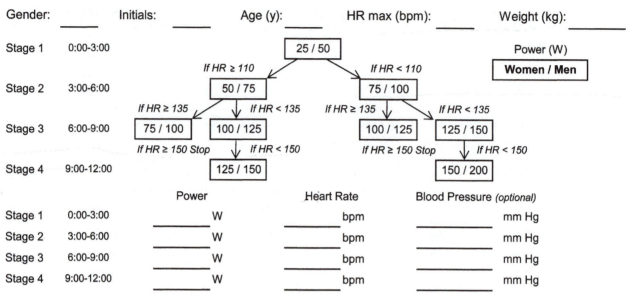

Stage 1   0:00-3:00   25 / 50   Power (W)

If HR ≥ 110   If HR < 110   Women / Men

Stage 2   3:00-6:00   50 / 75   75 / 100

If HR ≥ 135   If HR < 135   If HR ≥ 135   If HR < 135

Stage 3   6:00-9:00   75 / 100   100 / 125   100 / 125   125 / 150

If HR ≥ 150 Stop   If HR < 150   If HR ≥ 150 Stop   If HR < 150

Stage 4   9:00-12:00   125 / 150   150 / 200

		Power	Heart Rate	Blood Pressure *(optional)*
Stage 1	0:00-3:00	_____ W	_____ bpm	_____ mm Hg
Stage 2	3:00-6:00	_____ W	_____ bpm	_____ mm Hg
Stage 3	6:00-9:00	_____ W	_____ bpm	_____ mm Hg
Stage 4	9:00-12:00	_____ W	_____ bpm	_____ mm Hg

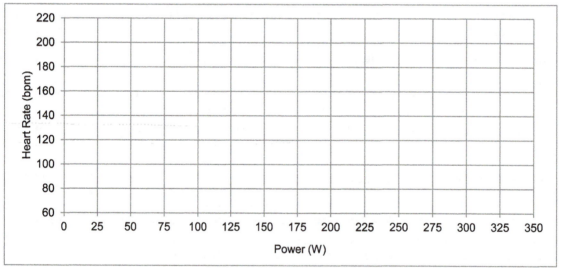

Pmax (W) = _____ $\dot{V}O_2$max (ml·kg^{-1}·min^{-1}) = [10.8 * Pmax / Body wt (kg)] + 7] = _____

Fitness category *(from Table 14.7)* _____

Evaluation / comments: _____

_____

_____

Maximal Test   Gender: _____   Pmax (W): _____   BW (kg): _____   Age (y): _____

$\dot{V}O_2$max = _____ + (_____ * _____) + (_____ * _____) - (_____ * _____) = _____ ml·min^{-1}

Pmax (W)   BW (kg)   Age (y)

$\dot{V}O_2$max = _____ ml·min^{-1} / _____ kg = _____ ml·kg^{-1}·min^{-1}

$\dot{V}O_2$max   BW

MAXIMAL OXYGEN CONSUMPTION

A test of aerobic fitness that truly qualifies as a laboratory test is the Maximal Oxygen Consumption ($\dot{V}O_2$max) Test. Although this test may involve a substantial anaerobic contribution to metabolism at the terminal portion of the test, it is primarily an aerobic test.

Whereas the run/jog/walk, step tests, and cycle tests attempt to estimate aerobic power as accurately as possible, the $\dot{V}O_2$max Test *measures* aerobic power. The run/jog/walk tests, for example, predict maximal oxygen consumption based on the relationship between maximal oxygen consumption and time or distance of running or walking; some run/jog/walk tests combine running or walking performance with heart rate. The step tests and cycle tests estimate the maximal oxygen consumption based on the relationship among heart rate, oxygen consumption, and power level. Because the $\dot{V}O_2$max Test directly measures oxygen consumption, it requires more expensive and sophisticated equipment than that required by field tests.

In this chapter, the direct measurement of oxygen consumption is described for submaximal and maximal exercise. Special importance is given to the latter stages of the exercise protocol, because that is when the *maximal* oxygen consumption typically occurs.

PURPOSE OF THE MAXIMAL OXYGEN CONSUMPTION TEST

The purpose of the Maximal Oxygen Consumption Test is to measure aerobic fitness. Aerobic fitness is synonymous with several other terms, such as aerobic power, cardiovascular fitness, cardiovascular endurance, circulorespiratory endurance, and cardiorespiratory endurance. Cardiovascular fitness, as characterized by $\dot{V}O_2$max, is inversely related to coronary heart disease and all-cause mortality.[6,28]

The Maximal Oxygen Consumption Test has received more recognition than any other exercise physiology laboratory test. Testimony to this is the fact that the purpose of many field tests is to predict maximal oxygen consumption—the variable that often has been used synonymously with aerobic fitness.[44,54,64] Traditionally, no other single laboratory test has been used as frequently to indicate a person's aptitude for success in events calling upon maximal efforts longer than 2 min. In addition, combined with some anaerobic tests, it helps indicate success for events lasting 1–3 min. In conjunction with measures of efficiency (economy), ventilatory threshold/breakpoint,

glycogen storage, acclimatization, and fractional utilization of maximal oxygen consumption, the $\dot{V}O_2$max Test is also an important indicator of success for all-out events lasting between 20 min and 4 h.[53]

Also, the Maximal Oxygen Consumption Test provides insight into the cardiorespiratory system. For example, the clinical severity of disease decreases with an increase in functional aerobic fitness.[11] Thus, the Maximal Oxygen Consumption Test has been used to assess not only aerobic fitness, but also the abilities of the cardiovascular and respiratory systems to transport and supply oxygen.

PHYSIOLOGICAL RATIONALE

The ability to consume oxygen is important for the metabolic function of body cells. Cellular activity is dependent upon oxygen because the cell derives its energy from adenosine triphosphate (ATP). Aerobic metabolism produces large volumes of ATP via the oxidative pathway. This pathway reflects the ability of the muscles' mitochondria to synthesize ATP.

The maximal consumption of oxygen depends not only upon the cells' ability to extract and use oxygen but also upon the ability of the cardiovascular and respiratory systems to transport this oxygen to the cells. Cardiovascularly, the transport of oxygen is represented by the cardiac output, the amount of blood pumped by the left ventricle per minute. Thus, a greater maximal cardiac output leads to a greater maximal oxygen consumption under normal conditions. The respiratory system's transport of oxygen is represented by ventilation, which is measured as liters of air per minute. A greater ventilation capacity is usually associated with a greater maximal oxygen consumption. It now appears that respiratory muscle work during heavy maximal exercise affects exercise performance by decreasing leg blood flow.[31]

The term **maximal oxygen consumption** is usually used to denote the *single highest oxygen consumption* elicited during graded exercise to exhaustion. Because oxygen consumption depends on the amount of muscle mass involved, exercise test modes like the treadmill and cross-country ski ergometer that use more muscle mass yield higher values than a cycle ergometer or step test. Specifically, when $\dot{V}O_2$ is measured in most people on the treadmill versus the cycle ergometer, the value is 5–10 % higher on a treadmill.[42] So, if one participant completes several exercise tests using different modes, the test that yields the highest $\dot{V}O_2$ value would be used as the true maximal oxygen consumption ($\dot{V}O_2$max). Another term often used is **peak oxygen consumption,** which is measured during a *specific test,* but it may not truly be the highest or maximal oxygen consumption possible. There are generally two different conditions where the term peak oxygen consumption ($\dot{V}O_2$peak) is used. The first is as described above, where exercise tests using different modes elicit different oxygen consumption values. The highest recorded value (recorded on the treadmill, for example) would be considered the *maximal* oxygen consumption, whereas any lower values (recorded on a cycle ergometer or step test, for example) would be considered *peak* oxygen consumptions. The second condition is where symptoms or a lack of motivation limit the participant's ability to reach a true physiological maximum. Participants may voluntarily stop during an exercise test due to leg pain, chest pain, dyspnea (a feeling of being unable to breathe enough air), or other symptoms prior to reaching a maximal effort. Or a participant simply may not be motivated sufficiently during the test, resulting in a less than maximal effort. Thus, *maximal oxygen consumption* is the term used for the highest possible value attained during a maximal-effort graded exercise test using a large muscle mass, and *peak oxygen consumption* can be used to describe any value attained during one particular test that may be lower than maximal oxygen consumption due to the mode of exercise, physical symptoms, or a lack of motivation. For simplicity, maximal oxygen consumption ($\dot{V}O_2$max) is used almost exclusively throughout this laboratory manual. It should be understood, however, that every graded exercise test does not necessarily yield a true maximal oxygen consumption, but it will always result in a peak oxygen consumption.

METHODS

The methods and procedures for the administration of oxygen consumption (metabolic) testing may seem complicated, especially for first-year exercise physiology students. However, it is certainly possible for novices to gain an appreciation and understanding of maximal oxygen consumption testing simply by observing the participant and by monitoring the instruments during the exercise test. The methods include a description of the equipment, the exercise protocol, the procedures, and the calculations. A description of the accuracy of the $\dot{V}O_2$max Test is in Box 15.1.

Equipment

Until the 1970s, the equipment used for measuring oxygen consumption consisted of several instruments purchased from separate manufacturers. The investigator then would interface the individual instruments so that online testing could be accomplished, or the investigator would collect

---

BOX 15.1 | Accuracy of the $\dot{V}O_2$max Test

The accuracy of the Maximal Oxygen Consumption Test is maximized by achieving the traditional criteria of the max test, such as (1) the plateau of the oxygen consumption despite an increase of power level, (2) the attainment of respiratory exchange ratios > 1.10, (3) the attainment of maximal heart rate, (4) high blood lactates, and (5) the exhaustion of the participant.

Reliability

The test-retest reliability of maximal oxygen consumption tests is high—about 0.95[46,64] to 0.99.[11] The intraclass correlation coefficient is 0.93 and the day-to-day variability is < 5 % or $\approx$ 2 ml·kg^{-1}·min^{-1}.[50] The standard error of estimate (*SEE*) of the $\dot{V}O_2$max Test may range from a low of about 2.5 %[64] to a high of about 5–6 %[37] of the mean score for an average person; it may extend up to about 8 % in aerobically trained males.[15] Thus, an individual would be expected to vary by about 2 to 4 ml·kg^{-1}·min^{-1}, even when tested weeks apart.[11,42,64] For example, if a person's maximal oxygen consumption is truly 40 ml·kg^{-1}·min^{-1}, then repeated tests with an *SEE* of 5 % would be expected to vary between 38.0 and 42.0 ml·kg^{-1}·min^{-1}. The $\dot{V}O_2$max is highly consistent even over four months, having an average coefficient of variation of about 4.3 %.[68]

Validity

The validity of any exercise test is partly dependent upon the exercise modality and the specific fitness of the participant. Although not supported by all physiologists,[19,46] most investigators and reviewers[2,44,54,64] have supported the maximal oxygen consumption value as the best single physiological indicator of a person's capacity for endurance activities dependent upon the cardiorespiratory system. High maximal oxygen consumptions, when expressed relative to body mass (ml·kg^{-1}·min^{-1}), are associated with successful running performance in events lasting more than a couple minutes. For example, correlations of 0.90 and 0.91 have been reported between $\dot{V}O_2$max and 12 min distance.[17,27] However, a lower correlation of −0.74 was reported between $\dot{V}O_2$max and 1.5 mile time.[40]

---

the exhaled air in special bags for post-test analysis of oxygen and carbon dioxide concentrations and ventilation volumes. Today a variety of manufacturers combine the individual components into a single package. These interfaced consoles include a computer to make all the calculations for deriving the metabolic and respiratory values (Ametec™; Consentius Technologies). Improved and consolidated instrumentation has led to portable and breath-by-breath capabilities in measuring oxygen consumption (Cosmed™; Sensor Medics).

Ergometers

It is best to use the type of ergometer that simulates the type of movement for which the participant has been training. For example, runners should be tested on treadmills, cyclists on cycle ergometers, rowers on rowing ergometers, wheelchair athletes on wheelchair or arm ergometers, cross-country skiers on ski ergometers, and swimmers in swim flumes, on swim benches, or in a pool while tethered to weighted pulleys. Another consideration is the norms by which the participant will be evaluated. The Maximal Oxygen Consumption Test should be performed on the same ergometer as that which was used by those performers whose scores generated the norms. A practical consideration is the cost and ancillary objectives of

the test. For example, a step bench is inexpensive but is not a specific mode for a swimmer. A cycle ergometer facilitates the measurement of blood pressure by clinicians but is not specific for walkers and joggers.

The treadmill has two basic units of measure: (1) speed and (2) slope or grade (Table 15.1). Maximal speeds (mph or km·h^{-1}) may vary with different treadmills from 12 mph (19.3 km·h^{-1}) to 15 mph (24 km·h^{-1}) to 25 mph (40.2 km·h^{-1}). The maximal slopes or grades of laboratory treadmills are about 25 %, but some can reach 40 % grade ($\approx$ 22°). Table 15.1 provides the equivalent speeds in the American and metric systems, along with the slopes in degrees and percent grade.

Table 15.1 Conversion Between Units for Treadmill Speed and Grade

Speed (Based on 1 mph = 1.609 km·h^{-1} = 26.8 m·min^{-1})

mph	km·h^{-1}	m·min^{-1}	mph	km·h^{-1}	m·min^{-1}
1.7	2.7	46	5.5	8.8	147
2.0	3.2	54	6.0	9.7	161
2.5	4.0	67	6.5	10.5	174
3.0	4.8	80	7.0	11.3	188
3.5	5.6	94	7.5	12.1	201
4.0	6.4	107	8.0	12.9	214
4.5	7.2	121	8.5	13.7	228
5.0	8.0	134	9.0	14.5	241

Grade or Slope (Based on slope = tangent of angle × 100)

%	degrees	%	degrees
1%	0.6°	9%	5.1°
2%	1.2°	10%	5.7°
3%	1.8°	11%	6.3°
4%	2.3°	12%	6.8°
5%	2.9°	13%	7.4°
6%	3.4°	14%	8.0°
7%	4.0°	15%	8.5°
8%	4.6°	16%	9.1°

Metabolic Measurement Equipment

Three variables—pulmonary ventilation ($\dot{V}_E$) and the fractions of exhaled oxygen (F_EO_2) and carbon dioxide (F_ECO_2)—need to be continuously measured throughout the test in order to determine oxygen consumption and a variety of related metabolic variables (e.g., CO_2 production, respiratory exchange ratio). The measurement of pulmonary ventilation requires an **air volume meter,** which can either be part of an automated system (e.g., pneumotachometer, turbine) or a nonautomated piece of equipment (e.g., dry gas meter, tissot spirometer). Figure 15.1 demonstrates the components of a typical metabolic measurement system. Ventilation is most often measured during exhalation and is designated as exhaled ventilation ($\dot{V}_E$). In some cases, usually when using a dry gas meter, it can also be measured during inhalation and is then referred to as inhaled ventilation ($\dot{V}_I$). The recorded unit of measure for pulmonary ventilation is liters per minute (L·min^{-1}).

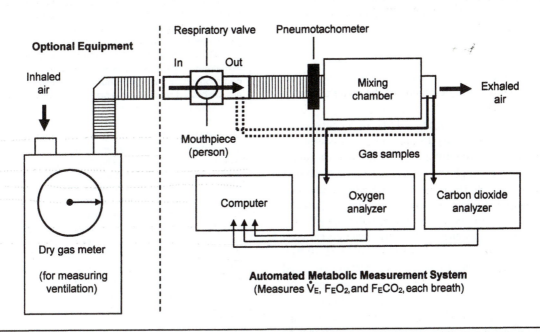

Figure 15.1 Schematic of the components of an automated (computerized) metabolic measurement system for measuring ventilation ($\dot{V}_E$) and the fractions of exhaled O_2 (F_EO_2) and CO_2 (F_ECO_2). In some cases, gas samples are drawn from the respiratory valve (instead of the mixing chamber) and $\dot{V}_E$ is measured with a turbine or spirometer (usually if non-automated). Optionally, a dry gas meter can be used to measure inhaled (or exhaled) ventilation.

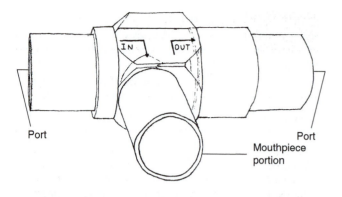

Figure 15.2 A two-way, non-rebreathing respiratory valve prevents air from exiting the same port that it entered.

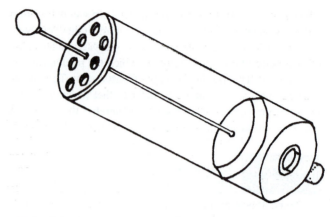

Figure 15.3 A 3 L syringe helps calibrate the ventilation volume measured by an air volume meter.

To collect and sample the exhaled air, several auxiliary pieces of equipment are necessary. A **respiratory valve** (Figure 15.2) is a two-way valve that allows inhaled air to enter through one port (inlet port), but then directs all of the exhaled air through the opposite port (outlet port), where it enters a **breathing tube** or **ventilatory hose.** This particular tube or hose is flexible yet is corrugated or contains metal wire so that it does not collapse. The respiratory valve can be outfitted with a **saliva trap** that prevents saliva from entering the breathing tube. Typically, support is provided for the respiratory valve through the use of special headgear, or it can be supported from above (from an overhead rail or from the ceiling). A **rubber mouthpiece** similar to a scuba mouthpiece attaches to the respiratory valve. The flanges of the mouthpiece prevent the leakage of air around the participant's mouth, while the protruding tabs allow gripping the mouthpiece with the teeth. A **noseclip** is worn to prevent inhalation and exhalation of air through the nose. Before the test, the air volume meter is calibrated with a special **calibration syringe** (Figure 15.3). The calibration syringe is specially designed and manufactured to provide an exact volume of air per stroke (e.g., 1 liter, 3 liters) and is used in the calibration of the metabolic measurement system (Box 15.2).

In addition to measuring the volume of air inhaled or exhaled, it is also necessary to measure the fractions of exhaled O_2 and CO_2, requiring an oxygen analyzer and a carbon dioxide analyzer. Many electronic **oxygen analyzers** are available, most of which use paramagnetic or galvanic fuel cell principles to determine the fractional (or percentage) concentration of oxygen in the exhaled air (F_EO_2). These analyzers are designed to be most accurate between oxygen concentrations of 15 % (0.15) and 21 % (0.21), which roughly corresponds to the values expected in exhaled air. Most **carbon dioxide analyzers** use an infrared principle to determine the fractional (or percentage) concentration of carbon dioxide (F_ECO_2). The reference standard for gas concentrations is the mass spectrometer, which can be used to analyze various gases. It is not frequently used in exercise physiology laboratories, however, because of its expense. A cylinder of **calibration gas** is used to regularly

---

BOX 15.2 | **Calibration of Metabolic Instruments**

Regular calibration of the metabolic instruments is essential for maintaining the reliability and validity of the $\dot{V}O_2$max Test. It is best to follow the specific calibration instructions provided by the manufacturer of the equipment. However, some general calibration guidelines can be recommended. The instruments should be powered up and allowed to warm up for at least 30 min (or longer) prior to beginning any calibration. The equipment used for measuring meteorological conditions (i.e., thermometer, barometer, and hygrometer) should also be periodically calibrated.

Calibration procedures typically call for the calibration of three instruments, the air volume meter, the oxygen analyzer, and the carbon dioxide analyzer. It is assumed in this manual that a metabolic measurement system (or metabolic cart) is being used, so the calibration procedures in this case apply to the system as a whole. However, laboratories without an automated system will need to calibrate each component individually.

The instrument for measuring air volume (pulmonary ventilation) differs from system to system, but the most common is the pneumotachometer or turbine. These devices are calibrated by passing a specific volume of air through them with the use of a calibration syringe (Figure 15.3). This syringe is carefully manufactured so that one stroke delivers an exact volume of air (i.e., 1, 3, or 5 liters). Calibration of the air volume meter typically need not be done prior to every test but should be done daily or at least weekly.

Calibration of the gas analyzers requires a standardized calibration gas with known concentrations of O_2 and CO_2 determined by mass spectrometry (the "gold standard"). These calibration gases typically come with the metabolic measurement system or are available from a commercial gas vendor. It is typical to calibrate both analyzers against these standard gases prior to each exercise test. A two-point calibration (zero or low range and high range) is most common, but some authorities recommend a three-point calibration (zero, midrange, and high range).[36]

---

check the calibration of the gas analyzers. A typical calibration gas might consist of 16 % oxygen and 4 % carbon dioxide to simulate the values observed in exhaled air. The gas sample used for analysis during the exercise test can be drawn directly from the respiratory valve, or it can be drawn from a **mixing chamber** (Figure 15.1). The mixing chamber, typically a Plexiglas™ cylinder or box with internal baffles, promotes mixing of the exhaled air such that a uniformly mixed sample of exhaled air can be drawn for analysis of F_EO_2 and F_ECO_2. Most automated systems draw the gas sample continuously from the exhaled air and then filter, dry, and warm it to account for the water vapor in the sample. The values of F_EO_2 and F_ECO_2 are then determined automatically and sent to the computer, where the metabolic variables are calculated and displayed at the desired time intervals (e.g., 15 s, 30 s, 1 min). When nonautomated systems are used, gas samples can be collected in small rubber bags (*aliquots*) or can be drawn from large collection bags (e.g., Douglas bag, meteorological balloon) for analysis.

Exercise Protocol

The Maximal Oxygen Consumption Test usually requires the participant to exercise to exhaustion, although it need not be quite so stressful as long as the other traditional criteria are met. The exercise may be performed on various modalities, such as (a) step bench, (b) cycle ergometer, (c) treadmill, (d) swim flume, (e) wheelchair ergometer, (f) rowing ergometer, (g) skiing ergometer, and others. The test protocol, which consists of the prescription for time spent at each power level, is often a continuous and progressive type that eventually exceeds the aerobic power of the exerciser. Thus, the test includes submaximal, maximal, and supramaximal exercise relative to $\dot{V}O_2$max. The supramaximal portion contributes highly to the participant's exhaustion.

Several protocols may be used to elicit peak or maximal oxygen consumption.[2] Some of these are described in Chapter 19 on the ECG Test, while two protocols are presented, one for the cycle ergometer and one for the treadmill, in this chapter.

Although it is possible to reach nearly the maximal oxygen consumption level in 1 min when performing an all-out 90 s cycling task,[59] the test (excluding warm-up) is seldom less than 5 min and often no longer than 9 min. Occasionally, it is as long as 20 min for aerobically fit individuals starting at low stages, or if a longer time for monitoring the electrocardiogram is desired, or if mechanical efficiency is being measured simultaneously. Some investigators recommend a continuous protocol that brings participants to their limit of tolerance in about 10 min ± 2 min.[13]

Cycling Protocols

Before the test, the estimated $\dot{V}O_2$max of the participant from previous field tests helps in determining the proper protocol. If no prior tests exist, then questioning the participant about training habits is helpful.

The cycle protocols presented in Table 15.2 are modifications of a former continuous protocol[39] and are based

Table 15.2	Cycle Ergometer Protocols for Measuring $\dot{V}O_2$max		
	Below average fitness	Average fitness	Above average fitness
Warm-up 0:00–5:00	25 W	75 W	150 W
Exercise			
0:00–2:00	50 W	100 W	175 W
2:00–4:00	75 W	125 W	200 W
4:00–6:00	100 W	150 W	225 W
6:00–8:00	125 W	175 W	250 W
8:00–10:00	150 W	200 W	275 W
10:00–12:00	175 W	225 W	300 W
12:00–14:00	200 W	250 W	325 W
Recovery 0:00–3:00	50–75 W	50–75 W	125–200 W

Table 15.3	Estimation of Relative Oxygen Consumption (ml·kg⁻¹·min⁻¹) from Cycle Power (W)					
Cycle Power	$\dot{V}O_2$ (ml·kg⁻¹·min⁻¹) Body Weight (kg)					
	50	60	70	80	90	100
50 W	18	16	15	14	13	12
75 W	23	21	19	17	16	15
100 W	29	25	22	21	19	18
125 W	34	30	26	24	22	21
150 W	39	34	30	27	25	23
175 W	45	39	34	31	28	26
200 W	50	43	38	34	31	29
225 W	56	48	42	37	34	31
250 W	61	52	46	41	37	34
275 W	66	57	49	44	40	37
300 W	72	61	53	48	43	39

Note: Estimated $\dot{V}O_2$ (ml·kg⁻¹·min⁻¹) is based on equation from American College of Sports Medicine (2000)[2] as follows: $\dot{V}O_2 = [(10.8*Power (W)) / Body weight (kg) + 7]$.

on the aerobic fitness status of the participant. They are for persons who are estimated to have below average, average, or above average aerobic fitness. For persons with below average fitness, the initial power level is 50 W and increases by 25 W for subsequent 2 min power intervals. A similar protocol is followed for persons with average levels of aerobic fitness, except that the initial power level is 100 W. For persons with suspected $\dot{V}O_2$max levels that are exceptionally high, the starting power level can be 175 W in order to keep the duration of the test close to a 9 min maximum. For some elite cyclists who could reach 450 W, the test duration would be 30 min if they started at 175 W; so an even higher starting power or a larger increase in power per stage may be appropriate. Oxygen consumption can be estimated for cycling as seen in Table 15.3. Although economy or efficiency of cycling may vary with pedal rpm during submaximal exercise,[16,29,48,49,58,63] it does not mean that rpm will necessarily alter the peak or maximal oxygen consumption.[51]

Treadmill Protocol

It appears that similar results are obtained with a variety of treadmill protocols, although some take less time than others.[25] One of the most popular treadmill tests is the Bruce Test, the earliest standard treadmill test.[42] Although it is often used for cardiovascular screening purposes,[12] it is also a common protocol for predicting[1,5,38] and directly measuring maximal oxygen consumption.[46]

The Bruce protocol (Table 15.4) consists of seven 3 min stages. Most participants should walk during the initial three stages in the first 9 min.[9] Although the initial stages are important for cardiovascular screening (e.g., ECG monitoring), they are sometimes deleted when the primary purpose is to measure maximal oxygen consumption; in these cases, the initial stage for $\dot{V}O_2$max testing is dependent upon the fitness level of the participant. Table 15.4 also lists the approximate oxygen costs for each completed stage of the Bruce protocol.[2] The oxygen cost of treadmill running is reduced if the participant relies on the handrails.[10] Therefore, tables and equations relating $\dot{V}O_2$ to exercise stages are not valid when the participant uses the handrails. While on the treadmill, the participant should look straight ahead to prevent possible nausea from viewing the moving belt. Both the speed and grade of the treadmill should be calibrated annually. Instructions for treadmill calibration are usually in the manufacturer's instruction manual or other sources.[39]

Criteria for Establishing Maximal Oxygen Consumption

Part of the protocol of the Maximal Oxygen Consumption Test is to establish whether the participant reached a maximal level of exertion. A number of criteria have been described that indicate a maximal test, including those of a *physiological* nature that are measured during or after the test and those of a *psychological* nature involving exertion and motivation.

It has been recommended that for the test to be considered maximal it should result in one or more of the following physiological observations: (1) a plateau in oxygen -consumption with increasing workload,[4,33,34,52,53,64] (2) a respiratory exchange ratio (RER) greater than 1.05–1.15,[2,3,22,34,41,53,55] (3) a blood lactate greater than 8–10 mM·L^{-1},[2,23,41,53] and/or (4) a heart rate within 10–12 beats of age-predicted maximal heart rate (HRmax = 220 – age).[24,43,53,67] The observation of a plateau in oxygen consumption (i.e., a $\dot{V}O_2$ below that predicted from the linear relationship observed at lower intensities) with an increase in workload is not without controversy. The concept has "historical roots" in the writings of Hill[33] and Taylor[64] and Åstrand[4] over the last 35–80 years. Oxygen consumption "traditionally" was described to increase linearly to a point where it would increase no further (i.e., plateau) despite a further increase in running speed or workload. The original criterion for the plateau, which is still frequently cited,[34,52,53] compared the results of two repeated tests both run at 7 mph, but with the second test run at a grade 2.5 % higher than the first. If the two oxygen consumptions differed by less than 150 ml·min^{-1} or 2.1 ml·kg^{-1}·min^{-1}, the test conditions were considered to yield a maximal oxygen consumption. If a larger difference was observed, the test was repeated one or more times with another 2.5 % increase in grade until the difference was less than the criterion.[64] This specific criterion, however, by itself has limited practical value. An alternative approach is to define the plateau as an increase in $\dot{V}O_2$ of less than half of the *expected* increase estimated from the treadmill running speed and grade[52] or cycle power. The major problem with applying any "plateau criterion" at all is that it is frequently *not observed* over the course of a graded exercise test to exhaustion. Studies have observed a plateau in $\dot{V}O_2$ in only 17 % (12 of 71 tests) of adult men,[21] 33 % (8 of 24 tests) of children,[56,57] and in general no more than about 50–60 % of graded exercise tests.[21,23,37,62] In fact, there are researchers who report a nonlinear *increase* in $\dot{V}O_2$ (i.e., the opposite of a plateau) during graded exercise at high power levels,[30,69,70] possibly due to increased lactate and hydrogen ion concentration, increased muscle temperature, and/or recruitment of less efficient fast-twitch muscle fibers.[69] In summary, the *presence* of a plateau (however defined) in $\dot{V}O_2$ at the end of a graded exercise test to exhaustion provides support for the test being maximal. However, the *absence* of a plateau does not necessarily discount the $\dot{V}O_2$ as maximal.

Several other "secondary" physiological criteria may be applied in the presence or absence of a plateau in oxygen consumption. The first is a *respiratory exchange ratio* (RER) in excess of 1.05,[22] 1.10,[34,41] or 1.15.[2,3,53,55] A high RER ($\geq$ 1.00) indicates an increase in carbon dioxide production proportionally greater than the related increase in

Table 15.4	Bruce Treadmill Protocol with Estimated $\dot{V}O_2$ (ml·kg^{-1}·min^{-1}) Based on Speed and Grade			

Modified Bruce	Stage	Speed (mph)	Grade (%)	Est'd $\dot{V}O_2$
0:00–3:00	0	1.7	0	8.1
3:00–6:00	0	1.7	5	12.2

Standard Bruce	Stage	(mph)	Grade (%)	Est'd $\dot{V}O_2$
0:00–3:00	1	1.7	10	16.3
3:00–6:00	2	2.5	12	24.7
6:00–9:00	3	3.4	14	35.6
9:00–12:00	4	4.2	16	47.2
12:00–15:00	5	5.0	18	52.0
15:00–18:00	6	5.5	20	59.5
18:00–21:00	7	6.0	22	67.5

Recovery		(mph)	Grade (%)	Est'd $\dot{V}O_2$
0:00–3:00		2.5	0	9.7

Note: Estimated $\dot{V}O_2$ (ml·kg^{-1}·min^{-1}) is based on equations from American College of Sports Medicine (2000)[2] as follows: $\dot{V}O_2$ = [(0.1* Speed(m·min^{-1})) + (1.8 * Speed * Grade (%) / 100) + 3.5] for walking; and $\dot{V}O_2$ = [(0.2 * Speed (m·min^{-1})) + (0.9 * Speed * Grade (%) / 100) + 3.5] for running (5 mph and over).

oxygen consumption. The accelerated CO_2 production is a result of the buffering of hydrogen ions produced near the end of a graded exercise test. At this point, aerobic metabolism nears its maximal rate and anaerobic energy production becomes necessary to maintain the very high intensity over the last several minutes of the test. In general, the higher the RER the more likely the effort was maximal, so it may be appropriate to use the highest criterion (RER ≥ 1.15). Another criterion is a venous *blood lactate* concentration in excess of 8 $mM \cdot L^{-1}$ [2,23,53] or 10 $mM \cdot L^{-1}$.[41] These values are 8–10 times the typical blood lactate concentration at rest (1 $mM \cdot L^{-1}$). Blood lactates this high indicate the intense nature of the exercise and the heavy contribution required of the lactic acid system. Because of the need for blood sampling, however, this specific criterion is more difficult to assess. A final physiological variable to -consider is *heart rate*. Although there is considerable variability in maximal heart rate, as indicated by a standard deviation of 10–12 bpm, it is reliable and reproducible within individuals. If during an exercise test where $\dot{V}O_2$ is being directly measured, the participant reaches a *previously measured* maximal heart rate, it can be assumed that the $\dot{V}O_2$ reached will also be maximal. In cases where maximal heart rate has not been previously determined, a maximal heart rate predicted from age (220 – Age) may be used. In assessing whether a test is maximal it is preferred that exercise heart rate meet this predicted HRmax, but other sources consider an exercise heart rate within 12 bpm[24] or 10 bpm[43,53,67] of predicted HRmax as evidence of maximal effort.

With regard to the psychological criteria, the participant is typically instructed to give a maximal effort, to exercise to exhaustion, to run or cycle until he or she can go no longer. This requires a high degree of motivation. To help quantify and allow for a more objective assessment of exertion, the participant typically provides a rating of perceived exertion (RPE) throughout the graded exercise test. The RPE scale (Table 15.5) integrates a variety of signals from the body—cardiovascular, respiratory, muscular, and nervous systems—into a general whole sensation that allows the participant to provide a perception of the intensity of exertion. The original Borg 15-category RPE scale,[7] ranging from the lowest level of exertion, 6, to the highest level of exertion, 20, is based on the linear relationship between exertion, power output, and heart rate.[7] It was later revised with ratio properties based on the nonlinear properties of psychophysical and some physiologic variables, such as blood lactate and ventilation,[2] and was renamed the Borg 10-category ratio (CR-10) RPE scale.[8] This newer category-ratio scale (CR-10) may be more suitable for determining subjective symptoms associated with breathing, aches, and pains and is highly correlated with blood lactate.[8,62] The choice of which scale to use is up to the tester. An RPE > 17[2] or an RPE of 19 or 20[41] have been recommended as indicating a maximal effort.

Sources: From Borg (1970)[7] and Borg (1982).[8]

Table 15.5	Borg Rating of Perceived Exertion (RPE) Scale	
Original 15-Category Scale (6–20)	**Modified Category-Ratio (CR-10) Scale (0–10)**	
6	0	Nothing at all
7 Very, very light	0.5	Very, very weak (*just noticeable*)
8		
9 Very light	1	Very weak
10	2	Weak
11 Light	3	Moderate
12	4	Somewhat strong
13 Somewhat heavy	5	Strong
14	6	
15 Heavy	7	Very strong
16	8	
17 Very heavy	9	
18	10	Very, very strong
19 Very, very heavy		(*almost maximal*)
20	10+	Maximal

Procedures for the Maximal Oxygen Consumption Test

The initial steps for the $\dot{V}O_2$max Test consist of calibrating the ergometer and metabolic instruments, selecting an exercise mode and protocol, and preparing the participant for the exercise test.

Preparation

As with the other aerobic tests, the participant should be well rested and refrain from prior exercise the day of testing, should not eat a large meal within 2–3 hours of the test, and should be normally hydrated and refrain from consuming or taking any stimulants. The technician (tester) prepares for the test by completing the following steps.

1. Periodically calibrate the ergometer being used (e.g., treadmill, cycle ergometer).
2. Calibrate the metabolic measurement system (review Box 15.2) according to the manufacturer's specifications.
3. Measure and record the participant's basic data (name, age, height, and body weight) along with the meteorological data (temperature, barometric pressure, and relative humidity) on Form 15.2.
4. Establish the desired exercise mode and protocol to be used during the test. Orient the participant by explaining the purpose and protocol of the Maximal Oxygen Consumption Test.
5. If heart rate is to be determined by electrocardiography (ECG) or heart-rate monitor, prepare and attach the required equipment (e.g., ECG electrodes, heart-rate transmitter). Likewise, if blood pressure is to be recorded, prepare and attach all necessary equipment. (*Note:* Blood drawing equipment would also be prepared at this point if blood lactate measurement is desired.)

6. Instruct the participant on the proper use of the ergometer (e.g., how to mount and dismount the moving treadmill belt, how to maintain pedaling form and rate on the cycle ergometer). If using a treadmill, it is especially important to prevent injury by instructing the participant on how to grab the rails and dismount the treadmill at the point of exhaustion.

7. Instruct the participant on proper use of the rating of perceived exertion (RPE) scale.

8. Instruct the participant on hand signals that may be used during the test (e.g., a thumbs-up sign indicating the desire to continue) due to the inability to speak because of the mouthpiece and respiratory equipment.

9. Have the participant complete an appropriate warm-up before the test. Little warm-up is needed if the protocol begins at a low level to allow the collection of submaximal data. More warm-up is indicated if the protocol starts at a higher level with less emphasis on submaximal data collection.

Procedures During the Exercise Test

Typically more than one technician is involved during the test. If this is the case, each technician needs to know his or her specific duties and responsibilities and carry them out correctly during the test. The procedures for the $\dot{V}O_2max$ test are as follows:

1. Attach all necessary equipment (e.g., headgear for support of respiratory valve) and optional equipment (e.g., heart-rate monitor, ECG lead wires); insert the mouthpiece of the respiratory valve into the participant's mouth; attach the breathing tube to the "out" port of the valve; and affix the noseclip to the participant's nose (do not forget the noseclip).

2. Instruct the participant to begin exercising at the initial stage of the exercise test protocol.

3. Simultaneously start all equipment (e.g., metabolic measurement system, ECG, heart-rate monitor) and timers.

4. If an automated metabolic measurement system is being used (which is assumed), all metabolic data are measured, displayed, and recorded automatically for the duration of the test. If a semiautomated or manual system is being used (for instructional purposes), each technician records a specific variable (e.g., ventilation, F_EO_2, F_ECO_2, heart rate) at specific intervals (e.g., 15 s, 30 s, 1 min) throughout the test.

5. Follow the test protocol by increasing treadmill speed and/or grade or cycle ergometer power at the appropriate times (if not done automatically by the ergometer). Record any desired data (not recorded automatically) at specific intervals. It is typical to record heart rate each minute; RPE at 1, 2, or 3 min intervals; and if recording the ECG or blood pressure, they are typically recorded at 3 min intervals (but this can vary based on the protocol).

6. Monitor the participant for any signs or symptoms that could warrant stopping the test prematurely (e.g., chest pain, leg pain, ECG changes, blood pressure changes, dizziness, nausea).

7. Determine when the participant is approaching a maximal effort through the use of heart rate (approaching a *previously measured* HRmax or within 10 beats of age-predicted HRmax); respiratory exchange ratio (approaching an RER of 1.15 or above); rating of perceived exertion (approaching an RPE of 18 or above); and other observations (e.g., participant no longer gives thumbs-up sign, changes in treadmill gait, changes in cycling mechanics).

8. When signs of maximal effort begin to appear, encourage the participant to continue as long as possible without jeopardizing safety. If the test is being done on a treadmill, a spotter should be used to assist the participant to reduce the likelihood of injury.

9. When the participant voluntarily stops at what is assumed to be the point of exhaustion, safely end the test. As quickly as possible, begin a cool-down. It is important that the participant spend minimal time standing still on the treadmill belt or sitting still on the cycle ergometer, because of the possibility of blood pooling in the legs.

10. Remove all equipment. Discard any disposable equipment (e.g., electrodes), and clean and sanitize all reusable equipment (e.g., mouthpiece, noseclip, respiratory valve, breathing tube, heart-rate monitor, blood pressure cuff) according to accepted practices. Various forms of disinfection (e.g., Cidex™, iodine, bleach, etc.) may be considered.

Calculation of Oxygen Consumption and Related Variables

It is assumed in this manual that in most cases an automated system will be used to measure, record, and display oxygen consumption and a variety of related variables throughout the exercise test, as seen in Figure 15.4. However, an important concept in this chapter is how the raw data ($\dot{V}_E$, F_EO_2, and F_ECO_2) are used mathematically to derive the desired physiological results. For this reason, what follows is a detailed discussion of the necessary mathematical calculations.

Ventilation and Ambient/Standard Conditions

The first variable of interest in calculating oxygen consumption is the pulmonary ventilation or, simply, ventilation. Ventilation is typically measured on exhalation by collecting all of the air exhaled or expired by the participant. When ventilation is measured during exhalation it is referred to as exhaled ventilation or the total volume of air exhaled from the lungs per minute (abbreviated as $\dot{V}_E$). Ventilation may also be measured by measuring the inhaled

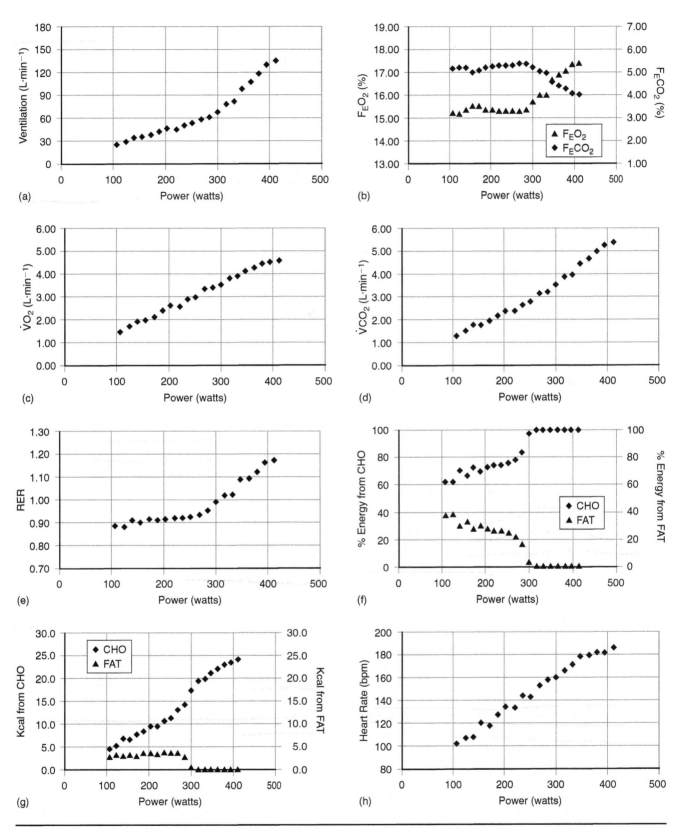

Figure 15.4 Sample data from graded exercise test showing: (*a*) ventilation, (*b*) F_EO_2 and F_ECO_2, (*c*) oxygen consumption, (*d*) CO_2 production, (*e*) respiratory exchange ratio, (*f*) % energy from carbohydrate and fat, (*g*) energy expenditure from carbohydrate and fat, and (*h*) heart rate.

ventilation or the total volume of air inspired into the lungs per minute ($\dot{V}_I$).

Ventilation ($\dot{V}_E$), like any other air volume or lung volume (e.g., vital capacity), is subject to the gas laws, meaning that it is affected by the ambient (surrounding) conditions. The two biggest factors that affect $\dot{V}_E$ are temperature and pressure (i.e., barometric pressure). Consider the effect that these two factors have on the volume (size) of a balloon. If a balloon is warmed, the movement of the air molecules inside the balloon increases and they exert more pressure on the walls of the balloon, causing it to increase in size (expand). If cooled, the molecular movement decreases, exerting less pressure and causing it to decrease in size (shrink). When the pressure surrounding the balloon changes, it inversely affects the volume. That is, a drop in surrounding (barometric) pressure allows the balloon to expand, while a rise in pressure squeezes the balloon, causing it to shrink.

Two specific sets of atmospheric conditions affecting ventilation and other air and lung volumes are referred to as **ambient conditions** and **standard conditions.** Ambient conditions are the surroundings under which air volumes are measured. The conditions apply to three variables: temperature, pressure, and saturation. For this reason, the abbreviation ATPS, for *ambient temperature, pressure, saturated,* is used for ambient conditions. Ambient (or room) temperature and barometric pressure vary and must be measured and recorded at the time of the exercise test to be used in the calculation of oxygen consumption. Air exhaled from the lungs is assumed to be fully saturated with water vapor; thus when V_E is measured under ATPS conditions, it is assumed to be saturated. Standard conditions refer to a universally designated set of conditions that have been determined to consist of a *standard temperature* of 0°C (or 273 K) and a *standard pressure* of 760 mm Hg (typical barometric pressure at sea level, also equal to 1013 hPa), with the air or gas assumed to be *dry;* hence, the abbreviation STPD, for *standard temperature, pressure, dry.*

Oxygen consumption is (nearly) always expressed under STPD conditions. This allows all $\dot{V}O_2$max values recorded under any ambient conditions, regardless of ambient temperature or barometric pressure, to be expressed in the same standard conditions, allowing for direct comparisons. An STPD correction factor (CF) can be calculated for a given set of ambient conditions, and then that STPD CF is used to correct $\dot{V}_E$ from ATPS to STPD conditions. The STPD CF is calculated taking into consideration ambient temperature, barometric pressure, the vapor pressure of water at ambient temperature (a lower temperature decreases the amount of water vapor pressure in the expired air), standard temperature (0°C or 273 K), and standard pressure (760 mm Hg or 1013 hPa). The vapor pressure of water (P_{H_2O}) varies with ambient temperature, as seen in Table 15.6. The STPD correction factor is calculated by using Equation 15.1. Note that 273 is added to each temperature (°C) to convert it into the Kelvin scale, which is necessary for the calculation.

Table 15.6	Water Vapor Pressure (P_{H_2O}) at 100 % Saturation at Given Temperatures				
Temperature		P_{H_2O}	Temperature		P_{H_2O}
°C	K	mm Hg	°C	K	mm Hg
20	293	18	26	299	25
21	294	19	27	300	27
22	295	20	28	301	28
23	296	21	29	302	30
24	297	22	30	303	32
25	298	24	37	310	47

$$\text{STPD CF} = \frac{[T_{STD} (°C) + 273 \text{ K}]}{[TA(°C) + 273 \text{ K}]}$$
$$* \frac{[P_B \text{ (mm Hg)} - P_{H_2O} \text{ at } T_A]}{[P_{STD}]}$$

Eq. 15.1

Where: T_{STD}: Standard temperature (0 °C)

Where: T_A: Ambient temperature (varies)

Where: P_B: Barometric pressure (varies)

Where: P_{H_2O} Vapor pressure of water at T_A (varies)

Where: P_{STD}: Standard pressure (760 mm Hg)

Example: If the ambient conditions are as follows: T_A = 24°C; P_B = 756 mm Hg; and P_{H_2O} = 22 mm Hg; then the STPD CF for correcting any volume from ambient conditions (ATPS) to standard conditions (STPD) would be 0.888, as seen in Equation 15.2a and Table 15.7. A pulmonary ventilation ($\dot{V}_{E \text{ ATPS}}$) of 100 L·min⁻¹ measured under ambient conditions (ATPS) is corrected to standard conditions (STPD) by multiplying by the STPD CF, with the result being $\dot{V}_{E \text{ STPD}}$ = **88.8** L·min⁻¹ (Eq. 15.2b).

$$\text{STPD CF} = \frac{[0°C + 273 \text{ K}]}{[\mathbf{24} °C + 273 \text{ K}]}$$
$$* \frac{[\mathbf{756} \text{ mm Hg} - \mathbf{22} \text{ mm Hg}]}{[760 \text{ mm Hg}]} = \mathbf{0.888}$$

Eq. 15.2a

$$\dot{V}_{E \text{ STPD}} \text{ (L·min}^{-1}) = \dot{V}_{E \text{ ATPS}} \text{ (L·min}^{-1}) * \text{STPD CF}$$
$$= \mathbf{100} * \mathbf{0.888} = \mathbf{88.8} \text{ L·min}^{-1}$$

Eq. 15.2b

Oxygen Consumption

Three specific variables—pulmonary ventilation expressed in STPD conditions ($\dot{V}_{E \text{ STPD}}$), and the fractions (or percentages) of exhaled or expired oxygen (F_EO_2) and carbon dioxide (F_ECO_2)—must be continuously measured and recorded throughout the exercise test for the purpose of calculating submaximal and maximal oxygen consumption and other related metabolic variables. Oxygen consumption, or the volume of oxygen being consumed by the body per minute ($\dot{V}O_2$), is literally the difference between the volume of oxygen being inhaled into the body ($\dot{V}_IO_2$) and the volume being exhaled from the body ($\dot{V}_EO_2$). This is

Table 15.7 Correction Factors for Reducing Volumes from Ambient to Standard Conditions

Barometric Pressure (mm Hg)	STPD Correction Factors Ambient Temperature (°C)								
	20	21	22	23	24	25	26	27	28
740	0.885	0.881	0.877	0.873	0.868	0.863	0.859	0.854	0.850
742	0.888	0.883	0.879	0.875	0.871	0.865	0.861	0.856	0.852
744	0.890	0.886	0.882	0.877	0.873	0.868	0.864	0.859	0.854
746	0.893	0.888	0.884	0.880	0.876	0.870	0.866	0.861	0.857
748	0.895	0.891	0.886	0.882	0.878	0.873	0.869	0.863	0.859
750	0.897	0.893	0.889	0.885	0.880	0.875	0.871	0.866	0.862
752	0.900	0.896	0.891	0.887	0.883	0.878	0.873	0.868	0.864
754	0.902	0.898	0.894	0.890	0.885	0.880	0.876	0.870	0.866
756	0.905	0.900	0.896	0.892	0.888	0.882	0.878	0.873	0.869
758	0.907	0.903	0.899	0.894	0.890	0.885	0.881	0.875	0.871
760	0.910	0.905	0.901	0.897	0.893	0.887	0.883	0.878	0.874
762	0.912	0.908	0.904	0.899	0.895	0.890	0.885	0.880	0.876
764	0.915	0.910	0.906	0.902	0.897	0.892	0.888	0.882	0.878

Note: STPD CF = [(273 K) / (T_A + 273 K) * [(P_B − P_{H_2O} at T_A) / (760 mm Hg)]; T_A = Ambient temperature; P_B = Barometric pressure; P_{H_2O} = Vapor pressure of water at ambient temperature.

the basis of the derivation of a mathematical equation to be used to calculate oxygen consumption beginning with Equations 15.3a and 15.3b. By knowing the fraction (or percentage) of a total volume that is made up by a particular gas (i.e., O_2, CO_2, or N_2), it is possible to determine the specific volumes of inspired and expired gasses. Given Equations 15.3c and 15.3d, substitution into Equation 15.3b yields Equation 15.3e.

Given: $\dot{V}O_2$ = Inspired] − [$\dot{V}O_2$ Expired]   Eq. 15.3a

Given: $\dot{V}O_2$ = [$\dot{V}_I O_2$] − [$\dot{V}_E O_2$]   Eq. 15.3b

   Where: $\dot{V}_I O_2$: Volume of inspired O_2

   Where: $\dot{V}_E O_2$: Volume of expired O_2

Given: $\dot{V}_I O_2 = \dot{V}_I * F_I O_2$ Eq. 15.3c

   Where: $\dot{V}_I$: Volume of inspired air

   Where: $F_I O_2$: Fraction of inspired O_2

Given: $\dot{V}_I O_2 = \dot{V}_E * F_E O_2$ Eq. 15.3d

   Where: $\dot{V}_E$: Volume of expired air

   Where: $F_E O_2$: Fraction of expired O_2

Substitution yields: $\dot{V}O_2 = [\dot{V}_I * F_I O_2]$
− [$\dot{V}_E * F_E O_2$]   Eq. 15.3e

The next step in the derivation of the desired mathematical equation is a brief comment on nitrogen and the relationship between the total volume of air inhaled into the lungs ($\dot{V}_I$) and that exhaled from the lungs ($\dot{V}_E$). It is commonly assumed that nitrogen (N_2) is neither consumed nor produced by humans. For this reason, it can also be assumed that the volume of nitrogen inhaled ($\dot{V}_I N_2$) is equal to the volume exhaled ($\dot{V}_E N_2$), as seen in Equation 15.4a. Based on the given values in Equations 15.4b and 15.4c, and again as

a product of substitution, the result is Equation 15.4d. Equation 15.4d can then be transposed to solve for $\dot{V}_I$ (Eq. 15.4e), which is important, because this allows the measurement of only exhaled or expired volumes ($\dot{V}_E$) and does not require the additional work of also measuring the inhaled or inspired volumes ($\dot{V}_I$).

Assume: $\dot{V}_I N_2 = \dot{V}_E N_2$ Eq. 15.4a

   Where: $\dot{V}_I N_2$: Volume of inspired N_2

   Where: $F_I N_2$: Fraction of inspired N_2

Given: $\dot{V}_I N_2 = \dot{V}_I * F_I N_2$ Eq. 15.4b

Given: $\dot{V}_I N_2 = \dot{V}_E * V_E N_2$ Eq. 15.4c

   Where: $\dot{V}_E N_2$: Volume of expired N_2

   Where: $F_E N_2$: Fraction of expired N_2

Substitution yields: $\dot{V}_I * F_I N_2 = \dot{V}_E * F_E N_2$ Eq. 15.4d

Transposition yields: $\dot{V}_I = (\dot{V}_E * F_E N_2) / F_I N_2$ Eq. 15.4e

The final steps involved in deriving the desired mathematical equation for calculating $\dot{V}O_2$max involve substituting Equation 15.4e into Equation 15.3e to yield Equation 15.5a. Then one final step, substituting the assumed values of $F_I N_2$ and $F_I O_2$ (Eq. 15.5b), yields the desired equation (Eq. 15.5c). Typically the calculation of $F_E N_2$ (Eq. 15.5d) is done separately, but can also be substituted into Equation 15.5c if desired, resulting in one combined equation.

Substitution yields: $\dot{V}O_2 = [(\dot{V}_E * F_E N_2 / F_I N_2) * F_I O_2]$
− [$\dot{V}_E * F_E O_2$]   Eq. 15.5a

Given: $F_I N_2 = 0.7903$, and $F_I O_2 = 0.2093$ Eq. 15.5b

Substitution yields: $\dot{V}O_2 = [(\dot{V}_{E\ STPD} * F_E N_2) * 0.2648]$
− [$\dot{V}_{E\ STPD} * F_E O_2$]   Eq. 15.5c

Where: $F_E N_2 = 1.00 - (F_E O_2 + F_E CO_2)$ Eq. 15.5d

Example: A person with a, $\dot{V}_{E\,STPD} = 100$ L·min^{-1}, $F_E O_2 = 0.1750$ (17.5 %), $F_E CO_2 = 0.0375$ (3.75 %), and therefore $F_E N_2 = 0.7875$ (78.75 %), would have an absolute $\dot{V}O_2$ of 3.35 L·min^{-1}, as seen in Equation 15.6.

$$\dot{V}O_2 = [\mathbf{100} * \mathbf{0.7875} * 0.2648] - [\mathbf{100} * \mathbf{0.1750}]$$
$$= 20.85 - 17.50 = \mathbf{3.35}\ \text{L·min}^{-1} \qquad \text{Eq. 15.6}$$

Relative Oxygen Consumption

The oxygen uptake calculated in Equation 15.6 is considered an *absolute oxygen uptake* (expressed in L·min^{-1}). This value is important because it is used to calculate respiratory exchange ratio and energy expenditure. However, when using $\dot{V}O_2$max to express someone's aerobic fitness, it is more common to express it on a relative basis per kg of body weight yielding a *relative oxygen consumption*. This is calculated by converting the absolute $\dot{V}O_2$ from liters to milliliters by multiplying by 1000 (ml·L^{-1}), then dividing by body weight (kg), as seen in Equation 15.7a.

Example: If the same participant above (with an absolute $\dot{V}O_2$ of 3.35 L·min^{-1}) weighs 80 kg, the relative $\dot{V}O_2$ would be 41.9 ml·kg^{-1}·min^{-1} (Eq. 15.7b).

Relative $\dot{V}O_2$ (ml·kg^{-1}·min^{-1})
= Absolute $\dot{V}O_2$ (L·min^{-1})
* 1000 / Body weight (kg)   Eq. 15.7a

Relative $\dot{V}O_2 = \mathbf{3.35}$ L·min^{-1} * 1000 / $\mathbf{80}$ kg
= $\mathbf{41.9}$ ml·kg^{-1}·min^{-1} Eq. 15.7b

Carbon Dioxide Production

With increasing exercise intensity, there is an increase not only in $\dot{V}O_2$, but also in carbon dioxide production ($\dot{V}CO_2$) as a by-product of elevated aerobic metabolism. The measurement of $\dot{V}CO_2$ is important because it allows for the subsequent calculation of the respiratory exchange ratio (RER). $\dot{V}CO_2$ is the difference between the volume of CO_2 exhaled from the lungs and the volume of CO_2 inhaled into the lungs (Eq. 15.8a), which can also be expressed as in Equation 15.8b. If it is assumed that the volume of CO_2 inhaled into the lungs is negligible (since $F_I CO_2 = 0.0003$), the equation reduces to Equation 15.8c. And finally, because the volume of exhaled CO_2 is the product of the exhaled ventilation and the fraction of CO_2 (Eq. 15.8d), this may be substituted to yield the equation used to mathematically calculate $\dot{V}CO_2$ (Eq. 15.8e).

Given: $\dot{V}CO_2 = [\dot{V}CO_2\ \text{Expired}]$
$- [\dot{V}CO_2\ \text{Inspired}]$ Eq. 15.8a

Given: $\dot{V}CO_2 = [\dot{V}_E CO_2] - [\dot{V}_I CO_2]$ Eq. 15.8b

Where: $\dot{V}_E CO_2$: Volume of expired CO_2

Where: $\dot{V}_I CO_2$: Volume of inspired CO_2

Assume: $\dot{V}_I CO_2$ is negligible ($F_I CO_2 = 0.0003$)

Given: $\dot{V}CO_2 = \dot{V}_E CO_2$ Eq. 15.8c

Given: $\dot{V}_E CO_2 = \dot{V}_E * F_E CO_2$ Eq. 15.8d

Substitution yields: $\dot{V}CO_2 = \dot{V}_{E\,STPD} * F_E CO_2$ Eq. 15.8e

Example: A person with a $\dot{V}_{E\,STPD} = 100$ L * min^{-1} and $F_E CO_2 = 0.0375$ (3.75 %), would have a $\dot{V}CO_2$ of 3.75 L·min^{-1}, as seen in Equation 15.9.

$$\dot{V}CO_2 = [\mathbf{100} * \mathbf{0.0375}] = \mathbf{3.75}\ \text{L·min}^{-1} \qquad \text{Eq. 15.9}$$

Respiratory Exchange Ratio

RER, the ratio of carbon dioxide production to oxygen consumption, is calculated by dividing $\dot{V}CO_2$ by $\dot{V}O_2$ (Eq. 15.10a). Based on the previous examples, if $\dot{V}CO_2 = 3.75$ L·min^{-1} and $\dot{V}O_2 = 3.35$ L·min^{-1}, then RER would be calculated as 1.12 (Eq. 15.10b).

$$\text{RER} = \dot{V}CO_2\ (\text{L·min}^{-1}) / \dot{V}O_2\ (\text{L·min}^{-1}) \qquad \text{Eq. 15.10a}$$

$$\text{RER} = \mathbf{3.75}\ \text{L·min}^{-1} / \mathbf{3.35}\ \text{L·min}^{-1} = \mathbf{1.12} \qquad \text{Eq. 15.10b}$$

RER reflects two important characteristics with regard to exercise, the *intensity* of the exercise and the *fuel being utilized* for energy production. RER increases during graded exercise in parallel with the increase in exercise intensity. It begins from a low of around 0.70–0.75 at rest; it increases to around 0.85–0.90 during moderate intensity exercise; then it peaks at around 1.10–1.20 during maximal intensity exercise. In fact, an RER in excess of 1.10 is one criterion to determine whether a person has reached a *maximal oxygen consumption*. Less importantly for this lab, but still important nutritionally, is the ability to use RER to determine the type of fuel being utilized. When RER = 0.70, the sole source of energy is fat (100 % of the energy is derived from fat). When RER = 1.00 or above, the sole source of energy is carbohydrate (100 % of the energy is derived from carbohydrate). This concept can be explained by reviewing two summary reactions (Eq. 15.11a and 15.11b), one for the complete aerobic breakdown of 1 mole of fat (palmitic acid) and the other for the aerobic breakdown of 1 mole of carbohydrate (glucose). The value of the RER can be used to determine the fractional utilization of fat or carbohydrate, and the actual energy expended from fat or carbohydrate for any exercise intensity, as seen in Table 15.8. RER rises in direct relation to exercise intensity, so it should be clear from Table 15.8 that fat is the primary energy source for lower intensity exercise (when RER < 0.85) and that carbohydrate is the preferred source for higher intensity exercise (when RER > 0.85).

1 Palmitic acid ($C_{16}H_{32}O_2$) + 23 O_2 → 16 CO_2 + 16 H_2O

Where: $CO_2 / O_2 = 16 / 23 = \mathbf{0.70}$ Eq. 15.11a

1 Glucose ($C_6H_{12}O_6$) + 6O_2 → 6 CO_2 + 6H_2O

Where: $CO_2 / O_2 = 6/6 = \mathbf{1.00}$ Eq. 15.11b

Table 15.8 Total Energy (kcal) Expended per Liter of Oxygen (kcal·L⁻¹ O₂) and Percent Contribution and Caloric Expenditure from Fat and Carbohydrate based on Respiratory Exchange Ratio (RER)

RER	Total kcal	Fat %	Fat kcal	Carbohydrate %	Carbohydrate kcal	RER	Total kcal	Fat %	Fat kcal	Carbohydrate %	Carbohydrate kcal
0.71	4.69	99	4.62	1	0.07	0.86	4.87	48	2.32	52	2.55
0.72	4.70	95	4.47	5	0.23	0.87	4.89	44	2.16	56	2.73
0.73	4.71	92	4.32	8	0.39	0.88	4.90	41	2.00	59	2.90
0.74	4.73	88	4.18	12	0.55	0.89	4.91	37	1.84	63	3.07
0.75	4.74	85	4.03	15	0.71	0.90	4.92	34	1.67	66	3.25
0.76	4.75	82	3.88	18	0.87	0.91	4.94	31	1.51	69	3.43
0.77	4.76	78	3.72	22	1.04	0.92	4.95	27	1.35	73	3.60
0.78	4.78	75	3.58	25	1.20	0.93	4.96	24	1.18	76	3.78
0.79	4.79	71	3.42	29	1.37	0.94	4.97	20	1.01	80	3.96
0.80	4.80	68	3.26	32	1.54	0.95	4.99	17	0.85	83	4.14
0.81	4.81	65	3.11	35	1.70	0.96	5.00	14	0.68	86	4.32
0.82	4.83	61	2.96	39	1.87	0.97	5.01	10	0.51	90	4.50
0.83	4.84	58	2.80	42	2.04	0.98	5.02	7	0.34	93	4.68
0.84	4.85	54	2.64	46	2.21	0.99	5.03	3	0.17	97	4.86
0.85	4.86	51	2.48	49	2.38	1.00	5.05	0	0.00	100	5.05

Note: Total caloric expenditure per liter of oxygen (Total kcal) can be estimated by kcal = (1.23 * RER) + 3.82. The percent contribution from fat (Fat %) can be estimated by Fat % = (−340 * RER) + 340. The percent contribution from carbohydrate (Carbohydrate %) is the remainder from 100%.
Source: Data from Carpenter (1948).[14]

Energy Expenditure

The final metabolic variable related to oxygen consumption to be calculated and discussed in this chapter is energy expenditure in kcal·min⁻¹. Energy expenditure can be estimated from oxygen consumption by the process of indirect calorimetry. The caloric equivalent of 1 liter of oxygen ranges from 4.67 to 5.05,[14] but is assumed to be 5 kcal for simplicity. That is to say, 5 kcal of energy is expended for every 1 liter of O_2 consumed. So energy expenditure can be calculated by multiplying the $\dot{V}O_2$ (L·min⁻¹) by the assumed caloric equivalent of 5.0 kcal·L⁻¹ (Eq. 15.12a). Although the metric unit for energy is the kilojoule (kJ), because kcal is still used so widely in the United States, it is used here. The conversion from kcal to kJ can be done simply by multiplying by 4.186 kJ·kcal⁻¹ if so desired, as seen in Equation 15.12b. Using the previously reported $\dot{V}O_2$ of 3.35 L·min⁻¹, energy expenditure is estimated to be 16.8 kcal·min⁻¹ (Eq. 15.12c) or 70.3 kJ·min⁻¹ (Eq. 15.12d).

$$\text{Energy (kcal·min}^{-1}) = \dot{V}O_2 \text{ (L·min}^{-1}) * 5.0 \text{ kcal·L}^{-1} \qquad \text{Eq. 15.12a}$$

$$\text{Energy (kJ·min}^{-1}) = \text{Energy (kcal·min}^{-1}) * 4.186 \text{ kJ·kcal}^{-1} \qquad \text{Eq. 15.12b}$$

$$\text{Energy (kcal·min}^{-1}) = \mathbf{3.35} \text{ L·min}^{-1} * 5.0 \text{ kcal·L}^{-1} = \mathbf{16.8} \text{ kcal·min}^{-1} \qquad \text{Eq. 15.12c}$$

$$\text{Energy (kJ·min}^{-1}) = \mathbf{16.8} \text{ kcal·min}^{-1} * 4.186 \text{ kJ·kcal}^{-1} = \mathbf{70.3} \text{ kJ·min}^{-1} \qquad \text{Eq. 15.12d}$$

RESULTS AND DISCUSSION

The emphasis in this chapter is on the measurement of maximal oxygen consumption ($\dot{V}O_2$max) as a measure of aerobic fitness. Because $\dot{V}O_2$max depends on the body's maximal ability to supply oxygen, it reflects the health and training status of the heart and lungs. And secondly, because it is also determined by the maximal ability to extract oxygen, it reflects the ability of the blood vessels to redistribute blood to the working muscle and the level of training of the skeletal muscle itself (i.e., capillary density, mitochondrial density, enzyme activity, etc.). In general, $\dot{V}O_2$max is found to be (1) higher in men than in women, (2) higher in younger adults than in older adults, (3) higher in aerobically trained persons than in anaerobically trained or in untrained persons, and (4) higher when tested using a mode of exercise that requires a larger muscle mass (e.g., cross-country skiing ergometer or treadmill) compared to a smaller muscle mass (e.g., cycle ergometer).

Fitness categories and comparative data for men and women over a wide range of age groups are provided in Table 15.9. It can be seen that relative $\dot{V}O_2$max in men averages about 10 ml·kg·min⁻¹ higher than women across all age groups. This is partly due to gender differences in cardiorespiratory factors (e.g., heart size, maximal cardiac output, etc.) but is also due in large part to the greater percent body fat characteristic of women compared to men. The decrease in $\dot{V}O_2$max with age apparent in Table 15.9 is possibly explained by a decrease in maximal heart rate due to changes in the autonomic nervous system and a decrease in maximal stroke volume due to reduced myocardial contractility and reduced vascular compliance, the combination of which results in a decrease in maximal cardiac output.[66] The data in Table 15.9 come from a study that compiled results from 62 different studies of healthy, untrained males and females ages 6–75 y from the United States, Canada, and Europe.[60] They found that *absolute* $\dot{V}O_2$max increased in male youths from about 1.0 L·min⁻¹ at age 6 y to over 3.0 L·min⁻¹ by age 18 y, then decreased to about

Table 15.9 Aerobic Fitness Category for Men and Women for Maximal Oxygen Consumption

	Maximal Oxygen Consumption (ml·kg^{-1}·min^{-1})							
	Men				Women			
Category	< 20 y	20–29 y	30–39 y	40–49 y	< 20 y	20–29 y	30–39 y	40–49 y
Excellent	> 62	> 61	> 55	> 50	> 53	> 49	> 45	> 39
Very Good	57–62	56–61	51–55	46–50	48–53	45–49	41–45	36–39
Good	51–56	50–55	46–50	41–45	43–47	41–44	36–40	32–35
Average	46–50	44–49	39–45	36–40	38–42	36–40	32–35	28–31
Fair	39–45	37–43	34–38	31–35	33–37	32–35	28–31	25–27
Poor	33–38	31–36	29–33	26–30	28–32	27–31	24–27	21–24
Very Poor	< 33	< 31	< 29	< 26	< 28	< 27	< 24	< 21

Source: Based on adaptation of data from Shvartz & Reibold (1990).[60]

1.5 L·min^{-1} by age 75 y. A similar trend was observed in females whose absolute $\dot{V}O_2$max was about 0.8 L·min^{-1} at age 6 y, peaked at about 2.2 L·min^{-1} at age 18 y, and decreased to about 1.0 L·min^{-1} by age 75 y. They further observed *relative* $\dot{V}O_2$max differences with age and gender and found smaller gender differences and a considerably smaller increase from 6 y to 18 y when compared with absolute $\dot{V}O_2$max. Relative $\dot{V}O_2$max decreased with age in males from a high of about 50 ml·kg^{-1}·min^{-1} during late adolescence (age 13–15 y) to about 25 ml·kg^{-1}·min^{-1} at age 75 y, or a rate of about 4 ml·kg^{-1}·min^{-1} per decade. Females demonstrated a high of about 40 ml·kg^{-1}·min^{-1} in late adolescence, which decreased to 17 ml·kg^{-1}·min^{-1} by age 75 y, at a rate similar to men.

Several investigators and reviewers support the use of $\dot{V}O_2$max as the best single indicator of a person's capacity for maintaining endurance-type activity.[44,54,64] A high relative $\dot{V}O_2$max reflects the ability to sustain a high percentage of absolute $\dot{V}O_2$max during aerobic activity. Relative $\dot{V}O_2$max may also be used as a predictor of endurance running performance because of its inverse relationship with 1.5 mile running time ($r = -0.74$).[40] Other investigators question the use of $\dot{V}O_2$max alone as an indicator of success in aerobic performance. They encourage the use of factors such as running economy,[20] the fractional utilization of $\dot{V}O_2$max,[18] and metabolic or ventilatory thresholds,[65] in addition to $\dot{V}O_2$max, to more accurately predict performance. For example, when aerobic performance is predicted with the addition of the fractional utilization of $\dot{V}O_2$max, the correlation with 1.5 mile run time is significantly improved from $r = -0.74$ to $r = -0.86$ compared to using $\dot{V}O_2$max alone.[40]

Aerobically trained athletes demonstrate very high $\dot{V}O_2$max values as a result of years of aerobic training. Representative ranges of $\dot{V}O_2$max values by sport are seen in Table 15.10. Sports characterized by continuous, long duration, aerobic activity such as Nordic (cross-country) skiing, distance running, rowing, and road cycling show the highest $\dot{V}O_2$max values ranging in men from 60 to 94 ml·kg^{-1}·min^{-1} and in women from 47 to 75 ml·kg^{-1}·min^{-1}.[66] Athletes who compete in more discontinuous, anaerobic sports like basketball, football, and volleyball still have good aerobic endurance, but have considerably lower $\dot{V}O_2$max values in the range of 40 to 60 ml·kg^{-1}·min^{-1}.

Treadmill protocols typically elicit $\dot{V}O_2$max values that range from 5 % to 14 % higher than cycle ergometry[22,32,35] because of the greater amount of muscle mass involved. The larger muscle mass requires greater energy demand that subsequently requires increased oxygen consumption and aerobic metabolism. The greater $\dot{V}O_2$max with treadmill running is likely to be more pronounced in those who are untrained or those who train by running. Trained cyclists however, because they spend so many hours training specifically on the bike, can elicit the same or higher $\dot{V}O_2$max on a cycle ergometer as on the treadmill. Arm ergometer protocols, which use considerably less muscle mass than leg ergometer or treadmill protocols, produce a $\dot{V}O_2$max 20–30 % lower when compared to the treadmill.[26] This is probably also due in part to the fact that most persons do not regularly aerobically train or even use their arms to the same degree as their legs, further supporting the specificity of training concept.

Table 15.10 Maximal Oxygen Consumption Values by Sport

Sport	Age (y)	$\dot{V}O_2$ (ml·kg^{-1}·min^{-1}) Men	Women
Skiing, Nordic	20–28	65–94	60–75
Running	18–39	60–85	50–75
Rowing	20–35	60–72	58–65
Cycling	18–26	62–74	47–57
Speed skating	18–24	56–73	44–55
Swimming	10–25	50–70	40–60
Canoeing	22–28	55–67	48–52
Soccer	22–28	54–64	50–60
Ice hockey	10–30	50–63	–
Wrestling	20–30	52–65	–
Basketball	18–30	40–60	43–60
Football	20–36	42–60	–
Volleyball	18–22	–	40–56
Gymnastics	18–22	52–58	36–50

Source: Data from Wilmore & Costill (2004).[67]

Summary

Maximal oxygen consumption ($\dot{V}O_2$max) is an important physiological variable that can be directly measured in the exercise physiology laboratory. It is highly dependent on the ability of the heart and lungs to supply oxygen and on the ability of the skeletal muscles to extract oxygen. For this reason, it reflects a person's overall aerobic or cardiorespiratory fitness very well. $\dot{V}O_2$max also determines a person's maximal aerobic power, which means that it contributes to sports and physical performances that rely predominantly on aerobic metabolism. The preferred method for determining $\dot{V}O_2$max is to directly measure it by exercising to exhaustion as evidenced by specific physiological and psychological criteria. However, numerous field tests involving walking, jogging, running, cycling, and stepping are also available that indirectly estimate $\dot{V}O_2$max through the use of submaximal exercise and the relationships observed between oxygen consumption, heart rate, running speed, cycle power level, and stepping rate and height. These indirect tests, because of the variability inherent in human physiology and performance, estimate $\dot{V}O_2$max with an error of $\pm 10 \%$. A comparison of the $\dot{V}O_2$max values derived from the aerobic tests described in the previous chapters with directly measured $\dot{V}O_2$max can be made.

References

1. Alexander, J. F., Liang, M. T. C., Stull, G. A., Serfass, R. C., Wolfe, D. R., & Ewing, J. L. (1984). A comparison of the Bruce and Liang equations for predicting $\dot{V}O_2$max in young adult males. *Research Quarterly for Exercise and Sport, 55,* 383–387.

2. American College of Sports Medicine (2010). *ACSM's guidelines for exercise testing and prescription, 8th ed.* Philadelphia: Lippincott Williams & Wilkins.

3. Andersen, K. L., Shephard, R. J., Denolin, H., Varnauskas, E., & Masironi, R. (Eds.). (1971). *Fundamentals of exercise testing.* Geneva: World Health Organization.

4. Åstrand, P. -O., & Rodahl, K. R. (1970). *Textbook of work physiology.* New York: McGraw-Hill.

5. Baumgartner, T. A., & Jackson, A. S. (1987). *Measurement for evaluation in physical education and exercise science.* Dubuque, IA: Wm. C. Brown.

6. Blair, S. N., Kohl, H. W., Paffenbarger, R. S., Clark, D. G., Cooper, K. H., & Gibbons, L. W. (1989). Physical fitness and all-cause mortality. *JAMA, 262,* 2395–2401.

7. Borg, G. A. (1970). Perceived exertion as an indicator of somatic stress. *Scandinavian Journal of Rehabilitative Medicine, 2,* 92–98.

8. Borg, G. A. (1982). Psychophysical bases of perceived exertion. *Medicine and Science in Sports and Exercise, 14,* 377–381.

9. Brooks, G. A., & Fahey, T. D. (1987). *Fundamentals of human performance.* New York: Macmillan.

10. Bruce, R. A. (1974). Methods of exercise testing. *The American Journal of Cardiology, 33,* 715–720.

11. Bruce, R. A., Kusumi, F., & Hosmer, D. (1973). Maximal oxygen intake and nomographic assessment of functional impairment in cardiovascular disease. *American Heart Journal, 85,* 546–562.

12. Bruce, R. A., & McDonough, J. R. (1969). Stress testing in screening for cardiovascular disease. *Bulletin of New York Academy of Medicine, 45,* 1288.

13. Buchfuhrer, M. J., Hansen, J. E., Robinson, T. E., Sue, D. Y., Wasserman, K., & Whipp, B. J. (1983). Optimizing the exercise protocol for cardiopulmonary assessment. *Journal of Applied Physiology, 55,* 1558–1564.

14. Carpenter, T. M. (1948). *Tables, factors, and formulas for computing respiratory exchange and biological transformations of energy* (4th ed.). Publication 303C. Washington, DC: Carnegie Institute of Washington.

15. Clear, M. S., & Frisch, F. (1984). Intra-individual biological variability in maximum aerobic power of trained and untrained individuals. *International Journal of Sportsmedicine, 5* (Abstract), 162.

16. Coast, J. R., & Welch, H. G. (1985). Linear increase in optimal pedal rate with increased power output in ergometry. *European Journal of Applied Physiology, 53,* 339–342.

17. Cooper, K. H. (1968). Testing and developing cardiovascular fitness within the United States Air Force. *Journal of Occupational Medicine, 10,* 636–639.

18. Costill, D. L., Thomason, H., & Roberts, E. (1973). Fractional utilization of the aerobic capacity during distance running. *Medicine and Science in Sports and Exercise, 5,* 248–252.

19. Cureton, T. K. (1973). Interpretation of the oxygen intake test—What is it? *American Corrective Therapy Journal, 27,* 17–23.

20. Daniels, J. T. (1985). A physiologist's view of running economy. *Medicine and Science in Sports and Exercise, 17,* 332–338.

21. Day, J. R., Rossiter, H. B., Coats, E. M., Skasick, A., & Whipp, B. J. (2003). The maximally attainable $\dot{V}O_2$ during exercise in humans: The peak vs. maximum issue. *Journal of Applied Physiology, 95,* 1901–1907.

22. deVries, H. A. (1986). *Physiology of exercise for physical education and athletics.* Dubuque, IA: Wm. C. Brown.

23. Duncan, G. E., Howley, E. T., & Johnson, B. N. (1997). Applicability of $\dot{V}O_2$max criteria: Discontinuous versus continuous protocols. *Medicine and Science in Sports and Exercise, 29,* 273–278.

24. Durstine, J. L., & Pate, R. R. (1988). Cardiorespiratory responses to acute exercise. In American College of Sports Medicine (Ed.), *Resource manual for guidelines for exercise testing and prescription* (pp. 38–54). Philadelphia: Lea & Febiger.

25. Falls, H. B., & Humphrey, D. H. (1973). A comparison of methods for eliciting maximum oxygen uptake from college women during treadmill walking. *Medicine and Science in Sports, 5,* 239–241.

26. Franklin, B. A. (1985). Exercise testing, training and arm ergometry. *Sports Medicine, 2,* 100–119.

27. Getchell, L. H., Kirkendall, D., & Robbins, G. (1977). Prediction of maximal oxygen uptake in young adult women joggers. *Research Quarterly, 48,* 61–67.

28. Gibbons, L. W., Blair, S. N., Cooper, K. H., & Smith, M. (1983). Association between coronary heart disease risk factors and physical fitness in healthy adult women. *Circulation, 67,* 977–983.

29. Hagberg, J. M., Mullin, J. P., Giese, M. D., & Spitznagel, E. (1981). Effect of pedaling rate on submaximal exercise responses of competitive cyclists. *Journal of Applied Physiology, 51,* 447–451.

30. Hansen, J. E., Casaburi, R., Cooper, D. M., & Wasserman, K. (1988). Oxygen uptake as related to work rate increment during cycle ergometer exercise. *European Journal of Applied Physiology, 57,* 140–145.

31. Harms, C. A., & Dempsey, J. A. (1999). Cardiovascular consequences of exercise hyperpnea. In J. O. Holloszy (Ed.), *Exercise and sport sciences reviews* (pp. 37–62). Philadelphia: Lippincott Williams & Wilkins.

32. Hermansen, L., & Saltin, B. (1969). Oxygen uptake during maximal treadmill and bicycle exercise. *Journal of Applied Physiology, 26,* 31–37.

33. Hill, A. V., & Lupton, H. (1923). Muscular exercise lactic acid and the supply and utilization of oxygen. *Quarterly Journal of Medicine, 16,* 135–171.

34. Holly, R. G. (1993). Fundamentals of cardiorespiratory exercise testing. In American College of Sports Medicine (Ed.), *Resource manual for guidelines for exercise testing and prescription* (pp. 247–257). Philadelphia: Lea & Febiger.

35. Horvath, S. M., & Yousef, M. K. (1981). *Environmental physiology: Aging, heat and altitude.* New York: Elsevier/North-Holland.

36. Howley, E. T., Bassett, D. R., & Welch, H. G. (1995). Criteria for maximal oxygen uptake: Review and commentary. *Medicine and Science in Sports and Exercise, 27,* 1292–1301.

37. Katch, V. L., Sady, S. S., & Freedson, P. (1982). Biological variability in maximum aerobic power. *Medicine and Science in Sports and Exercise, 14,* 21–25.

38. Liang, M. T. C., Alexander, J. F., Stull, G. A., & Serfass, R. C. (1982). The use of the Bruce equation for predicting $\dot{V}O_2$max in healthy young men. *Medicine and Science in Sports and Exercise, 14,* Abstract #129.

39. Luft, V. C., Cardus, D., Lim, T. P. K., Anderson, E. C., & Howarth, J. L. (1963). Physical performance in relation to body size and composition. *Annals of N.Y. Academy of Science, 110,* 795–808.

40. Mayhew, J. L., & Andrew, J. (1975). Assessment of running performance in college males from aerobic capacity percentage utilization coefficients. *Journal of Sports Medicine and Physical Fitness, 15,* 342–346.

41. McConnell, T. R. (1988). Practical considerations in the testing of $\dot{V}O_2$max in runners. *Sports Medicine, 5,* 57–68.

42. McDonough, J. R., & Bruce, R. A. (1969). Maximal exercise testing in assessing cardiovascular function. *Journal of South Carolina Medical Association, 65* (Suppl.), 26–33.

43. McMiken, D. F., & Daniels, J. T. (1976). Aerobic requirements and maximum aerobic power in treadmill and track running. *Medicine and Science in Sports and Exercise, 8,* 14–17.

44. Mitchell, J. H., Sproule, B. J., & Chapman, C. B. (1958). The physiological meaning of the maximal oxygen intake test. *Journal of Clinical Investigation, 37,* 538.

45. Noakes, T. D. (1988). Implications of exercise testing for prediction of performance: A contemporary perspective. *Medicine and Science in Sports and Exercise, 20,* 319–330.

46. Noble, B. J. (1986). *Physiology of exercise and sport.* Santa Clara, CA: Times Mirror/Mosby College.

47. Noble, B. J., Borg, G. A., Jacobs, I., Ceci, R., & Kaiser, P. (1983). A category-ratio perceived exertion scale: Relationship to blood and muscle lactates and heart rate. *Medicine and Science in Sports and Exercise, 15,* 523–528.

48. Patterson, R. P., & Moreno, M. I. (1990). Bicycle pedalling forces as a function of pedalling rate and power output. *Medicine and Science in Sports and Exercise, 22,* 512–516.

49. Patterson, R. P., & Pearson, J. L. (1983). The influence of flywheel weight and pedalling frequency on the biomechanics and psychological responses to bicycle exercise. *Ergonomics, 26,* 659–668.

50. Pivarnik, J. M., Dwyer, M. C., & Lauderdale, M. A. (1996). The reliability of aerobic capacity ($\dot{V}O_2$max) testing in adolescent girls. *Research Quarterly for Exercise and Sport, 67,* 345–348.

51. Pivarnik, J. M., Montain, S. J., Graves, J. E., & Pollock, M. L. (1988). Effects of pedal speed during incremental cycle ergometer exercise. *Research Quarterly for Exercise and Sport, 59,* 73–77.

52. Plowman, S. A., & Smith, D. L. (2003). *Exercise physiology for health, fitness and performance.* San Francisco: Benjamin Cummings.

53. Powers, S. K., & Howley, E. T. (2011). *Exercise physiology: Theory and application to fitness and performance, 8th ed.* New York: McGraw-Hill.

54. Robinson, S. (1938). Experimental studies of physical fitness in relation to age. *Arbeitsphysiologie, 10,* 251–323.

55. Rogers, M. A., Yamamoto, C., Hagberg, J. M., Martin, W. H., Ehsani, A. A., & Holloszy, J. O. (1988). Effect of six days of exercise training on responses to maximal and submaximal exercise in middle-aged men. *Medicine and Science in Sports and Exercise, 20,* 260–264.

56. Rowland, T. W. (1993). Does peak $\dot{V}O_2$ reflect $\dot{V}O_2$max in children? Evidence from supramaximal testing. *Medicine and Science in Sports and Exercise, 25,* 689–693.

57. Rowland, T. W., & Cunningham, L. N. (1992). Oxygen uptake plateau during maximal treadmill exercise in children. *Chest, 101,* 485–489.

58. Seabury, J. J., Adams, W. C., & Ramey, M. R. (1977). Influence of pedalling rate and power output on energy expenditure during bicycle ergometry. *Ergonomics, 20,* 491–498.

59. Serresse, O., Lortie, G., Bouchard, C., & Boulay, M. R. (1988). Estimation of the contribution of the various energy systems during maximal work of short duration. *International Journal of Sports Medicine, 9,* 456–460.

60. Shvartz, E., & Reibold, R. C. (1990). Aerobic fitness norms for males and females aged 6 to 75 years: A review. *Aviation, Space, and Environmental Medicine, 61,* 3–11.

61. St. Clair-Gibson, A., Lambert, M. I., Hawley, J. A., Broomhead, S. A., & Noakes, T. D. (1999). Measurement of maximal oxygen uptake from two different laboratory protocols in runners and squash players. *Medicine and Science in Sports and Exercise, 31,* 1226–1229.

62. Sylven, C., Borg, G., Holmgren, A., & Astrom, H. (1991). Psychophysical power functions of exercise limiting symptoms in coronary heart disease. *Medicine and Science in Sports and Exercise, 23,* 1050–1054.

63. Tanaka, H., Bassett, D. R., Swensen, T. C., & Sampredo, R. M. (1993). Aerobic and anaerobic power characteristics of competitive cyclists in the United States Cycling Federation. *International Journal of Sports Medicine, 14,* 334–338.

64. Taylor, H. L., Buskirk, E., & Henschel, A. (1955). Maximal oxygen intake as an objective measure of cardiorespiratory performance. *Journal of Applied Physiology, 8,* 73–80.

65. Vago, P., Mercier, J., Ramonatxo, M., & Prefant, C. (1987). Is ventilatory anaerobic threshold a good index of endurance capacity? *International Journal of Sports Medicine, 8,* 190–195.

66. Williams, J. H., Powers, S. K., & Stuart, M. K. (1986). Hemoglobin desaturation in highly trained athletes during heavy exercise. *Medicine and Science in Sports and Exercise, 18,* 168–173.

67. Wilmore, J. H., Costill, D. L., & Kenney, W. L. (2007). Physiology of exercise and sport, 4th ed. Champaign, IL: Human Kinetics.

68. Wyndham, C. H., Strydom, N. B., Maritz, J. S., Morrison, J. F., Peter, J., & Potgieter, Z. U. (1959). Maximum oxygen intake and maximum heart rate during strenuous work. *Journal of Applied Physiology, 14,* 927–936.

69. Zoladz, J. A., Duda, K., & Majerczak, J. (1998). Oxygen uptake does not increase linearly at high power outputs during incremental exercise test in humans. *European Journal of Applied Physiology, 77,* 445–451.

70. Zoladz, J. A., Rademaker, A. C., & Sargent, A. J. (1995). Non-linear relationship between O_2 uptake and power output at high intensities of exercise in humans. *Journal of Physiology, 488,* 211–217.

Form 15.1
MAXIMAL OXYGEN CONSUMPTION

NAME _____ DATE _____ SCORE _____

Homework

Gender: **M**   Initials: **AA**   Age (y): **22**   Height (cm): **170**   Weight (kg): **75.0**

T_A (°C): **23** P_B (mmHg): **756**   RH (%): **30**   STPD C.F. : _____ *(Table 15.7)*

Time	$\dot{V}_{E\,ATPS}$ (L·min^{-1})	$\dot{V}_{E\,STPD}$ (L·min^{-1})	F_EO_2	F_ECO_2	F_EN_2	HR (bpm)	RPE
6:00	56.1		0.1520	0.0518		130	11
9:00	105.7		0.1644	0.0439		170	14
11:00	120.0		0.1686	0.0429		182	17
12:00	146.0		0.1733	0.0401		195	19

$\dot{V}O_2$ (L·min^{-1})	$\dot{V}O_2$ (ml·kg^{-1}·min^{-1})	$\dot{V}CO_2$ (L·min^{-1})	RER	% Energy from Fat	% Energy from CHO	Energy (kcal·min^{-1})	Energy (kJ·min^{-1})
___	___	___	___	___	___	___	___
___	___	___	___	___	___	___	___
___	___	___	___	___	___	___	___
___	___	___	___	___	___	___	___

Equations:

$\dot{V}_{E\,STPD} = \dot{V}_{E\,ATPS} *$ STPD C.F.

$F_EN_2 = 1.0000 - (F_EO_2 + F_ECO_2)$

Absolute $\dot{V}O_2$ (L·min^{-1}) = [$\dot{V}_{E\,STPD} * F_EN_2 * 0.2648$] - [$\dot{V}_{E\,STPD} * F_EO_2$]

Relative $\dot{V}O_2$ (ml·kg^{-1}·min^{-1}) = Absolute $\dot{V}O_2$ (L·min^{-1}) * 1000 / Body wt (kg)

$\dot{V}CO_2$ (L·min^{-1}) = [$\dot{V}_{E\,STPD} * F_ECO_2$]

Respiratory exchange ratio (RER) = $\dot{V}CO_2$ (L·min^{-1}) / $\dot{V}O_2$ (·Lmin^{-1})   *(See Table 15.8 for fuel use)*

Energy (kcal·min^{-1}) = $\dot{V}O_2$ (L·min^{-1}) * 5 (kcal·L^{-1})   *(1 kcal = 4.186 kJ)*

Criteria for $\dot{V}O_2$max: ☐ Plateau in $\dot{V}O_2$ ☐ RER ≥ 1.10   ☐ HR within 10 bpm of HRmax   ☐ RPE ≥ 18

Absolute $\dot{V}O_2$max (L·min^{-1}) = _____   Relative $\dot{V}O_2$max (ml·kg^{-1}·min^{-1}) = _____

Fitness category *(from Table 15.9):* _____

Evaluation / comments: _____

_____

_____

_____

Form 15.2
MAXIMAL OXYGEN CONSUMPTION

NAME _____ DATE _____ SCORE _____

Lab Results

Gender: _____ Initials: _____ Age (y): _____ Height (cm): _____ Weight (kg): _____

T_A (°C): _____ P_B (mmHg): _____ RH (%): _____ STPD C.F. : _____ *(Table 15.7)*

Time	$\dot{V}_{E\,ATPS}$ (L·min⁻¹)	$\dot{V}_{E\,STPD}$ (L·min⁻¹)	F_EO_2	F_ECO_2	F_EN_2	HR (bpm)	RPE
___	___	___	___	___	___	___	___
___	___	___	___	___	___	___	___
___	___	___	___	___	___	___	___
___	___	___	___	___	___	___	___

$\dot{V}O_2$ (L·min⁻¹)	$\dot{V}O_2$ (ml·kg⁻¹·min⁻¹)	$\dot{V}CO_2$ (L·min⁻¹)	RER	% Energy from Fat	% Energy from CHO	Energy (kcal·min⁻¹)	Energy (kJ·min⁻¹)
___	___	___	___	___	___	___	___
___	___	___	___	___	___	___	___
___	___	___	___	___	___	___	___
___	___	___	___	___	___	___	___

Equations:

$\dot{V}_{E\,STPD} = \dot{V}_{E\,ATPS}$ * STPD C.F.

$F_EN_2 = 1.0000 - (F_EO_2 + F_ECO_2)$

Absolute $\dot{V}O_2$ (L·min⁻¹) = $[\dot{V}_{E\,STPD} * F_EN_2 * 0.2648] - [\dot{V}_{E\,STPD} * F_EO_2]$

Relative $\dot{V}O_2$ (ml·kg⁻¹·min⁻¹) = Absolute $\dot{V}O_2$ (L·min⁻¹) * 1000 / Body wt (kg)

$\dot{V}CO_2$ (L·min⁻¹) = $[\dot{V}_{E\,STPD} * F_ECO_2]$

Respiratory exchange ratio (RER) = $\dot{V}CO_2$ (L·min⁻¹) / $\dot{V}O_2$ (·Lmin⁻¹)   *(See Table 15.8 for fuel use)*

Energy (kcal·min⁻¹) = $\dot{V}O_2$ (L·min⁻¹) * 5 (kcal·L⁻¹)   *(1 kcal = 4.186 kJ)*

Criteria for $\dot{V}O_2$max: ☐ Plateau in $\dot{V}O_2$ ☐ RER ≥ 1.10   ☐ HR within 10 bpm of HRmax   ☐ RPE ≥ 18

Absolute $\dot{V}O_2$max (L·min⁻¹) = _____   Relative $\dot{V}O_2$max (ml·kg⁻¹·min⁻¹) = _____

Fitness category *(from Table 15.9):* _____

Evaluation / comments: _____

_____

_____

_____

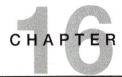

RESTING BLOOD PRESSURE

Numerous researchers have reported an inverse (negative) relationship between physical activity or fitness and morbidity (disease rate) or mortality (death rate), not only from coronary heart disease[5,6,13,32,42,44,46] but from all causes.[6,7] Thus, physical activity and fitness are associated with a reduced risk of cardiovascular disease (CVD), as well as reduced deaths from CVD and all causes. In light of such evidence it seems prudent that the student of exercise physiology be knowledgeable about cardiovascular tests.

Blood pressure measurement is one of the most common clinical tests. It is recommended that all persons over 3 y of age have their blood pressure checked annually.[47]

Because blood pressure screening or monitoring is such an important part of many physical fitness clinics, the technique of measuring blood pressure should be learned by many types of allied health personnel. Dr. Herman Hellerstein, a renowned cardiologist, speaking as a member of the American Medical Association's Committee on Exercise, said, "Certainly every physical educator should know how to take blood pressure and record it."[22] Additionally, every physical educator should know how to interpret blood pressure.

PURPOSE OF BLOOD PRESSURE MEASUREMENT

Millions of Americans are hypertensive. **Primary hypertension** means that the cause of hypertension is not known; **secondary hypertension** means that it is caused by known endocrine or structural disorders.[1] Although the cause of hypertension (high blood pressure) in at least 90 % of adults is unknown, it is associated with a high risk for future cardiovascular morbidity and mortality.[17] Hypertensive persons are more likely to accelerate atherosclerosis that may cause vascular occlusions and ruptures about 20 y earlier than in normotensives.[27] If there were obvious symptoms (e.g., pain, nausea) associated with high blood pressure, there would be less need to measure the actual pressure. However, high blood pressure may not be noticed outwardly until a fatal or near-fatal heart attack or stroke occurs. Thus, the primary clinical purpose of measuring blood pressure is to determine the potential risk of cardiovascular disease; if the pressure is high, then appropriate medications or lifestyle changes are recommended. Periodic monitoring of the blood pressure is done in order to check the efficacy of such recommendations.

Another purpose of measuring resting blood pressure is to establish a baseline by which to compare the effect of exercise on blood pressure. Thus, the effects of different types, intensities, or durations of exercise may be compared by noting their effects upon the baseline value. For example, blood pressure comparisons may be made between (1) static versus dynamic exercise, (2) different intensities of muscle actions (e.g., 30 % vs. 80 % maximal forces), and (3) short versus long durations of exercise.

PHYSIOLOGICAL RATIONALE

High blood pressure is unhealthy; blood pressure, per se, is not unhealthy. Without blood pressure there would be no blood flow. Blood pressure is primarily dependent upon the volume of blood and the resistance of the blood vessels. The blood pressure commonly measured is that of the arteries. Thus, blood pressure may be defined for laboratory purposes as the force of blood distending the *arterial* walls. Typically, the brachial artery is sampled because of convenience and its position at heart level. The brachial artery (Figure 16.1) is a continuation of the axillary artery and extends medially alongside the humerus; it gradually moves centrally as it nears the antecubital fossa (anterior crease of the elbow), where it divides into the radial and ulnar arteries.

Korotkoff Sounds

The determination of blood pressure in the typical laboratory setting is based upon the sounds made by the vibrations from the vascular walls. These sounds are referred to as Korotkoff sounds (named after their discoverer in 1905) (Figure 16.2). In brief, when there is no blood flow (as when a tourniquet is applied), there will be no vibrations and thus no sound. Paradoxically, when there is completely nonobstructed flow of the blood, there is also no vibration and thus no sound; this is due to the streamlined flow of the blood. When blood flow is restricted by the application of a tourniquet or by any kind of pressure, and then gradually released, a bolus of blood escapes at the peak point of blood pressure coinciding with left ventricular contraction (systole). This bolus of blood causes vascular vibrations that result in a faint sound (phase 1); this is **systolic pressure.** As the restriction or pressure continues to be released, more blood escapes, causing even greater vibration and louder sounds. Phases 2 and 3 are not commonly used in

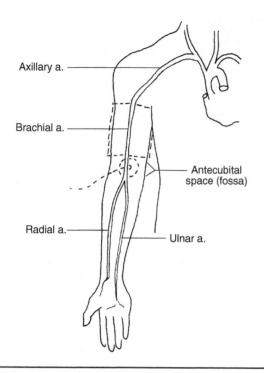

Figure 16.1 An internal view of the brachial artery and its origins and branches; the dotted diaphragm of the stethoscope is at the antecubital fossa (a. = artery).

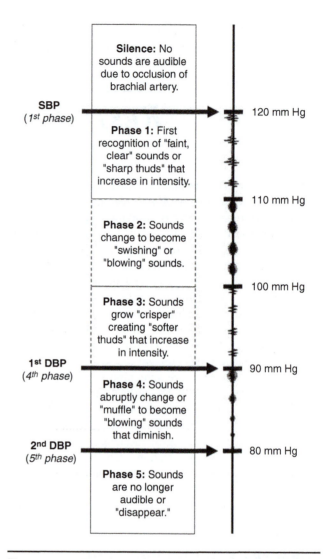

Figure 16.2 Demonstration of using Korotkoff sounds to auscultate arterial blood pressure. Systolic blood pressure (120 mm Hg) corresponds to Phase 1, with the first diastolic blood pressure (90 mm Hg) and second diastolic pressure (80 mm Hg) corresponding to Phase 4 and Phase 5, respectively.

recording blood pressures. More blood escapes as the cuff pressure continues to decrease. However, after phase 3, as the blood flow becomes more streamlined due to less compression, there is a reduction of vibrations, causing a muffling sound (phase 4). The fourth phase is sometimes difficult to distinguish. The American Heart Association describes it as ". . . a distinct, abrupt, muffling of sound (usually of a soft, blowing quality) . . .".[17] Identifying phase 4 is more difficult than identifying phase 5.[16] When blood flow is completely streamlined (laminar flow), there is a disappearance of sound (phase 5). The disappearance denotes **diastolic pressure, the lowest pressure that exists in the arteries.** However, the fourth phase is closer to the actual invasive diastolic pressure; hence, it is sometimes referred to as the true diastolic pressure. The fifth phase is often referred to as the clinical diastolic pressure because it is the reference for normative classification.

The Task Force on Blood Pressure Control in Children[47] recommends that both the point of muffling (phase 4) and the point of disappearance (phase 5) of the sound be recorded when taking blood pressure in children. Because of the frequency of these occurring simultaneously or of the fifth phase's not occurring at all in children, the Task Force and the American Heart Association use the fourth phase to interpret children's norms and the fifth phase for all persons above 12 y of age. Occasionally, phase 4 should be used for adults whose sounds remain very faint to near zero levels.[48] Usually, the fourth phase is significantly higher than the fifth phase by about 5 mm of mercury (Hg).[12] Rarely do

true diastolic pressures reach less than 40 mm Hg.[14] Thus, for any person whose sounds can be heard below this level, it seems logical to use the fourth phase instead of the fifth phase as the true diastolic pressure. Exercise technicians are encouraged to practice recording the fourth phase in all persons because of the fourth phase's importance during exercise (Chapter 17).

Pulse Pressure and Mean Arterial Pressure

In addition to systolic and diastolic pressure, two other pressures are frequently described: **pulse pressure (PP)** and **mean arterial pressure (MAP).** Pulse pressure is the difference between systolic and diastolic pressure (phase 5), as seen in Equation 16.1. High pulse pressures may indicate increased risk of myocardial infarction (heart attack).[36] Pulse pressure reflects the vascular compliance (distensibility) in large arteries. Pulse pressure is used to calculate mean arterial pressure.

$$\text{Pulse pressure (mm Hg)} = \text{SBP} - \text{DBP (5th)} \qquad \text{Eq. 16.1}$$

Where: SBP is systolic blood pressure (mm Hg)

Where: DBP is diastolic blood pressure (mm Hg) using the fifth-phase sound

Mean arterial pressure is based upon the actual pressure that the arteries would sustain if blood flow was constant and not pulsating. Because arterial blood pressure under resting conditions is at systolic level only about $\frac{1}{20}$ of the time during a cardiac cycle, MAP is always closer to diastolic pressure than it is to systolic pressure. Resting MAP is usually estimated as one-third the distance between systolic pressure and fifth-phase diastolic pressure,[45] as seen in Equation 16.2a. For example, a person with a systolic blood pressure of 120 mm Hg and a diastolic blood pressure of 80 mm Hg would have a pulse pressure of 40 mm Hg (Eq. 16.2b) and a mean arterial pressure of 93 mm Hg (Eq. 16.2c).

$$\text{Mean arterial pressure (mm Hg)} = \text{DBP} + (\text{PP} / 3) \qquad \text{Eq. 16.2a}$$

Where: DBP is diastolic blood pressure (mm Hg)

Where: PP is pulse pressure (mm Hg)

Assume: SBP is **120** mm Hg and DBP is **80** mmHg

$$\text{PP (mm Hg)} = \mathbf{120 - 80 = 40} \text{ mm Hg} \qquad \text{Eq. 16.2b}$$

$$\text{MAP (mm Hg)} = \mathbf{80 + (40 / 3) = 80 + 13} = \mathbf{93} \text{ mm Hg} \qquad \text{Eq. 16.2c}$$

METHODS

The accuracy of blood pressure measurements is described in Box 16.1. Many types of instruments exist for measuring blood pressure. The original instrument in 1733, water in a glass tube, was used to measure the blood pressure of a horse.[4] Due to water's light weight (lower density) in comparison with mercury, the liquid now being used, a ladder was needed to enable the investigator to read the water column, which had risen about 10 ft. Mercury, being nearly 14 times denser than water, enables the measurement of blood pressure with a glass tube, which can be about $\frac{1}{14}$ the length of the original water-filled glass tubes. If we still used water to measure human blood pressure, the tube would have to be a minimum of six feet tall, and the column of water would oscillate by more than one foot with each heartbeat.[23]

The International System's unit of measure for pressure is the hectopascal. However, due to the traditional use of mercury in blood pressure instrumentation, the unit of measure for blood pressure recordings is millimeters of mercury (mm Hg). Regardless of the type of blood pressure method or instrument, the unit of measure remains mm Hg.

<table>
<tr><td colspan="2">BOX 16.1   Accuracy of Blood Pressure Measurements</td></tr>
</table>

BOX 16.1   Accuracy of Blood Pressure Measurements

Reliability

The ability of the human ear to hear sounds depends upon the frequency (Hz) and decibels (dB) of the sounds. Unfortunately, Korotkoff sounds are neither of high frequency nor high decibel—both being less than the optimal hearing of the human ear.[34] Acceptable reliability coefficients can be obtained for the test-retest values of systolic ($r = 0.89$) and diastolic ($r = 0.83$) blood pressures.[a] The diastolic values of the fifth phase may be more repeatable than those of the fourth phase due to greater difficulty in determining muffling points of fourth phases versus disappearance points of fifth phases. In fact, one investigator encourages the use of the fifth phase for this reason, although it may not be hemodynamically justified for all persons.[29]

Validity

The cuff method of measuring systolic and fifth-phase diastolic blood pressure is usually lower than the more accurate invasive method of measuring blood pressure by about 10 mm Hg (8 %) and 5 mm Hg (6 %), respectively; the fourth phase, however, is not significantly different from the invasive measurement of diastolic pressure.[45] Thus, the fourth phase appears to be the most valid indicator of diastolic pressure, although the fifth phase is commonly used for calculating mean pressures during a resting body state.

Automated Blood Pressure Devices

Numerous automated blood pressure devices have been validated using the International Protocol of the European Society of Hypertension (ESH). In the process of this validation, SBP and DBP were measured simultaneously by the device and by two trained persons using standard BP measurement methods. The mean $\pm$ SD difference (mm Hg) between the device and standard method for SBP and DBP respectively for several devices were: -1.4 ± 5.5 and -0.4 ± 4.8 for the Omron™ HEM-4011C-E, -2.13 ± 7.37 and 0.09 ± 4.91 for the Omron™ HEM-7000-E, -1.4 ± 8.6 and -0.1 ± 3.5 for the Spengler™ KP7500D, and 1.6 ± 4.2 and 0.5 ± 2.8 for the Microlife™ BP A100 Plus.[3]

[a]Adams G. M. (1968). Blood pressure reliability in the elderly. Unpublished raw data.

The graduations on the sphygmomanometer gauge are in 2 mm divisions and extend to 300 mm Hg.

The methods of blood pressure measurement may be divided into two categories—invasive and noninvasive. The *invasive* method is the more valid of the two methods and is usually reserved for clinical settings or precise research investigations. A thin teflon tube, called an endhole catheter or cannula, is connected on one end to a pressure transducer. The sensor end of the catheter is inserted into the brachial artery or ascending aorta while the transducer end is connected to a recorder. Although the invasive method is accurate for mean and diastolic pressures in the ascending aorta,[18] it is expensive, elaborate, and traumatic, compared with the noninvasive method.

Two major methods are used to measure *noninvasive blood pressure*—cuff manometry and ultrasound Doppler. The more common cuff manometry method uses an instrument called a sphygmomanometer (*sphygmo* = pulse; pronounced sfig-mo-ma-nóm-a-ter); also referred to as a manometer. Pressure can be measured through the use of either an aneroid ("without fluid") or mercury manometer. The aneroid manometer includes an air bellows mechanism that expands or contracts as cuff pressure changes and displays pressure by movement of a needle on a round dial. Aneroid systems are less expensive and "safer" because they do not provide a threat of mercury exposure. They may be less accurate, they need to be calibrated frequently, and they are prone to damage if dropped. The mercury manometer displays pressure directly by observing the height of a column of mercury. Mercury systems are very accurate because they are essentially self-calibrating. Improper handling of the mercury manometer however, can result in accidental mercury leakage. Both aneroid and mercury methods of manometry require a cuff with an air bladder; thus, the method is sometimes referred to as the cuff method (Figure 16.3). Although aneroid manometers are not favored over mercury manometers,[1,24] if the aneroids are calibrated routinely (Box 16.2), they are acceptable.

Fully automated blood pressure devices are commercially available (e.g., Omron™, etc.) for monitoring blood pressure at home (Figure 16.4). Regular self-measurement of blood pressure (outside of the doctor's office) provides valuable information for hypertension diagnosis, assists in the treatment and control of hypertension, and improves patients' compliance with antihypertensive therapy.[40] Many of these devices have been validated using what is referred to as the International Protocol established by the European Society of Hypertension (ESH).[41] The protocol utilizes three experienced testers, two of whom simultaneously measure BP using a mercury sphygmomanometer, while the third measures BP with the device. Testing takes place in two phases. During the first phase, 15 participants (45 BP

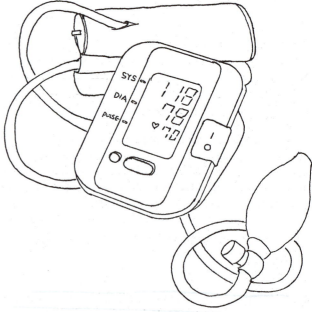

Figure 16.4 An example of a typical automated blood pressure device (Omron M1 Plus™) used to measure resting blood pressure.

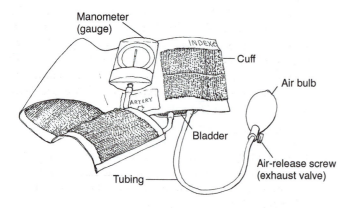

Figure 16.3 The main parts of an aneroid sphygmomanometer are the gauge, tubing, cuff, bladder, air bulb, and air-release screw.

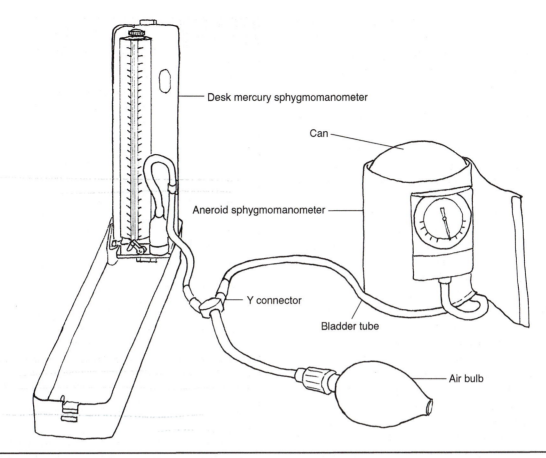

Figure 16.5 The configuration for aneroid sphygmomanometer calibration.

measurements) are tested. Provided the device passes the first phase, the second phase tests 18 more participants (54 BP measurements). The final results yield the accuracy of the device in measuring both systolic and diastolic blood pressure and determine whether it is valid. Specific devices that have been validated using this protocol include the Omron M1™ (HEM-4011C-E), Omron M6 Comfort™ (HEM-7000-E), Spengler™ (KP7500D), Microlife™ (BP A100 plus), and Oregon Scientific™ (BPU 330), among others.[3,33] The specific accuracy of some of these devices is described in Box 16.1.

Mercury and aneroid sphygmomanometers require a stethoscope to auscultate the Korotkoff sounds; when this is done, the noninvasive method may be referred to as the **auscultatory method.** Ambulatory blood pressure monitors can be programmed to take readings every 5 min to 120 min throughout a 24 h period. The pressures can be analyzed after being downloaded to a computer.[15]

Procedures

Certain preparations, such as calibration and participant orientation, should be made in order to facilitate blood pressure measurement. Calibration of aneroid manometers, using a mercury manometer, should be done at six-month[24,27] to annual[28,47] intervals (Box 16.2).

Participant orientation includes such preparatory rules as were suggested for the stepping test (Chapter 13) and cycling test (Chapter 14). Whereas those tests prescribed abstaining from smoking and caffeine for 3 h prior to testing, the Joint National Committee on Detection, Evaluation, and Treatment of High Blood Pressure prescribes only a 30 min abstention.[24] The participant should relax for at least five minutes in a comfortable environment prior to the blood pressure measurement.[17,24] Also, sleeveless shirts/blouses or loose-fitting sleeves are recommended attire; if the sleeve appears to fit tightly around the person's arm when the sleeve is rolled up, the shirt should be removed. The cuff and stethoscope should not be placed over cloth. Most of the following procedures for measuring blood pressure are the recommendations of the Joint National Committee on Detection, Evaluation, and Treatment of High Blood Pressure (1997).[24]

Procedural Steps

1. The participant should sit comfortably in a chair with a backrest for at least 5 min. The arm bared is at heart level and resting on the armrest of a chair or on a table (Figure 16.6).
2. The manometer should be clearly visible to the technician; mercury gauges should read so that the meniscus (top of mercury) is at eye level.

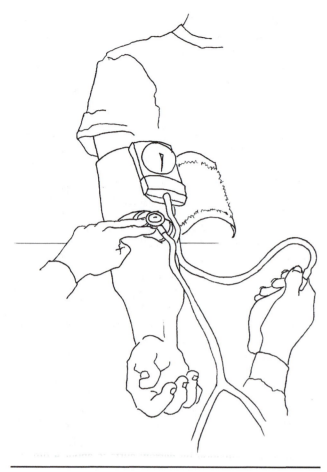

Figure 16.6   The bottom border of the cuff is placed about 1 in., or 2.5 cm, above the antecubital space and diaphragm of the stethoscope.

Table 16.1	Guidelines for Selecting Cuff Based on Limb Girth (cm)		
Limb Girth (cm)	Type of Cuff	Bladder Size (cm)	
		Length	Width
Upper arm			
18–24	Child	21.5	10
24–32	Adult	24	12.5
32–42	Large adult	33 or 42	15
Thigh			
42–50	Thigh	37	18.5

3. For persons with suspected small or large arm circumferences, the technician measures the circumference of the participant's upper arm.
   a. The appropriate cuff size is selected based on the arm circumference guidelines in Table 16.1.
   b. Some cuffs have index lines that indicate if the cuff is too small or too large (Figure 16.7). In general the *bladder* should wrap around at least 80 % of the arm.
4. The technician snugly places the blood pressure cuff so that the lower edge is approximately 2.5 cm (1 in.) above the antecubital space.[30]

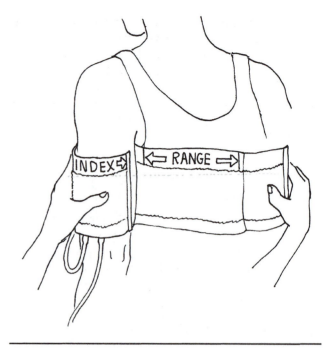

Figure 16.7   The cuff's index and range lines determine the appropriate cuff size for some sphygmomanometers.

   a. The center of the bladder should be over the brachial artery.
   b. Some cuffs have a mark to line up with the brachial artery. To assure alignment, it may be helpful to palpate the brachial artery along the medial side of the antecubital space.[17]
5. The technician places the diaphragm, or bell, of the stethoscope firmly, but not tight enough to indent the skin, over the brachial artery in the antecubital space.
6. After turning the air-release screw clockwise, the technician quickly inflates the cuff to any of the three following levels:
   a. 160 mm Hg
   b. 20 mm Hg above expected or known SP
   c. 20 mm Hg to 30 mm Hg above the disappearance of the palpated radial pulse[17]
7. The technician turns the air-release screw counterclockwise so that the cuff pressure decreases at a rate of about 2 mm Hg to 3 mm Hg per second.[24]
8. The technician listens carefully and mentally notes the first Korotkoff sound of two consecutive beats—systolic pressure (first phase)—then fourth phase (muffling)—then fifth phase (disappearance)—at the nearest 2 mm mark on the manometer, respectively.
9. The technician continues listening for 10 mm Hg to 20 mm Hg below the last sound heard to confirm disappearance.
10. The technician rapidly and fully deflates the cuff.
11. The technician records the values in even numbers onto Form 16.2 according to the accepted format: e.g., systolic/fourth phase DP/fifth phase DP. Thus, a hypothetical recording would appear as 128/92/86 mm Hg.

12. The technician repeats the measurement after 1–2 min, then averages the two readings unless they differ by more than 5 mm Hg—in which case, additional readings are made.[24,27] If more than two readings are necessary, the technician averages them all.

13. The technician uses the first and fifth phases to classify persons according to Tables 16.2 and 16.3 and records this on Form 16.2.

Comments on Blood Pressure Procedures

Body and Arm Position

There is no practical difference in blood pressure measured in the seated position versus that measured in the supine position. However, statistically, slightly higher values occur for systolic (6–7 mm Hg) and diastolic (1 mm Hg) in the supine position.[31,49] The standing position increases diastolic pressure but not systolic pressure.[20]

The sitting position should automatically place the person's antecubital space of the arm at heart level. Blood pressures are higher if the arm is below the heart versus above the heart (nearly 1 mm Hg for each centimeter above or below heart level). Erroneously higher systolic and diastolic pressures occur if the arm is allowed to hang at the person's side rather than supported at heart level.[49]

For best exposure of the antecubital position, it helps to have the person's palm upward with the thumb-side rotated outwardly (the anatomical position) and to have the arm nearly straight while resting on a platform (e.g., table). This provides the best contact with the brachial artery. The antecubital space should be left clear for the stethoscope.[8]

Various authorities recommend that the right arm be chosen for the blood pressure measurement.[9,47] This is partly because of the remote possibility that the genetic anomaly of coarctation (abnormal narrowing) between the aorta and subclavian artery will cause an elevated blood pressure. If the pressure in the right arm is normal, it is likely to be normal everywhere. However, higher right-arm values were not confirmed by some investigators,[12,19] nor did the investigators in the famous epidemiological study in Framingham, Massachusetts, measure blood pressure in the right arm.[26] In older patients, one group of investigators found that the systolic pressure in the right arm was not more than a few millimeters higher than in the left arm and that the diastolic pressure was virtually the same in both arms.[21] The American Heart Association recommends that both arms be measured at the initial examination and the arm with the higher pressure be measured in subsequent examinations.[17] Another consideration should be the comfort and convenience of both the technician and the participant.

Cuff Size

Special cuff sizes are available for small or large arms. Cuffs that are too small will over estimate blood pressure, where as cuffs that are too large will under estimate blood pressure. The average over estimation by narrow cuffs is about 9 mm Hg

Table 16.2 Percentile Category for Resting Blood Pressure for Men and Women by Age Group

	Resting Blood Pressure (mm Hg)							
	Men				Women			
	20–29 y		30–39 y		20–29 y		30–39 y	
Category (percentile)	SBP	DBP	SBP	DBP	SBP	DBP	SBP	DBP
Much lower than ave (> 90th)	< 110	< 70	< 108	< 70	< 99	< 63	< 100	< 65
Lower than ave (70th–90th)	111–118	70–78	108–116	70–78	99–106	63–70	100–110	65–70
Average (30th–70th)	119–130	79–84	117–130	79–85	107–120	71–80	111–120	71–80
Higher than ave (10th–30th)	131–140	85–90	131–140	86–92	121–130	81–82	121–130	81–90
Much higher than ave (< 10th)	> 140	> 90	> 140	> 92	> 130	> 82	> 130	> 90

Source: Based on data from Pollock, Wilmore, & Fox (1978).[43]

Table 16.3 Criteria for Blood Pressure (mm Hg) Categories with Follow-Up Recommendations

Category	Criteria Systolic		Diastolic	Follow-Up
Normal	< 120 mm Hg	*and*	< 80 mm Hg	Recheck in 2 years
Prehypertension	120–139 mm Hg	*or*	80–89 mm Hg	Recheck in 1 year (if SBP and DBP categories are different, follow shorter time follow-up)
Hypertension - Stage 1	140–159 mm Hg	*or*	90–99 mm Hg	Confirm within 2 months
Hypertension - Stage 2	≥ 160 mm Hg	*or*	> 100 (mm Hg)	Evaluate or refer to source of care within 1 month. For those with higher pressures (e.g., > 180/110 mm Hg), evaluate and treat immediately or within 1 week depending on clinical situation and complications.

Source: Joint National Committee on Prevention, Detection, Evaluation, and Treatment of High Blood Pressure (2003).[25]

and 5 mm Hg for SP and DP, respectively.[37] The ideal cuff size is when the cuff is 20 % wider than the diameter of the arm and bladder length is 80 % of arm girth.[24]

Some cuff manufacturers print a criterion index line by which to determine proper cuff size (review Figure 16.7). For example, the cuff is placed so that the vertical arrow printed on the cuff is over the brachial artery. After the cuff encircles the arm, the index line should fall within the two horizontal range lines; otherwise, the cuff is too small. These index lines can vary considerably among manufacturers. It has been recommended to mark a line on the interior surface of the cuff at a distance of 32 cm from the standard cuff's left border.[37] Table 16.1 provided the proper guidelines for cuff size. Either the larger or smaller cuff may be used for overlapping values found in that table. A distended, bulging, or ballooning bladder is a sign that something is wrong with the manometer.

Controlling the Manometer and Stethoscope

No air spaces should be allowed between the skin and the diaphragm of the stethoscope. By not pressing heavily on the bell or diaphragm, the technician can avoid turbulent blood flow induced by the diaphragm. Turbulence can lower the diastolic pressure reading but is unlikely to distort systolic pressure.[35] The technician should clear the cuff bladder's tubing away from the diaphragm because when they touch each other it sounds much like the Korotkoff sounds.

The technician should place the air bulb deep in the palm of the hand so that the thumb and index finger control the air-release screw. Although an effective method for knowing when to stop inflating the cuff is by palpating the person's radial artery, it can be an awkward procedure. The technician has to take one hand off the stethoscope's diaphragm while palpating the pulse. Often, technicians decrease the pressure too fast. Low systolic and high diastolic readings may occur when the rate of deflation is too fast.[17] Very slow deflation rates should be avoided in order to prevent prolonged discomfort, apprehensiveness, and fidgeting in the participant, all of which may increase the individual's blood pressure. If the person requires a repeated measurement for any reason, the pressure cuff should remain deflated for about 1–2 min between determinations.[24] This will allow the blood in the venous circulation to return to normal.[17]

The meniscus level (the peak of the "hump") at the top of the column of mercury is the measuring point when using *mercury* manometers. The indicating pointer is used for the *aneroid* gauge. If using the mercury manometer, the observer's eyes should be level with the meniscus in order to avoid parallax (angle distortion). When reading the aneroid dial, the observer's eyes should be directly in front of the gauge.

RESULTS AND DISCUSSION

The interpretation of blood pressure is based upon the criteria that have been established by various professional medical groups. These criteria are established from large-scale studies that indicate the norms for that particular population and/or subpopulation, such as African Americans, males, females, and children.

Blood pressure criteria are based upon the contribution of blood pressure to the risk of death from cardiovascular disease—heart attacks, strokes, and congestive heart failure—and kidney damage, blindness, and dementia.[24] The authoritative study groups on blood pressure such as the American Heart Association,[2] the Task Force on Blood Pressure,[47] the Joint National Committee,[24] and National High Blood Pressure Program[39] indicate that the criteria for systolic hypertension and diastolic hypertension are equally important. However, the Joint National Committee indicates that systolic pressure in older adults is a superior predictor of cardiovascular events.[24] Because blood pressure may be affected by nonpathological (nondisease) factors, such as emotions, it is recommended that no one be classified as hypertensive on the basis of only one day's measurements. A person should be classified as hypertensive only when measurements taken on two separate visits are over the established hypertension criteria.[24]

Normal blood pressure is considered systolic blood pressure (SBP) below 120 mm Hg and diastolic blood pressure (DBP) below 80 mm Hg. Typically, the lower the blood pressure, the better. However, if blood pressure gets too low (hypotension), symptoms may develop, including lightheadedness, dizziness, and/or faintness (syncope).[24] Therefore, identifying a particular "optimal blood pressure" is difficult.

The average blood pressure for over 5000 men, ages 20 y to 60 y, who were tested at a fitness clinic was 125/82 mm Hg.[43] These values are probably lower than in a random sample because the men were tested at a fitness clinic and presumably were healthier and more active than average. The average blood pressure for nearly 1000 women of the same age range at the same fitness clinic was 119/78 mm Hg. Descriptive categories for resting blood pressure based on percentile values are shown in Table 16.2. Assuming "average" blood pressure is described as the range of blood pressures from the 30th to the 70th percentile, the average blood pressure for men (age 20–29 y) is 119–130 mm Hg for systolic and 79–84 mmHg for diastolic. For women (age 20–29 y), the average systolic pressure is 107–120 mm Hg and diastolic pressure is 71–80 mm Hg.

The criteria for classifying hypertension in Table 16.3 are based on the Seventh Report of the Joint National Committee on Prevention, Detection, Evaluation and Treatment of High Blood Pressure (JNC7).[25] The values of blood pressure used to determine this classification are systolic and the second diastolic value (5th phase). A **pre-hypertension** category was added in this most recent report described as either a SBP of 120–139 mm Hg or a DBP of 80–89 mm Hg. About 28 % of American adults age 18 and older have prehypertension.[2] The prevalence is higher in men (39.0 %) than in women (23.1 %), and higher in 20–39-year-old African Americans (37.4 %) than in whites (32.2 %) and

Hispanics (30.9 %). **Hypertension** is defined as a SBP $\geq$ 140 mm Hg or a DBP $\geq$ 90 mm Hg.[25,50] All that is necessary to meet the criterion is for either systolic or diastolic pressure to reach the respective value, not necessarily both of them. When only one of the pressures exceeds the criterion it is often referred to as *isolated* systolic (or diastolic) hypertension. A person taking blood pressure medication whose blood pressure is controlled at a level lower than this criterion is still considered hypertensive. Hypertension is further divided into two categories or stages: Stage 1 hypertension is either a SBP of 140–159 mm Hg or a DBP of 90–99 mmHg, and Stage 2 hypertension is a SBP $\geq$ 160 mm Hg or a DBP $\geq$ 100 mmHg. The prevalence of hypertension in the United States by gender, age, and race/ethnicity is seen in Table 16.4. The largest disparity observed is by age group. The prevalence of hypertension increases from 6.7 % in young adults (20–39 y), to 29.1 % in middle-aged adults (40–59 y), to 65.2 % in older adults (> 60 y). Hypertension was considered the primary or contributing cause of death in 11.4 % of all deaths in the United States in 2003[2] mostly through the incidence of heart attack or stroke. About 69 % of people who have a first heart attack are hypertensive (BP > 140/90 mm Hg). Persons with a SBP $\geq$ 160 mm Hg and/or a DBP $\geq$ 95 mm Hg have a relative risk for stroke about four times greater than for those with normal blood pressure. And the economic impact of hypertension is staggering. The direct and indirect cost of hypertension was estimated to reach $63.5 billion in 2006.[2]

Numerous public health initiatives are directed at the detection, prevention, and treatment of high blood pressure, such as the National High Blood Pressure Education Program operated by the National Heart, Lung, and Blood Institute (www.nhlbi.nih.gov/about/nhbpep/). Persons with hypertension should consult with their primary care provider about treatment options, including medication

Table 16.4	Percentage of U.S. Adults with Hypertension by Gender, Age Group, and Race/Ethnicity	
Group	**%**	**(95%CI)**
Gender		
Men	27.8 %	(24.9–29.7)
Women	29.0 %	(27.3–30.8)
Age Group		
20–39 y	6.7 %	(5.3–8.2)
40–59 y	29.1 %	(25.9–32.4)
> 60 y	65.2 %	(62.4–68.0)
Race/Ethnicity		
Hispanic	25.1 %	(23.1–27.1)
White (Non-Hispanic)	27.4 %	(25.3–29.5)
Black (Non-Hispanic)	40.5 %	(38.2–42.8)
Total	28.6%	(26.8–30.4)

Note: Hypertension defined as SBP $\geq$ 140 mm Hg or DBP $\geq$ 90 mm Hg or on antihypertensive medication.
Source: Data from Centers for Disease Control and Prevention (2005).[10]

Table 16.5	Recommended Lifestyle Modifications to Manage Hypertension	
Modification	**Approximate Reduction in Systolic Blood Pressure**	
Weight reduction	5–20 mm Hg	
Adopt DASH eating plan	8–14 mm Hg	
Restrict dietary sodium	2–8 mm Hg	
Increase physical activity	4–9 mm Hg	
Moderate alcohol intake	2–4 mm Hg	

Note: See text for more detailed description of modifications. SBP reduction for weight reduction is per 10 kg weight loss. DASH, Dietary Approaches to Stop Hypertension.
Source: Joint National Committee on Prevention, Detection, Evaluation, and Treatment of High Blood Pressure (2003).[25]

and lifestyle modification. Specific lifestyle modifications that have been found to reduce blood pressure (Table 16.5) include (1) reducing body weight; (2) consuming a diet higher in fruits, vegetables, and low-fat dairy products (the DASH diet); (3) reducing dietary sodium intake to no more than 2.4 g of sodium or 6.0 g of sodium chloride (salt); (4) engaging in regular aerobic exercise and physical activity at least 30 min per day, most days of the week; and (5) limiting alcohol consumption to no more than 2 drinks (1 ounce or 30 ml of alcohol) per day in men and no more than 1 drink per day in women and lighter weight persons.[25]

There are no increased risks for cardiovascular disease in hypotensive persons; in fact, lower pressures reduce the cardiovascular risk.[17] A hypotension criterion of 90 mm Hg is meant only for systolic pressure; there is no accepted criterion for diastolic pressure with respect to hypotension, although less than 60 mm Hg is unusual.[38] As with optimal blood pressure, hypotensive criteria really should be based upon symptoms. Thus, if an individual is experiencing dizziness, syncope, coldness, pallor, nausea, low urine output, and high arterial blood lactates when blood pressure decreases to a certain point, then that point should be the criterion for hypotension for that person.[11]

BOX 16.3	Chapter Preview/Review

What is the purpose of measuring blood pressure?

In what blood vessel is BP most frequently measured?

What are the Korotkoff sounds and how do they relate to the identification of systolic and diastolic BP?

What is pulse pressure and how is it calculated?

What is mean arterial pressure and how is it calculated?

How does limb girth affect cuff size selection?

What are the categories of BP (e.g., normal, prehypertension, etc.) and what are the SBP and DBP criteria that define them?

How is the prevalence (percentage) of hypertension in the United States affected by age and race/ethnicity?

References

1. American College of Sports Medicine. (2000). *ACSM's guidelines for exercise testing and prescription.* Philadelphia: Lippincott Williams & Wilkins.
2. American Heart Association. (2006). Heart disease and stroke statistics—2006 update. A report from the American Heart Association Statistics Committee and Stroke Statistics Subcommittee. *Circulation, January 11, 2006,* epub ahead of print. Available at http://circ.ahajournals.org/cgi/reprint/ CIRCULATIONAHA.105.171600v1. Accessed on January 23, 2006.
3. Belghazi, J., El Feghali, R. N., Moussalem, T., Rejdych, M., & Asmar, R. G. (2007). Validation of four automatic devices for self-measurement of blood pressure according to the International Protocol of the European Society of Hypertension. *Vascular Health and Risk Management, 3,* 389–400.
4. Best, C. H., & Taylor, N. B. (1956). *The human body.* New York: Henry Holt & Co.
5. Blackburn, H., & Jacobs, D. R. (1988). Physical activity and the risk of coronary heart disease. *New England Journal of Medicine, 319,* 1217–1219.
6. Blair, S. N., Kampert, J. B., Kohl, H. W., Barlow, C. E., Paffenbarger, R. S., & Gibbons, L. W. (1996). Influences of cardiorespiratory fitness and other precursors on cardiovascular disease and all-cause mortality in men and women. *JAMA: The Journal of the American Medical Association, 276*(3), 205–210.
7. Blair, S. N., Kohl, H. W., Paffenbarger, R. S., Clark, D. G., Cooper, K. H., & Gibbons, L. W. (1989). Physical fitness and all-cause mortality. A prospective study of healthy men and women. *Journal of the American Medical Association, 262,* 2395–2401.
8. Boyer, J. (1976). Exercise and hypertension. *The Physician and Sportsmedicine, 4*(12), 35–49.
9. Burch, G. E. (1976). *Consultations in hypertension: A clinical symposium.* Rochester, NY: Pennwalt Prescription Products.
10. Centers for Disease Control and Prevention. (2005). Racial/ethnic disparities in prevalence, treatment, and control of hypertension—United States, 1999–2002. *Morbidity and Mortality Weekly Report, 54,* 7–8.
11. daLuz, P. L., Weil, M. H., Liu, V. Y., & Shubin, H. (1974). Plasma volume prior to and following volume loading during shock complicating acute myocardial infarction. *Circulation, 49,* 98–105.
12. Das, B. C., & Mukherjee, B. N. (1963). Variation in systolic and diastolic pressure with changes in age and weight. *Gerontologia, 8,* 92–104.
13. Ekelund, L.-G., Haskell, W. L., Johnson, J. L., Whaley, F. S., Criqui, M. H., & Sheps, D. S. (1988). Physical fitness as a predictor of cardiovascular mortality in asymptomatic North American men. The Lipid Research Clinics' mortality follow-up study. *New England Journal of Medicine, 319,* 1379–1384.
14. Engler, R. L. (1977). Historical and physical findings in patients with aortic valve disease. *Western Journal of Medicine, 126,* 463–467.
15. Estes, S. B. (1977, May). Putting the cuff on hypertensive patients. *Patient Care,* p. 25.
16. Freis, E. D., & Sappington, R. F. (1968). Dynamic reactions produced by deflating a blood pressure cuff. *Circulation, 38,* 1085–1096.
17. Frohlich, E. D., Grim, C., Labarthe, D. R., Maxwell, M. H., Perloff, D., & Weidman, W. H. (1987). *Recommendations for human blood pressure determination by sphygmomanometers: Report of a special task force appointed by the steering committee, American Heart Association.* Dallas: National Center, American Heart Association.
18. Griffen, S. E., Robergs, R. A., & Heyward, V. H. (1977). Blood pressure measurement during exercise: A review. *Medicine and Science in Sports and Exercise, 29,* 149–159.
19. Harrison, E. G., Foth, G. M., & Hines, E. A. (1960). Bilateral indirect and direct arterial pressures. *Circulation, 22,* 419–436.
20. Hasegawa, M., & Rodbard, S. (1979). Effect of posture on arterial pressures, timing of the arterial sounds, and pulse wave velocities in the extremities. *Cardiology, 64,* 122–132.
21. Hashimoto, F., Hunt, W. C., & Hardy, L. (1984). Differences between right and left arm blood pressures in the elderly. *Western Journal of Medicine, 141,* 189–192.
22. Hellerstein, H. K. (1976). Exercise and hypertension. *The Physician and Sportsmedicine, 4*(12), 35–49.
23. Hill, A. V. (1927). *Living machinery.* New York: Harcourt, Brace, & Co.
24. Joint National Committee on Detection, Evaluation, and Treatment of High Blood Pressure. (1997). The sixth report of the Joint National Committee on Detection, Evaluation, and Treatment of High Blood Pressure (JNC VI). NIH Publication No. 98-4080. Bethesda, MD.
25. Joint National Committee on Detection, Evaluation, and Treatment of High Blood Pressure. (2003). Seventh Report of the Joint National Committee on Prevention, Detection, Evaluation, and Treatment of High Blood Pressure (JNC7). *Hypertension, 42,* 1206–1252.
26. Kannel, W. B., Philip, A. W., McGee, D. L., Dawber, T. R., McNamara, P., & Castelli, W. P. (1981). Systolic blood pressure, arterial rigidity, and risk of stroke. *Journal of the American Medical Association, 245,* 1225–1229.
27. Kaplan, N. M. (1983). Hypertension. In N. Kaplan & J. Stannler (Eds.), *Prevention of coronary heart disease. Practical management of risk factors.* Philadelphia: W. B. Saunders.

28. Kaplan, N. M., Deveraux, R. B., Miller, H. S. (1994). Systemic hypertension. *Medicine and Science in Sports and Exercise, 26*(10), S268–S270.

29. King, G. E. (1969). Taking the blood pressure. *Journal of the American Medical Association, 209,* 1902–1904.

30. Kirkendall, W. M., Burton, A. C., Epstein, F. H., & Freis, E. D. (1967). Recommendations for human blood pressure determination by sphygmomanometry. *Circulation, 36,* 980.

31. Lategola, M. T., & Busby, D. E. (1975). Differences between seated and recumbent resting measurements of auscultative blood pressure. *Aviation, Space, & Environmental Medicine, 46,* 1027–1029.

32. Leon, A. S., Connett, J., Jacobs, D. R., & Rauramaa, R. (1987). Leisure time physical activity levels and risk of coronary heart disease and death: The multiple risk factor intervention trial. *Journal of the American Medical Association, 258,* 2388–2395.

33. Li, L., Zhang, X., Yan, C., & Liang, Q. (2008) Validation of the Oregon Scientific BPU 330 for self-monitoring of blood pressure according to the International Protocol. *Vascular Health and Risk Management, 4,* 1121–1125.

34. Lightfoot, J. T., Tuller, B., & Williams, D. F. (1996). Ambient noise interferes with auscultatory blood pressure measurement during exercise. *Medicine and Science in Sports and Exercise, 28,* 502–508.

35. Londe, S., & Klitzner, T. S. (1984). Auscultatory blood pressure measurement—Effect of pressure on the head of the stethoscope. *Western Journal of Medicine, 141,* 193–195.

36. Madhavan, S., Ooi, W. L., Cohen, H., & Alderman, M. H. (1994). Relation of pulse pressure reduction to the incidence of myocardial infarction. *Hypertension, 24,* 368.

37. Manning, D. M., Kuchirka, C., & Kaminski, J. (1983). Miscuffing: Inappropriate blood pressure cuff application. *Circulation, 68,* 763–766.

38. Milnor, W. R. (1968). Normal circulatory function. In V. B. Mountcastle (Ed.), *Medical physiology I* (pp. 118–133). St. Louis: Mosby.

39. National High Blood Pressure Education Program Working Group. (1993). Report on primary prevention of hypertension. *Archives of Internal Medicine, 153,* 186–208.

40. O'Brien, E., Asmar, R., Beilin, L., Imai, Y., Mancia, G., et al. (2005). European Society of Hypertension Working Group on Blood Pressure Monitoring. Practice guidelines of the European Society of Hypertension for clinic, ambulatory and self blood pressure measurement. *Journal of Hypertension, 23,* 697–701.

41. O'Brien E., Pickering, T., Asmar, R., Myers, M., Parati, G., et al. (2002). Working Group on Blood Pressure Monitoring of the European Society of Hypertension International Protocol for validation of blood pressure measuring devices in adults. *Blood Pressure Monitoring, 7,* 3–17.

42. Peters, R. K., Cady, L. D., Bischoff, D. P., Bernstein, L., & Pike, M. C. (1983). Physical fitness and subsequent myocardial infarction in healthy workers. *Journal of the American Medical Association, 249,* 3052–3056.

43. Pollock, M. L., Wilmore, J. H., & Fox, S. M. (1978). *Health and fitness through physical activity.* Santa Barbara, CA: John Wiley & Sons.

44. Powell, K. E., Thompson, P. D., Caspersen, C. J., & Kendrick, J. S. (1987). Physical activity and the incidence of coronary heart disease. *Annual Review of Public Health, 8,* 253–287.

45. Robinson, T. E., Sue, D. Y., Huszczuk, A., Weiler-Ravell, D., & Hansen, J. E. (1988). Intra-arterial and cuff blood pressure responses during incremental cycle ergometry. *Medicine and Science in Sports and Exercise, 20,* 142–149.

46. Slattery, M. L., Jacobs, D. R., & Nichaman, M. Z. (1989). Leisure time physical activity and coronary heart disease death: The U.S. railroad study. *Circulation, 79,* 304–311.

47. Task Force on Blood Pressure Control in Children. (1987). Report of the task force on blood pressure control in children. *Pediatrics, 79,* 1–25.

48. Walther, R. J., & Tifft, C. P. (1985). High blood pressure in the competitive athlete: Guidelines and recommendations. *The Physician and Sportsmedicine, 13*(3), 93–114.

49. Webster, J., Newnham, D., Petrie, J. C., & Lovell, H. G. (1984). Influence of arm position on measurement of blood pressure. *British Medical Journal, 288,* 1574–1575.

50. WHO/ISH. (1983). Guidelines for the treatment of mild hypertension. Memorandum from a WHO/ISH meeting. *Hypertension, 5,* 394–397.

Probably won't be much on resting blood pressure on the quiz

Form 16.1

NAME _____ DATE _____ SCORE _____

RESTING BLOOD PRESSURE

Homework

Gender: **M**   Initials: **AA**   Age (y): **22**   Height (cm): **175**   Weight (kg): **80.0**

Type of manometer: [X] Mercurial   [ ] Aneroid   Body position: [X] Seated   [ ] Stand   [ ] Supine

Limb: [X] R arm   [ ] L arm   Limb girth (cm): **30**   Cuff: [ ] Child [ ] Adult [ ] Large adult

	First tester, Initials: **BB**			Second tester, Initials: **CC**		
	SBP (1st)	DBP (4th)	DBP (5th)	SBP (1st)	DBP (4th)	DBP (5th)
Trial 1	132	82	74	124	86	80
Trial 2	136	82	78	132	82	74
Average *	/	/				

* Average of all measurements taken.

Pulse pressure (PP) = SBP (1st) - DBP (5th) = _____ - _____ = _____ mmHg

Mean arterial pressure (MAP) = DBP (5th) + (PP/3) = _____ + _____ = _____ mmHg

Percentile category (Table 16.2): SBP _____   DBP _____

BP category (Table 16.3): _____   Follow-Up: _____

Evaluation of resting blood pressure: _____

_____

_____

Gender: **F**   Initials: **DD**   Age (y): **22**   Height (cm): **155**   Weight (kg): **52.0**

Type of manometer: [X] Mercurial   [ ] Aneroid   Body position: [X] Seated   [ ] Stand   [ ] Supine

Limb: [X] R arm   [ ] L arm   Limb girth (cm): **23**   Cuff: [ ] Child [ ] Adult [ ] Large adult

	First tester, Initials: **EE**			Second tester, Initials: **FF**		
	SBP (1st)	DBP (4th)	DBP (5th)	SBP (1st)	DBP (4th)	DBP (5th)
Trial 1	118	72	72	120	80	80
Trial 2	112	76	70	116	78	74
Average *	/	/				

* Average of all measurements taken.

Pulse pressure (PP) = SBP (1st) - DBP (5th) = _____ - _____ = _____ mmHg

Mean arterial pressure (MAP) = DBP (5th) + (PP/3) = _____ + _____ = _____ mmHg

Percentile category (Table 16.2): SBP _____   DBP _____

BP category (Table 16.3): _____   Follow-Up: _____

Evaluation of resting blood pressure: _____

_____

_____

Form 16.2
RESTING BLOOD PRESSURE

NAME _____ DATE _____ SCORE _____

Lab Results

Gender: _____ Initials: _____ Age (y): _____ Height (cm): _____ Weight (kg): _____

Type of manometer: ☐ Mercurial ☐ Aneroid Body position: ☐ Seated ☐ Stand ☐ Supine

Limb: ☐ R arm ☐ L arm Limb girth (cm): _____ Cuff: ☐ Child ☐ Adult ☐ Large adult

First tester, Initials: _____   Second tester, Initials: _____

	SBP (1st)	DBP (4th)	DBP (5th)		SBP (1st)	DBP (4th)	DBP (5th)
Trial 1	_____	/ _____	/ _____		_____	/ _____	/ _____
Trial 2	_____	/ _____	/ _____		_____	/ _____	/ _____
Average *	_____	/ _____	/ _____				

* Average of all measurements taken.

Pulse pressure (PP) = SBP (1st) - DBP (5th) = _____ - _____ = _____ mmHg

Mean arterial pressure (MAP) = DBP (5th) + (PP/3) = _____ + _____ = _____ mmHg

Percentile category (Table 16.2): SBP _____ DBP _____

BP category (Table 16.3): _____ Follow-Up: _____

Evaluation of resting blood pressure: _____

_____

_____

Gender: _____ Initials: _____ Age (y): _____ Height (cm): _____ Weight (kg): _____

Type of manometer: ☐ Mercurial ☐ Aneroid Body position: ☐ Seated ☐ Stand ☐ Supine

Limb: ☐ R arm ☐ L arm Limb girth (cm): _____ Cuff: ☐ Child ☐ Adult ☐ Large adult

First tester, Initials: _____   Second tester, Initials: _____

	SBP (1st)	DBP (4th)	DBP (5th)		SBP (1st)	DBP (4th)	DBP (5th)
Trial 1	_____	/ _____	/ _____		_____	/ _____	/ _____
Trial 2	_____	/ _____	/ _____		_____	/ _____	/ _____
Average *	_____	/ _____	/ _____				

* Average of all measurements taken.

Pulse pressure (PP) = SBP (1st) - DBP (5th) = _____ - _____ = _____ mmHg

Mean arterial pressure (MAP) = DBP (5th) + (PP/3) = _____ + _____ = _____ mmHg

Percentile category (Table 16.2): SBP _____ DBP _____

BP category (Table 16.3): _____ Follow-Up: _____

Evaluation of resting blood pressure: _____

_____

_____

EXERCISE BLOOD PRESSURE

It is just as important to measure blood pressure at exercise as it is to measure heart rate. If only heart rate is measured, blood pressure is neglected as a contributor to the total power output of the heart. The consideration of both heart rate and blood pressure provides a better estimate of myocardial oxygen consumption than heart rate alone, and the calculation of the rate-pressure product provides an indication of the heart's power output.[10,37]

The measurement of systolic pressure during progressive exercise may provide input toward diagnosing heart disease[57] and may reveal potential problems in persons who show exaggerated increases in exercise blood pressure despite being normotensive in a resting state.[18,35,36] Conversely, decreases in systolic blood pressure, despite increases in exercise intensity, may be clinically significant if accompanied by cardiac ischemia or chest pain.[2]

The pulse pressure—the difference between systolic and diastolic pressure—provides the basis for calculating mean pressure at exercise. Lastly, the measurement of blood pressure during recovery from exercise may lead to the prevention of syncope (fainting) in the exercise participant.

PHYSIOLOGICAL RATIONALE

Numerous factors may affect blood pressure at exercise. These include characteristics of the exercise participants, such as their age, muscle mass, fitness level, and smoking status. Also, the type of exercise may affect blood pressure.[59] For example, weight lifting in five 22–28-year-old body builders increased intra-arterial blood pressure during leg presses to 355 mm Hg over 281 mm Hg.[11] This is 2–3 times higher than in rhythmical aerobic exercise, such as cycling or walking. Differences are found even among types of aerobic exercise; cycling, for example, elicits higher blood pressures than treadmill exercise.[31,48] Additionally, the exercise protocol itself may affect the rate of increase and absolute levels of blood pressure during exercise.

Pressure, in physics, is the product of flow and resistance. Blood pressure then is mainly a function of cardiac output (flow) and total peripheral resistance (resistance). As a result, blood pressure can be mathematically determined as the product of cardiac output (Q) and total peripheral resistance (TPR), as seen in Equation 17.1a. For example, a resting blood pressure of 120/80 mm Hg could be the product of Q (or blood flow) and TPR, as seen in Equations 17.1b

and 17.1c. An increase in either Q or TPR results in higher blood pressures, while a decrease in either results in a decrease in pressures.

Blood pressure = Cardiac output * Total
peripheral resistance   Eq. 17.1a

Assume: Cardiac output (flow) during systole = **6** L·min^{-1}

Assume: Cardiac output (flow) during diastole = **4** L·min^{-1}

Assume: Total peripheral resistance = **20** mm Hg^{-1}·L·min^{-1}

Systolic blood pressure = **6** L·min^{-1}
* **20** mm Hg^{-1}·L·min^{-1} = **120** mm Hg   Eq. 17.1b

Diastolic blood pressure = **4** L·min^{-1}
* **20** mm Hg^{-1}·L·min^{-1} = **80** mm Hg   Eq. 17.1c

Blood Pressure During Aerobic Exercise

Systolic blood pressure (SBP) increases linearly with increasing exercise intensity,[3,56] while diastolic blood pressure (DBP) changes very little,[9,13,16] when measured by noninvasive sphygmomanometry. The responses in SBP and DBP occur as a result of changes in Q and TPR. Cardiac output increases significantly during graded exercise as a result of increases in heart rate and stroke volume. The increase in Q leads to an increase in blood flow entering the arterial system. Much of the increase in flow (and pressure) is "absorbed" by the elasticity of the aorta and large arteries. These elastic vessels act to "dampen" the changes in blood flow and ultimately in blood pressure, which is sometimes referred to as the *Windkessel effect.* Table 17.1 and Figure 17.1 are included to explain why SBP rises and DBP remains unchanged in a "normal" person during graded exercise on a cycle ergometer. As the power increases, there is a significant rise in blood flow entering the arterial system. Most of this increase in flow occurs during systole. But even during diastole, there is a small increase in blood flow as a result of the recoil of the large arteries. The rise in systolic blood flow creates a rise in SBP even with the concurrent drop observed in TPR due to vasodilation of the large arteries (Table 17.1). The drop in TPR reduces or limits the maximal SBP reached during exercise. Theoretically, if the TPR remained *unchanged* at 20 units (*which it does not*), but blood flow could still increase from 6 L·min^{-1} to 42 L·min^{-1} during systole (*which it would not*), the SBP would increase to 840 mm Hg, likely resulting in a lot of burst blood vessels.

Table 17.1 **Cardiac Output (Q), Total Peripheral Resistance (TPR), and Blood Pressure Responses to Graded Exercise in Normal Persons and Persons with Higher Total Peripheral Resistance**

Status	SBP—Normal			DBP—Normal			SBP—High TPR			DBP—High TPR		
	Q	TPR	SBP	Q	TPR	DBP	Q	TPR	SBP	Q	TPR	SBP
Rest	6.0 *	20.0 =	**120**	4.0 *	20.0 =	**80**	6.0 *	25.0 =	**150**	4.0 *	25.0 =	**100**
50 W	15.0 *	10.0 =	**150**	8.0 *	10.0 =	**80**	15.0 *	12.5 =	**188**	8.0 *	12.5 =	**100**
100 W	24.0 *	7.0 =	**168**	11.5 *	7.0 =	**81**	24.0 *	8.8 =	**210**	11.5 *	8.8 =	**101**
150 W	33.0 *	5.5 =	**182**	14.5 *	5.5 =	**80**	33.0 *	6.9 =	**227**	14.5 *	6.9 =	**100**
200 W	42.0 *	4.5 =	**189**	18.0 *	4.5 =	**81**	42.0 *	5.6 =	**236**	18.0 *	5.6 =	**101**
Recovery	15.0 *	9.0 =	**135**	9.0 *	9.0 =	**81**	15.0 *	11.3 =	**169**	9.0 *	11.3 =	**101**

Note: Values are estimated and "idealized" for the purpose of illustration. Persons with elevated total peripheral (TPR) are assumed to have the same cardiac output (Q) and blood flow as "normal" persons but a 25 % higher TPR due to atherosclerosis.

The rise in blood flow during diastole (due to the Windkessel effect) is much less than during systole. In fact, the rise in diastolic blood flow is almost equally offset by the drop in TPR. Together this means that DBP remains virtually unchanged from rest to maximal aerobic exercise (Figure 17.1) in healthy people with normal vascular resistance.

Atherosclerosis is a disease process that slowly thickens arterial walls such that it starts to narrow the inside lumen of the vessel, resulting in an increase in vascular resistance or TPR. Therefore, persons with elevated TPR due to cardiovascular disease, assuming they still have the same Q, would be expected to have both a higher SBP and DBP (Table 17.1 and Figure 17.1). Blood pressure responses during graded exercise to maximum can provide important information relative to the status of the arterial system.

Another use of SBP is to combine it with heart rate to yield a variable referred to as double product or *rate-pressure product* (RPP). The power output or work required of the heart during exercise depends on both the rate of pumping (HR) and the load or resistance (SBP) against which it pumps. Therefore, the RPP reflects how hard the heart is working. The value of RPP is supported by its close correlation with measured myocardial oxygen consumption.[2,20,40] RPP is calculated as the mathematical product of HR and SBP (Eq. 17.2a). In this equation, the product is divided by 100 to reduce the value to a convenient unit[54] and so that it parallels the oxygen consumption (mL·min^{-1}) of the heart. For example, a heart rate of 150 bpm combined with an SBP of 200 mm Hg yields a RPP of 300 (Eq. 17.2b). Not all references, however, divide by 100. In numerous instances in the literature, RPP is expressed simply as the product of HR and SBP.

Rate-pressure product (RPP) = HR (bpm)
    * SBP (mm Hg) / 100   Eq. 17.2a

Assume: HR = **150** bpm and SBP = **200** mm Hg

RPP = **150** * **200** / 100 = **300**   Eq. 17.2b
(*Note:* RPP is usually "unitless.")

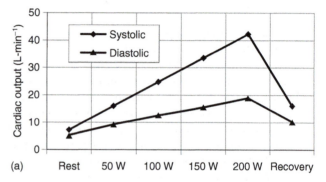

(a)

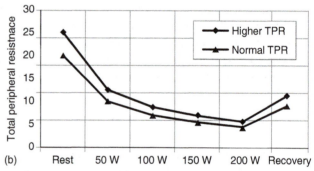

(b)

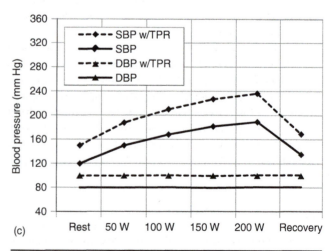

(c)

Figure 17.1 Responses in: (a), cardiac output (Q); (b), total peripheral resistance (TPR); and (c), systolic and diastolic blood pressure in "normal" persons and in persons with 25 % higher TPR.

As mentioned in Chapter 16, mean arterial pressure (MAP) is determined from DBP and pulse pressure (PP). It was calculated at rest as DBP + (PP/3) due to the time or fractions of the cardiac cycle spent in systole and diastole. The issue is more complicated during exercise due to the variations in the cardiac cycle causing the time spent in systole and diastole to vary widely. For this reason, some recommend that MAP not be determined during exercise or that it be determined differently. One study recommends that the calculation of MAP be modified during exercise as DBP + (PP/2), with the pulse pressure being calculated from either the first DBP (phase 4) or second DBP (phase 5) when using a cuff.[55]

METHODS

The measurement of blood pressure during exercise is a common measurement in an exercise laboratory. However, the technique is one of the most difficult to master, requiring many trials before the technician becomes confident. Although standards exist for measuring *resting* blood pressure, no such standards exist for *exercise* blood pressure.[25]

As expected, there are many similarities between the measurement of blood pressure at rest and at exercise. The differences include minor adjustments to the blood pressure technique and a more intense concentration on the fourth phase (muffling). During exercise it is not unusual for the vibrations to be heard even near zero levels[43] due to enhanced vasodilation at exercise.[22] Thus, the fifth phase is not a valid indicator of diastolic pressure during exercise tests in some people. For this reason, the American Heart Association recommends the recording of the fourth phase for exercise testing.[23] See Box 17.1 for a discussion on the accuracy of exercise blood pressure measurements.

If the participant tenses the arm while the technician is taking the blood pressure, it will cause large oscillations in the aneroid pointer or the mercury column. Presumably, this is due to the changes in upper arm circumference as the muscles contract and relax. Thus, it is very important to promote muscle relaxation of the participant's arm (Figure 17.2). Also, it is important to clear the antecubital space for the placement of the stethoscope's diaphragm. Sometimes the cuff will slide toward the elbow during exercise, or the bladder's rubber tubes will interfere with the antecubital space. Some researchers advise placing the cuff so that the tubing runs along the back of the upper arm rather than the front, especially during treadmill exercise.

Contraindicative Blood Pressure

Another consideration in measuring blood pressure at exercise is whether to perform the exercise test in the first place. The term *contraindicative* means that for some people "the risks of exercise testing outweigh the potential benefits."[2] For example, the risk is greater than the benefit

---

BOX 17.1 | **Accuracy and Calibration of Exercise Blood Pressure Measurements**

Reliability

Although various investigators have not supported high reliabilities in automated blood pressure methods,[4,5,41,50] including the measurement of diastolic blood pressure during recovery,[36] some have concluded that a few automated devices are a suitable alternative to human auscultatory methods.[25,42]

Validity

The ability to measure exercise blood pressure accurately is complicated by the noise of the equipment and movement of the participant. Although the indirect noninvasive measurement of systolic pressure has been reported to be satisfactory,[47] it appears that the noninvasive cuff method of measuring systolic pressure underestimates the invasive direct measure of systolic pressure anywhere from 8 mm Hg[30,45] up to 11 mm Hg[55] or 15 mm Hg[30] during aerobic exercise.

One group of investigators[55] found that the intra-arterial diastolic pressures exceeded the noninvasive fourth and fifth phases for diastolic pressure by 5 mm Hg and 13 mm Hg, respectively. This supports the use of the indirectly measured fourth phase as the most valid diastolic pressure during exercise. Their correlations between intra-arterial pressures and cuff pressures were 0.95 and 0.84 for systolic and diastolic (fourth phase) pressures, respectively. However, the fourth phase is not as clearly distinguishable as the fifth phase.

One group of reviewers recommended manual or automated sphygmomanometry to measure systolic pressure if the goal is to estimate the rate-pressure product.[25]

---

of exercise testing for someone who has just had a heart attack or someone with uncontrolled erratic heart rhythm accompanied by disturbing symptoms. Some authorities suggest that exercise testing is contraindicated if resting systolic BP is greater than 165–180 mm Hg or diastolic BP is greater than 95–100 mm Hg.[51] The American College of Sports Medicine (2000) takes a more liberal view by having no *absolute* contraindication criteria for blood pressure but providing *relative* contraindicative criteria. This means that if resting systolic pressure is greater than 200 mm Hg or diastolic pressure is greater than 110 mm Hg, the risk-benefit ratio must be evaluated before exercise testing.[2]

Protocol for Exercise Blood Pressure

Two multistage cycling protocols are presented in Table 17.2. Technicians usually find it easier to measure blood pressure when participants cycle than when they walk or run on a treadmill. In order to prescribe an appropriate exercise protocol, consideration should be given to the participant's fitness level. An exercise interval of at least 3 min should assure a steady state at each stage.[43] The exercise period starts at 25 or 50 W, depending upon the fitness level of the participant. Power levels are increased by 25–50 W after each 3 min interval. Until the technician gains considerable confidence, repeated measures should be taken throughout the test; only the pressures measured within the last 30–60 s of each power level, however, need to be recorded. In order to calculate the rate-pressure product (RPP), the heart rate must be measured by either another technician with a stethoscope or by a heart-rate monitor.

Summary of Procedures

The major differences in the technique for measuring blood pressure at exercise versus at rest are the following: (a) the technician must support the exerciser's arm; (b) greater listening concentration is required due to the noise of the ergometer; and (c) the muffling point (phase 4) is used

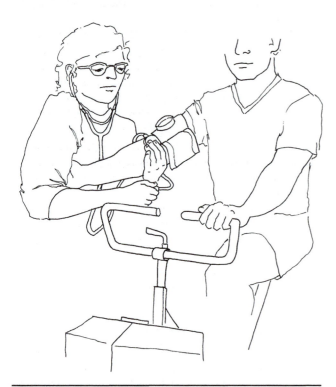

Figure 17.2 An appropriate position for the technician and participant while blood pressure is being measured at pre-exercise or during exercise.

| Table 17.2 | Cycle Ergometer Protocols for Measuring Exercise Blood Pressure |

Status	Time (min)	Average Fitness	Above-Average Fitness
Exercise			
Stage 1	0:00–3:00	25 W	50 W
Stage 2	3:00–6:00	75 W	100 W
Stage 3	6:00–9:00	100 W	150 W
Stage 4	9:00–12:00	125–150 W	200 W
Recovery	0:00–3:00	25–50 W	25–50 W

sometimes as the primary indicator of diastolic pressure at exercise.[55,60] The procedural steps for measuring blood pressure are as follows.

Pre-Exercise

1. With the participant seated on the cycle ergometer, place the participant's arm between your elbow and the side of your body (Figure 17.2) to provide support and maintain the arm in an extended position. If using the treadmill, assume a similar position with the participant's arm between your elbow and side of the body.
2. Follow the procedural steps in Chapter 16 to obtain resting or baseline blood pressures (with the participant seated on the ergometer or standing on the treadmill) as summarized below.

   a. Choose the appropriate cuff based on limb girth.
   b. Place the cuff snugly around the arm above the antecubital space.
   c. Increase the pressure in the cuff to 160 mm Hg, or 20 mm Hg above the expected value, or 20–30 mm Hg above the disappearance of the palpated radial pulse.
   d. Allow the cuff pressure to decrease at a rate of 2–3 mm Hg per second.
   e. Record in even numbers the values for SBP, DBP (phase 4), and DBP (phase 5).

   Note: It is not necessary to record DBP (phase 4), it is frequently difficult to distinguish.

Exercise

3. If resting blood pressure is elevated, it should be determined whether exercise is contraindicated.
4. Begin the exercise protocol. (*Note:* The stages are described as 3 min in duration, but they can be extended in this case to allow the tester, especially if inexperienced, more time to complete the measurement of blood pressure, and to allow for a second tester.)
5. Have the participant exercise for about 2 min at each stage to allow blood pressure to stabilize before taking the measurement.
6. Use the same procedural steps as described in Step 2 for resting blood pressure with the following modifications.
   a. Increase the pressure in the cuff to 200 mm Hg (or higher), or 20–40 mm Hg above the expected value. (*Note:* Because SBP increases with exercise, the pressure in the cuff must be increased sufficiently to occlude the brachial artery.)
   b. Allow the cuff pressure to decrease at a faster rate of 5–6 mm Hg per second.[49] (*Note:* The rate of cuff deflation is important. If deflated too rapidly, the values may be underestimated. If deflated too slowly, too many extraneous sounds may be heard and it is uncomfortable for the participant.)

7. Record in even numbers the values for SBP, DBP (phase 4), and DBP (phase 5) obtained within the last portion (30–60 s) of each exercise stage.
   Note: It is not necessary to record DBP (phase 4), it is frequently difficult to distinguish.

8. If rate-pressure product (RPP) is to be determined, HR and SBP must be recorded simultaneously.

9. Continue the exercise protocol for as many stages (up to four) as the participant can comfortably complete. If exercise blood pressure is elevated, or if signs of exertional intolerance are observed (e.g., dizziness, nausea), stopping the exercise at that point may be indicated.

Recovery

10. Measure blood pressures for several minutes (or as long as necessary) into recovery to ensure that the participant is recovering appropriately.

11. Record in even numbers the values for SBP, DBP (phase 4), and DBP (phase 5) obtained during recovery.
    Note: This is where students should concentrate on listening for and recording DBP (phase 4).

Graph

12. On Form 17.2, graph SBP and the first DBP (phase 4) and/or second DBP (phase 5) against power level (W) at each stage to observe how blood pressure responds to graded exercise.

RESULTS AND DISCUSSION

The responses of systolic and diastolic blood pressure to submaximal and maximal graded exercise reveal a lot about the physical nature of the participant's arterial system. Whenever possible, blood pressure should be measured during any graded exercise test. Abnormal or unexpected changes (e.g., exaggerated rise in SBP or DBP) can occur in persons without prior warning or symptoms.

Blood Pressure at Submaximal Aerobic Exercise

Even before exercise begins, persons anticipating the exercise test may have a systolic pressure about 10 mm Hg higher than their normal resting pressure.[14] Theoretically, systolic pressure is expected to increase somewhat linearly during aerobic cycling by approximately 10 mm Hg[44] or 15 mm Hg[3] for each 50 W increase in cycling power level. One group of investigators reported a rate of increase of 18 mm Hg per 50 W based on a 30 mm Hg increase per liter increase in oxygen consumption on less active persons monitored by intra-arterial catheter.[55]

During treadmill exercise, one might expect a 10 mm Hg ($\pm$ 2) increase per MET increase.[2] One MET corresponds to a relative oxygen consumption of 3.5 ml·kg^{-1}·min^{-1}.

It would be unusual for exercise heart rate to exceed systolic pressure in young adults. A hypertensive response in treadmill exercise may be indicated when systolic pressure increases at a rate greater than 20 mm Hg per MET,[19] or per 0.25 L·min^{-1} oxygen consumption. If systolic pressure fails to increase at all with progressive exercise, or actually decreases, it may be a sign of coronary artery disease[57] or a high risk indication.[1,2,21]

More variability exists regarding diastolic pressure changes than systolic pressure changes during exercise. Fifth-phase diastolic pressure usually decreases or stays the same in healthy persons.[2] Part of this variability may be attributed to the method of measuring diastolic pressure. One group concluded that the noninvasive fifth-phase diastolic pressure decreases slightly from rest to heavy cycling by only 3 mm Hg, but the fourth-phase cuff pressure and intra-arterial diastolic pressure increases from rest through maximal cycling by about 7–11 mm Hg per liter of oxygen consumed.[55]

Some researchers report decreases in fifth-phase diastolic pressure with progressive exercise in highly fit persons.[9,46] Others claim that a normal fifth-phase diastolic pressure response to exercise is one that does not increase by more than 10 mm Hg[18] to 15 mm Hg.[57] During treadmill exercise, many healthy persons show slight increases in diastolic pressure of no more than 10 mm Hg during the first couple of minutes, followed by a progressive reduction into the peak exercise period.[12] Others report a slight decrease or no change in diastolic pressure in healthy men during treadmill exercise.[62]

The mean arterial pressures (MAP) of healthy sedentary males and females (17–29 y) were determined at 50 W and 60 % $\dot{V}O_2$max, respectively. The 95 males averaged a MAP of 94 ($\pm$ 9.1) mm Hg and 105 ($\pm$ 9.9) mm Hg, respectively. The 134 females' MAPs were 90 ($\pm$ 9.7) mm Hg and 101 ($\pm$ 12.0) mm Hg, respectively.[61]

Blood Pressure at Maximal Aerobic Exercise

Quite often it is impossible to get a technically reliable blood pressure measurement while the participant is exercising at or near maximal intensity. In these cases, the blood pressure should be taken immediately after exercise with precautions taken to avoid postural (orthostatic) syncope in the participant; usually, this would mean easy walking on the treadmill or easy pedaling on the ergometer. The peak blood pressure may be slightly underestimated by waiting to take blood pressure immediately after exercise, rather than during exercise.[32]

Maximal systolic pressure can be quite variable, ranging from 150 mm Hg to 250 mm Hg in men and women,[9] with an average in a normal young adult of about 182 mm Hg[15] up to 200 mm Hg.[28] This concurs with other investigators who reported a maximal systolic pressure of 194 ($\pm$ 20) mm Hg for running on the treadmill.[17] Normotensive middle-aged persons reach maximal systolic pressures

Table 17.3	Peak Blood Pressure in Healthy Men and Women During Maximal Treadmill Testing				
	Men (N = 7863)		Women (N = 2406)		
	SBP	DBP	SBP	DBP	
Age (y)	M (SD)	M (SD)	M (SD)	M (SD)	
20–29	182 (21)	71 (12)	156 (20)	70 (12)	
30–39	184 (20)	76 (12)	160 (22)	74 (11)	
40–49	188 (21)	80 (12)	167 (23)	78 (11)	
50–59	193 (23)	83 (12)	177 (24)	81 (12)	
60–69	197 (24)	84 (12)	186 (24)	81 (13)	

Source: Data from Daida, et al. (1996).[15]

between 180 mm Hg and 190 mm Hg.[10] Table 17.3 provides the mean systolic and diastolic pressures at peak exercise during treadmill testing of males and females 18–69 y of age. Men's pressures were higher than women's pressures and were directly related to age.[15] If systolic blood pressure exceeds 240 mm Hg, it may indicate a susceptibility for developing resting hypertension.[38]

Sometimes during an exercise test, the blood pressure reaches a level that calls for termination of the test. A systolic pressure greater than 260 mm Hg is a general indication by ACSM for stopping the test in a low-risk person.[2] Ruptures have occurred in the blood vessels of experimental animals when systolic pressures were between 260 and 280 mm Hg.[29] Others suggest caution and consider it a hypertensive response if the systolic pressure exceeds 220 mm Hg.[8,12] Some consider the exercise response as hypertensive if the systolic pressure increases by more than 96 mm Hg from the resting level, and as hypotensive if the systolic pressure does not increase more than 33 mm Hg at maximal exercise.[52]

Caution may be prudent when the participant's exercise diastolic pressure reaches 95 mm Hg.[8] However, the ACSM's indication for halting the test for low-risk adults is when DP exceeds 115 mm Hg.[2]

Typical mean arterial pressures at maximal exercise are approximately 130 mm Hg, but may reach as high as 155 mm Hg.[9] A large group (*n* = 95) of 17–29-year-old males' MAP averaged 122 mm Hg at maximal cycling exercise. The average MAP for the females (*n* = 134) of the same age was 117 mm Hg.[61]

Blood Pressure During Recovery from Aerobic Exercise

Blood pressure often returns to the pre-exercise level within 5–8 min after the cessation of moderate exercise.[34,44,56] It is not unusual for systolic pressure to drop slightly lower than the pre-exercise systolic pressure[6,27,28,39] and remain lower for several hours.[2] For example, from the 5th to the 60th,[38] or up to the 90th min[6] of recovery from treadmill walking, systolic blood pressure was slightly lower (8–12 mm Hg)

than it was preceding exercise, possibly due to endorphin-like (opioid) effects.[7]

Usually, diastolic pressure during recovery remains similar to pre-exercise. The return of blood pressure to resting levels is affected by the type, intensity, and duration of the original exercise in addition to the type of recovery. For example, it requires more than 3 min for blood pressure to return to normal after heavy cycling exercise (85 % $\dot{V}O_2max$) if the cyclist recovers with unloaded pedaling at a slow rate.[55] However, if the participant were to stand upright immediately after the same exercise, it is quite possible that blood pressure would drop rapidly and drastically. Venous pooling of blood in the legs would reduce the blood flow to the brain and possibly lead to syncope. Postexercise hypotensive symptoms are most likely after bouts of exercise lasting 30 min or more. Recovery hypotension is due to various factors besides venous pooling, such as cessation of muscle pump during passive recovery, loss of plasma volume due to sweating, reduced venous return, and reduced vasoconstriction.[26]

Rate-Pressure Product

Rate-pressure product (RPP), the mathematical product of HR and SBP, as mentioned previously, provides an estimate or prediction of myocardial oxygen consumption[2,10,20,37,40] and reflects the metabolic load on the heart. A study of 1623 healthy men and women ranging in age from 20–70 y reported mean RPP values at rest of 75.2 ± 17.5, and for maximal treadmill exercise (using a Bruce protocol) of 328.0 ± 44.7.[33] This 4-fold increase in RPP implies a 4-fold increase in myocardial oxygen consumption at maximal exercise. Comparative data for RPP in healthy men and women can be found in Table 17.4. Similar values for RPP during maximal exercise have been reported in men (341 ± 55) and in women (281 ± 37).[10] RPP is believed to be related to physical fitness in healthy persons. Fit persons have been found to have a lower resting RPP and a higher maximal RPP.[33]

Rate-pressure product is used in clinical settings to assess myocardial perfusion and to monitor exercise intensity in persons who experience chest pain (angina) or significant daily fluctuations in blood pressure. RPP at peak exercise in patients with heart disease and coronary ischemia (insufficient blood flow) is lower than expected and is related to an increased risk of mortality.[53] Many patients with heart disease who experience chest pain do so at a repeatable RPP.[24] This allows appropriate exercise intensity to be determined and monitored by the use of RPP. On the other hand, RPP at peak exercise can be much higher than expected in persons with hypertension when they work at high exercise intensities. The RPP attained during exercise can be used to determine and monitor exercise intensity, especially in persons where exercise BP fluctuates from day to day. For example, if an RPP of 200 is desired and prescribed for a workout, the participant would be limited to

Table 17.4
Table 17.4 Comparative Data for Rate Pressure Product (RPP), Maximal Heart Rate (MHR), and Systolic Blood Pressure (SBP) during Treadmill Exercise

| | At Rest | | During Maximal Exercise | | | | | |
| | Men | Women | Men | | | Women | | |
Category	RPP	RPP	MHR	SBP	RPP	MHR	SBP	RPP
Much higher than ave	> 103	> 108	> 197	> 225	> 404	> 198	> 210	> 376
Higher than average	87 – 103	93 – 108	187 – 197	204 – 225	363 – 404	188 – 198	188 – 210	335 – 376
Average	63 – 86	70 – 92	171 – 186	173 – 203	305 – 362	171 – 187	155 – 187	275 – 334
Lower than average	45 – 62	53 – 69	160 – 170	151 – 172	263 – 304	160 – 170	132 – 154	232 – 274
Much lower than ave	< 45	< 53	< 160	< 151	< 263	< 160	< 132	< 232
Mean	**74.2**	**80.4**	**177.8**	**187.5**	**333.1**	**178.5**	**170.4**	**303.6**

Source: Data from Hui, Jackson & Wier (2000).[33] *Note:* Based on 1341 men and 282 women. RPP, rate pressure product; MHR, maximal heart rate (bpm); SBP, systolic blood pressure (mmHg). Maximal exercise values were recorded during treadmill exercise using a Bruce protocol.

a HR of 100 bpm if simultaneously the SBP was measured at 200 mmHg. However, on another day, if SBP remained lower at 180 mmHg, HR could be allowed to increase to 111 bpm, also resulting in an RPP of 200. Theoretically, the heart would be stressed to the same degree on each day, working at the same myocardial oxygen uptake, as indicated by the same RPP.

BOX 17.2 Chapter Preview/Review

How is blood pressure defined mathematically?

How does systolic blood flow and SBP respond to graded exercise? Why does it respond this way?

How does diastolic BP respond to graded exercise? Why does it respond this way?

What is the effect of increased TPR on SBP and DBP during graded exercise?

What levels of SBP and DBP contraindicate exercise?

How is rate-pressure product (RPP) calculated? What does it represent? How does it respond to graded exercise?

References

1. American Association of Cardiovascular and Pulmonary Rehabilitation. (1999). *Guidelines for cardiac rehabilitation and secondary prevention programs.* Champaign, IL: Human Kinetics.

2. American College of Sports Medicine (2009). *ACSM's guidelines for exercise testing and prescription, 8th ed.* Philadelphia: Lippincott Williams & Wilkins.

3. Andersen, K. L., Shephard, R. J., Denolin, H., Varnauskas, E., & Masironi, R. (1971). *Fundamentals of exercise testing.* Geneva: World Health Organization.

4. Barker, W. F., Hediger, M. L., Katz, S. H., & Bowers, E. J. (1984). Concurrent validity studies of blood pressure instrumentation. *Hypertension, 6,* 85–91.

5. Becque, M. D., Katch, V., Marks, C., & Dyer, R. (1993). Reliability within subject variability of VE, V̇O₂, heart rate and blood pressure during submaximum cycle ergometry. *International Journal of Sports Medicine, 14,* 220–223.

6. Bennett, T., Wilcox, R. G., & MacDonald, I. A. (1984). Postexercise reduction of blood pressure in hypertensive men is not due to an acute impairment of baroreflex function. *Clinical Science, 67,* 97–103.

7. Boone, J. B., Levine, M., Flynn, M. G., Przza, F. Y., Kubitz, E. R., & Andres, F. F. (1992). Opioid receptor modulation of postexercise hypotension. *Medicine and Science in Sports and Exercise, 24,* 1108–1113.

8. Boyer, J. (1976). Exercise and hypertension. *The Physician and Sportsmedicine, 4*(12), 35–49.

9. Brooks, G. A., & Fahey, T. D. (1984). *Exercise physiology: Human bioenergetics and its application.* New York: John Wiley & Sons.

10. Bruce, R. A. (1977). Current concepts in cardiology: Exercise testing for evaluation of ventricular function. *New England Journal of Medicine, 296,* 671–675.

11. Carswell, H. (1984). Brief reports. Headaches: A weighty problem for lifters? *The Physician and Sportsmedicine, 12*(7), 23.

12. Chung, E. K. (1983). *Exercise electrocardiography—A practical approach.* Baltimore: Waverly Press.

13. Clarke, D. H. (1975). *Exercise physiology.* Englewood Cliffs, NJ: Prentice-Hall.

14. Cooper, C. B. (2000). Blood pressure measurement, hypertension and endurance exercise. *ACSM's Health and Fitness Journal, 4,* 32–33.

15. Daida, H., Allison, T. G., Squires, R. W., Miller, T. D., & Gau, G. T. (1996). Peak exercise blood pressure stratified by age and gender in apparently healthy subjects. *Mayo Clinic Proceedings, 71,* 445–452.

16. deVries, H. A. (1986). *Physiology of exercise for physical education and athletics.* Dubuque, IA: Wm. C. Brown.

17. Dishman, R. K., Patton, R. W., Smith, J., Weinberg, R., & Jackson, A. (1987). Using perceived exertion to prescribe and monitor exercise training heart rate. *International Journal of Sports Medicine, 8,* 208–213.

18. Dlin, R. A., Hanne, N., Silverberg, D. S., & Bar-Or, O. (1983). Follow-up of normotensive men with exaggerated blood pressure response to exercise. *American Heart Journal, 106,* 316–320.

19. Dressendorfer, R. H. (1980, July). *ACSM workshop manual,* p. 110.

20. Edington, D. W., & Cunningham, L. (1975). *Biological awareness.* Englewood Cliffs, NJ: Prentice-Hall.

21. Fletcher, G. F., Balady, G., Froelicher, V. F., Hartley, L. H., Haskell, W. L., & Pollock, M. L. (1995). Exercise standards: A statement for health care professionals from the American Heart Association. *Circulation, 91,* 580–615.

22. Frohlich, E. D., Grim, C., Labarthe, D. R., Maxwell, M. H., Perloff, D., & Weidman, W. H. (1987). *Recommendations for human blood pressure determination by sphygmomanometers: Report of a special task force appointed by the steering committee, American Heart Association.* Dallas: National Center, American Heart Association.

23. Frohlich, E. D., Grim, C., Labarthe, D. R., Maxwell, M. H., Perloff, D., & Weidman, W. H. (1988). Recommendations for human blood pressure determination by sphygmomanometers: Report of a special task force appointed by the steering committee. *Hypertension, 11,* 210A–222A.

24. Gobel, F. L., Nordstrom, L. A., Nelson, R. R., Jorgensen, C. R., & Wang, Y. (1977). The rate-pressure product as an index of myocardial oxygen consumption during exercise in patients with angina pectoris. *Circulation, 57,* 549–556.

25. Griffin, S. A., Robergs, R. A., & Heyward, V. H. (1997). Blood pressure measurement during exercise: A review. *Medicine and Science in Sports and Exercise, 29,* 149–159.

26. Halliwill, J. R. (2001). Mechanisms and clinical implications of post-exercise hypotension in humans. *Exercise and Sport Sciences Reviews, 29,* 65–70.

27. Hannum, S. M., & Kasch, F. W. (1981). Acute postexercise blood pressure response of hypertensive and normotensive men. *Scandinavian Journal of Sport Science, 3,* 11–15.

28. Hayberg, J. M., Montain, S. J., & Martin, W. H. (1987). Blood pressure and hemodynamic responses after exercise in older hypertensives. *Journal of Applied Physiology, 63,* 270–276.

29. Hellerstein, H. K. (1976). Exercise tests inadequate for cardiac patients. *The Physician and Sportsmedicine, 4*(8), 58–62.

30. Henschel, A., De la Vega, F., & Taylor, H. L. (1954). Simultaneous direct and indirect blood pressure measurements in man at rest and work. *Journal of Applied Physiology, 6,* 506–512.

31. Hermansen, L., Ekblom, B., & Saltin, B. (1970). Cardiac output during submaximal and maximal treadmill and bicycle exercise. *Journal of Applied Physiology, 29,* 82–86.

32. Hollingsworth, V., Bendick, P., & Franklin, B. (1988). Validity of postexercise arm ergometer blood pressures? *Medicine and Science in Sports and Exercise, 20* (Suppl. 2), Abstract #435, S73.

33. Hui, S. C., Jackson, A. S., & Wier, L. T. (2000). Development of normative values for resting and exercise rate pressure product. *Medicine and Science in Sports and Exercise, 32,* 1520–1527.

34. Hyman, A. S. (1971). Cardiorespiratory endurance. In ACSM (Eds.), *Encyclopedia of sport sciences and medicine* (pp. 1067–1070). New York: Macmillan.

35. Jette, M., Landry, F., Sidney, K., & Blumchen, G. (1988). Exaggerated blood pressure response to exercise in the detection of hypertension. *Journal of Cardiopulmonary Rehabilitation, 8,* 171–177.

36. Jette, M., Landry, F., Tiemann, B., & Blumchen, G. (1991). Ambulatory blood pressure and Holter monitoring during tennis play. *Canadian Journal of Sport Science, 16,* 40–44.

37. Jorgensen, C. R. (1972). Physical training and myocardial function. *New England Journal of Medicine, 287,* 104–105.

38. Kaplan, N. M., Deveraux, R. B., & Miller, H. S. (1994). Systemic hypertension. *Medicine and Science in Sports and Exercise, 26*(10), S268–S270.

39. Kaufman, F. L., Hughson, R. L., & Schaman, J. P. (1987). Effect of exercise on recovery blood pressure in normotensive and hypertensive subjects. *Medicine and Science in Sports and Exercise, 19,* 17–20.

40. Kitamura, K., Jorgensen, C. R., Gobel, F. L., Taylor, H. L., & Wang, Y. (1972). Hemodynamic correlates of myocardial oxygen consumption during upright exercise. *Journal of Applied Physiology, 32,* 516–522.

41. Labarthe, D. R. (1976). New instruments for measuring blood pressure. *Drugs, 11* (Suppl. I), 48–51.

42. Lightfoot, J. T., Tankersley, C., Rowe, S. A., Freed, A. N., & Fortney, S. M. (1989). Automated blood pressure measurements during exercise. *Medicine and Science in Sports and Exercise 21,* 698–707.

43. Lightfoot, J. T., Tuller, B., & Williams, D. F. (1996). Ambient noise interferes with auscultatory blood pressure measurement during exercise. *Medicine and Science in Sports and Exercise, 28,* 502–508.

44. Michael, E. D., Burke, E. J., & Avakian, E. V. (1979). *Laboratory experiments in exercise physiology.* Ithaca, NY: Mouvement.

45. Morehouse, L. E., & Miller, A. T. (1976). *Physiology of exercise.* St. Louis: Mosby.

46. Nagle, F. J. (1975, May). *Conducting the progressive exercise test.* Symposium at the 22nd Annual American College of Sports Medicine Convention, New Orleans.

47. Nagle, F. J., Naughton, J., & Balke, B. (1966). Comparison of direct and indirect blood pressure with pressure-flow dynamics during exercise. *Journal of Applied Physiology, 21,* 317–320.

48. Niederberger, M., Bruce, R., Kusumi, F., & Whitkanack, S. (1974). Disparities in ventilatory and circulatory responses to bicycle and treadmill exercise. *British Heart Journal, 36,* 377–382.

49. Nieman, D. C. (1995). *Fitness and sports medicine: A health-related approach.* Palo Alto, CA: Bull.

50. O'Brien, E., Fitzgerald, D., & O'Malley, K. (1985). Blood pressure measurement: Current practice and future trends. *British Medical Journal, 290,* 729–733.

51. Pollock, M. L., Wilmore, J. H., & Fox, S. M. (1978). *Health and fitness through physical activity.* Santa Barbara, CA: John Wiley & Sons.

52. Pyfer, H. R., Mead, W. F., Frederick, R. C., & Doane, B. L. (1976). Exercise rehabilitation in coronary heart disease: Community group programs. *Archives of Physical Medicine and Rehabilitation, 57,* 335–342.

53. Rasmussen, K., Juul, S., Bagger, J. P., & Henningsen, P. (1987). Usefulness of ST deviation induced by pronlonged hyperventilation as a predictor of cariac death in angina pectoris. *American Journal of Cardiology, 59,* 763–768.

54. Robinson, B. F. (1967). Relation of heart rate and systolic blood pressure to the onset of pain in angina pectoris. *Circulation, 35,* 1073–1083.

55. Robinson, T. E., Sue, D. Y., Huszczuk, A., Weiler-Ravell, D., & Hansen, J. E. (1988). Intra-arterial and cuff blood pressure responses during incremental cycle ergometry. *Medicine and Science in Sports and Exercise, 20,* 142–149.

56. Ruddell, H., Berg, K., Todd, G. L., McKinney, M. E., Buell, T. C., & Eliot, R. S. (1985). Cardiovascular reactivity and blood chemical changes during exercise. *Journal of Sports Medicine, 25,* 111–119.

57. Sheps, D. S., Ernst, J. C., Briese, F. W., & Myerburg, R. J. (1979). Exercise-induced increase in diastolic pressure: Indicator of severe coronary artery disease. *The American Journal of Cardiology, 43,* 708–712.

58. Singh, J. P., Larson, M. G., Manolio, T. A., O'Donnell, C. J., Lauer, M., Evans, J. C., & Levy, D. (1999). Blood pressure response during treadmill testing as a risk factor for new-onset hypertension. *Circulation, 99,* 1831–1836.

59. Tuxen, D. V., Sutton, J., Upton, A., Sexton, A., McDougal, D., & Sale, D. (1983). Brainstem injury following maximal weight lifting attempts. *Medicine and Science in Sports and Exercise, 15* (Abstract), 158.

60. Walther, R. J., & Tifft, C. P. (1985). High blood pressure in the competitive athlete: Guidelines and recommendations. *The Physician and Sportsmedicine, 13*(3), 93–114.

61. Wilmore, J. H., Stanforth, P. R., Gagnon, J., Rice, T., Mandel, S., Leon, A. S., Rao, D. C., Skinner, J. S., & Bouchard, C. (2001). Heart rate and blood pressure changes with endurance training: The HERITAGE Family Study. *Medicine and Science in Sports and Exercise, 33,* 107–116.

62. Wolthius, R. A., Froelicker, V. F., Fischer, J., & Triehwasser, J. H. (1977). The response of healthy men to treadmill exercise. *Circulation, 55,* 153–157.

Form 17.1

EXERCISE BLOOD PRESSURE

NAME _____ DATE _____ SCORE _____

Homework (Done)

Record blood pressure at rest, in response to increasing power levels, and during recovery.

Gender: **M**   Initials: **AA**   Age (y): **22**   Height (cm): **178**   Weight (kg): **81.0**

Power (W)		HR (bpm)	SBP (1st)		DBP (4th)		DBP (5th)	RPP
			Tester Initials		**BB**			
	Resting BP	78	110	/	80	/	70	
50	(25-50 W)	102	122	/	82	/	70	
100	(75-100 W)	130	140	/	80	/	66	
150	(100-150 W)	164	166	/	80	/	70	
200	(150-200 W)	185	184	/	84	/	70	
	Recovery BP	126	110	/	74	/	50	

Plot blood pressure versus power level. Label SBP and DBP (4th) and/or DBP (5th).

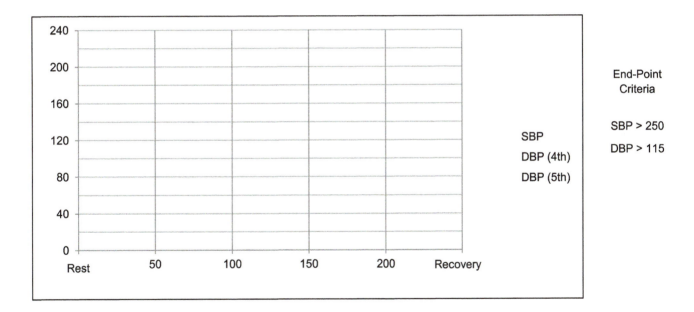

SBP
DBP (4th)
DBP (5th)

End-Point Criteria

SBP > 250
DBP > 115

Category for: Resting RPP _____   Maximal RPP _____   *(Table 17.4)*

Evalution of exercise blood pressure: _____

_____

_____

_____

_____

Form 17.2

NAME _____ DATE _____ SCORE _____

EXERCISE BLOOD PRESSURE

Lab Results

Record blood pressure at rest, in response to increasing power levels, and during recovery.

Gender: _____ Initials: _____ Age (y): _____ Height (cm): _____ Weight (kg): _____

Tester Initials
_____

Power (W)		HR (bpm)	SBP (1st)	DBP (4th)	DBP (5th)	RPP
	Resting BP	_____	____ / ____	____ / ____	_____
_____	(25-50 W)	_____	____ / ____	____ / ____	_____
_____	(75-100 W)	_____	____ / ____	____ / ____	_____
_____	(100-150 W)	_____	____ / ____	____ / ____	_____
_____	(150-200 W)	_____	____ / ____	____ / ____	_____
	Recovery BP	_____	____ / ____	____ / ____	_____

Plot blood pressure versus power level. Label SBP and DBP (4th) and/or DBP (5th).

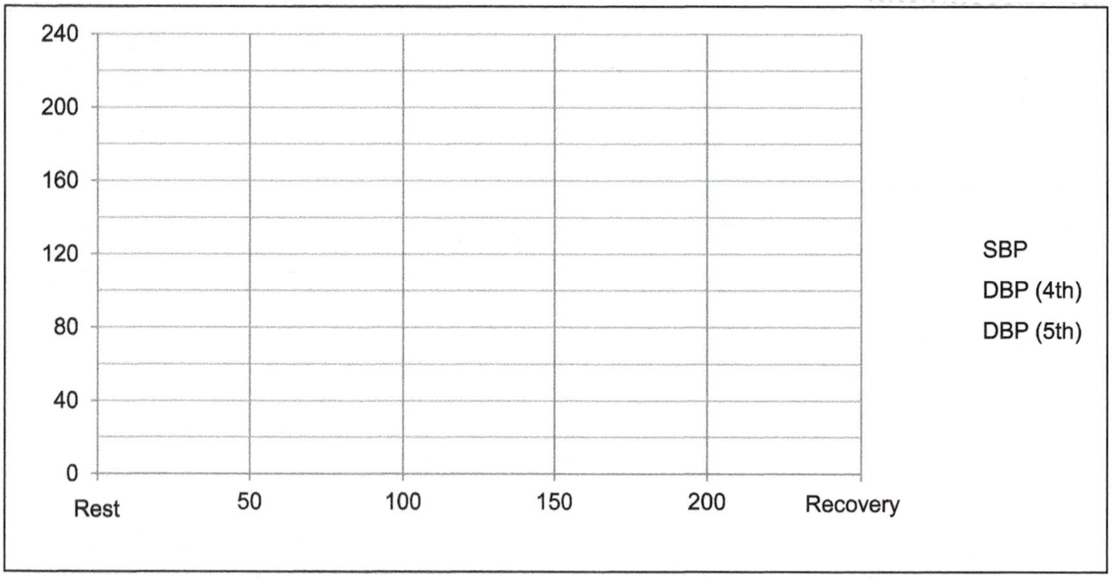

SBP
DBP (4th)
DBP (5th)

End-Point Criteria

SBP > 250
DBP > 115

Category for: Resting RPP _____   Maximal RPP _____   (Table 17.4)

Evelution of exercise blood pressure: _____

_____

_____

_____

_____

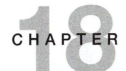

RESTING ELECTROCARDIOGRAM

The diagnosis of the electrocardiogram (ECG) is one of the most important and accurate evaluations of the quantity and quality of heartbeats. Although 4 million electrocardiograms may have been interpreted by computer in the United States in 1975, that still leaves 76 million that were interpreted by the human brain.[8] An Englishman was the first (1887) to record electrical current from the human body's surface,[1,3] but it was a Dutchman, Willem Einthoven, who received the Nobel Prize in 1924 for his 1901 "elektrokardiograph" (EKG) because of his more sophisticated instrument and his publications on electrocardiography.[5] Although the electrocardiogram is widely known as a clinical test, it has been used numerous times by physiologists and kinesiologists to quantify resting and exercise heart rates accurately.

PHYSIOLOGICAL RATIONALE

The **electrocardiogram** is a graphical recording of the electrical current generated in the electrical conductive system of the heart (Figure 18.1). Each electrical signal or impulse originates in the sinus node, also called the sinoatrial (SA) node. This signal electrically stimulates (depolarizes) the atria and passes into the atrioventricular (AV) node, where it is delayed for about 0.1 s. It then passes rapidly down the left and right bundle branches, which terminate in the Purkinje fibers that carry the signals into the myocardium (heart muscle), where they lead to the depolarization and contraction of the ventricles. These electrical signals or electrical currents can be detected by attaching electrodes to the surface of the chest. The voltage from an ordinary flashlight battery is about 1500 times greater than the skin's voltage.[9] Voltage is an electromotive force that causes a current to flow between two points (electrodes). The electrodes transfer the current from the skin to the **electrocardiograph,** where it is graphically recorded as the electrocardiogram.

Three characteristics of the electrical signals can be determined based on the size and shape of the deflections

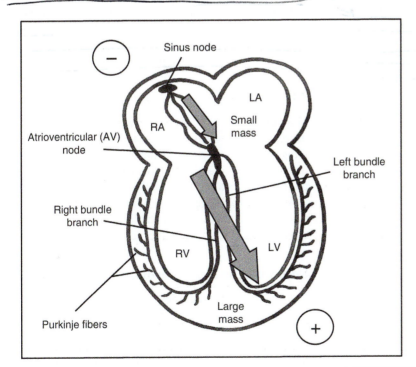

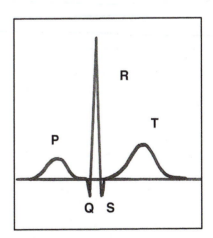

P wave: Atrial depolarization
QRS complex: Ventricular depolarization
T wave: Ventricular repolarization

Figure 18.1 Conduction of electrical signals through the electrical conductive system of the heart. The signals move slowly through a small mass in the atria, creating a small, round, upright wave (P wave) representing atrial depolarization. The signals move rapidly through a large mass in the ventricles, creating a large, upright spike (R wave) representing ventricular depolarization. The final large, rounded upright wave (T wave) represents ventricular repolarization.

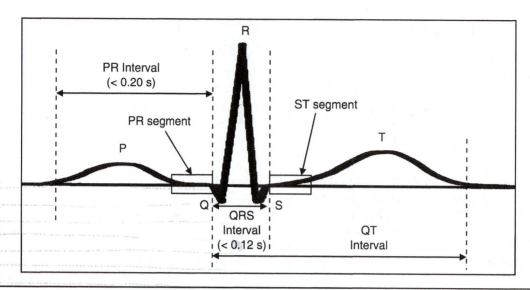

Figure 18.2 Demonstration of ECG intervals including PR interval (< 0.20 s), QRS interval (< 0.12 s), and QT interval, which vary depending on heart rate; and ECG segments including PR segment and ST segment.

on the ECG: (1) the *direction* in which the signal is moving, (2) the *speed* at which the signal is moving, and (3) the *mass* of the tissue through which the signal is moving. When the signal is moving toward the positive electrode, it creates an upright deflection (wave) on the ECG. When it is moving away from the positive electrode, it creates an inverted deflection. When there is no movement of the current, there is neither an upright nor inverted deflection; thus the tracing remains at baseline and is termed isoelectric.[14] A slow-moving signal creates a rounded wave, whereas a fast-moving signal creates a sharp wave or spike. And in general, small waves are generated when the signal is moving through a small mass (i.e., the atria); large waves are generated when it passes through a large mass (i.e., the ventricles). Therefore, in Figure 18.1, as the initial signal passes slowly through the atria (represented by the arrow) toward the positive electrode, it creates a small, rounded upright wave (the P wave) that represents atrial depolarization. Next there is a brief pause as the signal is delayed inside the AV node. The signal then very rapidly passes down the bundle branches and out the Purkinje fibers. This rapid signal moving through the large ventricles toward the positive electrode creates a large, upright spike (the R wave). On either side of the R wave, there are typically small downward deflections, referred to as the Q wave and the S wave, that represent early and late ventricular depolarization. The three waves (Q, R, and S waves) are usually referred to collectively as the QRS complex, which represents ventricular depolarization. The ventricles then repolarize (T wave) back to their original conditions so that they can subsequently depolarize and contract again.

Other important characteristics of the ECG are shown in Figure 18.2. The height of the deflections can be measured to help determine whether any hypertrophy (enlargement) of the heart exists. Tall P waves can indicate atrial

hypertrophy, and tall R waves can indicate ventricular hypertrophy. Also of interest are specific time intervals that can be measured and interpreted. The PR interval (normally < 0.20 s in duration) indicates the time for atrioventricular conduction; the QRS interval (normally < 0.12 s in duration) indicates the time for intraventricular conduction; and the QT interval is related to the length of time required for the ventricles to repolarize. The ST segment is also of importance because its displacement above or below the isoelectric baseline can be clinically significant. ST segment depression is potentially indicative of myocardial ischemia (lack of blood flow) and hypoxia (lack of oxygen).

METHODS

This section not only describes the methods used to record the electrocardiogram, but provides further detail on identifying and explaining the 12 standard ECG leads, determining heart rate, identifying sinus rhythms, and screening the ECG for ectopic beats and ST segment changes. The information in this chapter is limited and is intended only to gain a fundamental understanding of the electrical events occurring in a healthy heart.

Recording the Electrocardiogram

The ECG can be recorded for various reasons, and as such, the complexity with which it is recorded varies. The simplest ECG records only a single lead (or one view) by attaching two or three electrodes to the torso of the participant. Originally, reusable silver electrodes were placed on the limbs (wrists and ankles). Although this can still be done today, the more common practice is to place disposable electrodes (to limit infection or the transmission of disease) on the torso instead of the limbs (so as not to interfere

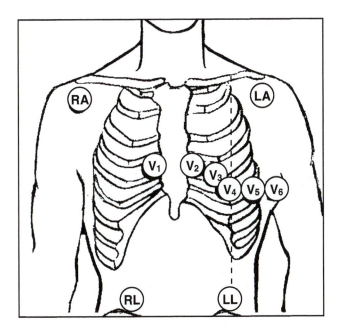

Anatomical sites for location of electrodes:

V₁	Fourth intercostal space, right sternal border
V₂	Fourth intercostal space, left sternal border
V₃	Midway between V₂ and V₄
V₄	Fifth intercostal space, midclavicular line
V₅	Level with V₄, anterior axillary line
V₆	Level with V₅, midaxillary line

Figure 18.3 Typical placement of the 10 electrodes necessary to record the standard 12-lead ECG, with description of anatomical sites for electrode location.

with the ability to exercise). The single-lead ECG is adequate in apparently healthy participants to monitor and record heart rate, to screen for ectopic beats, and to look for signs of ischemia. The ECG becomes more diagnostic and more useful in persons suspected to have coronary heart disease (CHD) if a full 12-lead ECG is recorded. This requires placing 10 electrodes at specific locations on the torso of the participant (Figure 18.3).

Identifying the ECG Leads

If the full 12-lead ECG is recorded, the leads are described as follows. Four of the 10 electrodes attached to the torso (or attached to the actual four limbs) are used to record the **limb leads,** or extremity leads. These electrodes are referred to by the limb to which they attach (or that they represent if attached to the torso), including the right arm (RA), left arm (LA), right leg (RL), and left leg (LL). The right leg electrode acts as a ground to eliminate electrical interference from the ECG. The limb leads can be further distinguished as *standard* limb leads and *augmented* limb leads. The three standard limb leads (designated I, II, and III) are bipolar leads that use the combination of the RA, LA, and LL electrodes to sense differences in electric potential

between two limbs or two points on the torso. The three augmented limb leads (designated aVR, aVL, aVF) compare a central point of the standard limb leads to the RA, LA, and LL electrodes, creating unipolar augmented voltage (aV) leads. In doing so, the voltage or amplitude of these leads is about 50 % greater than the standard limb leads.[5] So, the augmented lead using the RA electrode is aVR, and the lead using the LA electrode is aVL. The lead using the LL electrode is called aVF ("F" stands for "foot" represented by the left leg, since the "L" abbreviation was already taken). These six leads provide six different views (all rotated 30° from one another) of the electrical activity of the heart in a frontal plane (Figure 18.4). The remaining six standard leads are referred to as the **chest leads,** or precordial leads, because the six electrodes used to record them are placed on the precordium, the surface of the chest overlying the heart. Chest electrodes are positioned vertically relative to intercostal spaces (between ribs) and horizontally according to the sternum, clavicle, and axilla (armpit). The six unipolar chest leads are referred to as V₁ through V₆ (Figure 18.4) and provide a cross-sectional, or transverse, view of the electrical activity of the heart. An example of what each of the 12 leads looks like in a standard 12-lead ECG is seen in Figure 18.5.

The 12-lead ECG is used primarily in clinical situations where there is interest in helping identify myocardial ischemia, atrial and/or ventricular hypertrophy, atrial and/or ventricular rhythm, conduction disturbances, and more. If the main purpose of the ECG is simply to monitor and record heart rate in apparently healthy (or low-risk) adults, then recording a single-lead ECG using only two or three electrodes is sufficient. One of the more commonly used leads is Lead II because it typically yields the largest deflections. Even when using only one lead, it is still possible to screen for ectopic beats and ST segment depression. A sample of a single-lead ECG is shown in Figure 18.6. Pay particular attention to the details of the ECG paper. Each small square is 1 mm, and each large square (identified by the darker, thicker line) is 5 mm. When the ECG paper is run at 25 mm·s⁻¹, which is standard, each 1 mm square is 0.04 s and each 5 mm square is 0.20 s. Vertically, each 1 mm square is 0.1 mV, so that two 5 mm squares (or 10 small squares) combined is 1.0 mV. A 12-lead ECG may be used for this lab, but Form 18.2 is designed to use a single-lead ECG recording.

Determining Heart Rate

In most situations where an electrocardiograph is being used, heart rate (HR) will be displayed digitally. When a digital display is not available, heart rate can be determined by different methods. Some brands of ECG paper have short vertical "tick marks" across the top of the paper, spaced 75 mm apart, so that when the paper is run at 25 mm·s⁻¹, the marks are 3 s apart. To determine HR, count the number of R waves that occur within the

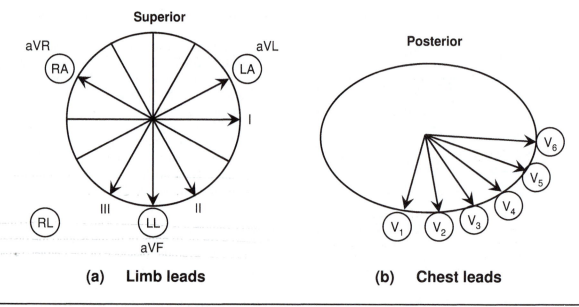

Superior

aVR
aVL

RA
LA

I

III
II

RL
LL

aVF

(a) Limb leads

Posterior

V₆
V₅
V₄
V₁ V₂ V₃

(b) Chest leads

Figure 18.4 Demonstration of (a) six limb leads (three standard leads, I, II, and III; and three augmented leads, aVR, aVL, and aVF) and (b) six chest leads (V_1, V_2, V_3, V_4, V_5, and V_6).

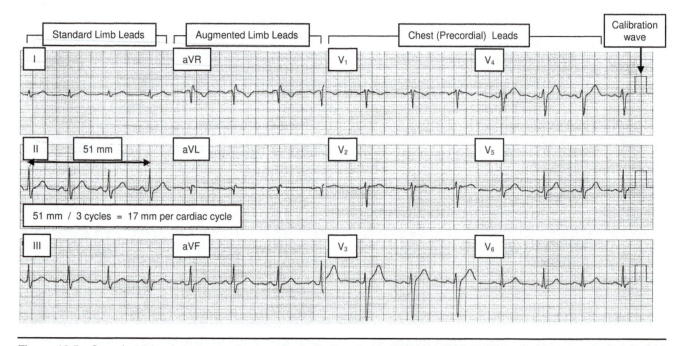

Standard Limb Leads   Augmented Limb Leads   Chest (Precordial) Leads   Calibration wave

I   aVR V_1 V_4

II   51 mm   aVL V_2 V_5

51 mm / 3 cycles = 17 mm per cardiac cycle

III   aVF V_3 V_6

Figure 18.5 Sample 12-lead electrocardiogram. Typically the standard limb leads (I, II, III) are the first recorded, followed by the augmented limb leads (aVR, aVL, aVF), followed by the first three chest leads (V_1–V_3), the last three chest leads (V_4–V_6), and finally by a calibration wave. Notice in Lead II, the distance between four consecutive R waves is measured at 51 mm, which means the average distance for one cardiac cycle is 17 mm. This means that the heart rate in this ECG is 1500 mm·min^{-1} / 17 mm·beat^{-1}, or 88 bpm (rounded to the nearest whole number).

3 s time interval and then multiply this number by 20 to convert it into a HR in beats·min^{-1} (bpm). It is also appropriate (and probably preferred) to count the number of R waves in double the time (6 s) and multiply by 10 to convert it into a HR (Figure 18.6). This is directly analogous to palpating a radial or carotid pulse and counting the

number of pulses that occur in 3 s or 6 s and multiplying by 20 or 10, respectively.

Another method to determine HR involves measuring the average distance (in mm) of one cardiac cycle. This can be done using any number of cardiac cycles. In the ECG shown in Figure 18.6, the average of three cardiac cycles was

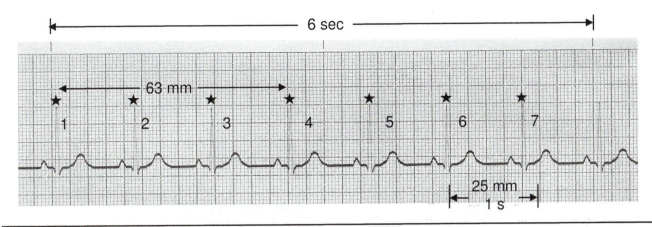

Figure 18.6 Heart rate (HR) can be determined in various ways. In this example it is determined by counting 7 R waves in 6 s (denoted by the vertical "tick" marks) and multiplying by 10 to yield a HR of 70 bpm; or by measuring the distance between 4 R waves (3 cardiac cycles) as 63 mm, dividing this by 3 to give the "average" distance of the cardiac cycle (21 mm), which can then be used to calculate HR as 1500 / 21 = 71 bpm.

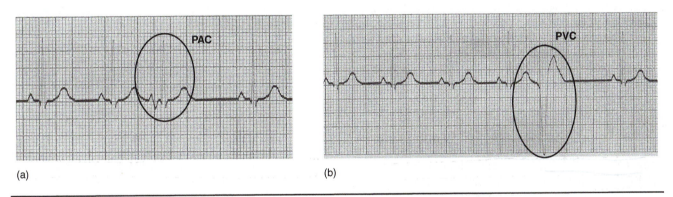

Figure 18.7 ECG demonstrating two ectopic beats that arise from outside the sinus node as seen in (a) premature atrial contraction (PAC) arises from the atria; and (b) premature ventricular contraction (PVC) arises from the ventricles, causing a "wide, bizarre" QRS complex.

determined by measuring the distance between four consecutive R waves, 63 mm, and dividing by 3 to yield an average of 21 mm. This average distance is then used to calculate HR, as seen in Equation 18.1a. The 1500 value is the horizontal length (mm) of a 1 min section of the ECG; so there are 1500 mm·min^{-1}. The R–R distance is the average time required for one beat—in mm·beat^{-1}. So, for this example, since the average distance of one cardiac cycle is 21 mm, then by Equation 18.1b, the HR would be 71 bpm. This method, because it uses only three cardiac cycles, is susceptible to error when the heart rate is variable (i.e., quickly speeds up and slows down) or the person has an irregular heart rhythm.

Heart rate (bpm) = 1500 mm·min^{-1}
  / R–R distance (mm·beat^{-1})

Where: 1500 is the horizontal length in mm of a
  1 min section (1500 mm·min^{-1})

Assume: R–R distance = **21** mm   Eq. 18.1a

Heart rate (bpm) = 1500 / **21** = **71** bpm
  (*rounded to the nearest whole beat*)   Eq. 18.1b

Normal Sinus Rhythm and Ectopic Beats

When all beats come from the sinus node, a person is said to be in a **sinus rhythm**. It is further referred to as normal sinus rhythm if the heart rate is between 60 and 100 bpm. A sinus rhythm with HR < 60 bpm is classified as a sinus **bradycardia** (slow HR), whereas a sinus rhythm with HR > 100 bpm is labeled a sinus **tachycardia** (high HR). Sinus bradycardia is common for trained persons whose resting HR is below 60 bpm. Sinus tachycardia occurs every time a person exercises and the heart rate exceeds 100 bpm, assuming it is still a sinus rhythm.

Occasionally, a beat can originate from somewhere outside the sinus node, and when it does it is referred to as an **ectopic beat.** Typically these beats occur prematurely, before the normal sinus beat, and are therefore referred to as premature beats or contractions. In most cases, it is possible to distinguish whether the ectopic beat arose from the atria (or AV node) or from the ventricles. Look carefully at Figure 18.7 for any beats that appear to occur earlier than expected. Then look at the

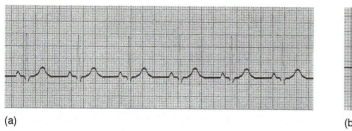

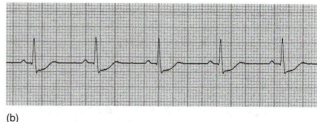

(a)   (b)

Figure 18.8 ECG demonstrating the difference between (a) a normal ST segment and (b) ST segment depression.

shapes of the P wave and the QRS complex of any prematurely occurring beats. If the P wave is abnormally shaped (or missing), but the shape of the QRS complex is normal, it indicates that the beat came from the atria (or AV node) and is known as a **premature atrial contraction (PAC)** or an atrial premature beat (APB). The abnormal P wave is created by the electrical signal passing through the atria in an abnormal direction, because it did not originate in the sinus node. Because the signal then goes through the AV node and down the bundle branches in a normal fashion, the QRS complex still looks normal. When the signal originates in a ventricle, it no longer follows the electrical conductive system, but instead is transmitted across the cardiac cells. This leads to a "wide, bizarre" QRS complex for that one ectopic beat, which is called a **premature ventricular contraction (PVC),** or a ventricular premature beat (VPB). When the number of ectopic beats begins to exceed the number of sinus beats, the person is no longer in a sinus rhythm but is in an atrial or ventricular rhythm (which will not be explained further in this laboratory manual).

ST Segment Changes

The last characteristic of the ECG discussed in this manual is related to the ST segment, that portion of the ECG from the end of the QRS complex to the beginning of the T wave. Myocardial injury (which occurs during an acute heart attack) can displace the ST segment above the isoelectric and lead to *ST elevation.* Myocardial ischemia (lack of blood flow to the heart) displaces the ST segment downward, causing *ST depression.* The more severe the ST depression gets, the more likely it is that the participant truly does have ischemia and coronary heart disease. ST segment changes can be observed in Figure 18.8.

Procedures for Recording the ECG

The procedures described here for recording the electrocardiogram are general. Because of the wide variety of electrocardiographs available, it is not practical to give specific directions regarding one particular ECG. A brief description of the procedures for calibrating the ECG

| BOX 18.1 | Calibration of the Electrocardiograph |

The electrocardiograph (*the instrument*) is used to produce the electrocardiogram (*the printed result*) or the ECG. The ECG is printed on special paper which allows the technician to check the calibration of the ECG machine. ECG paper consists of small (1 mm) boxes that are "grouped" into large (5 mm) boxes, with a large box consisting of 25 small boxes. When the paper is run at the standard speed (25 mm·s^{-1}), 1 small box represents 0.04 s and 1 large box represents 0.20 s in duration. The height of the boxes represents the voltage recorded on the ECG paper. A deflection that is 1 mm tall (one small box) represents a 0.1 millivolt (mV) input signal, while a deflection 5 mm tall (one large box) represents a 0.5 mV input signal.

Most ECG machines are calibrated at the factory prior to delivery and are expected to maintain that calibration through the lifetime of the machine. The calibration can be checked however each time an ECG is recorded. Typically each recorded ECG has a "calibration wave" embedded into it. The calibration wave visible in Figure 18.5 is typical. This specific wave, generated by a 1 mV signal of 0.2 s in duration, should result in a "calibration wave" that is 5 mm wide (0.2 s) and 10 mm high (1 mV).

The purpose of checking the calibration is to ensure that the ECG deflections are being recorded correctly. The height of specific ECG deflections relates to the diagnosis of atrial or ventricular hypertrophy for example. If the height of the R wave or the depth of the S wave is recorded incorrectly, ventricular hypertrophy may be incorrectly diagnosed. ST segment depression (a horizontal displacement of the ST segment) can only be correctly assessed if the ECG is properly calibrated. The "calibration wave" also ensures that the time duration of the ECG deflections is correct. When checking conduction times, atrioventricular conduction (PR interval) should occur within 0.2 s, while intraventricular conduction (QRS interval) should occur within 0.12 s.

---

is seen in Box 18.1. The procedures for recording the ECG include (1) preparing the participant for the ECG, (2) applying the electrodes, (3) recording the ECG for a single-lead ECG and for a standard 12-lead ECG, and (4) screening the ECG for heart rate, ectopic beats, and ST segment changes.

Preparing the Participant

1. The participant can be prepped in either a seated position or in a supine position.
2. For a single-lead ECG, where only 3 electrodes are applied, participants do not need to remove any clothing. However, if 10 electrodes are being applied to record a 12-lead ECG, it is best to remove the participant's shirt. Women should be instructed ahead of time to wear a sports bra or swimsuit top if completing a 12-lead ECG.

Applying the Electrodes

3. Identify the sites at which the electrodes will be attached. For a single-lead ECG (Lead II), identify the RA, LL, and RL sites (Figure 18.3). Many other combinations of electrode placements are possible for a single-lead ECG that are not described here. For a 12-lead ECG, identify all 10 sites at which electrodes will be applied.
4. Any body hair at the sites of electrode application, because it prevents good skin contact and reduces the adhesion of the electrode, must be removed. An electric shaver or a disposable razor may be used. The entire chest need not be shaved, but the 3 or 10 sites at which the electrodes will be applied need to be free of body hair.
5. Clean the desired sites with an alcohol swab (or other mild cleaner). Rub each site with an abrasive pad to remove dead skin cells. This improves contact with the skin and allows for a better ECG signal.
6. Apply a disposable electrode to each of the desired sites. Press on the borders of the electrodes to help seal them against the skin. Pressing in the middle of the electrode before the borders sometimes squeezes electrolyte gel from the electrode that can reduce the adhesion of the electrode to the skin.
7. Attach the wires from the ECG to the electrodes.
8. Instruct the person to relax in general, and specifically to relax all muscles near the sites of the electrodes. Electrical activity from contracting skeletal muscles can cause interference or artifacts that make it difficult to read the ECG.

Recording the ECG

9. Turn on the power to the ECG machine.
10. If using a single-lead ECG, record Lead II for 10–15 s. If using a 12-lead ECG, record one standard 12-lead ECG and record a rhythm trace for 10–15 s.
11. If only a resting ECG is to be recorded, and there will be no exercise test, remove all electrodes and wipe the sites clean of gel.

Screening the ECG

12. Determine heart rate and screen the ECG for intervals, ectopic beats, and ST depression, and record on Form 18.2.

RESULTS AND DISCUSSION

The surgeon general and others have declared that daily moderate physical activity is protective against cardiovascular disease and all-cause mortality.[4,12] Clinical exercise physiologists often administer ECG tests to high-risk persons in the United States who may be following the advice of the surgeon general's *Physical Activity and Health* report[12] to initiate or increase their physical activity level. Three of the most basic variables encountered on an electrocardiogram are (1) heart rate, (2) heart rhythm, and (3) ST depression.

Heart Rate

Persons with resting heart rates over 100 b·min^{-1} are in a state of tachycardia, whereas those with resting heart rates less than 60 b·min^{-1} are in bradycardia. Further divisions of bradycardia may be designated arbitrarily, as depicted in Table 18.1.[7] Sinus bradycardia often does not indicate a clinically abnormal state. Table 18.1 indicates that rates between 40 b·min^{-1} and 49 b·min^{-1} are categorized as moderate bradycardia.[9,13] However, reports[9] of trained distance runners having heart rates of 43 ($\pm$ 5 b·min^{-1}) during waking hours indicate a bradycardiac condition that is normal.

The seated heart rates for men and women from the ages of 18 y to over 65 y are presented in Table 18.2. Because heart rate is not known to differ with age in adult persons, the original tables[6] are reduced to a single age group. In general, the average man's heart rate (ranging from 66 to 71 bpm) is slightly less than the average woman's heart rate (68 to 72 bpm). Although the original tables of the YMCA publication attach qualitative ("excellent," etc.) fitness categories to each heart-rate range, Table 18.2 simply provides nonqualitative categories.

Table 18.1 Clinical Types of Bradycardia

Bradycardia Type	Heart Rate
Mild	50–59
Moderate	40–49
Severe (pathologic)	< 40

Source: Based on statements by Kammerling (1988).[7]

Table 18.2 Norms for Resting Heart Rate (HR) in Men and Women, Ages 18 y to 65+ y

Heart-Rate Category	Heart Rates (b·min^{-1})	
	Men	Women
Low	35–56	39–58
Moderately low	57–61	59–63
Lower than average	62–65	64–67
Average	66–71	68–72
Higher than average	72–75	73–77
Moderately high	76–81	78–83
High	82–103	84–104

Source: Based on data from Golding (2000).[6]

Heart Rhythm

Irregular rhythm of the heartbeats is referred to as **arrhythmia.** One author noted an arrhythmic criterion as a difference > 0.12 s (3 mm) between two adjacent cycle times (lengths).[11] Usually, premature ventricular contractions (PVCs) are of greater concern than premature atrial (supraventricular) contractions (PACs). Usually, a PVC has no P wave.[2] One hierarchy of PVC severity ranges from an absence of severity if no PVCs occur in one hour to a high severity if more than 30 PVCs occur per hour. Also, the severity increases in level from (1) PVCs vary in shape, then (2) repetitive couplets (e.g., bigeminy), then (3) ventricular tachycardia (> 3 consecutive PVCs).[10]

ST Depression

The ST portion (Figure 18.2) of the ECG is a segment that is often used to diagnose coronary heart disease. It is measured from the baseline (isoelectric). If the whole segment is more than 1 mm below the isoelectric line, it could indicate ischemic heart disease, depending upon other factors, such as angina and other ECG abnormalities. The final diagnosis should be made by a cardiologist.

BOX 18.2 | **Chapter Preview/Review**

What are the structures that make up the electrical conductive system in the heart?

What electrical events in the heart are represented by the P wave, QRS complex, and T wave?

How are the PR interval and QRS interval defined?

What are the limb leads and chest leads on the ECG?

What does ST segment depression indicate?

How are bradycardia and tachycardia defined?

What is an ectopic beat?

How do you distinguish between a premature atrial contraction (PAC) and a premature ventricular contraction (PVC)?

References

1. Adrian, R. H., Channell, R. C., Cohen, L., & Noble, D. (1976, July). The Einthoven string galvanometer and the interpretation of the T-wave of the electrocardiogram. *Physiological Society,* pp. 67–70.
2. American College of Sports Medicine. (2009). *ACSM's guidelines for exercise testing and prescription, 8th ed.* Philadelphia: Lippincott Williams & Wilkins.
3. Besterman, E., & Creese, R. (1979). Waller—Pioneer of electrocardiography. *British Heart Journal, 42,* 61–64.
4. Blair, S. N., Kampert, J. B., Kohl, H. W., Barlow, C. E., Macera, C. A., Paffenbarger, R. S., & Gibbons, L. W. (1996). Influences of cardiorespiratory fitness and other precursors on cardiovascular disease and all-cause mortality in men and women. *JAMA, 276,* 205–210.
5. Brailey, A. G. (1975). Basic electrocardiography. In P. K. Wilson (Ed.), *Cardiac rehabilitation and adult fitness* (pp. 69–83). Baltimore: University Park Press.
6. Golding, L. A. (2000). *YMCA fitness testing and assessment manual.* Champaign, IL: Human Kinetics.
7. Kammerling, J. M. (1988). Sinus node dysfunction. In D. P. Zipes & D. J. Rowlands (Eds.), *Progress in cardiology* (pp. 205–230). Philadelphia: Lea & Febiger.
8. Laks, M. M., & Ginzton, L. (1979). Computerized ECG interpretation. *Practical Cardiology, 5,* 127–149.
9. Lemish, M. G. (1979, June). Trouble-free cardiac monitoring. *Emergency,* pp. 58–59.
10. Lown, B., & Wolf, M. (1971). Approaches to sudden death from coronary heart disease. *Circulation, 44,* 130–142.
11. Nieman, D. C. (1995). *Fitness and sports medicine: A health-related approach.* Palo Alto, CA: Bull.
12. United States Surgeon General's Office. (1996). *Physical activity and health: A report of the Surgeon General Executive Summary.* Washington, DC: U.S. Government Printing Office.
13. Viitasalo, M. T., Kala, R., & Eisalo, A. (1982). Ambulatory electrocardiographic recording in endurance athletes. *British Heart Journal, 47,* 213.
14. Winsor, T. (1968). The electrocardiogram in myocardial infarction. *Clinical Symposia, 20.*

Form 18.1
RESTING ELECTROCARDIOGRAM

NAME _____ DATE _____ SCORE _____

Homework

Gender: **M**   Initials: **AA**   Age (y): **22**   Height (cm): **175**   Weight (kg): **80.0**

Below is a sample resting single-lead ECG.

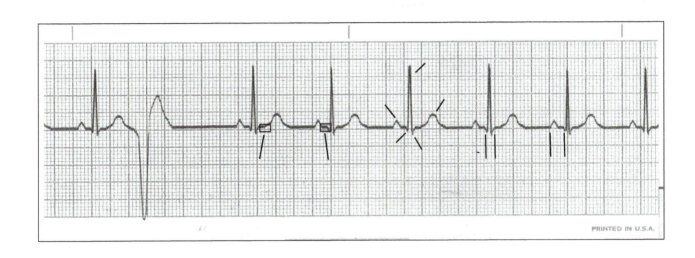

Label all waves (P,Q,R,S,T), segments (PR,ST), and intervals (PR,QRS) in one cardiac cycle.

Determine HR: HR = number of R waves within 6 s _____ x 10 = _____ bpm

and/or   Average R-R distance (mm) _____   HR = 1500 / _____ = _____ bpm

Assess HR: ☐ bradycardia (< 60 bpm)   ☐ normal sinus rhythm (60-100 bpm)   ☐ tachycardia (> 100 bpm)

Assess PR interval: ☐ normal (< 0.20 s)   ☐ prolonged (> 0.20 s)   Note: 0.20 s = 5 small squares

Assess QRS interval: ☐ normal (< 0.12 s)   ☐ prolonged (> 0.12 s)   Note: 0.12 s = 3 small squares

Screen for ectopic beats: ☐ none observed   ☐ PAC   ☐ PVC   Circle and label any ectopic beats

Screen for ST changes: ☐ none observed   ☐ ST elevation   ☐ ST depression

Evaluation of resting ECG: _____

_____

_____

_____

_____

Form 18.2

RESTING ELECTROCARDIOGRAM

Lab Results

Gender: _____ Initials: _____ Age (y): _____ Height (cm): _____ Weight (kg): _____

Cut and paste a sample resting single-lead ECG below.

Label all waves (P,Q,R,S,T), segments (PR,ST), and intervals (PR,QRS) in one cardiac cycle.

Determine HR: HR = number of R waves within 6 s _____ x 10 = _____ bpm

and/or   Average R-R distance (mm) _____   HR = 1500 / _____ = _____ bpm

Assess HR: ☐ bradycardia (< 60 bpm)   ☐ normal sinus rhythm (60-100 bpm)   ☐ tachycardia (> 100 bpm)

Assess PR interval: ☐ normal (< 0.20 s)   ☐ prolonged (> 0.20 s)   Note: 0.20 s = 5 small squares

Assess QRS interval: ☐ normal (< 0.12 s)   ☐ prolonged (> 0.12 s)   Note: 0.12 s = 3 small squares

Screen for ectopic beats: ☐ none observed ☐ PAC ☐ PVC   Circle and label any ectopic beats

Screen for ST changes: ☐ none observed ☐ ST elevation ☐ ST depression

Evaluation of resting ECG: _____

_____

_____

_____

_____

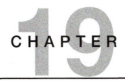
EXERCISE ELECTROCARDIOGRAM

The Exercise ECG Test is often a part of the stress test, also known as the Graded Exercise Test (GXT) and the Exercise Tolerance Test (ETT). These tests usually include the measurements of heart rate, blood pressure and ratings of perceived exertion (RPE). Sometimes, oxygen consumption is measured or predicted. The primary distinction of this test is the recording of the electrical conductivity of the heart—the electrocardiogram (ECG). The Exercise ECG Test has the advantage over some other evaluations of the cardiovascular system in that it is noninvasive, nonradiative, and relatively inexpensive.

Objectives There are at least three objectives in monitoring the electrocardiogram during the exercise test: (1) to assure the safety of the participant during exercise testing and training, (2) to measure accurate heart rates, and (3) to diagnose the participant or patient for cardiovascular disease.

The first two objectives—safety and accurate heart-rate recordings—may be accomplished by nonmedical personnel. However, the Exercise ECG may not be warranted for all asymptomatic—no cardiovascular disease (CVD) symptoms—and apparently healthy persons. The American College of Cardiology and the *American Heart Association Guidelines* state that the Exercise ECG Test is not warranted unless "healthy" people have two or more major risk-factors—smoking, hypertension, hypercholesterolemia, and family history of CVD.[3] The American College of Sports Medicine does not consider an annual medical examination and the clinical Exercise ECG Test prerequisites if apparently healthy persons of any age at low or moderate risk perform only moderate exercise ($\leq 60 \%$ $\dot{V}O_2max$; 3–6 MET) during recreation or testing. The same holds true for vigorous exercise in low-risk persons.[4] Some believe that the exercise ECG is beneficial for all persons because it provides a baseline by which to compare their future Exercise ECG Tests.

The third objective—diagnosis of cardiovascular disease—is the primary responsibility of the physician, who may seek input from the allied health staff, which may include a clinical exercise physiologist and/or exercise technologist. Thus, the ECG Exercise Test is often an interdisciplinary test between medical and allied health personnel.[2] Although it is not within the role of an exercise laboratory technician to serve as a cardiologist, it is important for the technician to understand the basic concepts of electrocardiography and to recognize the most critical ECG abnormalities encountered in exercise testing.[23] For persons with angina pectoris, the Exercise ECG Test is often the precursor test to one or more of the following tests: (1) angiography, which requires an X-ray-visible dye to be injected into the coronary arteries; (2) exercise scintigraphy, whereby radionuclide thallium allows the blood flow to be followed in the myocardium; (3) echocardiography, which provides views of the heart produced by ultrasound waves; and (4) calcium scanning of the arteries by electron-beam computed tomography. However, the Exercise ECG Test, using the exercise time, ST displacement, and angina index together, can be as accurate as these sophisticated tests in predicting the risk of future cardiovascular events.[19]

PHYSIOLOGICAL RATIONALE

The exercise electrocardiogram is more apt to reveal latent (previously hidden) cardiovascular problems than the resting electrocardiogram.[15] For example, 10.2 % of 7023 normal resting ECG exams were deemed abnormal on maximal treadmill ECG tests.[12] Of those persons with known coronary heart disease, 30 % may not be revealed by resting ECG, but, if an exercise ECG is administered, 70 % of these will be revealed.[28]

METHODS

The Exercise ECG Test is usually preceded by a resting electrocardiogram in order to screen persons for whom exercise may be contraindicated and to enhance the interpretation of the exercise electrocardiogram. The Exercise ECG Test always includes measurements of heart rate and blood pressure periodically throughout the test. Often, a prediction of aerobic power ($\dot{V}O_2max$) is made on the basis of heart rate or exercise duration. Sometimes a scale for rating perceived exertion (RPE) is used to monitor the participant's perception of the exercise stress. See Box 19.1 for a discussion of the accuracy of the Exercise ECG and predictive $\dot{V}O_2max$ Test.

The Exercise Electrocardiogram (ECG)

Using an Exercise ECG Test, or stress test, to help diagnose coronary heart disease (CHD) can only be done by a physician and is beyond the scope of this laboratory manual. The purposes of recording the exercise ECG here are (1) to observe changes between

BOX 19.1 — Accuracy of Exercise ECG Test in Diagnosing CHD and Estimating VO_2max

The accuracy of the Exercise ECG Test in diagnosing coronary heart disease (CHD) is described in terms of its sensitivity and specificity. The *sensitivity* of the test is its ability to correctly identify those persons who have CHD. A test is considered "positive" for CHD if the person shows ≥ 1 mm of horizontal or downsloping ST depression, develops chest pain during or after exercise, or if the test is stopped for other related complications. ST changes and chest pain are more likely to occur when coronary artery occlusion exceeds 70 %.[4] Studies in men report a mean sensitivity of 72 % (range 45–92 %),[22,37] meaning the Exercise ECG Test correctly identifies 72 out of 100 persons who have CHD. That means, however, that 28 persons (28 %) with CHD who were tested will be missed. These tests are labeled "false negative" and may be due to monitoring an insufficient number of ECG leads, CHD limited to just one coronary vessel, inability of the participant to reach an exercise intensity where ST changes or chest pain would appear, or observer error.[4] Other sources report lower sensitivities in men of 60 %[20] and 45 %[21] when applying stricter criteria. In women, sensitivity is reported at 62 %.[22] Sensitivity may be lower in women due to lower exercise capacity, the effect of estrogen on ST-segment changes, or smaller coronary vessel size.[22]

The *specificity* of the Exercise ECG Test is its ability to correctly identify those who do not have CHD. The studies cited previously reporting a sensitivity of 72 %, report a specificity for exercise testing of 77 % (range 17–92 %).[22,37] In this case, 23 persons out of 100 (23 %) without CHD who were tested will show a "false positive" test possibly due to cardiac hypertrophy, coronary artery spasm, abnormal myocardial perfusion, or other causes.[4] Women are also more likely to show a "false positive" test thus demonstrating a lower specificity.[22]

Provided that data are recorded during the stress test regarding treadmill speed and grade, cycling power, heart rate, and exercise duration, these results can be used to estimate the maximal oxygen consumption (VO_2max) and/or functional capacity of the participant. The validity of the maximal treadmill stress test is quite high. A correlation of 0.90 between maximal treadmill time and measured VO_2max with a standard error of estimate (SEE) of less than 2 ml·kg⁻¹·min⁻¹ was reported when using the Bruce protocol.[10] Other reported correlations for treadmill testing range from 0.88 (Balke protocol) to 0.97 (Bruce protocol) with SEEs of about 3 ml·kg⁻¹·min⁻¹, which is somewhere in the range of 4 to 6 %.[6]

or a failure of heart rate or blood pressure to rise with increasing exercise intensity.[4] These criteria are summarized in Table 19.1.

Procedures for Recording the Exercise ECG

The initial procedures for recording the exercise ECG are identical to those for recording the resting ECG described in Chapter 18. They involve preparing the participant, applying the ECG electrodes, and recording the resting ECG. Either a single-lead ECG (Lead II or equivalent) or the full 12-lead ECG can be used. The ECG is typically recorded at rest (often in a supine position), pre-exercise (seated on the cycle ergometer or standing on the treadmill belt), at regular intervals (e.g., 3 min) throughout the exercise test, and during recovery. The person's name, date, body position (e.g., supine), status (e.g., resting), exercise stage, and heart rate should be labeled appropriately on the ECG. If the particular ECG machine does not automatically print this information, it should be recorded by hand on the ECG.

Resting and/or Pre-Exercise ECG

Ideally, a resting 12-lead ECG should be taken before administering the Exercise ECG Test. It should be required for persons who are at greater risk based on their medical

Table 19.1 — Potential Indications for Terminating Exercise (End-Point Criteria for Exercise)

Signs or Symptoms of Exertional Intolerance
1. Onset of moderate to severe angina (chest pain)
2. Signs of poor perfusion (blood flow) including pallor, cyanosis, cold/clammy skin
3. Unusual or severe shortness of breath (SOB), dyspnea, or wheezing
4. CNS symptoms including ataxia (incoordination), vertigo (dizziness), visual or gait problems, or confusion
5. Manifestations of severe fatigue
6. Leg cramps or intermittent claudication
7. Participant requests to stop at any time

Blood Pressure Changes
1. Systolic blood pressure, SBP ≥ 250 mm Hg
2. Diastolic blood pressure, DBP ≥ 115 mm Hg
3. Drop in SBP of 10 mm Hg from baseline despite an increase in exercise intensity

Electrocardiographic (ECG) Changes
1. Sustained ventricular tachycardia (V tach)
2. ST segment depression (> 2 mm of horizontal or downsloping ST depression)
3. ST segment elevation (> 1 mm of ST elevation in leads other than V_1 or aVF)
4. Significant ectopic beats (multifocal PVCs, coupled PVCs, R on T PVC)
5. Ventricular bigeminy, trigeminy, or frequent unifocal PVCs (> 6–10 per minute)
6. Supraventricular tachycardia (SVT)
7. Development of bundle branch block (BBB) or intraventricular conduction disturbance that cannot be distinguished from V tach
8. Failure of ECG monitoring system

Source: Adapted from information in ACSM (2006).[4]

the resting ECG and exercise ECG (e.g., changes in R–R distance, changes in HR) and (2) to increase the safety of the graded exercise test by watching for the appearance of ectopic beats, ST segment depression, or other ECG criteria that might warrant stopping the test prematurely. In addition to the ECG criteria, other potential indications for terminating a graded exercise test include signs of exertional intolerance (e.g., chest pain, leg pain, shortness of breath, dizziness); hypertensive responses (e.g., SBP ≥ 250 mm Hg, DBP ≥ 115 mm Hg);

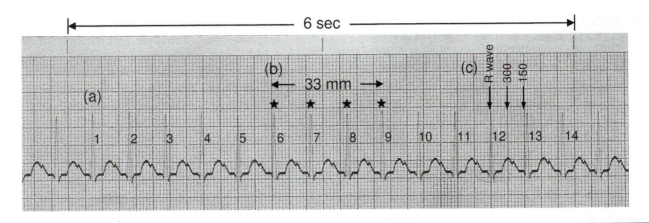

Figure 19.1 Sample of a single-lead ECG recorded during exercise. Heart rate (HR) can be determined as (a) *140 bpm* by counting 14 R waves in 6 s and multiplying by 10; or (b) *136 bpm* by dividing 1500 by the average R–R distance, which is 11 mm; or (c) about *140 bpm* by counting the number of 5 mm boxes between two consecutive R waves and estimating HR based on Table 19.2.

history or risk factor analysis. Although some laboratories include a pre-exercise hyperventilation recording, some authorities do not recommend it because of reducing the test's specificity (i.e., the ability to detect true normals).[14] After taking the resting ECG, a pre-exercise recording should be taken while the participant is seated on the cycle or standing on the treadmill.

Exercise and Recovery ECG

During exercise and recovery, the ECG is monitored on screen constantly, but is typically only printed out once per stage; more frequent recordings may be made if so indicated. A recording should be taken immediately after the last stage of exercise. A recording should be taken during active recovery at 1 min or 2 min, as well as at passive recovery at the 5th min of post-exercise. The participant should not be released from monitoring until at least 5 min and all subjective and physiological (e.g., ECG baseline) symptoms have stabilized at a reasonable level.

Uses of the ECG During Exercise

The exercise ECG is used during the exercise test to determine heart rate (HR) and screen for ectopic beats and signs of ischemia. Heart rate can be determined in various ways, as described in Chapter 18 and reviewed here. The exercise ECG is also used to screen for ectopic beats, which in some cases are associated with CHD, but may also be due to other causes unrelated to CHD. Changes in the displacement of the ST segment (either ST elevation or ST depression) are also monitored during exercise because of their potential relationship to myocardial injury or ischemia.

Determining Heart Rate

As described previously, if the particular ECG machine being used does not display HR, there are simple ways to manually determine HR. The first is to count the number of R waves (cardiac cycles) in 6 s and multiply by 10 to convert to the HR. The second is to determine the average R–R distance (mm) and divide this value into 1500 to convert to HR. Both methods are reviewed in Figure 19.1. By counting 14 R waves in 6 s, the HR is determined to be 140 bpm. By dividing 1500 by the average R–R distance (11 mm), the HR in the same trace is determined to be 136 bpm. Although there is a small difference in HR between the two methods (i.e., 4 bpm), this difference is considered insignificant and either HR can be used. This second method is sometimes altered slightly to estimate HR more easily and quickly without the need for calculation. Instead of calculating the average R–R distance, a single R–R distance (or the distance between two consecutive R waves) is observed. If the distance between two consecutive R waves is one 5 mm box (indicated by the thicker, bold lines on the ECG paper), then HR can be estimated as 300 bpm (1500 / 5 mm per cardiac cycle). If the distance is two 5 mm boxes (10 mm), then HR is 150 (1500 / 10 mm). So by counting the number of 5 mm boxes between two consecutive R waves, HR may be estimated (Table 19.2).

Screening for Ectopic Beats

It is anticipated that apparently healthy adults—those free of heart disease, with no signs or symptoms of heart disease, and no more than one major CHD risk factor—will typically remain in a sinus rhythm throughout the exercise test. However, it is not uncommon to observe ectopic beats in these same persons. The exercise ECG, if recorded during exercise, should be constantly monitored throughout for any ectopic beats. The occurrence of premature ventricular contractions (PVCs) during exercise is of particular interest. Figure 19.2 demonstrates the recording of two premature ventricular contractions during exercise. This particular ECG recording is typical of an exercise "lead group" in which three ECG leads are recorded simultaneously,

Table 19.2	Rapid Estimation of Heart Rate (HR) from the Number of 5 mm Boxes (R–R Distance) Between Two Consecutive R Waves		
Number of 5 mm Boxes	R–R Distance (mm)	R–R Interval (s)	Heart Rate (bpm)
1.5	7.5	0.30	200
2.0	10.0	0.40	150
2.5	12.5	0.50	120
3.0	15.0	0.60	100
4.0	20.0	0.80	75
5.0	25.0	1.00	60
6.0	30.0	1.20	50

Note: Heart rate (bpm) can be determined by dividing 300 by the number of 5 mm boxes between two consecutive R waves; by dividing 1500 by R–R distance (mm); or by dividing 60 by R–R interval (s).

healthy adult will show no ST segment changes at rest. However, during exercise, when a greater load is placed on the heart, the blood flow to the heart may become insufficient, leading to myocardial ischemia and resulting in the appearance of ST segment depression (described in Chapter 18). Figure 19.4 is a printout from an automated ECG machine that shows a summary of the maximal ST segment changes observed in all 12 ECG leads during an exercise test. Note that in leads II, III, and aVF, a significant amount of ST segment depression (1.8–4.2 mm) was observed, and because of this, the exercise test was terminated. ST segment depression of 2 mm or more, because it is assumed to be due to myocardial ischemia, is frequently used as an end point to exercise due to the threat of developing an abnormal heartbeat. However, in some cases when persons with ST segment depression are subjected to further diagnostic testing, no coronary heart disease is found, indicating that in some specific cases it can be a "false" sign of CHD.

Uses of Blood Pressure and RPE During Exercise

In addition to recording the ECG during the exercise test to determine heart rate and screen for ectopic beats and signs of ischemia, it is also common to monitor exercise blood pressure and the participant's rating of perceived exertion (RPE).

Blood Pressure

The American College of Sports Medicine recommends that blood pressure be measured with the participant in the supine, sitting, and standing positions prior to exercise.[4]

including anterior (V_1), lateral (V_5), and inferior (aVF) views of the heart. A high frequency of PVCs (6–10 per minute) is considered significant and may warrant stopping the exercise test in certain situations. Figure 19.3 shows an exercise ECG with a high frequency of PVCs (> 10 per minute). Other forms of PVCs and other ECG criteria, as listed in Table 19.1, are also significant, but are not defined or discussed in this laboratory manual.

Screening for Signs of Ischemia

Monitoring the exercise ECG for changes in the ST segment during exercise is also important. Frequently an apparently

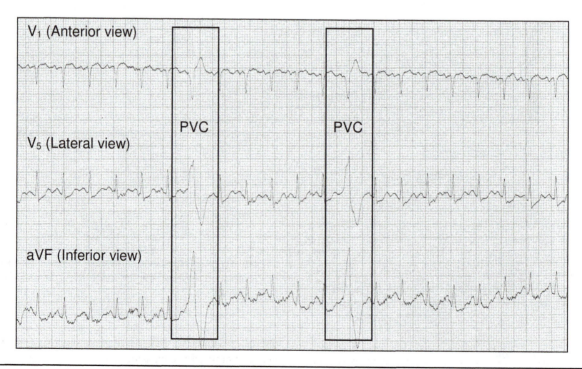

Figure 19.2 Example of an ECG rhythm strip recorded during exercise showing how the three leads are recorded simultaneously. Two premature ventricular contractions (PVCs) are visible within the boxes.

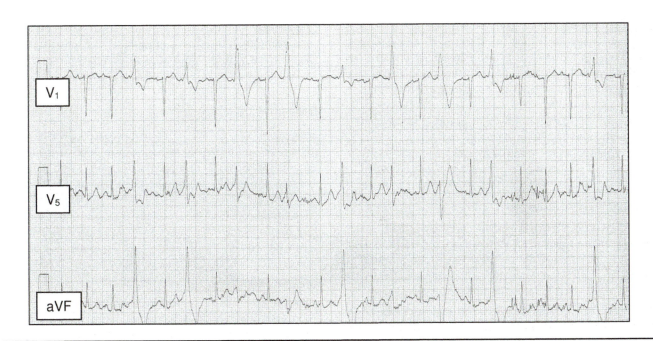

Figure 19.3 Frequent ectopic beats (PVCs) recorded during treadmill exercise in a 25-year-old, trained female. Subsequent diagnostic testing revealed no significant coronary heart disease.

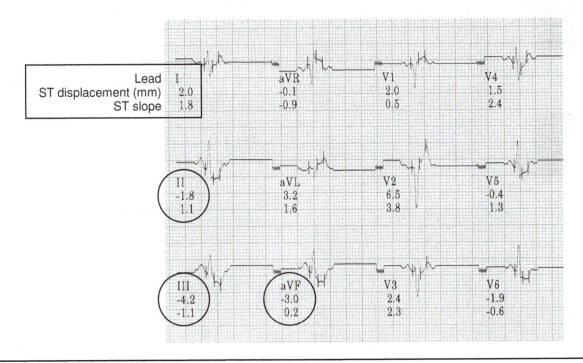

Lead	I	aVR	V1	V4
ST displacement (mm)	2.0	-0.1	2.0	1.5
ST slope	1.8	-0.9	0.5	2.4
	II	aVL	V2	V5
	-1.8	3.2	6.5	-0.4
	1.1	1.6	3.8	1.3
	III	aVF	V3	V6
	-4.2	-3.0	2.4	-1.9
	-1.1	0.2	2.3	-0.6

Figure 19.4 ST segment summary showing lead, ST displacement (mm), and ST slope (negative sign indicates "downsloping" ST depression). Results were recorded within the last minute of an exercise test at a heart rate of 163 bpm in a 50-year-old man with no previous history of coronary heart disease. Significant ST depression (2–4 mm) can be seen in leads II, III, and aVF. Subsequent diagnostic testing revealed significant coronary blockages (> 90 % occlusion), leading to balloon angioplasty and coronary artery stenting.

Presumably, these measures are taken under relaxed conditions. Additional resting measures may be taken when the participant is prepared to exercise while seated on the cycle ergometer, standing on the treadmill, or in front of the step bench. These last measurements are referred to as the anticipatory or pre-exercise measures.

At exercise the blood pressure should be taken during the last minute of each stage or interval of the exercise protocol.[4] Usually, the technician starts pumping the sphygmomanometer's air bulb at the 30th s of the last minute of each stage. In recovery, it is taken immediately after exercise and at 1–2 min intervals for at least 5 min. The first few measurements of recovery blood pressure may be taken during *active* recovery (e.g., low-intensity cycling or walking slowly on the treadmill or in place), and subsequent measurements may be made while the person is *passive* (e.g., seated in a chair) until the pressure returns nearly to baseline.

Rate of Perceived Exertion (RPE)

You may need to refresh your memory about RPE scales by referring to Chapter 15. Before the Exercise ECG Test, the participant should be instructed as to the meaning of the RPE scale. The revised RPE scale with ratio properties may be more suitable for determining subjective symptoms associated with breathing, aches, and pains.[7] A large RPE poster should be prominently placed or held so that the exerciser has no trouble viewing the RPE scale. The tester should read aloud the instructions as printed in Chapter 15. Thumb signals may be necessary if the participant is using a respiratory valve and is therefore unable to speak. During the last 15 s of each stage, the tester asks the participant to indicate by pointing to the number on the poster (if using the respiratory valve) or saying the RPE number. The thumbs-up ("I'm OK"), sideways ("I'm tired"), down ("I'm quitting soon") signals can be used anytime during the test if the participant is using the respiratory valve. The technician confirms the participant's RPE number by stating it aloud. Either the 6–20 or the category-ratio scale from 0–10 monitor the participant's stress. The authors of ACSM's guidelines state that the participants understand the 0–10 scale better than the 6–20 scale.[6] When participants indicate ratings between 18 and 19 ("very, very hard") and 9 to 10 ("extremely strong"; "strongest intensity") for either of the two scales, the testers will know that the participants are near exhaustion.[4]

Exercise Protocols

Although the first popular Exercise ECG Test used a step bench,[27] the most common protocols for these tests use either cycle ergometers or treadmills. The protocols for the Exercise ECG Test are usually continuous and progressive types. *Continuous,* as opposed to *intermittent,* is a term used to characterize a test in which the participant does not stop exercising until the end of the test. An intermittent, or noncontinuous, test has rest intervals between exercise bouts. *Progressive* simply means that the exercise intensity is graded—that is, the exercise bouts increase in intensity at periodic intervals.

Continuous-progressive protocols can be subdivided into two types based upon submaximal or maximal exercise. Submaximal tests are often targeted to a specified percentage of heart-rate reserve (e.g., 85 % HRR) or to symptom-limited end points. If the participant is healthy and willing, however, it is preferable to perform a maximal test.

Cycling Protocols

In general, the continuous cycling protocols provide either 3 min or 4 min periods at each power level if the power increments are 50 W or greater. Less time (1 min or 2 min) permits reasonable steady-state heart rates if the power increments are 25 W or less[26] (Table 19.3). A suggested criterion for the achievement of steady-state heart rate is obtaining heart rates at each end of two consecutive minutes that are within 6 b·min^{-1} of each other.[5] Equation 19.1 enables the prediction of the gross steady-state oxygen cost for any given power (W) (*SEE* = 7 % ml·kg^{-1}·min^{-1}).[4]

$$\dot{V}O_2 \ (\text{ml·kg}^{-1}\text{·min}^{-1}) = [10.8 * \text{Power (W)} \\ / \text{ Body weight (kg)}] + 7 \ \text{ml·kg}^{-1}\text{·min}^{-1} \qquad \text{Eq. 19.1}$$

Where: 7 ml·kg^{-1}·min^{-1} is the combined $\dot{V}O_2$ for the rest and unloaded cycling

A recovery period of 2–4 min should be allotted for no-load or minimal-load cycling. The quality of the electrocardiogram and the ease of measuring blood pressure are usually better during the cycling mode than during the treadmill mode of exercise.[4]

Treadmill Protocols

The treadmill is the most commonly used ergometer for graded exercise testing,[11,38] primarily because the general public is more used to walking than any other exercise mode (e.g., cycle ergometry, stepping). Several treadmill protocols are available, including the Bruce,[31] Ellestad,[16] and Stanford[4] protocols described in Table 19.4. The Bruce protocol is the most popular for exercise testing in healthy, active adults. The *standard* Bruce protocol (beginning at 1.7 mph and 10 % grade) is fairly rigorous and may not be appropriate for deconditioned persons. A *modified* Bruce protocol is also described which adds two additional stages[31] of a lower intensity to the beginning of the protocol (Table 19.4) that makes it more suitable for less fit persons and older adults. The modified Bruce is also beneficial if submaximal values of heart rate, blood pressure, and oxygen consumption are of particular interest. The Ellestad protocol is a rigorous protocol that may be better suited for more fit and/or younger persons. The original goal of the protocol was to have the participant exercise to 95 % of age-predicted maximal heart rate.[16] The Stanford protocol progresses at a considerably lower rate[4] than the Bruce or Ellestad protocols, making it more appropriate for less fit persons. The Balke protocol[36] and Naughton protocol[33] are also popular when testing less fit or older persons. A more complete summary of treadmill protocols is available by reviewing other references.[4,9,29,35,39]

Table 19.3 Cycle Ergometer Protocol with Estimated Oxygen Consumption (ml·kg⁻¹·min⁻¹) Based on Body Weight (lb; kg)

Time (min)	Power (W)	(lb) (kg)	99 45	110 50	121 55	132 60	143 65	154 70	165 75	176 80	187 85	198 90	209 95
			\multicolumn{11}{c}{Oxygen Consumption (ml·kg⁻¹·min⁻¹) Estimated from Body Weight}
0.00–1:59	50		19.0	17.8	16.8	16.0	15.3	14.7	14.2	13.8	13.4	13.0	12.7
2:00–3:59	75		25.0	23.2	21.7	20.5	19.5	18.6	17.8	17.1	16.5	16.0	15.5
4:00–5:59	100		31.0	28.6	26.6	25.0	23.6	22.4	21.4	20.5	19.7	19.0	18.4
6:00–7:59	125		37.0	34.0	31.5	29.5	27.8	26.3	25.0	23.9	22.9	22.0	21.2
8:00–9:59	150		43.0	39.4	36.5	34.0	31.9	30.1	28.6	27.3	26.1	25.0	24.1
10:00–11:59	175		49.0	44.8	41.4	38.5	36.1	34.0	32.2	30.6	29.2	28.0	26.9
12:00–13:59	200		55.0	50.2	46.3	43.0	40.2	37.9	35.8	34.0	32.4	31.0	29.7
14:00–15:59	225		61.0	55.6	51.2	47.5	44.4	41.7	39.4	37.4	35.6	34.0	32.6
16:00–17:59	250			61.0	56.1	52.0	48.5	45.6	43.0	40.8	38.8	37.0	35.4
18:00–19:59	275				61.0	56.5	52.7	49.4	46.6	44.1	41.9	40.0	38.3
20:00–21:59	300					61.0	56.8	53.3	50.2	47.5	45.1	43.0	41.1

Note: Estimated V̇O₂ (ml·kg⁻¹·min⁻¹) = [10.8 * Power (W) / Body wt (kg) + 7]. Most accurate for power outputs from 50–200 W. MET values can be calculated by dividing the values in the table by 3.5.
Source: Based on equations in ACSM (2006).[4]

Estimation of Oxygen Consumption

Approximate relative oxygen consumptions for cycle ergometry (by power level) are included in Table 19.3. Relative oxygen consumptions and MET (metabolic equivalent) values for each stage of the three treadmill protocols are included in Table 19.4. MET values are more commonly included in treadmill protocols, especially when they are done for clinical or diagnostic purposes. One MET is equivalent to resting metabolic rate (or a V̇O₂ = 3.5 ml·kg⁻¹·min⁻¹). So if a woman is working at 10 METs on the treadmill, she is assumed to be working at 10 times her resting metabolic rate, or a relative V̇O₂ of 35 ml·kg⁻¹·min⁻¹.

The oxygen cost or relative oxygen consumption of any cycle power level or treadmill speed and grade can be estimated (*SEE* = 7 %). One method of estimation is the use of the ACSM equations.[4] The equation for estimating relative oxygen consumption during cycle ergometry was previously given (Eq. 19.1). Equations are also available for estimating relative oxygen consumption while walking (Eq. 19.2) and running (Eq. 19.3).

$$\dot{V}O_2 \text{ (ml·kg}^{-1}\text{·min}^{-1}) = [0.1 * \text{Speed (m·min}^{-1})]$$
$$+ [1.8 * \text{Speed (m·min}^{-1}) * \text{Grade (decimal)}]$$
$$+ 3.5 \text{ ml·kg}^{-1}\text{·min}^{-1} \qquad \text{Eq. 19.2}$$

Where: Walking is typically considered up to 10 m·min⁻¹ (3.7 mph)

Where: Grade is percent treadmill grade (written as a decimal), 10 % = 0.10

Where: The 3.5 ml·kg⁻¹·min⁻¹ is resting V̇O₂

The difference between walking and running can be defined by speed, with walking speed typically considered up to 100 m·min⁻¹ (3.7) mph and running speed over

100 m·min⁻¹. But the real criterion is whether the person is truly walking or running at any speed. A person is considered walking if one foot is in contact with the ground (or treadmill belt) at all times. Running involves a "flight phase" where a portion of the time is spent in the air.

$$\dot{V}O_2 \text{ (ml·kg}^{-1}\text{·min}^{-1}) = [0.2 * \text{Speed (m·min}^{-1})]$$
$$+ [0.9 * \text{Speed (m·min}^{-1}) * \text{Grade (decimal)}]$$
$$+ 3.5 \text{ ml·kg}^{-1}\text{·min}^{-1} \qquad \text{Eq. 19.3}$$

Where: Running is typically considered over 100 m·min⁻¹ (3.7 mph)

Where: Grade is percent treadmill grade (written as a decimal), 10 % = 0.10

Where: The 3.5 ml·kg⁻¹·min⁻¹ is resting V̇O₂

Examples of estimating oxygen cost for cycling, treadmill walking, and treadmill running are given below (Eq. 19.4a, 19.4b, and 19.4c). This is followed by the estimated MET value for the treadmill running example (Eq. 19.4d).

Cycling: Assume a **70** kg person is cycling at **150** W.

$$\dot{V}O_2 = [10.8 * \mathbf{150} / \mathbf{70}] + 7 = \mathbf{30.1} \text{ ml·kg}^{-1}\text{·min}^{-1} \quad \text{Eq. 19.4a}$$

Walking: Assume a person is walking 3 mph (**80.4** m·min⁻¹) up a **10** % grade

$$\dot{V}O_2 = [0.1 * \mathbf{80.4}] + [1.8 * \mathbf{80.4} * \mathbf{0.10}] + 3.5$$
$$= \mathbf{26.0} \text{ ml·kg}^{-1}\text{·min}^{-1} \qquad \text{Eq. 19.4b}$$

Running: Assume a person is running 6 mph (**160.8** m·min⁻¹) up a **6** % grade

$$\dot{V}O_2 = [0.2 * \mathbf{160.8}] + [0.9 * \mathbf{160.8} * \mathbf{0.06}] + 3.5$$
$$= \mathbf{44.3} \text{ ml·kg}^{-1}\text{·min}^{-1} \qquad \text{Eq. 19.4c}$$

Table 19.4 — Sample Treadmill Protocols, Including Estimated Metabolic Values

Modified and Standard Bruce Protocol

Stage	Time	Speed (mph)	Grade (%)	Rel $\dot{V}O_2$	METs
0	0:00–2:59	1.7	0	8.1	2.3
0	3:00–5:59	1.7	5	12.2	3.5
1	0:00–2:59	1.7	10	16.3	4.6
2	3:00–5:59	2.5	12	24.7	7.0
3	6:00–8:59	3.4	14	35.6	10.2
4	9:00–11:59	4.2	16	42.2	12.1
5	12:00–14:59	5.0	18	52.0	14.9
6	15:00–17:59	5.5	20	59.5	17.0
7	18:00–20:59	6.0	22	67.5	19.3

Ellestad Protocol

Stage	Time	Speed (mph)	Grade (%)	Rel $\dot{V}O_2$	METs
1	0:00–2:59	1.7	10.0	16.3	4.6
2	3:00–4:59	3.0	10.0	26.0	7.4
3	5:00–6:59	4.0	10.0	34.6	9.9
4	7:00–11:59	5.0	10.0	42.4	12.1
5	12:00–15:59	6.0	15.0	57.4	16.4

Stanford Protocol

Stage	Time	Speed (mph)	Grade (%)	Rel $\dot{V}O_2$	METs
1	0:00–2:59	3.0	0.0	11.5	3.3
2	3:00–5:59	3.0	2.5	15.2	4.3
3	6:00–8:59	3.0	5.0	18.8	5.4
4	9:00–11:59	3.0	7.5	22.4	6.4
5	12:00–14:59	3.0	10.0	26.0	7.4
6	15:00–17:59	3.0	12.5	29.6	8.5
7	18:00–20:59	3.0	15.0	33.2	9.5
8	21:00–23:59	3.0	17.5	36.9	10.5
9	24:00–26:59	3.0	20.0	40.5	11.6

Note: Rel $\dot{V}O_2$: relative $\dot{V}O_2$ (ml·kg^{-1}·min^{-1}). Walking (< 4.0 mph) Rel $\dot{V}O_2$ = [(0.1 * Speed (m·min^{-1})) + (1.8 * Speed (m·min^{-1}) * Grade (%) / 100) + 3.5]. Running (≥ 4.0 mph) Rel $\dot{V}O_2$ = [(0.2 * Speed (m·min^{-1})) + (0.9 * Speed (m·min^{-1}) * Grade (%) / 100) + 3.5]. 1 mph = 26.8 m·min^{-1}
Source: Details of treadmill protocols from ACSM (2006).[4]

MET value: Assume the estimated relative $\dot{V}O_2$ is **44.3** ml·kg^{-1}·min^{-1}

$$\text{MET} = 44.3 \text{ ml·kg}^{-1}\text{·min}^{-1} / 3.5 \text{ ml·kg}^{-1}\text{·min}^{-1}$$
$$= \textbf{12.7 METs} \qquad \text{Eq. 19.4d}$$

Time to exhaustion on the Bruce treadmill protocol can also be used to assess aerobic power. Regression equations have been developed for men and women,[10] and for young men,[25] that estimate maximal oxygen consumption ($\dot{V}O_2$max) from exercise time, as seen in Equations 19.5a, 19.5b, and 19.5c.

Men: $\dot{V}O_2$ (ml·kg^{-1}·min^{-1}) = [(2.94
     * Exercise time (min)) + 7.65]   Eq. 19.5a

Women: $\dot{V}O_2$ (ml·kg^{-1}·min^{-1}) = [(2.94
     * Exercise time (min)) + 3.74]   Eq. 19.5b

Young men: $\dot{V}O_2$ (ml·kg^{-1}·min^{-1}) = [(3.62
     * Exercise time (min)) + 3.91]   Eq. 19.5c

Where: Exercise time (min) is time to exhaustion on on Bruce treadmill protocol

For example, if a woman completed Stage 2 of the Bruce protocol, with a time to exhaustion of 6.0 min, her $\dot{V}O_2$max would be 21.4 ml·kg^{-1}·min^{-1}, as seen in Equation 19.6. If using the oxygen cost data from Table 19.4, her estimated $\dot{V}O_2$max would be slightly higher, at 24.7 ml·kg^{-1}·min^{-1}.

Assume: A **woman** reaches exhaustion on the Bruce protocol at **6.0** min

$$\text{Estimated } \dot{V}O_2\text{max} = [(2.94 * \textbf{6.0}) + 3.74]$$
$$= \textbf{21.4} \text{ ml·kg}^{-1}\text{·min}^{-1} \qquad \text{Eq. 19.6}$$

RESULTS AND DISCUSSION

The main purpose of the Exercise ECG Test as described in this chapter is to look for changes in the ECG from rest to exercise and to use the ECG during exercise to determine heart rate and screen for ectopic beats and ST segment changes. When the exercise ECG is combined with the measurement of blood pressure and RPE, it can be used to increase the safety of the graded exercise test and to screen for changes that may indicate coronary heart disease. The test is diagnostic of CHD only when administered and interpreted by a physician. The secondary purpose of the ECG Exercise Test is to assess the metabolic response to exercise and to estimate maximal oxygen consumption.

A typical increase in heart rate during a graded exercise test is about 10 bpm (± 2 bpm) for each MET increase. Therefore, if an exercise stage increases in intensity 2–3 METs, heart rate would be expected to increase 20–30 bpm (± 4–6 bpm). Heart rate is expected to increase linearly with work load, and assuming the test is done to maximal effort, heart rate should reach near to the age-predicted maximum (220 – age). If the peak exercise heart rate attained during a voluntary maximal effort is more than 20 bpm lower than the age-predicted HR$_{max}$, it can be identified as chronotropic incompetence.[4] However, cautious interpretation of any criterion using age-predicted maximal heart rate is advised due to its high variability.[17]

It is not uncommon for apparently healthy persons to have occasional ectopic beats throughout the day.[32] The prevalence and frequency of ectopic beats is likely to increase with age and with duration of monitoring. Studies of PVC prevalence have found about 3 % of those completing a resting ECG will have ectopic beats during the recording of the ECG,[34] about 5 % of middle-aged men had PVCs when monitored for 2 min,[13] and 50 % of young adults had incidents of ectopic beats when monitored for 24 hours.[8] The chances of recording ECG abnormalities during exercise are greater than at rest.[24,30] During maximal exercise testing in normal men, younger men average close to 30 % incidence of PVCs, while middle-aged men average close to 43 %

incidence.[18] Forty-four percent of normal men in another study experienced PVCs during maximal exercise.[30] Older adults showed a prevalence of premature ventricular contractions of 16 % at rest and of 55 % during the combined exercise and recovery periods.[1]

ST segment depression is believed to be associated with myocardial ischemia due to changes in the repolarization of the ventricles, thereby causing changes in the ST segment.[5] Ischemia is also likely to increase the prevalence of ectopic beats, including premature ventricular contractions.[39] ST depression as a true sign of ischemia may not be evident unless a major coronary artery is at least 60% occluded.[9] When ST depression of at least 1 mm continues for 0.06 s in the lateral ECG leads, I, V_4, V_5, and V_6, it is considered especially significant.[4,14] The American Association of Cardiovascular and Pulmonary Rehabilitation (AACVPR)[2] classifies persons with 1–2 mm of exercise-induced ST depression as having moderate risk of CHD, while those with greater than 2 mm are considered high risk, especially if in combination with CHD symptoms (e.g., chest pain). If clinically significant ST segment changes are observed during a graded exercise test, a follow-up diagnostic test (e.g., thallium-imagery technique) is sometimes advised to validate the findings of the stress test.

References

1. Ambe, K. S., Adams, G. M., & de Vries, H. A. (1973). Exercising the aged. *Medicine and Science in Sports, 5*(Abstract), 63.

2. American Association of Cardiovascular and Pulmonary Rehabilitation. (1994). *Guidelines for cardiac rehabilitation programs.* Champaign, IL: Human Kinetics.

3. American College of Cardiology/American Heart Association Subcommittee on Exercise Testing. (1986). Guidelines for exercise testing: A report of the American College of Cardiology/American Heart Association Task Force on Assessment of Cardiovascular Procedures. *Journal of American College of Cardiology, 8,* 725–738.

4. American College of Sports Medicine. (2006). *ACSM's guidelines for exercise testing and prescription* (7th ed.). Philadelphia: Lippincott Williams & Wilkins.

5. Aslanidi, O. V., Clayton, R. H., Lambert, J. L., & Holden, A. V. (2005). Dynamical and cellular electrophysiological mechanisms of ECG changes during ischaemia. *Journal of Theoretical Biology, 237,* 369–81.

6. Baumgartner, T. A., Jackson, A. S., Mahar, M. T., & Rowe, D. A. (2003). *Measurement for evaluation in physical education & exercise science, 7th ed.* New York: McGraw-Hill Companies, Inc.

7. Borg, G. A. V. (1982). Psychophysical bases of perceived exertion. *Medicine and Science in Sports and Exercise, 14,* 377–381.

8. Brodsky, M., Wu, D., Denes, P., Kanakis, C., & Rosen, K. (1977). Arrhythmias documented by 24-hour continuous electrocardiographic monitoring in 50 male medical students without apparent heart disease. *The American Journal of Cardiology, 39,* 390–395.

9. Brooks, G. A., Fahey, T. D., White, T. P., & Baldwin, K. M. (2000). *Exercise physiology: Human bioenergetics and its applications, 3rd ed.* Mountain View, CA: Mayfield Publishing Co.

10. Bruce, R. A. (1972). Multi-stage treadmill test of submaximal and maximal exercise. In American Heart Association's Committee on Exercise (Ed.), *Exercise testing and training of apparently healthy individuals: A handbook for physicians* (pp. 32–34). New York: American Heart Association.

11. Chung, E. K. (1983). *Exercise electrocardiography: Practical approach.* Baltimore, MD: Williams & Wilkins.

12. Cooper, K. H. (1977). The treadmill re-examined. *American Heart Journal, 94,* 811–812.

13. Crow, R. S., Pineas, R. J., Dias, V., Taylor, H. L., Jacobs, D., & Blackburn, H. (1975). Ventricular premature beats in a population sample. *Circulation, 51*(Suppl.), III-211–III-215.

14. Dubach, P., & Froelicher, V. F. (1991). Recent advances in exercise testing. *Journal of Cardiopulmonary Rehabilitation, 11,* 29–38.

15. Duda, M. (1984). Basketball coaches guard against cardiovascular stress. *The Physician and Sportsmedicine, 12,* 193–194.

16. Ellestad, M. H. (1980). *Stress testing. Principles and practice.* Philadelphia: F. A. Davis.

17. Engels, H.-J., Zhu, W., & Moffatt, R. J. (1998). An empirical evaluation of the prediction of maximal heart rate. *Research Quarterly for Exercise and Sport, 69,* 94–98.

18. Faris, J. V., McHenry, P. L., Jordan, J. W., & Morris, S. N. (1976). Prevalence and reproducibility of exercise-induced ventricular arrhythmias during maximal exercise testing in normal men. *The American Journal of Cardiology, 37,* 617–622.

19. Franklin, B. A. (2000). Treadmill scores to diagnose heart disease and assess prognosis. *ACSM's Health and Fitness Journal, 4,* 29–31.

20. Froelicher, V. F., Lehmann, K. G., Thomas, R., Goldman, S., Morrison, D., Edson, R., Lavori, P., Myers, J., Dennis, C., Shabetai, R., Do, D., & Fronig, J. (1998). The electrocardiographic exercise test in a population with reduced workup bias: diagnostic performance, computerized interpretation, and multi-variable prediction. *Annals of Internal Medicine, 128,* 965–974.

21. Gianrossi, R., Detrano, R., Mulvihill, D., Lehmann, K., Dubach, P., Colombo, A., McArthur, D., & Froelicher, V. (1989). Exercise-induced ST depression in the diagnosis of coronary artery disease. A meta-analysis. *Circulation, 80,* 87–98.

22. Higgins, J. P., & Higgins, J. A. (2007). Electrocardiographic exercise stress testing: an update beyond the ST-segment. *International Journal of Cardiology, 116,* 285–299.

23. Knight, J. A., Laubach, C. A., Butcher, R. J., & Menapace, F. J. (1995). Supervision of clinical exercise testing by exercise physiologists. *The American Journal of Cardiology, 75,* 390–391.

24. Kosowsky, B. D., Lown, B., Whiting, R., & Guiney, T. (1971). Occurrence of ventricular arrhythmias with exercise as compared to monitoring. *Circulation, 46,* 826–832.

25. Liang, M. T. C., Alexander, J. F., Stull, G. A., & Serfass, R. C. (1982). The use of the Bruce equation for predicting VO2max in healthy young men. *Medicine and Science in Sports and Exercise, 14*(Abstract), 129.

26. Luft, V. C., Cardus, D., Lim, T. P. K., Anderson, E. C., & Howarth, J. L. (1963). Physical performance in relation to body size and composition. *Annals of New York Academy of Science, 110,* 795–808.

27. Master, A. M., & Oppenheimer, E. J. (1929). A simple exercise tolerance test for circulatory efficiency with standard tables for normal individuals. *American Journal of Medical Sciences, 177,* 223–243.

28. McArdle, W. D., Katch, F. I., & Katch, V. L. (1991). *Exercise physiology: Energy, nutrition, and human performance.* Philadelphia: Lea & Febiger.

29. McArdle, W. D., Katch, F. I., & Katch, V. L. (1994). *Essentials of exercise physiology.* Philadelphia: Lea & Febiger.

30. McHenry, P. L., Morris, S. N., Kavalier, M., & Jordan, J. W. (1976). Comparative study of exercise-induced ventricular arrhythmia in normal subjects and patients with documented coronary artery disease. *The American Journal of Cardiology, 37,* 609–616.

31. McInnis, K. J., & Balady, G. J. (1994). Comparison of submaximal exercise responses using the Bruce vs. modified Bruce protocols. *Medicine and Science in Sports and Exercise, 26,* 103–107.

32. Misner, J. E., Bloomfield, D. K., & Smith, L. (1975). Periodicity of premature ventricular contractions (PVC) in healthy, active adults. *Medicine and Science in Sports, 7*(Abstract), 72.

33. Naughton, J. (1977). Stress electrocardiography in clinical electrocardiographic correlations. In J. C. Rios (Ed.), *Cardiovascular Clinics, 8,* 127–139. Philadelphia: F. A. Davis.

34. Okajuma, M., Scholmerich, P., & Simonson, E. (1960). Frequency of premature beats. *Minnesota Medicine, 43,* 751.

35. Pollock, M. L., Bohannon, R. L., Cooper, K. H., Ayres, J. J., Ward, A., White, S. R., & Linnerud, A. C. (1976). A comparative analysis of four protocols for maximal treadmill stress testing. *American Heart Journal, 92,* 39–46.

36. Pollock, M. L., Foster, C., Schmidt, D. H., Hellman, C., Linnerud, A. C., & Ward, A. (1982). Comparative analysis of physiological responses to three different maximal graded exercise test protocols in healthy women. *American Heart Journal, 103,* 363.

37. San Roman, J. A., Vilacosta, I., Castillo, J. A., Rollan, M. J., Hernandez, M., Peral, V., Garcimartin, I., de la Torre, M. M., & Fernandez-Aviles, F. (1998). Selection of the optimal stress test for the diagnosis of coronary artery disease. *Heart, 80,* 370–376.

38. Thacker, S. B., & Berkelman, R. L. (1988). Public health surveillance in the United States. *Epidemiological Reviews, 10,* 164.

39. Wasserman, K., Hansen, J. E., Sue, D. Y., Whipp, B. J., & Casaburi, R. (1994). *Principles of exercise testing and interpretation.* Philadelphia: Lea & Febiger.

Form 19.1

EXERCISE ELECTROCARDIAOGRAM

Homework

Gender: **M**   Initials: **AA**   Age (y): **22**   Height (cm): **175**   Weight (kg): **80.0**

Below is a sample *resting* single-lead ECG.

Determine HR: HR = number of R waves within 6 s _____ x 10 = _____ bpm

Assess HR: ☐ bradycardia (< 60 bpm)   ☐ normal sinus rhythm (60-100 bpm)   ☐ tachycardia (> 100 bpm)

Screen for ectopic beats: ☐ none observed ☐ PAC ☐ PVC   Circle and label any ectopic beats

Screen for ST changes: ☐ none observed ☐ ST elevation ☐ ST depression

Evaluation of resting ECG: _____

_____

Below is a sample *exercise* single-lead ECG.

Determine HR: HR = number of R waves within 6 s _____ x 10 = _____ bpm

Assess HR: ☐ bradycardia (< 60 bpm)   ☐ normal sinus rhythm (60-100 bpm)   ☐ tachycardia (> 100 bpm)

Screen for ectopic beats: ☐ none observed ☐ PAC ☐ PVC   Circle and label any ectopic beats

Screen for ST changes: ☐ none observed ☐ ST elevation ☐ ST depression

Evaluation of exercise ECG: _____

_____

Form 19.2

EXERCISE ELECTROCARDIAOGRAM

Lab Results

Gender: _____   Initials: _____   Age (y): _____   Height (cm): _____   Weight (kg): _____

Cut and paste a **resting** single-lead ECG below.

Determine HR: HR = number of R waves within 6 s _____ x 10 = _____ bpm

Assess HR: ☐ bradycardia (< 60 bpm)   ☐ normal sinus rhythm (60-100 bpm)   ☐ tachycardia (> 100 bpm)

Screen for ectopic beats: ☐ none observed ☐ PAC ☐ PVC   Circle and label any ectopic beats

Screen for ST changes: ☐ none observed ☐ ST elevation ☐ ST depression

Evaluation of resting ECG: _____

_____

_____

Cut and paste an **exercise** single-lead ECG below.

Determine HR: HR = number of R waves within 6 s _____ x 10 = _____ bpm

Assess HR: ☐ bradycardia (< 60 bpm)   ☐ normal sinus rhythm (60-100 bpm)   ☐ tachycardia (> 100 bpm)

Screen for ectopic beats: ☐ none observed ☐ PAC ☐ PVC   Circle and label any ectopic beats

Screen for ST changes: ☐ none observed ☐ ST elevation ☐ ST depression

Evaluation of exercise ECG: _____

_____

_____

Form 19.3

NAME _____ DATE _____ SCORE _____

GRADED EXERCISE TEST (*OPTIONAL*)

Homework

Gender: **M**   Initials: **AA**   Age (y): **22**   Height (cm): **175**   Weight (kg): **80.0**

Exercise mode (T or C) :   **T**   (Treadmill / Cycle)   Exercise protocol: __**Bruce**__

Time	Cycling Power (W)	Treadmill * Speed (mph)	Grade (%)	HR (bpm)	Estimated VO$_2$ (ml·kg^{-1}·min^{-1})	Estimated METS
3:00		1.7	10	114		
6:00		2.5	12	135		
9:00		3.4	14	160		
12:00		4.2	16	178		
15:00		5.0	18	194		

Estimated HRmax = 220 - Age = 220 - _____ = _____ bpm   Selected HRmax = **194** bpm

Average increase in HR per MET =   (_____ - _____) / (_____ - _____) = _____ bpm per MET *
                                       HR$_{max}$ HR$_{min}$ MET$_{max}$ MET$_{min}$ * Average 10 bpm per MET

Relative VO$_{2max}$ from max time on Bruce = (2.94 * **15.0** min) + 7.65 = _____ ml·kg^{-1}·min^{-1}

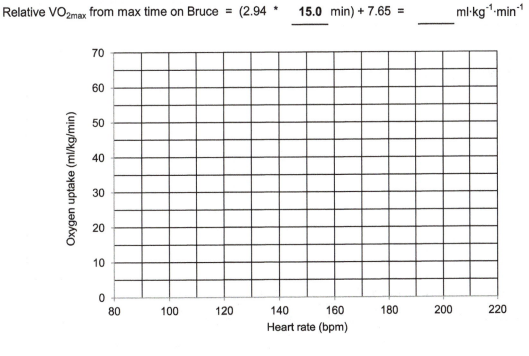

Estimated or measured HRmax = _____ bpm

Estimated relative VO$_2$max = _____ ml·kg^{-1}·min^{-1}

Category for aerobic fitness: _____   (*From Table* _____)

Form 19.4

NAME _____ DATE _____ SCORE _____

GRADED EXERCISE TEST (*OPTIONAL*)

Lab Results

Gender: _____   Initials: _____   Age (y): _____   Height (cm): _____   Weight (kg): _____

Exercise mode (T or C) : _____ (Treadmill / Cycle)   Exercise protocol: _____

Time	Cycling Power (W)	Treadmill * Speed (mph)	Grade (%)	HR (bpm)	Estimated VO_2 ($ml \cdot kg^{-1} \cdot min^{-1}$)	Estimated METS
____	____	____	____	____	____	____
____	____	____	____	____	____	____
____	____	____	____	____	____	____
____	____	____	____	____	____	____
____	____	____	____	____	____	____

Estimated HRmax = 220 - Age = 220 - _____ = _____ bpm   Selected HRmax = _____ bpm

Average increase in HR per MET = (_____ - _____) / (_____ - _____) = _____ bpm per MET *

HR_{max} HR_{min} MET_{max} MET_{min} * Average 10 bpm per MET

Relative VO_{2max} from max time on Bruce = (2.94 * _____ min) + 7.65 = _____ $ml \cdot kg^{-1} \cdot min^{-1}$

Estimated or measured HRmax = _____ bpm

Estimated relative VO_2max = _____ $ml \cdot kg^{-1} \cdot min^{-1}$

Category for aerobic fitness: _____   (*From Table _____*)

CHAPTER

RESTING LUNG VOLUMES

Measurement of lung volumes during rest enhances the interpretation of these volumes during exercise. Measurement of each of the four lung volumes demonstrates the physiology of respiration and tests for respiratory disease. For example, vital capacity, a composite of three lung volumes, has been used frequently for diagnosing lung disease.[29]

Physiologically, all four lung volumes are nonoverlapping divisions of the lungs at potentially different stages of breathing (Figure 20.1). For example, the **inspiratory reserve volume (IRV)** is the volume of air that can be inspired maximally at the end of a normal inspiration. The volume of air in a normal breath is the **tidal volume (TV or V_T)**. The volume of air that can be expired maximally after a normal expiration is the **expiratory reserve volume (ERV)**. The **residual volume (RV)** is the volume of air remaining in the lungs after a maximal expiration. The capacities are combinations of the different individual volumes. The **vital capacity (VC)** is the sum of three volumes, IRV, TV, and ERV, as seen in Equation 20.1a. The **total lung capacity (TLC)** is the sum of the vital capacity and residual volume (Eq. 20.1b), or it can also be described as the sum of all four volumes combined (Eq. 20.1c).

Vital capacity (VC) = Inspiratory reserve volume (IRV)
   + Tidal volume (TV) + Expiratory reserve
   volume (ERV)   Eq. 20.1a

Total lung capacity (TLC) = Vital capacity (VC)
   + ResidualVolume (RV)   Eq. 20.1b

Total lung capacity (TLC) = IRV + TV + ERV
   + RV   Eq. 20.1c

FORCED VITAL CAPACITY AND FORCED EXPIRATORY VOLUME

The vital capacity test is one of the oldest[16] and most common respiratory tests. The measurement of vital capacity (VC) simply requires that an individual blow as large a breath of air as possible into a spirometer. Thus, the person expels three of the four components of the total lung volume—the inspiratory reserve volume (IRV), the tidal volume (TV), and the expiratory reserve volume (ERV)—when performing the vital capacity test. It provides an indirect indication of the size of the lungs, although it is not a complete measure of the entire lung size because it does not include the residual volume. It is often measured in fitness and/or health clinics in order to assess the effects of smoking, disease, or environment, or as a part of the hydrostatic weighing test for body composition.

Inhalation is restricted by changes with aging leading to stiffness in the chest wall, thus older adults have lower vital capacities than younger people. Inhalation is restricted by respiratory muscle weakness, which can again be due to aging, but is also likely in younger persons who do insufficient amounts of sustained aerobic exercise to strengthen their respiratory muscles. Vital capacity is reduced clinically with *restrictive lung diseases* including pneumonia and fibrosis and with thoracic deformities such as pectus excavatum (a "sunken" chest). All of these conditions lead to a reduced FVC due to the limited ability to take a deep inhalation.

In general, vital capacity relates to three uncontrolled characteristics: (1) age, (2) height, and (3) gender. The older a person becomes, the less elastic (less compliant) become both the thoracic cage and respiratory muscles. The reduced expansion of the chest restricts lung expansion, which, along with reduced respiratory muscle strength, reduces vital capacity. The vital capacity is typically higher in taller people. This is basically a function of lung size, taller people having larger lungs. Chest circumference is not as closely related to lung size because chest muscle hypertrophy has little or nothing to do with lung size. Finally,

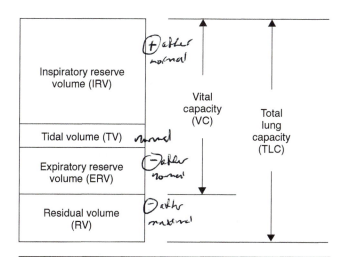

Figure 20.1 The four lung volumes (IRV, TV, ERV, and RV) are added together to form the two lung capacities (VC and TLC).

with respect to gender, men have larger lungs than women, even when corrected for body size.

The exhalation of the full vital capacity when measuring FVC may take well over 4–6 seconds. Another lung function test measures the ability to maximally exhale over a much shorter time, referred to as the **forced expiratory volume (FEV).** When FEV is measured over 1 s it is referred to as FEV_1. FEV can also be measured over 3 s (FEV_3), over 6 s (FEV_6), or other durations. The ability to exhale is reduced by numerous *obstructive lung diseases* including asthma, asthmatic bronchitis, chronic bronchitis, emphysema, and chronic obstructive pulmonary disease (COPD) which is combinations of all of the previous diseases. All of these conditions lead to a reduced FEV_1 due to the limited ability to exhale air from the lungs. The severity of some of these conditions can be at least partially alleviated with the use of inhaled bronchodilators.

METHODS

The equipment and procedures for measuring the four lung volumes and vital capacity have many similarities. Depending upon the type of equipment, some of these measures can be taken sequentially without changing the instrumentation. Many of the procedures described here are those recommended by the American Thoracic Society's Committee on Proficiency Standards.[2] The accuracy of measuring vital capacity and residual volume is presented in Box 20.1.

Equipment for Measuring Vital Capacity and Timed Volumes

Spirometer is the name of an instrument for measuring lung volumes and ventilation. These may have a mechanical

basis (volume-type spirometer), an electronic basis (flow-type spirometer) or a combination of both. Electronic (flow-type) spirometers have transducers of various types: (1) pneumotach, (2) turbine, (3) variable orifice, (4) hot wire, and (5) ultrasonic.[25] These have the advantage over traditional mechanical-based spirometers by providing (1) visual displays on monitor and printout, (2) computerized calculations, and (3) direct comparison with computer-stored norms.

Vital capacity and timed volumes can be measured with a variety of different spirometers. A typical electronic spirometer is the Spirolab™ (SDI Diagnostics, Eaton, MA) as seen in Figure 20.2. It measures flow ($0–16$ $L \cdot s^{-1}$) and volume ($0–10$ L) using a digital turbine with accuracies of 5 % (200 $mL \cdot s^{-1}$) for flow and 3 % (50 ml) for volume and with very low resistance (< 0.8 cm $H_2O \cdot L^{-1} \cdot s^{-1}$). Traditionally, prior to the popularity of electronic flow meters, lung function was measured using a wet spirometer. Examples of wet spirometers are the Collins 9 L Vitalometer™ and 13.5 L Respirometer™ (Warren E. Collins, Braintree, MA). These spirometers are still in use today in laboratories as teaching instruments, but are no longer commercially available. The SciEd™ 9 L wet spirometer, similar to the Vitalometer™, is available through various online vendors. The Vitalometer™ consists of a 9 L container filled with water with a tube running through the middle that extends above the water level inside the container and connects outside the container to a respiratory tube and mouthpiece (Figure 20.3). A lightweight plastic bell inside the container rises to capture the volume of air being exhaled by the participant. Two different pointers on the Vitalometer™ indicate the total volume of air exhaled (vital capacity) and the volume exhaled in a specific time, such as 1 second (FEV_1). The Vitalometer™ does not meet the American Thoracic Society (ATS) clinical requirement of providing a digital or graphic recording.[2] To meet all ATS

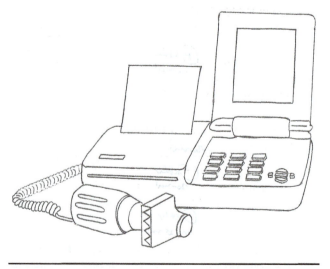

Figure 20.2 A typical electronic spirometer (Spirolab™, SDI Diagnostics) used to measure lung function (FVC, FEV_1, etc.).

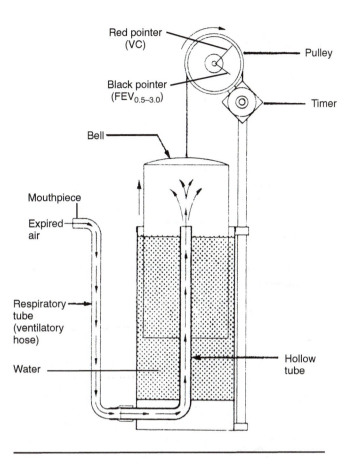

Red pointer (VC)

Pulley

Black pointer (FEV$_{0.5-3.0}$)

Timer

Bell

Mouthpiece

Expired air

Respiratory tube (ventilatory hose)

Water

Hollow tube

Figure 20.3 This diagram of an automated wet spirometer (e.g., Vitalometer™) shows the upward movement of the bell as the person exhales through the respiratory tube into the water-filled container.

requirements for clinical use, a spirometer must be capable of accumulating volume for ≥ 15 s, measuring volumes of ≥ 8 L (BTPS) with an accuracy of $\pm 3 \%$ (or ± 50 ml), and measuring flows of 0–14 L·s^{-1} with an accuracy of $\pm 5 \%$ (or 200 mL·s^{-1}), all with a total resistance to flow of < 1.5 cm H$_2$O·L^{-1}·s^{-1}.[22]

Regardless of which instrument is used to measure vital capacity, the methods are similar. The pretest preparations should ensure that the equipment is ready for use and is properly sanitized and calibrated, in addition to ensuring that the participant is prepared.

Procedures for Measuring Lung Volumes

The following procedures apply specifically to the measurement of lung volumes, vital capacity, and forced expiratory volumes using the Vitalometer™ and Respirometer™. However, most of the steps can be applied to all instruments.

Preparation for Lung Volumes, Vital Capacity, and Timed Volumes

Some researchers are very strict regarding abstention from exercise within 12 h of pulmonary function testing.[8] This is partly because the vital capacity has been shown to be reduced temporarily after exercise.[20] However, 12 h may be overly restrictive because both vital capacity and FEV$_1$ may be decreased significantly at the 5th and 10th min but not at the 30th min after varying intensities of exercise.[27] In addition, participants should not smoke within 1 h of the test, should not eat a large meal within 2 h of the test, should not consume alcohol within 4 h of the test, and should not wear clothing that restricts full chest and abdominal expansion.[21]

Testing may be performed either in the sitting or standing position, with sitting preferable to avoid falling due to syncope. The standing position, however, does in some cases yield larger values.[31] Obese persons, especially those with excessive weight around the midsection, frequently obtain a deeper inspiration when tested in the standing position.[21]

Participants should wear noseclips if they are inexperienced in the vital capacity test or if the data are to be used for research. The technician should ask the person if it is possible to breathe with the mouth closed when wearing the noseclip. If the person can still breathe, the noseclip should be readjusted until he or she cannot breathe with the mouth closed. Valid tests of vital capacity in experienced persons are possible by simply having them pinch the nose with the fingers during the test.

In order to ensure that the participant knows exactly what to do, the technician and participant should rehearse the commands and practice the breathing maneuvers. The technician should demonstrate the maneuvers,[2] but need not use the spirometer. The participant can also practice the maneuver without actually exhaling into the mouthpiece. The calibration of respiratory instruments is presented in Box 20.2.

Measuring IRV, TV, and ERV Using the Respirometer™

1. In preparation for the test, prepare the Respirometer™ (or pulmonary function system) by checking the operation of the kymograph (rotating, recording drum) and

---

BOX 20.2 **Calibration of Respiratory Instruments**

Manufacturers should testify that their instruments meet the recommendations of the American Thoracic Society.[2] To assure accurate volumes of spirometers or pneumotachs, the technician should pump air through the instrument using a calibrated syringe (≥ 3 L).

The residual volume analyzers require calibration with certified test gases—oxygen, nitrogen, helium, or carbon dioxide.

The steps for calibrating modern electronic spirometers vary with the type of device. Often, the computer monitor leads the technician through the steps. In general, make sure that both slow strokes and fast strokes are made with the calibrating syringe when calibrating the flowmeter. It is advisable to repeat the calibration to ensure its accuracy.

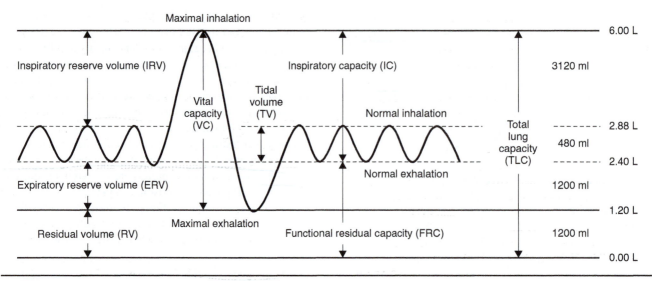

Figure 20.4 Spirogram demonstrating identification of lung volumes (IRV, TV, ERV, and RV) and lung capacities (IC, FRC, and TLC) with values representative of a young male.

status of the recording pens, and advancing the recording paper on the drum to an unmarked position.

2. Before the participant begins the test, the tester or technician pulls up on the bell of the spirometer such that 3–5 L of room air are drawn into the bell of the spirometer. The participant attaches the noseclip and seals the lips around the disposable cardboard mouthpiece. The power to the drum is turned on, and the speed indicator is set to the appropriate speed (typically the slowest speed).

3. The participant inhales and exhales normally for several breaths. At this point the participant inhales as deeply as possible (maximal inspiration), holds it for just a second, and then exhales all air from the lungs (maximal expiration). The participant should be specifically told to concentrate on inhaling and exhaling as much air as possible. The participant returns to normal breathing and inhales and exhales 2–3 more normal breaths.

4. This procedure (measuring IRV, TV, and ERV) may be repeated if desired. The test provides results similar to those shown in Figure 20.4. The technician determines the IRV, TV, and ERV from the results of the

test, corrects them to body (BTPS) conditions, and records them on Form 20.2. If these volumes are not measured, they may be estimated based on data found in Table 20.1.

Measuring FVC and FEV₁ Using the Vitalometer™

1. In preparation for the test, prepare the Vitalometer™ (or pulmonary function system). For theVitalometer™ this means pushing the bell down to the lowest position and setting the indicators to the starting position. The timing knob should also be set to the desired duration (to 1.0 s if measuring FEV₁).

2. The participant attaches the noseclip and inhales as deeply as possible (maximal inspiration), seals the lips around the disposable cardboard mouthpiece, and forcefully exhales all air from the lungs (maximal expiration) as quickly as possible. The participant should be specifically told to concentrate on blowing as fast as possible ("blasting" the air out of the lungs) for the first second and then to continue to exhale for as long as necessary ("keep going") to empty the lungs as much as possible.

Table 20.1 **Typical Respiratory Lung Volumes and Capacities**

| Lung Volume | % VC | Volumes (ml) | | | Capacities (ml) | | |
		Lung Volume	Men	Women	Lung Capacity	Men	Women
IRV	65 %	IRV	3120	2080	VC	4800	3200
TV	10 %	TV	480	320	IC	3600	2400
ERV	25 %	ERV	1200	800	FRC	2400	1800
RV	25 %	RV	1200	800	TLC	6000	4200

Note: See text for meaning of lung volume and capacity abbreviations. IRV, TV, ERV, and RV are estimated based on % VC; IC = IRV + TV; FRC + ERV + RV; TLC = VC + RV.

Source: Data from Comroe, et al. (1962).[6]

3. The entire exhalation should last about 5–10 s,[2] although most persons will exhale their entire VC within 4 s.[15] End of trial (EOT) criteria include (1) the participant cannot exhale further, or (2) the volume-time curve (if using a flow-type system) shows no change in volume for > 1 s.[22] It has been recommended that a shorter FVC maneuver of 6 s (FEV_6) could be better in young adults because it would be less effort for the participant, provides a more explicit EOT criterion, and does not differ significantly from FVC measured for longer durations.[11] Older adults, however, require expiratory times greater than 6 s to reach their FVC.

4. This procedure (measuring FVC and FEV_1) is typically done a minimum of three times in an attempt to get three acceptable trials and to measure the highest value possible. If the participant continues to improve on the third attempt (trial exceeds previous trial by 0.15 L[22]), more subsequent attempts (usually up to a maximum of eight) can be performed until a maximal value is attained for both volumes. The maximal values for FVC and FEV_1 do not need to occur on the same trial.

5. When using the Vitalometer™, each trial is done independently with a break in between to reset the spirometer. With most automated systems, however, multiple trials can be performed continuously without the need for a break.

6. The highest value for FVC and FEV_1 of all of the trials is recorded on Form 20.2. These two values (which were recorded under ATPS conditions if using the Vitalometer™ or any other volume-type spirometer) are then corrected to BTPS and recorded as actual FVC and FEV_1. Typical values for FVC and FEV_1 are given in Table 20.2.

7. At the conclusion of the test, dispose of the mouthpiece and lift and lower the Vitalometer™ bell at least five times to flush the bell with room air to promote clearance of water droplets and enhance decontamination of the Vitalometer™.

Procedures for Measuring Residual Volume (RV)

The residual volume is the only lung volume that cannot be measured directly; measuring it is also the most complicated and expensive method. Depending upon the chosen method and instrumentation, the reader may have to consult additional sources.[7,9,34,35]

Residual volume has been shown to increase temporarily after exercise.[10] It should not be measured for at least 30 min after exercise.[4]

Traditional methods to measure residual volume require expensive gas analyzers. The **nitrogen washout** method requires a nitrogen or oxygen analyzer, depending upon the use of the traditional or simplified version. The two **helium dilution methods** (multiple breath and single breath) require a helium analyzer, but neither is discussed here.

The rationale for using the nitrogen washout method of estimating residual volume is based upon the measurement of the functional residual capacity (FRC; see Figure 20.4). This is because residual volume cannot be measured directly but can be derived by subtracting the known expiratory reserve volume (ERV) from the FRC.

The **simplified O_2 dilution** method can eliminate the need for a nitrogen or helium analyzer but requires rapid-responding carbon dioxide and oxygen analyzers.[35] Fortunately, the analyzers are common in exercise physiology laboratories. A 5 L neoprene or rubber bag (anesthesia bag) filled with oxygen is used to determine the extent of its dilution after the participant breathes into it.

The calculation of residual volume from the simplified oxygen dilution technique[35] is based on the volume of oxygen in the bag to begin the test and the percentage of nitrogen in the mixed air at equilibrium at the end of the test, as seen in Equation 20.2a. If instead of a N_2 analyzer, combined O_2 and CO_2 analyzers are being used, then N_2 % is determined from O_2 % and CO_2 % and the calculation is made using Equation 20.2b.

$$\text{Residual volume (L)} = \frac{\text{Volume of } O_2(L) * N_2 \%}{79.8\% - N_2\%} \quad \text{Eq. 20.2a}$$

Where: Volume of O_2 is initial volume of O_2 in the bag

Where: N_2 % is percentage of N_2 in the mixed air at equilibrium

Where: 79.8 % is percentage of N_2 in alveolar air − 0.2 %[35]

Table 20.2	Typical Values for Forced Vital Capacity (FVC) and Forced Expiratory Volume (FEV_1) by Gender and Age					
	Men			**Women**		
Lung Volume	< 20 y (N = 1575)	20–40 y (N = 928)	> 40 y (N = 528)	< 20 y (N = 1725)	20–40 y (N = 1389)	> 40 y (N = 1320)
FVC (L)	3.22	4.93	4.34	2.82	3.53	2.99
FEV_1 (L)	2.77	4.10	3.37	2.51	3.02	2.36
FEV_1/FVC	86.10	83.20	77.60	89.10	85.50	78.90

Source: Data from Hankinson, Crapo, & Jensen (2003).[11]

Given: $N_2 \% = (100 \% - O_2 \% - CO_2 \%)$

By substitution:

Residual volume (L)

$$= \frac{\text{Volume of } O_2 (L) * (100 \% - O_2 \% - CO_2 \%)}{79.8 \% - (100 \% - O_2 \% - CO_2 \%)} \quad \text{Eq. 20.2b}$$

For example, if the initial volume of 100 % oxygen in the bag is 4.00 L, and the final percentage of N_2 in the mixed air in the bag at equilibrium is 19.0 %, then residual volume would be calculated as 1.25 L, as seen in Equation 20.3. Residual volume may also be estimated using Table 20.3.[35]

$$\text{Residual volume (RV)} = \frac{4.00 \text{ L} * (19.0 \%)}{79.80 \% - (19 \%)} = 1.25 \text{ L}$$

Eq. 20.3

Preparation for Measuring Residual Volume

Several preparations are necessary before measuring the residual volume using the simplified method.

1. Measure the participant's vital capacity before the RV test.
2. Set up the instrumentation as follows:
   a. Attach a 5 L anesthesia bag to a two-way syringe stopcock.
   b. Attach the other end of the bag to a three-way breathing valve that can be opened to room air or the bag.
   c. Manually push the bell of a spirometer that has been filled with 100 % oxygen so that the oxygen flows into the bag.
   d. Flush the bag with pure oxygen about three times.
   e. Fill the bag with an accurately measured volume of oxygen that is 80–90 % of the participant's vital capacity; measure the volume of oxygen, for example, by calculating the amount taken from the spirometer.

Measuring RV Using the Oxygen Dilution Method

The technician and participant interaction occurs during the following procedures:

1. The participant, wearing a noseclip and in the sitting position, breathes normally via the mouthpiece attached to the three-way breathing valve opened to room air. However, if the main purpose of measuring RV is subsequently to measure body density by underwater weighing, then RV should be measured in the same position as the one in the water.
2. The technician instructs the participant to perform a maximal expiration after a normal breath.
3. At the end of the maximal expiration, the technician turns the three-way valve open to the 5 L bag of oxygen.
4. The technician instructs the participant to breathe deeply (but not depleting the oxygen volume in the bag) five to seven times at about one breath per 2 s.
5. Following the five to seven breaths, the technician instructs the participant to exhale to maximal expiration.
6. The technician turns the valve to close the 5 L bag, thus opening the valve to room air.
7. The technician asks the participant to breathe normally, then removes the noseclip.
8. The participant removes his or her mouth from the mouthpiece.
9. The technician removes about 1 L of air from the bag; the remaining contents are analyzed using the carbon dioxide and oxygen analyzers.
10. A technician uses Equation 20.2a or 20.2b to find residual volume.
11. The technician repeats the procedure until readings are within 200 ml (a strict criterion may be 100 ml) of each other; the average of these is the participant's RV.
12. The technician corrects the volume to BTPS.
13. The total lung volume (TLV) or capacity (TLC) can be derived easily from a combination of lung volumes or capacities that are now known.

Calculations and Corrections for Lung Volumes and Vital Capacity

Certain calculations are made in order to correct respiratory volumes to conventional units of measure. Additionally,

Table 20.3 Calculation of Residual Volume (L) by Simplified Oxygen Dilution Technique from Volume of O_2 in Bag (L) and % N_2 in Mixed Air with Estimated RV (L)

	Vol O_2 in Bag (L)	Residual Volume (L) % N_2 or $(100 - \% O_2 - \% CO_2)$ in Mixed Air at Equilibrium							Estimated RV (L)
VC_{BTPS}	(80 % VC)	22.0	21.0	20.0	19.0	18.0	17.0	16.0	(25 % VC)
3.00	2.40	0.91	0.86	0.80	0.75	0.70	0.65	0.60	0.75
3.50	2.80	1.07	1.00	0.94	0.88	0.82	0.76	0.70	0.88
4.00	3.20	1.22	1.14	1.07	1.00	0.93	0.87	0.80	1.00
4.50	3.60	1.37	1.29	1.20	1.13	1.05	0.97	0.90	1.13
5.00	4.00	1.52	1.43	1.34	1.25	1.17	1.08	1.00	1.25
5.50	4.40	1.67	1.57	1.47	1.38	1.28	1.19	1.10	1.38
6.00	4.80	1.83	1.71	1.61	1.50	1.40	1.30	1.20	1.50
6.50	5.20	1.98	1.86	1.74	1.63	1.51	1.41	1.30	1.63

Note: RV = [(Volume of O_2) * N_2 %] / (79.8 % − N_2 %).

Source: Based on data from Wilmore et al. (1980).[35]

simple calculations are necessary in some instances in order to allow for easier interpretation of the norms; an example of the latter is the conversion of the FEV values to a percentage of the VC value.

The final recorded respiratory lung volumes are expressed in terms of BTPS, where the BT represents resting body temperature, the P represents the barometric pressure at the test site, and the S represents the saturation level of the air volume. However, the vital capacity value (liters or milliliters) that is read on the spirometer is in terms of ATPS. The ATPS abbreviation means that the volume of ambient (A) air is at laboratory pressure, at or near laboratory temperature, and is saturated. Some commercial metabolic systems use 31 °C and assume the expired air is saturated with water vapor. In other words, the air that is expired from the person's lungs decreases from the typical body temperature of 37 °C to 33 °C at the mouth exit[23] to that near the laboratory or spirometer temperature, usually 20 °C to 25 °C. The air remains saturated in a wet spirometer because of the water surrounding its bell. Even electronic spirometers sample exhaled air that is 100 % saturated. The barometric pressure is read from the laboratory barometer or weather station.

Calculation of BTPS Correction Factor

A correction must be made because of the temperature difference between the warm air in the lungs (body) and that of the cooler air being measured in the ambient environment (spirometer). Air molecules slow down at cooler (lower) temperatures; as a result, the volume of air exhaled from the lungs shrinks as it enters the cooler spirometer. To correct the lung volume back to the volume it actually occupied in the lungs, a BTPS correction factor must be determined. This correction factor depends on ambient temperature and barometric pressure, as seen in Equation 20.4a. Temperatures are converted to the Kelvin scale by adding 273. Differences in pressure depend mainly on differences in pressure exerted by the water vapor in the exhaled air. The vapor pressure of water (P_{H_2O}) is 47 mm Hg in the lungs when body temperature (T_B) is assumed to be 37 °C. The vapor pressure of water in the atmosphere varies in direct proportion to the ambient temperature and can be determined using Table 20.4. A BTPS correction factor can be calculated by using Equation 20.4a, which can be further simplified to Equation 20.4b.

$$\text{BTPS CF} = \frac{[T_B \,(^\circ C) + 273 \, K]}{[T_A \,(^\circ C) + 273 \, K]}$$

$$* \frac{[P_B \,(mm \, Hg) - P_{H_2O} \, at \, T_A]}{[P_B \,(mm \, Hg) - P_{H_2O} \, at \, T_B]} \qquad \text{Eq. 20.4}$$

Where: T_B: Body temperature (37 °C or 310 K)
Where: T_A: Ambient temperature (varies)
Where: P_B: Barometric pressure (varies)
Where: P_{H_2O} at T_A: Vapor pressure of water at T_A (varies)

Table 20.4 — Water Vapor Pressures (P_{H_2O}) at 100 % Saturation at Given Temperatures (°C; K)

Temperature		P_{H_2O}	Temperature		P_{H_2O}
°C	K	(mm Hg)	°C	K	(mm Hg)
20	293	18	26	299	25
21	294	19	27	300	27
22	295	20	28	301	28
23	296	21	29	302	30
24	297	22	30	303	32
25	298	24	37	310	47

Where: P_{H_2O} at T_B: Vapor pressure of water at T_B (47 mm Hg)

By substitution:

$$\text{BTPS CF} = \frac{[310 \, K]}{[T_A \,(^\circ C) + 273 \, K]}$$

$$* \frac{[P_B \,(mm \, Hg) - P_{H_2O} \, at \, T_A]}{[P_B \,(mm \, Hg) - 47 \, mm \, Hg]} \qquad \text{Eq. 20.4b}$$

Where: T_A: Ambient temperature (varies)

Where: P_B: Barometric pressure (varies)
Where: P_{H_2O} at T_A: Vapor pressure of water at T_A (varies)

For example, if ambient temperature (T_A) is 24 °C, whereby P_{H_2O} at 24 °C is 22 mm Hg (from Table 20.4), and barometric pressure (P_B) is 760 mm Hg, then the BTPS correction factor would be 1.080, as calculated in Equation 20.5. This value, the BTPS correction factor, may also be estimated from Table 20.5. The values in Table 20.5 assume a P_B of 760 mm Hg.

$$\text{BTPS CF} = \frac{[310 \, K]}{[24 \,^\circ C + 273 \, K]}$$

$$* \frac{[760 \, mm \, Hg - 22 \, mm \, Hg]}{[760 \, mm \, Hg - 47 \, mm \, Hg]} = 1.080 \qquad \text{Eq. 20.5}$$

Table 20.5 — Correction Factors (CF) for Converting Volumes from ATPS to BTPS Conditions

Ambient T (°C)	CF	Ambient T (°C)	CF
20	1.102	27	1.063
21	1.096	28	1.057
22	1.091	29	1.051
23	1.085	30	1.045
24	1.080	31	1.039
25	1.075	32	1.032
26	1.068	33	1.026

Note: Correction factors (CF) are calculated assuming a P_B of 760 mm Hg and a RH of 100 %.

This BTPS correction factor is then used to correct any measured lung volume from ATPS (ambient) conditions to BTPS (body) conditions. For example, if a person's vital capacity is measured under ambient conditions (T_A = 24 °C and P_B = 760 mm Hg) at 4.55 L, it would be corrected to BTPS by multiplying by 1.080 to yield 4.92 L. In other words, as the vital capacity is exhaled from the warm body (37 °C) into the cooler spirometer (24 °C) it shrinks from 4.92 L to 4.55 L. So to correct it back to the actual volume it occupied inside the lungs, the VC_{ATPS} must be multiplied by 1.080 or increased by 8 % to convert it into the VC_{BTPS}.

Predicting and Evaluating FVC and FEV$_1$

The actual or observed forced vital capacity (FVC) and forced expiratory volume (FEV$_1$) can be interpreted more meaningfully if they are compared to predicted or estimated values. The predicted FVC (PFVC) and predicted FEV$_1$ (PFEV$_1$) are based on the race, gender, height, and age of the participant. As mentioned previously, lung function is higher in men than in women, in taller than shorter persons, and in younger than older persons. Differences have also been observed in persons of different ethnicities (comparing Caucasians, African Americans, and Hispanics). FVC can be predicted for Caucasian men and women using Equations 20.6a, 20.6b, and 20.6c. FEV$_1$ can be predicted using Equations 20.6d, 20.6e, and 20.6f. These equations are based on a sample of over 7000 asymptomatic, lifelong nonsmoking participants who completed at least two acceptable lung function trials.[14] Spirometric reference equations for Caucasians, African Americans, Mexican Americans, and Asian Americans can be found in Table 20.6 and Table 20.7.

Men (Caucasian, < 20 y): PFVC$_{BTPS}$ (L) = −0.2585
$$- [0.20415 * \text{Age (y)}] + [0.010133 * \text{Age (y)}^2]$$
$$+ [0.00018642 * \text{Ht (cm)}^2] \qquad \text{Eq. 20.6a}$$

Men (Caucasian, ≥ 20 y): PFVC$_{BTPS}$ (L) = −0.1933
$$+ [0.00064 * \text{Age (y)}] - [0.000269 * \text{Age (y)}^2]$$
$$+ [0.00018642 * \text{Ht (cm)}^2] \qquad \text{Eq. 20.6b}$$

Women (Caucasian): PFVC$_{BTPS}$ (L) = −0.356
$$+ [0.0187 * \text{Age (y)}] - [0.000382 * \text{Age (y)}^2]$$
$$+ [0.00014815 * \text{Ht (cm)}^2] \qquad \text{Eq. 20.6c}$$

Men (Caucasian, < 20 y): PFEV$_{1\,BTPS}$ (L) = −0.7453
$$- [0.04106 * \text{Age (y)}] + [0.004477 * \text{Age (y)}^2]$$
$$+ 0.000140982 * \text{Ht (cm)}^2 \qquad \text{Eq. 20.6d}$$

Men (Caucasian, ≥ 20 y): PFEV$_{1\,BTPS}$ (L) = −0.5536
$$- [0.01303 * \text{Age (y)}] + [0.000172 * \text{Age (y)}^2]$$
$$+ [0.00014098 * \text{Ht (cm)}^2] \qquad \text{Eq. 20.6e}$$

Women (Caucasian): PFEV$_{1\,BTPS}$ (L) = 0.4333
$$- [0.00361 * \text{Age (y)}] - [0.000194 * \text{Age (y)}^2]$$
$$+ [0.00011496 * \text{Ht (cm)}^2] \qquad \text{Eq. 20.6f}$$

Where: PFVC$_{BTPS}$ is predicted forced vital capacity

Where: PFEV$_{1\,BTPS}$ is predicted forced expiratory volume

Where: Ht is height (cm)

For example, a 42-year-old Caucasian man who is 177 cm tall would have a predicted FVC of 5.20 L, as calculated in Equation 20.7a. A 22-year-old Caucasian woman who is 167 cm tall would have a predicted FEV$_1$ of 3.47 L, as calculated in Equation 20.7b. Both of these values may also be determined by using Tables 20.6 and 20.7.

PFVC$_{BTPS}$ (L) = − 0.1933 + [0.00064 * **42**]
$$- [0.000269 * \mathbf{42}^2] + [0.00018642 * \mathbf{177}^2]$$
$$= \mathbf{5.20}\,\text{L} \qquad \text{Eq. 20.7a}$$

PFEV$_{1\,BTPS}$ (L) = 0.4333 − [0.00361 * **22**]
$$- [0.000194 * \mathbf{22}^2] + [0.00011496 * \mathbf{167}^2]$$
$$= \mathbf{3.47}\,\text{L} \qquad \text{Eq. 20.7b}$$

Finally, to evaluate a person's lung function, the actual or observed values of FVC and FEV$_1$ are compared to the predicted values. A value is calculated to reflect the percentage of the predicted value by dividing the actual FVC (FVC) by the predicted FVC (PFVC) to yield % PFVC, as seen in Equation 20.8a. This same calculation can be done for the actual and predicted FEV$_1$ to yield % PFEV$_1$ (Eq. 20.8b). And one other ratio is also frequently calculated, that being the ratio of the actual FEV$_1$ to the actual FVC (FEV$_1$/FVC), as seen in Equation 20.8c.

% PFVC = [Actual FVC$_{BTPS}$ (L)
$$/ \text{Predicted FVC}_{BTPS}\,(\text{L})] * 100 \qquad \text{Eq. 20.8a}$$

% PFEV$_1$ = [Actual FEV$_{1\,BTPS}$ (L)
$$/ \text{Predicted FEV}_{1\,BTPS}\,(\text{L})] * 100 \qquad \text{Eq. 20.8b}$$

FEV$_1$ / FVC ratio = [FEV$_{1\,BTPS}$ (L)
$$/ \text{FVC}_{BTPS}\,(\text{L})\,] * 100 \qquad \text{Eq. 20.8c}$$

For example, a 27-year-old Caucasian man who is 182 cm tall, with an actual FVC$_{BTPS}$ of 4.85 L and an actual FEV$_{1\,BTPS}$ of 3.95 L, compared to his predicted values, a PFVC$_{BTPS}$ of 5.80 L and a PFEV$_{1\,BTPS}$ of 4.75 L, would yield a % PFVC of 84 %, a % PFEV$_1$ of 83 %, and an FEV$_1$ / FVC ratio of 81 %, as seen in Equations 20.9a, 20.9b, and 20.9c. In comparison with the results found in Table 20.8, this participant's actual FVC and FEV$_1$ would both be considered "normal" because the values fall between 80 and 99 % of the values predicted from his race, gender, age, and height.

% PFVC = [4.85 L / 5.80 L] * 100 = **84** %   Eq. 20.9a

% PFEV$_1$ = [3.95 L / 4.75 L] * 100 = **83** %   Eq. 20.9b

% FEV$_1$ / FVC = [3.95 L / 4.85 L] * 100 = **81** %   Eq. 20.9c

RESULTS AND DISCUSSION

When discussing the results of the tests the focus is on interpretation of test scores. The tests for the four lung volumes are of physiological significance and when interpreted in conjunction with vital capacity and FEV tests add a clinical significance. Although the norms are helpful for interpreting the results of a person's pulmonary test, serial test comparisons on a single person over a period of years can be even more helpful.[25]

Table 20.6 **Prediction of Forced Vital Capacity (PFVC$_{BTPS}$) in Men and Women Based on Race (Caucasian, African-American, Mexican-American, or Asian-American), Gender, Age (y) and Height (cm)**

Height (cm)	Caucasian Men Age (y)						Caucasian Women Age (y)					
	18–19	20–24	25–29	30–34	35–39	40–44	18–19	20–24	25–29	30–34	35–39	40–44
155 – 159	4.03	4.29	4.22	4.15	4.06	3.95	3.51	3.52	3.52	3.50	3.46	3.41
160 – 164	4.33	4.58	4.52	4.44	4.35	4.25	3.75	3.76	3.76	3.74	3.70	3.64
165 – 169	4.63	4.89	4.83	4.75	4.66	4.56	3.99	4.00	4.00	3.98	3.94	3.89
170 – 174	4.95	5.21	5.14	5.07	4.98	4.87	4.24	4.25	4.25	4.23	4.20	4.14
175 – 179	5.27	5.53	5.47	5.39	5.30	5.20	4.50	4.51	4.51	4.49	4.45	4.40
180 – 184	5.61	5.87	5.80	5.73	5.64	5.53	4.77	4.78	4.78	4.76	4.72	4.66
185 – 189	5.95	6.21	6.15	6.07	5.98	5.88	5.04	5.05	5.05	5.03	4.99	4.94
190 – 194	6.31	6.56	6.50	6.42	6.33	6.23	5.32	5.33	5.33	5.31	5.27	5.22

Note: Men (< 20 y), PFVC = −0.2584 − 0.20415 * Age + 0.010133 * Age^2 + 0.00018642 * Ht^2; Men (≥ 20 y), PFVC = −0.1933 + 0.00064*Age − 0.000269 * Age^2 + 0.00018642 * Ht^2; Women, PFVC = −0.3560 + 0.0187 * Age − 0.000382 * Age^2 + 0.00014815 * Ht^2

Height (cm)	African-American Men Age (y)						African-American Women Age (y)					
	18–19	20–24	25–29	30–34	35–39	40–44	18–19	20–24	25–29	30–34	35–39	40–44
155 – 159	3.37	3.55	3.46	3.37	3.28	3.19	3.06	3.04	3.00	2.95	2.89	2.81
160 – 164	3.64	3.82	3.72	3.63	3.54	3.45	3.28	3.26	3.22	3.17	3.10	3.02
165 – 169	3.91	4.09	4.00	3.91	3.82	3.73	3.50	3.48	3.44	3.39	3.33	3.25
170 – 174	4.20	4.37	4.28	4.19	4.10	4.01	3.73	3.71	3.67	3.62	3.56	3.48
175 – 179	4.49	4.66	4.57	4.48	4.39	4.30	3.97	3.95	3.91	3.86	3.79	3.72
180 – 184	4.78	4.96	4.87	4.78	4.69	4.60	4.21	4.19	4.15	4.10	4.04	3.96
185 – 189	5.09	5.27	5.18	5.09	4.99	4.90	4.46	4.44	4.41	4.35	4.29	4.21
190 – 194	5.41	5.58	5.49	5.40	5.31	5.22	4.72	4.70	4.66	4.61	4.55	4.47

Note: Men (< 20 y), PFVC = −0.4971 − 0.15497 * Age + 0.007701 * Age^2 + 0.00016643 * Ht^2; Men (≥ 20 y), PFVC = −0.1517 − 0.01821 * Age + 0.00016643 * Ht^2; Women, PFVC = −0.3039 + 0.00536 * Age − 0.000265 * Age^2 + 0.00013606 * Ht^2

Height (cm)	Mexican-American Men Age (y)						Mexican-American Women Age (y)					
	18–19	20–24	25–29	30–34	35–39	40–44	18–19	20–24	25–29	30–34	35–39	40–44
150 – 154	3.86	4.07	3.98	3.88	3.78	3.66	3.39	3.37	3.32	3.27	3.20	3.12
155 – 159	4.14	4.35	4.26	4.16	4.05	3.94	3.61	3.59	3.54	3.49	3.42	3.34
160 – 164	4.42	4.63	4.54	4.44	4.34	4.22	3.84	3.81	3.77	3.72	3.65	3.57
165 – 169	4.72	4.92	4.84	4.74	4.63	4.51	4.07	4.05	4.00	3.95	3.88	3.80
170 – 174	5.02	5.23	5.14	5.04	4.93	4.82	4.31	4.29	4.25	4.19	4.12	4.05
175 – 179	5.33	5.54	5.45	5.35	5.24	5.13	4.56	4.54	4.49	4.44	4.37	4.30
180 – 184	5.65	5.86	5.77	5.67	5.56	5.45	4.82	4.79	4.75	4.70	4.63	4.55
185 – 189	5.98	6.19	6.10	6.00	5.89	5.77	5.08	5.06	5.01	4.96	4.89	4.81

Note: Men (< 20 y), PFVC = −0.7571 − 0.0952 * Age + 0.006619 * Age^2 + 0.00017823 * Ht^2; Men (≥ 20 y), PFVC = 0.2376 − 0.00891 * Age − 0.000182 * Age^2 + 0.00017823 * Ht^2; Women, PFVC = 0.121 + 0.00307 * Age − 0.000237 * Age^2 + 0.00014246 * Ht^2

Height (cm)	Asian-American Men Age (y)						Asian-American Women Age (y)					
	18–19	20–24	25–29	30–34	35–39	40–44	18–19	20–24	25–29	30–34	35–39	40–44
150 – 154	3.29	3.52	3.46	3.40	3.32	3.23	2.89	2.90	2.90	2.88	2.85	2.80
155 – 159	3.54	3.77	3.72	3.65	3.57	3.48	3.09	3.10	3.10	3.08	3.05	3.00
160 – 164	3.81	4.03	3.98	3.91	3.83	3.74	3.30	3.31	3.31	3.29	3.26	3.21
165 – 169	4.08	4.30	4.25	4.18	4.10	4.01	3.51	3.52	3.52	3.51	3.47	3.42
170 – 174	4.35	4.58	4.53	4.46	4.38	4.29	3.73	3.74	3.74	3.73	3.69	3.64
175 – 179	4.64	4.87	4.81	4.75	4.67	4.58	3.96	3.97	3.97	3.95	3.92	3.87
180 – 184	4.93	5.16	5.11	5.04	4.96	4.87	4.19	4.20	4.20	4.19	4.15	4.10
185 – 189	5.24	5.46	5.41	5.34	5.26	5.17	4.44	4.45	4.44	4.43	4.39	4.34

Note: Asian-Americans are predicted based on Caucasian values corrected by a factor of 0.88.

Source: Spirometric reference equations for Caucasians, African-Americans, and Mexican-Americans from Hankinson, Odencrantz & Fedan (1999).[14] Values for Asian-Americans based on Hankinson et al. (2010).[12]

Height (cm)	Caucasian Men Age (y)						Caucasian Women Age (y)					
	18–19	20–24	25–29	30–34	35–39	40–44	18–19	20–24	25–29	30–34	35–39	40–44
155 – 159	3.50	3.66	3.55	3.44	3.31	3.18	3.13	3.09	3.03	2.95	2.87	2.77
160 – 164	3.73	3.88	3.78	3.66	3.54	3.40	3.32	3.28	3.21	3.14	3.05	2.96
165 – 169	3.96	4.12	4.01	3.89	3.77	3.63	3.51	3.47	3.40	3.33	3.24	3.15
170 – 174	4.20	4.35	4.25	4.13	4.01	3.87	3.70	3.66	3.60	3.52	3.44	3.34
175 – 179	4.44	4.60	4.49	4.38	4.25	4.12	3.90	3.86	3.80	3.72	3.64	3.54
180 – 184	4.70	4.85	4.75	4.63	4.51	4.37	4.11	4.07	4.00	3.93	3.84	3.75
185 – 189	4.96	5.11	5.01	4.89	4.77	4.63	4.32	4.28	4.21	4.14	4.05	3.96
190 – 194	5.22	5.38	5.27	5.16	5.03	4.90	4.54	4.50	4.43	4.36	4.27	4.18

Note: Men (< 20 y), PFEV$_{1.0}$ = −0.7453 − 0.04106 ∗ Age + 0.004477 ∗ Age^2 + 0.00014098 ∗ Ht^2; Men (≥ 20 y), PFEV$_{1.0}$= 0.5536 − 0.01303 ∗ Age − 0.000172 ∗ Age^2 + 0.00014098 ∗ Ht^2; Women, PFEV$_{1.0}$ = 0.4333 − 0.00361 ∗ Age − 0.000194 ∗ Age^2 + 0.00011496 ∗ Ht^2

Height (cm)	African-American Men Age (y)						African-American Women Age (y)					
	18–19	20–24	25–29	30–34	35–39	40–44	18–19	20–24	25–29	30–34	35–39	40–44
155 – 159	2.51	3.09	2.97	2.85	2.74	2.62	2.18	2.12	2.03	1.94	1.84	1.74
160 – 164	2.69	3.30	3.18	3.06	2.95	2.83	2.32	2.26	2.17	2.08	1.98	1.88
165 – 169	2.87	3.51	3.40	3.28	3.17	3.05	2.46	2.40	2.31	2.22	2.12	2.02
170 – 174	3.06	3.74	3.62	3.51	3.39	3.27	2.60	2.54	2.45	2.36	2.26	2.16
175 – 179	3.26	3.97	3.85	3.74	3.62	3.50	2.75	2.69	2.60	2.51	2.41	2.31
180 – 184	3.47	4.20	4.09	3.97	3.86	3.74	2.90	2.84	2.76	2.66	2.57	2.46
185 – 189	3.67	4.45	4.33	4.22	4.10	3.99	3.06	3.00	2.91	2.82	2.72	2.62
190 – 194	3.89	4.70	4.58	4.47	4.35	4.24	3.22	3.16	3.08	2.98	2.89	2.78

Note: Men (< 20 y), PFEV$_{1.0}$ = −0.7048 − 0.05711 ∗ Age + 0.004316 ∗ Age^2 + 0.00013194 ∗ Ht^2; Men (≥ 20 y), PFEV$_{1.0}$ = 0.3411 − 0.02309 ∗ Age + 0.00013194 ∗ Ht^2; Women, PFEV$_{1.0}$ = 0.3433 − 0.01283 ∗ Age − 0.000097 ∗ Age^2 + 0.00008546 ∗ Ht^2

Height (cm)	Mexican-American Men Age (y)						Mexican-American Women Age (y)					
	18–19	20–24	25–29	30–34	35–39	40–44	18–19	20–24	25–29	30–34	35–39	40–44
150 – 154	3.35	3.48	3.33	3.18	3.04	2.89	3.00	2.95	2.86	2.77	2.67	2.57
155 – 159	3.58	3.71	3.56	3.42	3.27	3.12	3.19	3.13	3.05	2.96	2.86	2.75
160 – 164	3.82	3.95	3.80	3.66	3.51	3.36	3.39	3.33	3.24	3.15	3.05	2.95
165 – 169	4.07	4.20	4.05	3.91	3.76	3.61	3.59	3.53	3.44	3.35	3.25	3.15
170 – 174	4.33	4.45	4.31	4.16	4.02	3.87	3.79	3.73	3.65	3.56	3.46	3.35
175 – 179	4.59	4.72	4.57	4.43	4.28	4.13	4.00	3.95	3.86	3.77	3.67	3.57
180 – 184	4.86	4.99	4.84	4.70	4.55	4.40	4.22	4.16	4.08	3.99	3.89	3.78
185 – 189	5.14	5.27	5.12	4.98	4.83	4.68	4.45	4.39	4.30	4.21	4.11	4.01

Note: Men (< 20 y), PFEV$_{1.0}$ = −0.8218 − 0.04248 ∗ Age + 0.004291 ∗ Age^2 + 0.00015104 ∗ Ht^2; Men (≥ 20 y), PFEV$_{1.0}$ = 0.6306 − 0.02928 ∗ Age + 0.00015104 ∗ Ht^2; Women, PFEV$_{1.0}$ = 0.4529 − 0.01178 ∗ Age − 0.000113 ∗ Age^2 + 0.00012154 ∗ Ht^2

Height (cm)	Asian-American Men Age (y)						Asian-American Women Age (y)					
	18–19	20–24	25–29	30–34	35–39	40–44	18–19	20–24	25–29	30–34	35–39	40–44
150 – 154	2.89	3.03	2.93	2.83	2.72	2.60	2.60	2.57	2.51	2.44	2.37	2.28
155 – 159	3.08	3.22	3.13	3.02	2.91	2.80	2.76	2.72	2.66	2.60	2.52	2.44
160 – 164	3.28	3.42	3.32	3.22	3.11	2.99	2.92	2.88	2.83	2.76	2.69	2.60
165 – 169	3.48	3.62	3.53	3.43	3.32	3.20	3.09	3.05	2.99	2.93	2.85	2.77
170 – 174	3.69	3.83	3.74	3.64	3.53	3.41	3.26	3.22	3.16	3.10	3.02	2.94
175 – 179	3.91	4.05	3.95	3.85	3.74	3.63	3.43	3.40	3.34	3.27	3.20	3.12
180 – 184	4.13	4.27	4.18	4.07	3.97	3.85	3.62	3.58	3.52	3.46	3.38	3.30
185 – 189	4.36	4.50	4.41	4.30	4.19	4.08	3.80	3.77	3.71	3.64	3.57	3.48

Note: Asian-Americans are predicted based on Caucasian values corrected by a factor of 0.88.

Source: Spirometric reference equations for Caucasians, African-Americans, and Mexican-Americans from Hankinson, Odencrantz & Fedan (1999).[14] Values for Asian-Americans based on Hankinson et al. (2010).[12]

Table 20.8 Classification of Lung Function Including Degrees of Lung Restriction or Obstruction

Classification	% Predicted
High (well above predicted) lung function	≥ 120 %
Good (above predicted) lung function	100–119 %
Normal (within predicted) lung function	80–99 %
Mild restriction (FVC) or obstruction (FEV)	65–79 %
Moderate restriction (FVC) or obstruction (FEV)	50–64 %
Severe restriction (FVC) or obstruction (FEV)	35–49 %
Very severe restriction (FVC) or obstruction (FEV)	< 35 %

Note: FVC, forced vital capacity; FEV, forced expiratory volume; predicted function based on race, age, height, and gender in nonsmokers.

Source: Adapted from Morris (1976).[25]

Respiratory Lung Volumes

Some typical values for three respiratory volumes[6] have been converted to percentages of vital capacity and total lung volume in Table 20.2. As long as a person's respiratory values are normal, they are not good predictors of fitness or performance in a normal environment. This is especially true when such values are adjusted for body size, gender, and age. The approximated percentages for IRV, TV, and ERV are based on the assumption that the percentages do not vary with total lung volume. Absolute values for residual volume and total lung volume in a typical 20- to 30-year-old man and woman are also presented in Table 20.1. A slightly higher value for residual volumes in adult men (1300 ml) has been reported.[26]

Lung Function Tests (FVC and FEV$_1$)

More than 20 "norms" for FVC are commonly used by various laboratories.[2] The valid interpretation of FVC should consider the person's age, height, gender, race and smoking status. The values in Tables 20.6 and 20.7 that provide predicted values for lung function are based on nearly 7000 non-smoking men and women.[14] The fact that they are non-smokers equates to a lung function equivalent to smokers who are 10 years younger[24], compared with some traditional norms that included smokers.[16,17] This is attributed to smoking causing the destruction of the alveoli and pulmonary tissue, which can subsequently lead to chronic obstructive pulmonary disease (COPD). Interestingly, the "vital" in forced vital capacity, has been associated with "vitality" or living capacity. Investigators in the famous epidemiological heart study done in Framingham, MA, indicated that FVC and FEV$_1$ were associated with living capacity, suggesting that the lower the FVC and FEV$_1$, the greater the risk of death.[3]

The results of both lung function tests, FVC and FEV$_1$, are most often interpreted by comparing the actual values recorded with the values predicted from a person's gender, age, height and race. As mentioned, Tables 20.6 and 20.7 provide predicted values of FVC (PFVC) and FEV$_1$ (PFEV$_1$) based on gender, age, height and race.[12,14] By dividing the actual measured value (FVC or FEV$_1$) by the predicted value (PFVC or PFEV$_1$) yields a % predicted value (% PFVC or % PFEV$_1$). The % predicted values can be used to classify the participant's lung function and assess any degree of restriction or obstruction using Table 20.8. Normal lung function is typically defined by a % PFVC or % PFEV1 of at least 80 % of the predicted value.[25] Values above 100 % can be interpreted as being good (100–119 %) or high (≥ 120 %) lung function. Values below 80 % indicate a mild, moderate or severe restrictive (if FVC is reduced) or obstructive (if FEV$_1$ is reduced) disease or condition. Clinically, the calculated ratio of FEV$_1$ divided by FVC (% FEV$_1$/FVC) and the actual FEV$_1$ divided by the predicted FEV$_1$ (% PFEV$_1$) are most often used to identify and classify COPD[33] as seen in Table 20.9. Normal lung function is characterized by % FEV$_1$/FVC ≥ 70 % and % PFEV1 ≥ 80 %. COPD, including stages of severity, is identified by a % FEV$_1$/FVC < 70 % along with a reduced % PFEV$_1$. A decrease in post-exercise FEV$_1$ versus pre-exercise FEV$_1$ of 10 % or greater following strenuous exercise might suggest exercise-induced bronchospasm.[18,19,28,32] This bronchospasm in most chronic asthmatics is usually maximal between 5 min and 15 min after exercise.

Racial differences in lung function have been investigated. African-American and Mexican-American men and women all have lower FEV$_1$ values than Caucasian men and women. The lower FEV$_1$ values in Mexican-Americans are explained by the fact that they are shorter than Caucasians. The lower FEV$_1$ values in African-Americans, however, are observed at the same height as Caucasians.[14] This may be explained by a difference in body build. African-Americans have a smaller trunk length to leg length ratio than Caucasians, meaning that their trunk and presumably their torso and chest cavity, make up a smaller portion of their entire height.[1] Even though most racial groups when compared to Caucasians show a lower FEV$_1$, they do not demonstrate a lower % FEV$_1$/FVC ratio.[1,13] Not until recently have studies of lung function been done on large samples of Asian-Americans. FEV$_1$ values in

Table 20.9 Classification of Stages of Chronic Obstructive Pulmonary Disease (COPD)

Classification	Criterion 1 % FEV$_1$/FVC	Criterion 2 % PFEV$_1$
Normal	≥ 70 %	≥ 80 %
Stage 1 (Mild)	< 70 %	≥ 80 %
Stage 2 (Moderate)	< 70 %	50–79 %
Stage 3 (Severe)	< 70 %	30–49 %
Stage 4 (Very Severe)	< 70 %	< 30 %

Note: % FEV$_1$/FVC = FEV$_1$ (forced expiratory volume in 1 s) divided by FVC (forced vital capacity); % PFEV$_1$ = Actual FEV$_1$/Predicted FEV$_1$

Source: Criteria from Vollmer et al. (2009).[33]

Asian-Americans, like most other racial groups, are lower than in Caucasians. A large multiethnic lung study of 1068 healthy non-smokers, 32 % of whom were Asian-American, suggested that a correction factor of 0.94 times the reference equations for Caucasians for FVC and FEV_1 provides a good overall prediction of lung function in Asian-Americans.[12]

BOX 20.3   Chapter Preview/Review

What four lung volumes make up total lung capacity?

How is VC defined functionally and mathematically?

What three body characteristics determine VC?

What is the difference between VC and FVC?

What is meant by restrictive and obstructive lung conditions?

How are FVC and FEV1 affected by restrictive and obstructive lung conditions?

How can static lung volumes be predicted from VC?

What is RV and how is it measured?

What is meant by ATPS and BTPS conditions?

What are % PFVC and % $PFEV_1$, and how are they used to classify lung function?

References

1. American Thoracic Society (1991). Lung function testing: selection of reference values and interpretative strategies. *American Review of Respiratory Disease, 144,* 1202–1218.

2. American Thoracic Society. (1995). Standardization of spirometry: 1994 update. *American Journal of Respiratory and Critical Care Medicine, 152,* 1107–1136.

3. Ashley, F., Kannel, W. B., Sorlie, P. D., & Masson, R. (1975). Pulmonary function: Relation to aging, cigarette habit, and mortality. *Annals of Internal Medicine, 82,* 736–745.

4. Buono, M. J., Constable, S. H., Morton, A. R., Rotkis, T. C., Stanforth, P. R., & Wilmore, J. H. (1981). The effect of an acute bout of exercise on selected pulmonary function measurements. *Medicine and Science in Sports and Exercise, 13,* 290–293.

5. Cissik, J. H., & Louden, J. A. (1979). Measurement precision of screening spirometry in normal adult men. *Cardiovascular Practice (CVP), 63,* 65–68.

6. Comroe, J. H., Forster, R. E., Dubois, A. B., Briscoe, W. A., & Carlsen, E. (1962). *The lung.* Chicago: Year Book Medical Publishers.

7. Cooper, C. B. (1995). Determining the role of exercise in patients with chronic pulmonary disease. *Medicine and Science in Sports and Exercise, 27,* 147–157.

8. Cordain, L., Tucker, A., Moon, D., & Stager, J. M. (1990). Lung volumes and maximal respiratory pressures in collegiate swimmers and runners. *Research Quarterly for Exercise and Sport, 61,* 70–74.

9. Enright, P. L., & Hyatt, R. E. (1987). *Office spirometry.* Philadelphia: Lea & Febiger.

10. Girandola, R., Wiswell, R., Mohler, J., Romero, G., & Barnes, W. (1977). Effects of water immersion on lung volumes: Implications for body compositional analysis. *Journal of Applied Physiology, 43,* 276–279.

11. Hankinson, J. L., Crapo, R. O., & Jensen, R. L. (2003). Spirometric reference values for the 6-s FVC maneuver. *Chest, 124,* 1805–1811.

12. Hankinson, J. L., Kawut, S. M., Shahar, E., Smith, L. J., Stukovsky, K. H., & Barr, R. G. (2010). Performance of American Thoracic Society-recommended spirometry reference values in a multiethnic sample of adults: The multi-ethnic study of atherosclerosis (MESA) lung study. *Chest, 137,* 138–145.

13. Hankinson, J. L., Kinsley, K. B., & Wagner, G. R. (1996). Comparison of spirometric reference values for Caucasian and African-American non-exposed blue-collar workers. *Journal of Occupational and Environmental Medicine, 38,* 137–143.

14. Hankinson, J. L., Odencrantz, J. R., & Fedan, K. B. (1999). Spirometric reference values from a sample of the general U.S. population. *American Journal of Respiratory and Critical Care Medicine, 159,* 179–187.

15. Hodgkin, J. E., Balchum, O. J., Kass, I., Glaser, E. M., Miller, W. F., Haas, A., Shaw, D. B., Kimbel, P., & Petty, T. L. (1975). Chronic obstructive airway diseases—Current concept in diagnosis and comprehensive care. JAMA: *The Journal of the American Medical Association, 232,* 1243.

16. Hutchinson, J. (1846). On capacity of lungs and on respiratory functions with view of establishing a precise and easy method of detecting disease by spirometer. *Tr. Med.-Chir. Society of London, 29,* 137.

17. Kory, R. C., Callahan, R., Boren, H. G., & Syner, J. C. (1961). The Veterans Administration-Army cooperative study of pulmonary function. *American Journal of Medicine, 30,* 243–258.

18. Kyle, J. M., Walker, R. B., Hanshaw, S. L., Leaman, J. R., & Frobase, J. K. (1992). Exercise-induced bronchospasms in the young athlete: Guidelines for routine screening and initial management. *Medicine and Science in Sports and Exercise, 24,* 856–859.

19. Mahler, D. A. (1993). Exercise-induced asthma. *Medicine and Science in Sports and Exercise, 25,* 554–561.

20. Maron, M., Hamilton, L., & Maksud, M. (1979). Alterations in pulmonary function consequent to competitive marathon running. *Medicine and Science in Sports and Exercise, 11,* 244–249.

21. Miller, M. R., Hankinson, J., Brusasco, V., Burgos, F., Casaburi, R., et al. (2005). ATS/ERS task force: Standardisation of lung function testing, number 1 in

series. General considerations for lung function testing. *European Respiratory Journal, 26,* 153–161.

22. Miller, M. R., Hankinson, J., Brusasco, V., Burgos, F., Casaburi, R., et al. (2005). ATS/ERS task force: Standardisation of lung function testing, number 2 in series. Standardisation of spirometry. *European Respiratory Journal, 26,* 319–338.

23. Miller, M. R., & Pincock, A. C. (1986). Linearity and temperature control of the Fleisch pneumotachograph. *Journal of Applied Physiology, 60,* 710–715.

24. Mohler, S. R. (1981). Reasons for eliminating the "age 60" rule. *Aviation, Space, and Environmental Medicine, 52,* 445–454.

25. Morris, J. F. (1976). Spirometry in the evaluation of pulmonary function. *The Western Journal of Medicine, 125,* 110–118.

26. National Academy of Sciences. (1958). *Handbook of respiration.* Philadelphia: W. B. Saunders.

27. O'Krory, J. A., Loy, R. A., & Coast, J. R. (1992). Pulmonary function changes following exercise. *Medicine and Science in Sports and Exercise, 24,* 1359–1364.

28. Scoggin, C. (1985). Exercise-induced asthma. *Chest, 87* (Suppl.), 48S–49S.

29. Sobol, B. J., & Emirgil, C. (1977). Clinical significance of pulmonary function tests. *Chest, 72,* 81–85.

30. Thorland, W. G., Johnson, G. O., Cisar, C. J., & Housh, T. J. (1987). Estimation of minimal wrestling weight using measures of body build and body composition. *International Journal of Sports Medicine, 8,* 365–370.

31. Townsend, M. C. (1984). Spirometric forced expiratory volumes measured in the standing versus the sitting posture. *American Review of Respiratory Disease, 130,* 123–124.

32. Virant, F. S. (1992). Exercise-induced bronchospasm—Epidemiology, patho-physiology, and therapy. *Medicine and Science in Sports and Exercise, 24,* 851–855.

33. Volmer, W. M., Gislason, P., Burney, P., Enright, P. L., Gulsvik, A., Kocabas, A., & Buist, A. S. (2012). Comparison of spirometry criteria for the diagnosis of COPD: results from the BOLD study. *European Respiratory Journal, 34,* 588–597.

34. Wilmore, J. H. (1969). A simplified method for determination of residual lung volume. *Journal of Applied Physiology, 27,* 96–100.

35. Wilmore, J. H., Vodak, P. A., Parr, R. B., Girandola, R. N., & Billing, J. E. (1980). Further simplification of a method for determination of residual lung volume. *Medicine and Science in Sports and Exercise, 12,* 216–218.

Form 20.1

NAME _____ DATE _____ SCORE _____

RESTING LUNG VOLUMES

Homework

Gender: **M**   Initials: **AA**   Age (y): **20**   Height (cm): **173**   Race: * **1**   (* See below)

T_A (°C): **23** P_B (mmHg): **760**   RH (%): **30**   BTPS CF: _____   (Table 20.5)

IRV (L) = _____   TV (L) = _____   ERV (L) = _____   RV (L) = _____   (Estimated from Table 20.1)

	T1	T2	T3	Highest FVC $_{ATPS}$	Actual FVC $_{BTPS}$		
FVC (L) =	**4.60**	**4.70**	**4.75**			Pred FVC $_{BTPS}$ (L) = ___	(Table 20.6)
	T1	T2	T3	Highest FEV$_1$ $_{ATPS}$	Actual FEV$_1$ $_{BTPS}$		
FEV$_1$ (L) =	**3.70**	**3.80**	**3.80**			Pred FEV$_1$ $_{BTPS}$ (L) = ___	(Table 20.6)

Evaluation   **Descriptive Evaluation** (Table 20.8)

% PFVC = _____ / _____ * 100 = _____ %   _____
              Actual   Predicted

% PFEV$_1$ = _____ / _____ * 100 = _____ %   _____
              Actual   Predicted

% FEV$_1$ / FVC = _____ / _____ * 100 = _____ %   _____
                 Act FEV$_1$ Act FVC

Gender: **F**   Initials: **BB**   Age (y): **20**   Height (cm): **167**   Race: * **1**   (* See below)

T_A (°C): **23** P_B (mmHg): **760**   RH (%): **30**   BTPS CF: _____   (Table 20.5)

IRV (L) = _____   TV (L) = _____   ERV (L) = _____   RV (L) = _____   (Estimated from Table 20.1)

	T1	T2	T3	Highest FVC $_{ATPS}$	Actual FVC $_{BTPS}$		
FVC (L) =	**4.15**	**4.10**	**4.10**			Pred FVC $_{BTPS}$ (L) = ___	(Table 20.6)
	T1	T2	T3	Highest FEV$_1$ $_{ATPS}$	Actual FEV$_1$ $_{BTPS}$		
FEV$_1$ (L) =	**3.30**	**3.35**	**3.30**			Pred FEV$_1$ $_{BTPS}$ (L) = ___	(Table 20.6)

Evaluation   **Descriptive Evaluation** (Table 20.8)

% PFVC = _____ / _____ * 100 = _____ %   _____
              Actual   Predicted

% PFEV$_1$ = _____ / _____ * 100 = _____ %   _____
              Actual   Predicted

% FEV$_1$ / FVC = _____ / _____ * 100 = _____ %   _____
                 Act FEV$_1$ Act FVC

* Race: 1 Caucasian, 2 African-American, 3 Mexican-American, 4 Asian-American, 5 Other

Form 20.2

NAME _____ DATE _____ SCORE _____

RESTING LUNG VOLUMES

Lab Results

Gender: _____ Initials: _____ Age (y): _____ Height (cm): _____ Race: * _____ (* See below)

T_A (°C): _____ P_B (mmHg): _____ RH (%): _____ BTPS CF: _____ (Table 20.5)

IRV (L) = _____ TV (L) = _____ ERV (L) = _____ RV (L) = _____ (Estimated from Table 20.1)

	T1	T2	T3	Highest FVC $_{ATPS}$	Actual FVC $_{BTPS}$		
FVC (L) =	_____	_____	_____	_____	_____	Pred FVC $_{BTPS}$ (L) = _____	(Table 20.6)

	T1	T2	T3	Highest FEV$_1$ $_{ATPS}$	Actual FEV$_1$ $_{BTPS}$		
FEV$_1$ (L) =	_____	_____	_____	_____	_____	Pred FEV$_1$ $_{BTPS}$ (L) = _____	(Table 20.6)

Evaluation   **Descriptive Evaluation** (Table 20.8)

% PFVC = _____ / _____ * 100 = _____ % _____
        Actual   Predicted

% PFEV$_1$ = _____ / _____ * 100 = _____ % _____
         Actual   Predicted

% FEV$_1$ / FVC = _____ / _____ * 100 = _____ % _____
            Act FEV$_1$ Act FVC

Gender: _____ Initials: _____ Age (y): _____ Height (cm): _____ Race: * _____ (* See below)

T_A (°C): _____ P_B (mmHg): _____ RH (%): _____ BTPS CF: _____ (Table 20.5)

IRV (L) = _____ TV (L) = _____ ERV (L) = _____ RV (L) = _____ (Estimated from Table 20.1)

	T1	T2	T3	Highest FVC $_{ATPS}$	Actual FVC $_{BTPS}$		
FVC (L) =	_____	_____	_____	_____	_____	Pred FVC $_{BTPS}$ (L) = _____	(Table 20.6)

	T1	T2	T3	Highest FEV$_1$ $_{ATPS}$	Actual FEV$_1$ $_{BTPS}$		
FEV$_1$ (L) =	_____	_____	_____	_____	_____	Pred FEV$_1$ $_{BTPS}$ (L) = _____	(Table 20.6)

Evaluation   **Descriptive Evaluation** (Table 20.8)

% PFVC = _____ / _____ * 100 = _____ % _____
        Actual   Predicted

% PFEV$_1$ = _____ / _____ * 100 = _____ % _____
         Actual   Predicted

% FEV$_1$ / FVC = _____ / _____ * 100 = _____ % _____
            Act FEV$_1$ Act FVC

* Race: 1 Caucasian, 2 African-American, 3 Mexican-American, 4 Asian-American, 5 Other

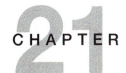

CHAPTER

EXERCISE VENTILATION

Justification for exercise testing is based on the nonlinear relationship between functional capacity and symptoms.[19] Thus, it is not unusual to find persons who function nonsymptomatically under resting conditions but have debilitating symptoms under exercise conditions. Combining the Exercise Ventilation Test with other measures, including maximum voluntary ventilation and oxygen consumption, is an effective, inexpensive, and noninvasive method for diagnosing exercise intolerance.[36]

The purpose of the Exercise Ventilation Test is to examine the influence of exercise upon such dynamic parameters as (a) pulmonary ventilation, (b) breathing rate, (c) tidal volume, (d) ventilatory equivalent, and (e) ventilatory threshold. A secondary purpose is to relate a measurement at rest—maximal voluntary ventilation—to exercise ventilation in determining ventilatory capacity, ventilatory reserve, and ventilatory constraint.

PHYSIOLOGICAL RATIONALE

Measurable differences exist in exercise respiratory parameters between aerobically fit and unfit people. In brief, fit people are expected to have lower ventilations, breathing rates, and ventilatory equivalents at any submaximal exercise intensity (power). The dynamics of the various respiratory parameters for both fit and unfit persons are the following: (a) a positive linear relationship between ventilation and power level except for the change in linearity at the ventilatory threshold, (b) a positive curvilinear relationship between both breathing rate and tidal volume versus power level, and (c) a horizontal (nonchanging) relationship between ventilatory equivalent and power levels below the ventilatory threshold. The kinetics of most ventilatory variables are similar to those of oxygen consumption, heart rate, and blood pressure. Thus, the time required to achieve steady state usually occurs within 2 min to 6 min, depending primarily upon the intensity of the power level.

Pulmonary Ventilation ($\dot{V}_E$)

The amount of air expired (E) in one minute is termed pulmonary ventilation ($\dot{V}_E$; L·min^{-1}). Typical pulmonary ventilations at rest range from 5 L·min^{-1} to 10 L·min^{-1} and at exhaustive exercise from 70 L·min^{-1} to 125 L·min^{-1}, with the lower ventilations in women. Ventilation increases linearly with increased exercise intensity in order to rid

the body of carbon dioxide and provide more oxygen. The increase in ventilation changes disproportionately at a point usually between 50 % and 75 % of maximal oxygen consumption,[29] with less fit persons closer to the 50 % value.

Breathing Rate (BR)

The number of breaths taken each minute is referred to as **breathing rate.** At rest, typical breathing rates range from 10 to 20 breaths per minute (br·min^{-1}), whereas at maximal exercise they typically range from 40 br·min^{-1} to 55 br·min^{-1}. The disproportionate rise in breathing rate with increased power levels is gradual at low and moderate power levels but rapid at high power levels.[26]

Tidal Volume (TV)

The volume of air expired with each breath is called the tidal volume (TV; V_T). It may be expressed either in milliliters or liters and sometimes as a percentage of the vital capacity (VC). At rest, typical tidal volumes are about 350–500 ml (about 10 % VC), whereas at maximal aerobic exercise they may reach about 1600 ml and 2400 ml for the typical woman and man, respectively (about 50–60 % VC). The curvilinear rise in tidal volume with increased power levels is opposite that of breathing rate; there is a rapid increase in TV when progressing from low to moderate power levels and smaller increases from moderate to high power levels. The larger tidal volume is due to both greater inspirations and expirations, thus encroaching upon the resting inspiratory and expiratory reserve volumes.[24] Typical responses for ventilation, breathing rate, and tidal volume are shown in Figure 21.1.

Ventilatory Equivalent ($\dot{V}_E/\dot{V}O_2$)

The ratio of ventilation to oxygen consumption is referred to as the oxygen ventilatory equivalent ($\dot{V}_E/\dot{V}O_2$). Typical oxygen ventilatory equivalents at rest are about 20–25 L of air for each liter of oxygen consumed, thus 20:1 to 25:1 ratios. The $\dot{V}_E/\dot{V}O_2$ remains relatively constant during subventilatory threshold exercise. Usually, the $\dot{V}_E/\dot{V}O_2$ exceeds 25:1 above the ventilatory threshold; it exceeds 30:1 at and above maximal oxygen consumption. The ventilatory equivalent for carbon dioxide ($\dot{V}_E/\dot{V}O_2$) is sometimes combined with $\dot{V}_E/\dot{V}O_2$ to determine the ventilatory threshold.

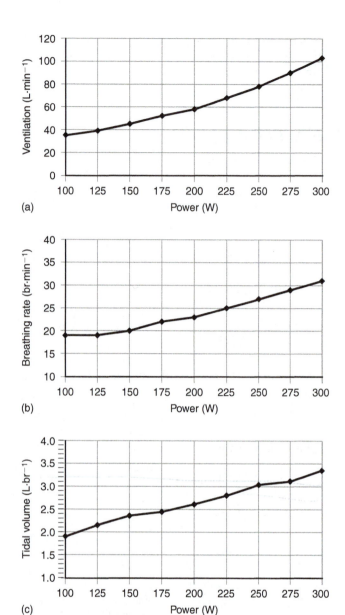

(a)

(b)

(c)

Figure 21.1 The responses of (a) ventilation, (b) breathing rate, and (c) tidal volume to graded exercise on a cycle ergometer in trained cyclists. Ventilation and breathing rate increase more rapidly with higher intensity exercise, while tidal volume increases faster initially with lower intensity exercise.

Ventilatory Threshold

Ventilation increases during exercise as a result of the increases in breathing rate and tidal volume. During submaximal exercise ($< 50 \%$ $\dot{V}O_2$ max), ventilation increases linearly with exercise intensity, as do most other physiological variables including heart rate, cardiac output and oxygen consumption. However, as seen in Figure 21.2, ventilation shows a nonlinear increase or exponential rise with increasing exercise intensity. This occurs at about 50 to 60 % of maximal oxygen consumption in most persons, but

may actually vary from 40 to 85 % of $\dot{V}O_2$ max max.[5,6,15,20] The point at which ventilation increases nonlinearly can be identified as the *ventilatory threshold*. This accelerated ventilation is believed to be due to the excess carbon dioxide produced due to the buffering of lactic acid that begins to appear in increasing amounts as a result of the stimulation of anaerobic metabolism. As exercise intensity progressively increases, a gradual change occurs in the conditions in the muscle. This starts to stimulate an increase in the rate of ATP formation by fast glycolysis in addition to the ATP that was heretofore being produced predominantly through aerobic metabolism.[33] With the increased activity of fast glycolysis, there is an increase in lactic acid within the working muscle. As lactic acid is produced, it dissociates (loses) a hydrogen ion (H^+) and becomes lactate as seen in Reaction 21.1a. Hydrogen ions are also produced in greater amounts during this increasing exercise intensity by dissociation from ammonium ions (NH_4^+) resulting in simultaneous ammonia production (Rx. 21.1b). The H^+ made from both sources is buffered by bicarbonate ions (HCO_3^-) found in the skeletal muscles and blood creating carbonic acid (Rx. 21.1c). The carbonic acid then circulates to the lungs where it is split by the enzyme carbonic anhydrase into carbon dioxide and water (Rx. 21.1d) whereby the increased CO_2 stimulates a non-linear increase in ventilation.[5,12,30,35]

Lactic acid $\rightarrow$ Lactate$^-$ +
    H^+ (hydrogen ion)   Rx. 21.1a

NH_4^+ (ammonium ion) $\rightarrow$ NH_3 (ammonia)
    + H^+ Rx. 21.1b

$H^+ + HCO_3^-$ (bicarbonate ion) $\rightarrow$
    H_2CO_3 (carbonic acid)   Rx. 21.1c

$H_2CO_3 \rightarrow CO_2$ (carbon dioxide) + H_2O (water)   Rx. 21.1d

Much of the increase in ventilation below the ventilatory threshold is due to an increase in tidal volume (an increased depth of ventilation) while the increase in ventilation above the ventilatory threshold is due more to an increase in breathing rate. The ventilatory threshold has practical implications because fatigue occurs sooner at power levels above that point than at power levels below it.[35] The point at which the ventilatory threshold occurs is believed to be similar to the point at which blood lactate increases nonlinearly as well, referred to by some as the *lactate threshold*. Others however have found the ventilatory threshold and lactate threshold to occur at significantly different exercise intensities.[8] Attempts have been made to use the ventilatory threshold to predict or estimate the lactate threshold. A significant correlation ($R = 0.67$) exists between heart rates at the ventilatory and lactate thresholds.[28] To actually identify and study lactate threshold requires multiple lactate values determined from blood samples, taken throughout the exercise from an indwelling catheter, the methods for which are not described in this laboratory manual.

Maximal Voluntary Ventilation

Maximal voluntary ventilation (MVV), also sometimes referred to as maximal breathing capacity (MBC), is the maximal volume of air that can be inhaled and exhaled from the lungs over a sustained time, typically 10–15 s. MVV is not measured for a full minute, because it would lead to extreme pH changes and most likely to dizziness and fainting. It is measured instead for 10–15 s, as seen in Figure 21.3, then calculated as the rate of air flow per minute ($L \cdot min^{-1}$). The highest MVV is usually attained by the person taking breaths of an average depth (about 30–50 % of vital capacity) at the highest rate possible (> 100 br$\cdot$min^{-1}). The measurement of MVV requires a high level of motivation and is not possible in all persons. When measuring MVV is not possible or desirable, it may be estimated from FEV_1 due to the high correlation ($r = 0.90$) between the two lung function variables.[24] Various references estimate MVV as anywhere from 35 to 50 times the FEV_1.[4,18,24,32]

MVV is a measure of the overall capacity of the respiratory system to move air, as it depends on the strength of the respiratory muscles, the compliance of the lung-thorax system, and the resistance of the airways.[24] MVV is typically high in aerobically fit persons and shows some correlation ($r = -0.49$) with distance-run time in trained middle-distance runners.[10] MVV is reduced in persons with lung conditions that restrict inhalation or obstruct exhalation. MVV can be used in conjunction with the measurement of exercise ventilation ($\dot{V}_E$) to determine a ventilatory or breathing reserve and to determine whether a person has a ventilatory or breathing limitation (constraint) during exercise. Ventilatory reserve or breathing reserve can be expressed either as (1) the absolute difference (in $L \cdot min^{-1}$) between the MVV and $\dot{V}_E$,[36] or (2) the ratio of $\dot{V}_E$/MVV, which is called the ventilatory reserve index (VRI) or breathing reserve index (BRI).[32] $\dot{V}_E$ max values are about 70 % of MVV values.[3] The maximum tolerable steady-state exercise ventilation is about 64 % of MVV.[13] And

persons with chronic lung conditions (e.g., asthma, cystic fibrosis) nearly always experience dyspnea (breathlessness) when the ventilation required of exercise exceeds 50 % of MVV.[14]

METHODS

The Exercise Ventilation Test demonstrates the effect of exercise upon such respiratory variables as ventilation, breathing rate, tidal volume, ventilatory equivalent, and ventilatory threshold. The procedures and calculations are described. The equipment is the same as that used to directly measure oxygen consumption, described in Chapter 15. Maximal voluntary ventilation can be measured with an automated system equipped with a pulmonary function testing module or a manual system utilizing a dry gas meter. Procedures for measuring MVV and calculations for related measures of ventilatory reserve are described. The accuracy of measuring ventilation and MVV is described in Box 21.1.

Measuring Exercise Ventilation and MVV

The measurement of pulmonary ventilation during exercise requires an air volume meter that can either be part of an automated system (e.g., pneumotachometer, turbine) or a nonautomated piece of equipment (e.g., dry gas meter, tissot spirometer). Ventilation is most often measured during exhalation and is designated as exhaled ventilation ($\dot{V}_E$). In some cases, usually when using a dry gas meter, it can also be measured during inhalation and is then referred to as inhaled ventilation ($\dot{V}_I$). To collect and measure the exhaled air, several auxiliary pieces of equipment are necessary (as described in Chapter 15). A respiratory valve with a rubber mouthpiece attached to a breathing tube is used to collect all exhaled air. A noseclip is worn to prevent inhalation and exhalation of air through the nose. Before the test, the air volume meter is calibrated with a special calibration syringe

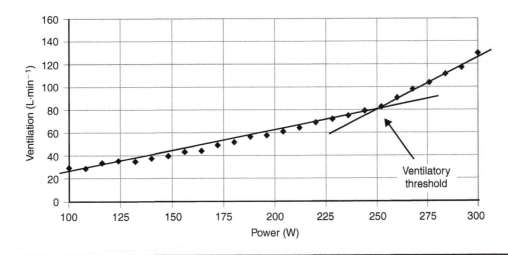

Figure 21.2 Ventilation increases linearly with a linear increase in power on the cycle ergometer until the ventilatory threshold, at which point there is a faster, nonlinear increase in ventilation.

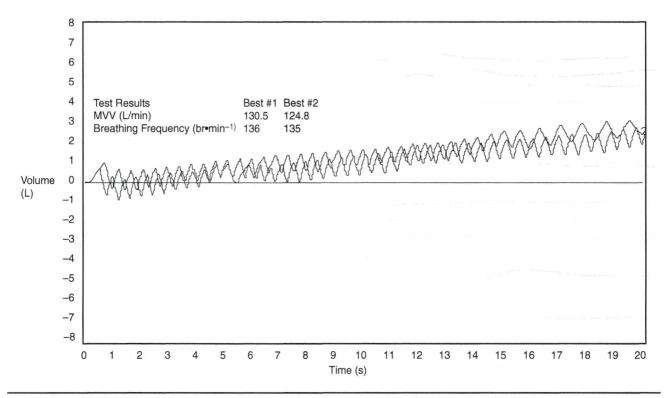

Figure 21.3 The printed graph from an automated computerized measurement of a 45-year-old man, who is 162.5 cm tall, shows two superimposed trials of maximal voluntary ventilation (MVV). Although each trial lasted 20 s, only 12 s of each trial was used to calculate the projected MVV (L/min) and breathing frequency per minute. Courtesy of Parvo-Medic, Consentius Technologies, Sandy, UT.

of at least 3 L according to the manufacturer's specifications.[2] In addition to measuring the volume of air inhaled or exhaled, it is also necessary to measure the fractions of exhaled O_2 and CO_2 using an oxygen analyzer and a carbon dioxide analyzer. The gas sample used for analysis during the exercise test can be drawn directly from the respiratory valve, or it can be drawn from a mixing chamber. Most automated systems draw the gas sample continuously from the exhaled air and then filter, dry, and warm it to account for the water vapor in the sample. When nonautomated systems are used, gas samples can be collected in small rubber bags (aliquots) or drawn from large collection bags (e.g., Douglas bag, meteorological balloon) for analysis.

Maximal voluntary ventilation (MVV) can be measured using the same automated system as is used to measure pulmonary ventilation during exercise. In most cases, these automated metabolic systems have a pulmonary function test (PFT) module that typically uses a separate airflow meter (i.e., pneumotachometer). A dry gas meter used to measure MVV manually is virtually identical to the meter used to measure the volume of natural gas you would find at your house or apartment. It has various dials that show the volume of air that passes through the dry gas meter. By knowing the numbers before and after the MVV test, one can determine the MVV. It is possible to interface the

---

BOX 21.1 **Accuracy of the MVV and Exercise Ventilation Tests**

Dry airflow meters with bellows (e.g., Parkinson-Cowan) are not recommended for research studies that measure online high-flow rates. This means that pulmonary tests, such as vital capacity and forced expiratory volumes, and exercise ventilations should not utilize the bellows type of dry spirometer. The only precise way that they could be used for heavy exercise purposes is to collect the air in Douglas bags, meteorological balloons, or anesthetic bags and then pump the air at a slow rate of flow through the meter.

Pneumotachometers and turbines are accurate to ± 2 % or about ± 50 ml of air. Instruments that measure inspiratory air instead of expiratory air are accurate to ± 1.0 %. One guideline is to try obtaining MVV volumes that are reproducible within 5 % of each other.[16]

Oxygen and carbon dioxide analyzers are accurate to volume fractions of about 0.1 %. Probably the best that can be expected from the automated devices is an accuracy of ± 2 % for measuring oxygen consumption. Although knowing the oxygen consumption permits the determination of ventilatory threshold, there still may remain about 30 % of the cases where no deflection point can be deciphered.[10] Although some evidence[7,17] supports the use of breathing frequency to determine accurately the ventilatory threshold, more confirmation is needed.

---

dry gas meter with a computer or connect it to a strip chart recorder and record a graphical representation of the MVV test. This manual method is useful when demonstrating MVV for teaching purposes, but it is not described further in this laboratory manual.

Preparation for Measuring Exercise Ventilation

As with the aerobic fitness tests, the participant should be well rested, should refrain from prior exercise the day of testing, should not eat a large meal 2–3 hours before the test, and should be normally hydrated and refrain from consuming or taking any stimulants. The technician (tester) prepares for the test by completing the following steps.

1. Periodically calibrate the ergometer being used (e.g., treadmill, cycle ergometer).
2. Calibrate the metabolic measurement system according to the manufacturer's specifications.
3. Measure and record the participant's basic data (name, age, height, and body weight) along with the meteorological data (temperature, barometric pressure, and relative humidity) on Form 21.2.
4. Establish the desired exercise mode and protocol to be used during the test. Orient the participant by explaining the purpose and protocol of the Exercise Ventilation Test.
5. Instruct the participant on the proper use of the ergometer (e.g., how to maintain pedaling form and rate on the cycle ergometer).
6. Instruct the participant on hand signals that may be used during the test (e.g., a thumbs-up indicating the desire to continue) due to the inability to speak because of the mouthpiece and respiratory equipment.

Procedures for Measuring Exercise Ventilation

The procedures for the Exercise Ventilation Test are as follows:

1. Attach all necessary equipment (e.g., headgear for support of respiratory valve) and insert the mouthpiece of the respiratory valve into the participant's mouth, attach the breathing tube to the "out" port of the valve, and affix the noseclip to the participant's nose (*do not forget the noseclip*).
2. Instruct the participant to begin exercising at the initial stage of the exercise test protocol.
3. Assuming an automated metabolic measurement system is being used, all metabolic data are measured, displayed, and recorded automatically for the duration of the test. If a semiautomated or manual system is being used (for instructional purposes), each technician records a specific variable (e.g., ventilation, F_EO_2, F_ECO_2, heart rate) at specific intervals (e.g., 15 s, 30 s, 1 min) throughout the test.

4. Follow the test protocol (Table 21.1) by increasing cycle ergometer power at the appropriate times (if not done automatically by the ergometer). Record any desired data (not recorded automatically) at specific intervals.
5. Monitor the participant for any signs or symptoms that could warrant stopping the test prematurely (e.g., chest pain, leg pain, dizziness, nausea).
6. At the conclusion of the test, begin a cool-down as quickly as possible. It is important that the participant spend minimal time sitting still on the cycle ergometer because of the possibility of blood pooling in the legs.
7. Remove all equipment. Discard any disposable equipment and clean and sanitize all reusable equipment (e.g., mouthpiece, noseclip, respiratory valve, breathing tube) according to accepted practices.

Preparation for Maximal Voluntary Ventilation

1. In preparation for the test, prepare and calibrate the pulmonary function testing (PFT) system according to the manufacturer's specifications.
2. Measure and record the participant's basic data (name, age, height, and body weight) on Form 21.2.
3. Instruct the participant on the proper procedures to be used for the MVV test.

Procedures for Measuring Maximal Voluntary Ventilation

1. The participant attaches the noseclip and breathes normally for two or three breaths.
2. The technician instructs the participant to inhale and exhale deeply (30–50 % of VC) as rapidly as possible (> 100 br·min^{-1}) for 20 s.
3. The participant should be specifically told to concentrate on inhaling and exhaling as fast as possible and to "keep going" for the full duration of the test. The entire MVV test may last for a total of 20 s, but the MVV is actually only recorded for 12 s.

Table 21.1 Cycle Ergometer Protocols for Measuring Exercise Ventilation

Status	Time	Average fitness	Above average fitness
Exercise			
Stage 1	0:00–1:59	50 W	100 W
Stage 2	2:00–3:59	75 W	125 W
Stage 3	4:00–5:59	100 W	150 W
Stage 4	6:00–7:59	125 W	175 W
Stage 5	8:00–9:59	150 W	200 W
Stage 6	10:00–11:59	175 W	225 W
Stage 7	12:00–13:59	200 W	250 W
Recovery	0:00–3:00	25–50 W	25–50 W

4. At the conclusion of the test, the calculated MVV ($L \cdot min^{-1}$, BTPS) is displayed. The test trial can be accepted if it appears to be a good test, or rejected if the participant was unable to complete the full test with a good effort.

5. Repeat the test at least one more time. Record the highest MVV value obtained on Form 21.2. Typical values for $\dot{V}_E$, BR, TV, TV/VC, and $\dot{V}_E/\dot{V}O_2$ are given in Table 21.2.

Calculations

The variables of concern are ventilation, breathing rate, tidal volume, TV/VC ratio, the ventilatory equivalent for oxygen, maximal voluntary ventilation, and ventilatory reserve. Equations are provided for performing the necessary calculations with numerous sample calculations.

Ventilation, the total volume of air exhaled from the lungs per minute, is the product of breathing rate and tidal volume as in Equation 21.1. For example, if during exercise a person is breathing at a rate of 30 $br \cdot min^{-1}$ and the average volume of each breath or tidal volume is 2 $L \cdot br^{-1}$, then the ventilation is 60 $L \cdot min^{-1}$. Provided any two of the three variables are known, the third can always be derived mathematically.

$$\dot{V}_E \ (L \cdot min^{-1}) = BR \ (br \cdot min^{-1})$$
$$* \ TV \ (L \cdot br^{-1}) \qquad \text{Eq. 21.1}$$

Where: $\dot{V}_E$ is ventilation, BR is breathing rate, and TV is tidal volume

In some cases, it is not possible or desirable to measure maximal voluntary ventilation. Instead, MVV can be estimated from FEV_1 if it is known (Eq. 21.2a), or from gender and age if no previous lung function test results

are known, as seen in Equation 21.2b (men) and 21.2c (women). A person with a measured FEV_1 of **4.50** L would have an estimated MVV of (4.50 * 37.5) + 15.8 or **185** $L \cdot min^{-1}$. If this same person was a **25-year-old male**, his MVV estimated from age alone would be 199.1 − (1.12 * 25) or **171** $L \cdot min^{-1}$.

$$\text{Estimated MVV } (L \cdot min^{-1}) = (FEV_1 * 37.5)$$
$$+ \ 15.8 \qquad \text{Eq. 21.2a}$$

Where: MVV is maximal voluntary ventilation, and FEV_1 is forced expiratory volume

$$\text{Estimated MVV } (L \cdot min^{-1}) = 199.1 − (1.12 * \text{Age}) \qquad \text{Eq. 21.2b}$$

$$\text{Estimated MVV } (L \cdot min^{-1}) = 147.4 − (0.76 * \text{Age}) \qquad \text{Eq. 21.2c}$$

The four remaining variables all relate in some way to the fitness level and ventilatory efficiency of the individual. The TV/VC ratio describes the depth of the breath (tidal volume) relative to the maximal breath (vital capacity) and is calculated as shown in Equation 21.3a. The ventilatory equivalent for oxygen ($\dot{V}_E/\dot{V}O_2$) reflects the ventilation needed for each liter of oxygen consumed, or the metabolic cost of breathing, and is calculated as in Equation 21.3b. The values obtained on a person for MVV and $\dot{V}_E$ can be used together to determine what has been termed the ventilatory or breathing reserve. It can be expressed as either the difference between these two values, as seen in Equation 21.3c, or it can be expressed as the ventilatory or breathing reserve index by calculating the ratio of $\dot{V}_E$ to MVV as in Equation 21.3d.

$$\text{TV/VC ratio } (\%) = \text{Tidal volume } (L)$$
$$/ \text{ Vital capacity } (L) * 100 \qquad \text{Eq. 21.3a}$$

$$\text{Ventilatory equivalent for } O_2 \ (\dot{V}_E/\dot{V}O_2)$$
$$= \dot{V}_E \ (L \cdot min^{-1}) / \dot{V}O_2 \ (L \cdot min^{-1}) \qquad \text{Eq. 21.3b}$$

Table 21.2	Estimated Values for Oxygen Consumption ($\dot{V}O_2$), Ventilation ($\dot{V}_E$), Breathing Rate (BR), Tidal Volume (TV), Tidal Volume/Vital Capacity Ratio (TV/VC), and Ventilatory Equivalent for Oxygen ($\dot{V}_E/\dot{V}O_2$) in Trained Cyclists

Power (W)	$\dot{V}O_2$ ($L \cdot min^{-1}$)	$\dot{V}_E$ ($L \cdot min^{-1}$)	BR ($br \cdot min^{-1}$)	TV ($L \cdot br^{-1}$)	TV/VC (%)	$\dot{V}_E/\dot{V}O_2$
25	0.50–0.70	12–15	12–19	0.90–1.40	23–33	15–20
50	0.75–1.05	15–23	13–20	1.00–1.50	26–36	15–20
75	1.00–1.40	24–34	15–21	1.30–1.70	27–37	15–20
100	1.29–1.75	28–42	15–22	1.51–2.28	28–42	17–20
125	1.59–1.87	33–46	15–23	1.75–2.52	33–47	17–20
150	1.84–2.20	37–53	15–25	1.88–2.83	35–53	17–20
175	2.05–2.56	42–62	17–26	2.09–2.81	39–52	17–20
200	2.42–2.77	49–68	18–28	2.23–2.99	41–55	17–20
225	2.79–3.17	57–78	19–31	2.33–3.27	43–61	17–21
250	3.08–3.70	60–96	20–33	2.63–3.43	49–63	17–22
275	3.35–4.13	68–112	23–35	2.85–3.38	53–63	17–23
300	3.80–4.43	81–126	24–38	2.96–3.73	55–69	18–23

Source: Data from Soungatoulin, Beam, Kersey, & Peterson (2003).[34]

Where: $\dot{V}_E$ is ventilation and $\dot{V}O_2$ is oxygen consumption

$$\text{Ventilatory reserve (L·min}^{-1}) = \text{MVV (L·min}^{-1}) - \dot{V}_E \text{ (L·min}^{-1}) \qquad \text{Eq. 21.3c}$$

$$\text{Ventilatory reserve index} = \dot{V}_E \text{ (L·min}^{-1}) / \text{MVV (L·min}^{-1}) \qquad \text{Eq. 21.3d}$$

Where: MVV is maximal voluntary ventilation and $\dot{V}_E$ is ventilation

For example, given a person with the following values: TV = 3.02 L, VC = 5.30 L, $\dot{V}_E$ = 122 L·min^{-1}, $\dot{V}O_2$ = 3.38 L·min^{-1}, and MVV = 175 L·min^{-1}, the calculated values would be as seen in Equations 21.4a through 21.4d.

$$\text{TV/VC ratio} = \textbf{3.02 L} / \textbf{5.30 L} * 100 = \textbf{57} \% \qquad \text{Eq. 21.4a}$$

$$\dot{V}_E / \dot{V}O_2 = \textbf{122 L·min}^{-1} / \textbf{3.38 L·min}^{-1} = \textbf{36} \qquad \text{Eq. 21.4b}$$

$$\text{Ventilatory reserve} = \textbf{175 L·min}^{-1} - \textbf{122 L·min}^{-1} = \textbf{53 L·min}^{-1} \qquad \text{Eq. 21.4c}$$

$$\text{Ventilatory reserve index} = \textbf{122 L·min}^{-1} / \textbf{175 L·min}^{-1} = \textbf{0.70 (70} \%) \qquad \text{Eq. 21.4d}$$

RESULTS AND DISCUSSION

With exercise comes an increased demand for pulmonary ventilation ($\dot{V}_E$). The movement of a greater volume of air through the lungs provides the added oxygen required of the exercising muscles and helps to clear from the body the carbon dioxide produced as a by-product of aerobic metabolism. This increase in $\dot{V}_E$ is a result of increases in breathing rate (BR) and tidal volume (TV). The majority of studies show that TV increases linearly for the most part throughout graded exercise.[21,25,26] The TV of trained cyclists is around 1.5 L·br^{-1} at 50 W and increases to about 3.0 L·br^{-1} by 300 W.[21,26] This is about 55–60 % of VC, compared to untrained men whose TV reaches 50–55 % of VC and untrained women who reach 40–45 % of VC.[36] However, BR increases only moderately with low- to moderate-intensity exercise, then shows an accelerated increase at higher intensity. The BR of trained cyclists increases from 18–20 br·min^{-1} at 50 W to only 25–30 br·min^{-1} at 250 W, but increases to 35–40 br·min^{-1} by 300 W and can approach or exceed 50 br·min^{-1} by 350–400 W. The increased BR and $\dot{V}_E$ during higher intensity exercise (above the ventilatory threshold) help compensate for the changes in acid–base balance associated with the increased production of hydrogen ions. The ventilatory threshold may be closely related to an RPE of 12 to 15 on the 6–20-point RPE scale.[31] This translates to exercise intensities described as "somewhat heavy" to "heavy." When running or cycling for 3 hours, the sustained intensity of exercise roughly coincides with the $\dot{V}O_2$ at the ventilatory threshold.[11]

Aerobically fit persons have lower ventilations for any given level of submaximal exercise than unfit persons. Trained male cyclists on a cycle ergometer at 200 W have breathing rates of 18–28 br·min^{-1}, tidal volumes of 2.23–2.99 L·br^{-1} (41–55 % of VC), and ventilations of 49–68 L·min^{-1} (Table 21.2). It appears that trained persons adopt a breathing pattern of a low breathing rate and high tidal volume.[21] Untrained males at a similar mean peak power level (185 W) show a considerably greater mean peak $\dot{V}_E$ of 119.6 ± 28.3 L·min^{-1}, as seen in Table 21.3,[25] nearly twice that of the trained cyclists. Because the mean $\dot{V}O_2$ values for each group were similar (untrained, $\dot{V}O_2$ = 2.62 ± 0.36; trained, $\dot{V}O_2$ = 2.42 − 2.77 L·min^{-1}), the ventilatory equivalent for oxygen is also about twice as high in the untrained males (mean $\dot{V}_E$ / mean $\dot{V}O_2$ = 46) compared to the trained cyclists ($\dot{V}_E$ / $\dot{V}O_2$ = 17 − 20). This indicates that aerobic training improves ventilatory efficiency, likely by reducing the metabolic cost of breathing and improving the diffusion of oxygen through the lungs.

Maximal voluntary ventilation (MVV) is not the same value as the maximal ventilation recorded during exercise ($\dot{V}_E$ max). MVV is intended to be a dynamic measure of maximal breathing capacity, but it is not measured during exercise. It is somewhat analogous to "revving" your car engine while the car is parked. This may reflect your car engine's maximum speed (rpm), but does not necessarily indicate how fast your car can go (mph). MVV is typically highest in young, aerobically trained athletes, who have no restrictive or obstructive lung conditions and whose respiratory muscles are well trained. One group of trained middle-distance runners is reported to have a mean MVV of 189 L·min^{-1}, with the highest being 252 L·min^{-1}.[10] Another group of high school athletes is reported to have a mean MVV of 146 ± 21 L·min^{-1}.[27] From the data presented in Table 21.4, it appears MVV peaks somewhere between age 20 and 40 y, then declines about 20 L·min^{-1} per decade in men and 10 L·min^{-1} per decade in women.[24] As mentioned previously, MVV is a difficult variable to measure because it requires a very high level of

Table 21.3	Peak Ventilatory Responses to Graded Exercise in Untrained Adults Age 20–39 y (M ± SD)	
Peak values	Men (*N* = 60)	Women (*N* = 60)
Power (W)	185 ± 32	116 ± 19
$\dot{V}O_2$ (L·min^{-1})	2.62 ± 0.36	1.68 ± 0.23
$\dot{V}_E$ (L·min^{-1})	119.6 ± 28.3	75.8 ± 13.7
$\dot{V}_E$/$\dot{V}O_2$	46*	45*
MVV (L·min^{-1})	168.5 ± 25.6	124.2 ± 12.1
MVV − $\dot{V}_E$	48.9*	48.4*
$\dot{V}_E$ / MVV	0.69 ± 0.12	0.60 ± 0.11

Note: Value determined from means, not individually measured.
Source: Data from Neder, et al. (2003).[25]

Table 21.4 — Category for Maximum Voluntary Ventilation (L·min⁻¹) by Gender and Age Group

Category (percentile)	Men (N = 50) Age (y)				Women (N = 50) Age (y)			
	20–29	30–39	40–49	50–59	20–29	30–39	40–49	50–59
Well above ave (> 95th)	> 200	> 219	> 208	> 178	> 147	> 142	> 128	> 140
Above ave (75th–95th)	181–200	190–219	175–208	151–178	135–147	131–142	121–128	120–140
Average (25th–74th)	153–180	150–189	128–174	114–150	116–134	116–130	110–120	92–119
Below ave (5th–24th)	134–152	121–149	94–127	87–113	104–115	105–115	102–109	72–91
Well below ave (< 5th)	< 134	< 121	< 94	< 87	< 104	< 105	< 102	< 72
Mean	167	170	151	132	126	124	116	106

Note: Values for percentiles are estimated using the reported means and standard deviations assuming the data are normally distributed.
Source: Data from Neder, Andreoni, Lerario, & Nery (1999).[24]

motivation. If a value for MVV is desired, but it is not possible to measure directly, several studies have recommended methods for estimating it. MVV (L·min⁻¹) can be estimated from FEV_1 (L·s⁻¹) by either: MVV = FEV_1 * 37.5[23]; or MVV = (FEV_1 * 37.5) + 15.8[24]; or MVV = FEV_1 * 40.[36] It can also be estimated from age alone by using Equation 21.2a for men and Equation 21.2b for women.

The usefulness of measuring MVV is related to its use in combination with $\dot{V}_E$ to identify something referred to as *ventilatory reserve*.[4,18,23,36] Theoretically, $\dot{V}_E$ during exercise represents the *ventilatory demand,* and MVV represents the *ventilatory capacity*—the maximum flow rate of air through the lungs. During maximal aerobic exercise, it would be logical to think that $\dot{V}_E$ max may approach this maximal flow rate (i.e., MVV). In Table 21.3, although not calculated individually for each person, the difference between the peak $\dot{V}_E$ during exercise and the mean MVV is nearly 50 L·min⁻¹ in both the men and the women.[25] In other studies, the difference between $\dot{V}_E$ max and MVV is also about 50 L·min⁻¹.[23] Interestingly, this ventilatory reserve (MVV − $\dot{V}_E$) may be reduced not only in persons with chronic obstructive lung disease but also in highly trained athletes with high maximal exercise ventilations. In some cases, a person whose $\dot{V}_E$ max is within 15 L·min⁻¹ of the MVV may have a clinically significant ventilatory problem.[9] But it is also observed in highly competitive cyclists that the mean $\dot{V}_E$ max (172 L·min⁻¹) comes within 26 L·min⁻¹ of the MVV (198 L·min⁻¹).[21] So, the ventilatory limitation or constraint in the case of the chronic lung condition is due to a reduced MVV, but the reduced ventilatory reserve in the trained cyclists is due more to the very high ventilations achieved during maximal exercise.

Another way to describe ventilatory reserve is not based on the absolute difference between $\dot{V}_E$ and MVV, but to calculate the ratio of $\dot{V}_E$ / MVV, referred to as the ventilatory reserve index (VRI) or breathing reserve index (BRI). For example, if $\dot{V}_E$ during exercise is 75 L·min⁻¹ and MVV in the same person is 150 L·min⁻¹, then VRI (or BRI) would be 0.50. In most persons, $\dot{V}_E$ max reaches only about 50–70 % of the measured MVV (indicated by a VRI of 0.50–0.70),[1,23] implying that the remaining 30 % is available *in reserve*. A ratio greater than 0.70 may indicate a ventilatory limitation.[1] The mean ventilatory reserve indexes at peak exercise for untrained adults free of chronic lung problems observed in Table 21.3 are 0.69 ± 0.12 for men and 0.60 ± 0.11 for women.[25] These fall within the normal range ($\dot{V}_E$ / MVV < 0.70). Although a high VRI (> 0.70) may indeed indicate a ventilatory "limitation," one must still be careful to interpret whether it is a *clinical limitation* brought on by some chronic lung condition or a *functional limit* that may be characteristic of highly trained athletes. Maximal exercise ventilations in highly competitive cyclists reach 86.9–90.0 % of MVV,[21] which may not be interpreted as a limitation, but that their ventilatory reserve is being reduced to the minimum due to their ability to reach such high exercise ventilations. It should also be noted, however, that using $\dot{V}_E$ and MVV alone to identify ventilatory reserve ignores the effect of breathing strategy and the degree of flow constraints. For this reason, other more sophisticated techniques (not described in this manual) involving the measurement and plotting of exercise tidal flow-volume (FV) loops should be considered in an attempt to better assess expiratory flow limitation and the degree of ventilatory constraint during exercise in various populations.[18]

BOX 21.2 Chapter Preview/Review

How is pulmonary ventilation ($\dot{V}_E$) defined functionally and mathematically?

How are breathing rate and tidal volume defined and how do they respond to graded exercise?

What is meant by the term ventilatory equivalent?

How is the ventilatory threshold identified and to what physiological responses does it relate?

What is MVV and how is it measured and/or predicted?

How do $\dot{V}_E$ max and MVV differ?

What is meant by TV/VC ratio and how does it respond to graded exercise of increasing intensity?

How are ventilatory reserve and ventilatory reserve index (VRI) calculated and interpreted?

References

1. American College of Sports Medicine. (2000). *ACSM's guidelines for exercise testing and prescription.* Philadelphia: Lippincott Williams & Wilkins.

2. American Thoracic Society. (1995). Standardization of spirometry—1994 update. Official Statement of the American Thoracic Society, *American Journal of Respiratory Critical Care Medicine, 152,* 1107–1136.

3. Åstrand, P. O., & Rodahl, K. (1986). *Textbook of work physiology.* New York: McGraw-Hill.

4. Babb, T. G., & Rodarte, J. R. (1993). Estimation of ventilatory capacity during submaximal exercise. *Journal of Applied Physiology, 74,* 2016–2022.

5. Brooks, G. A., Fahey, T. D., & Baldwin, K. M. (2005). *Exercise physiology: Human bioenergetics and its applications, 4th ed.* New York: McGraw-Hill.

6. Casaburi, R., Storer, T. W., Sullivan, C. S., & Wasserman, K. (1995). Evaluation of blood lactate elevation as an intensity criterion for exercise training. *Medicine and Science in Sports and Exercise, 27,* 852–862.

7. Cheng, B., Kuipers, H., Snyder, A. C., Keizer, H. A., Jeukendrup, A., & Hesseluk, M. (1992). A new approach for the determination of ventilatory and lactate thresholds. *International Journal of Sports Medicine, 13,* 518–522.

8. Chicharro, J. L., Perez, M., Vaquero, A. F., Lucia, A., & Legido, J. C. Lactic threshold versus ventilatory threshold during a ramp test on a cycle ergometer. *Journal of Sports Medicine and Physical Fitness, 37,* 117–171.

9. Cooper, C. B. (1995). Determining the role of exercise in patients with chronic pulmonary disease. *Medicine and Science in Sports and Exercise, 27,* 147–157.

10. Costill, D. L. (1971). Endurance running. In ACSM (Ed.), *Encyclopedia of sport science and medicine* (p. 338). New York: Macmillan.

11. Coyle, E. F. (1995). Integration of the physiological factors determining endurance performance ability. In J. O. Holloszy (Ed.), *Exercise and sport science reviews 23* (pp. 25–63). Baltimore: Williams & Wilkins.

12. Davis, J. A. (1985). Anaerobic threshold: Review of the concept and directions for future research. *Medicine and Science in Sports and Exercise, 17,* 6–18.

13. Freedman, S. (1970). Sustained maximum voluntary ventilation. *Respiratory Physiology, 3,* 230–244.

14. Gaensler, E. A., & Wright, G. W. (1966). Evaluation of respiratory impairment. *Archives of Environmental Health, 12,* 146–189.

15. Gollnick, P. W., Bayly, W., & Hodgson, D. (1986). Exercise intensity, training, diet, and lactate concentration in muscle and blood. *Medicine and Science in Sports and Exercise, 18,* 334-340.

16. Hill, N. S., Jacoby, C., & Farber, H. W. (1991). Effect of an endurance triathlon on pulmonary function. *Medicine and Science in Sports and Exercise, 23,* 1260–1264.

17. James, N. W., Adams, G. M., & Wilson, A. F. (1989). Determination of anaerobic threshold by ventilatory frequency. *International Journal of Sports Medicine, 10,* 192–196.

18. Johnson, B. D., Weisman, I. M., Zeballos, R. J., & Beck, K. C. (1999). Emerging concepts in the evaluation of ventilatory limitation during exercise: The exercise tidal flow-volume loop. *Chest, 116,* 488–503.

19. Jones, N. L. (1975). Exercise testing in pulmonary evaluation: Rationale, methods, and the normal respiratory response to exercise. *New England Journal of Medicine, 293,* 541–544.

20. Jones, N. L., & Ehrsam, R. E. (1982). The anaerobic threshold. In R. Terjung (Ed.), *Exercise and sport sciences review* (pp. 49–83). New York: Franklin Institute Press.

21. Lucia, A., Carvajal, A., Calderón, F. J., Alfonso, A., & Chicharro, J. L. (1999). Breathing pattern in highly competitive cyclists during incremental exercise. *European Journal of Applied Physiology, 79,* 512–521.

22. McArdle, W. D., Katch, F., & Katch, V. (1996). *Exercise physiology, energy, nutrition, and human performance.* Philadelphia: Williams & Wilkins.

23. Melissant, C. F., Lammers, L.-W. J., & Demedts, M. (1998). Relationship between external resistances, lung function changes and maximal exercise capacity. *European Respiratory Journal, 11,* 1369–1375.

24. Neder, J. A., Andreoni, S., Lerario, M. C., & Nery, L. E. (1999). Reference values for lung function tests. II. Maximal respiratory pressure and voluntary ventilation. *Brazilian Journal of Medical and Biological Research, 32,* 719–727.

25. Neder, J. A., Dal Corso, S., Malaguti, C., Reis, S., DeFuccio, M. B., Schmidt, H., Fuld, J. P., & Nery, L. E. (2003). The pattern and timing of breathing during incremental exercise: A normative study. *European Respiratory Journal, 31,* 530–538.

26. Origenes, M. M., Blank, S. E., & Schoene, R. B. (1993). Exercise ventilatory response to upright and aero-posture cycling. *Medicine and Science in Sports and Exercise, 25,* 608–612.

27. Pease, G. F. (1961). *Maximum breathing capacity in high school boys.* Unpublished master's thesis, San Diego State University, California.

28. Plato, P. A., McNulty, M., Crunk, S. M., & Tug Ergun, A. (2008). Predicting lactate threshold using ventilatory threshold. *International Journal of Sports Medicine, 28,* 732–737.

29. Powers, S. K., & Beadle, R. E. (1985). Onset of hyperventilation during incremental exercise: A brief review. *Research Quarterly for Exercise and Sport, 56,* 352–360.

30. Powers, S. K., & Howley, E. T. (2009). *Exercise physiology: Theory and application to fitness and performance, 7th ed.* New York: McGraw-Hill.

31. Prusacyzk, W. K., Cureton, K. J., Graham, R. E., & Ray, C. A. (1992). Differential effects of dietary carbohydrate on RPE at the lactate and ventilatory thresholds. *Medicine and Science in Sports and Exercise, 24,* 568–575.

32. Sexauer, W. P., Cheng, H.-K., & Fiel, S. B. (2003). Utility of the breathing reserve index at the anaerobic threshold in determining ventilatory-limited exercise in adult cystic fibrosis patients. *Chest, 124,* 1469–1475.

33. Skinner, J., & McLellan, T. (1980). The transition from aerobic to anaerobic metabolism. *Research Quarterly, 51,* 234–248.

34. Soungatoulin, V., Beam, W., Kersey, R., & Peterson, J. (2003). Comparative effects of traditional versus periodized intensity training on cycling performance. *Medicine and Science in Sports and Exercise, 35*(Suppl.), S35.

35. Wasserman, K. (1986). Anaerobiasis, lactate and gas exchange during exercise: The issues. *Federation Proceedings, 45,* 2904–2909.

36. Wasserman, K., Hansen, J. E., Sue, D. Y., Whipp, B. J., & Casaburi, R. (1994). *Principles of exercise testing and interpretation.* Philadelphia: Lea & Febiger.

Form 21.1

NAME _____ DATE _____ SCORE _____

EXERCISE VENTILATION

Homework

Gender: **M**   Initials: **AA**   Age (y): **35**   Height (cm): **180**   Weight (kg): **76.3**

FVC $_{BTPS}$ = **6.20** L   FEV$_{1\ BTPS}$ = **4.96** L   MVV $_{BTPS}$ = **202** L·min^{-1} ☐ Measured   ☒ Estimated

Power (W)	$\dot{V}O_2$ (L·min^{-1})	$\dot{V}_{E\ BTPS}$ (L·min^{-1}) *	Breathing rate (br·min^{-1})	Tidal volume (L·br^{-1})	TV / VC ratio (%) *	$\dot{V}_E/\dot{V}O_2$ equivalent *
100	1.40	28 ( )	16		( )	( )
150	2.02	44 ( )	19		( )	( )
200	2.72	62 ( )	20		( )	( )
250	3.63	84 ( )	23		( )	( )
300	4.40	115 ( )	30		( )	( )

Note: Estimated values from Table 21.2.

Category for MVV: _____ *(Table 21.4)*   *Possibly significant if :*

Ventilatory reserve: MVV - $\dot{V}_E$ max = _____ – _____ = _____ L·min^{-1} Vent reserve < 15 L·min^{-1}

Vent reserve index: $\dot{V}_E$ max / MVV = _____ / _____ = _____   VRI > 0.70 (70%)

Plot ventilation ($\dot{V}_E$) versus power and identify ventilatory threshold (V$_T$).   Power at V$_T$ = _____ W

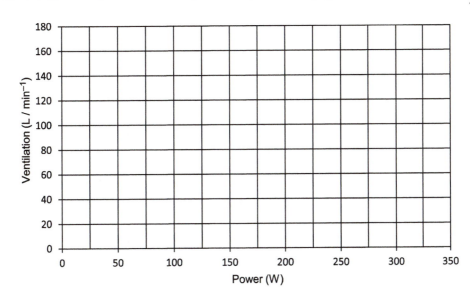

Comments: _____

_____

_____

_____

Form 21.2

EXERCISE VENTILATION

NAME _____ DATE _____ SCORE _____

Lab Results

Gender: _____ Initials: _____ Age (y): _____ Height (cm): _____ Weight (kg): _____

FVC_{BTPS} = _____ L $FEV_{1\ BTPS}$ = _____ L MVV_{BTPS} = _____ $L \cdot min^{-1}$ ☐ Measured   ☐ Estimated

Power (W)	$\dot{V}O_2$ ($L \cdot min^{-1}$)	$\dot{V}_{E\ BTPS}$ ($L \cdot min^{-1}$) *	Breathing rate (br·min⁻¹)	Tidal volume ($L \cdot br^{-1}$)	TV / VC ratio (%) *	$\dot{V}_E / \dot{V}O_2$ equivalent *
_____	_____	_____ ( )	_____	_____	_____ ( )	_____ ( )
_____	_____	_____ ( )	_____	_____	_____ ( )	_____ ( )
_____	_____	_____ ( )	_____	_____	_____ ( )	_____ ( )
_____	_____	_____ ( )	_____	_____	_____ ( )	_____ ( )
_____	_____	_____ ( )	_____	_____	_____ ( )	_____ ( )
_____	_____	_____ ( )	_____	_____	_____ ( )	_____ ( )

*Note: Estimated values from Table 21.2.

Category for MVV: _____ (Table 21.4)   Possibly significant if :

Ventilatory reserve: $MVV - \dot{V}_E$ max = _____ − _____ = _____ $L \cdot min^{-1}$ Vent reserve < 15 $L \cdot min^{-1}$

Vent reserve index: $\dot{V}_E$ max / MVV = _____ / _____ = _____   VRI > 0.70 (70%)

Plot ventilation ($\dot{V}_E$) versus power and identify ventilatory threshold ($\dot{V}_T$).   Power at $\dot{V}_T$ = _____ W

Comments: _____

_____

_____

_____

CHAPTER 22

FLEXIBILITY

Flexibility, an important fitness component, is described as the ability of a joint or combination of joints to move through a range of motion (ROM). A person who scores poorly on a flexibility test, such as the sit-and-reach test, or demonstrates poor ROM around a joint, has reduced flexibility. Indirectly, poor flexibility in school children in the mid-1950s was responsible for the formation of the President's Council on Physical Fitness and Sports (PCPFS) by President Dwight Eisenhower. He was stirred to action when investigators reported that American children from 6 to 16 y of age compared poorly with European children of the same age.[36] More than half (57 %) of the American children had failed a fitness battery composed of six tests, compared to only 8 % of European children who failed. Most of the American children failed due to poor flexibility, specifically the Kraus-Weber "floor touch" test, which 44 % of American children failed. Lower body flexibility is measured in children and adults using a variety of sit-and-reach tests. These tests typically look at the flexibility of a combination of joints acting at the same time. The range of motion of specific joint actions (e.g., hip flexion) can be measured using a goniometer. This chapter describes numerous sit-and-reach flexibility tests and also the measurement of ROM in a variety of upper and lower body joints using goniometry.

SIT-AND-REACH (SR) TEST

Most Americans will suffer from low-back pain at least once in their lifetime. Although never documented by the Sit-and-Reach (SR) Test, poor flexibility of low-back extensors and hamstrings has often been suggested to be associated with, or contribute to, muscular low-back pain.[5,32] In addition, poor hamstring flexibility may predispose injury to the hamstrings.[52,54] Tests for these two muscle groups (lower back muscles and hamstring muscles) have received the most attention. For example, the Sit-and-Reach Test has been incorporated as a health-related physical fitness item into such national fitness batteries as *AAHPERD Physical Best,*[4] the President's Council on Physical Fitness and Sports,[46] the Fitnessgram,[29] the AAHPERD Functional Fitness Assessment for Adults over 60 years,[10,43] and the American Alliance for Health, Physical Education, Recreation and Dance Health-Related Test.[2]

Despite the positive claims supporting flexibility as a health-related fitness component, *hypermobility* in static flexibility tests does not appear to be associated with a reduced risk of injury.[47] Furthermore, the data are not convincing in connecting a reduced injury risk to a stretching regimen prior to exercise.[35,45,50] More studies are needed before definitive conclusions can be made—especially randomized prospective studies that include large numbers of participants and control groups. A variety of stretching regimens should be studied, and distinctions should be made between regimens that include warm-up with the stretching regimen. For the present, it appears that participants will continue to stretch prior to exercise based on nearly universal beliefs, their habitual routines, and their own intuitions regarding the safety of their musculoskeletal system during exercise. This is probably their most prudent course of action until evidence is strong enough to call for a modification of their present pre-exercise regimen.

GONIOMETRY

Goniometry is a technique for measuring the range of motion (ROM) of a joint. It can be used to describe the flexibility of a healthy young child, college student or older adult. It is used more often in a clinical setting to assess musculoskeletal injuries, neurological disorders, and to look at the effect of aging in patients. Most ROM measurements are made with what is referred to as a *universal goniometer.* It is a plastic or metal device consisting of two "arms." The arms are connected within a protractor that can measure the position of the arms relative to one another on a full 360° circle. One of the arms, the "stationary arm" is placed on the proximal side of the joint. The "moving arm" is placed on the distal side of the joint. In most cases, the ROM of the joint is measured relative to 0° (no bend) or to "anatomical position" which in the ankle is 90°. For example, to measure plantarflexion in the ankle, the stationary arm of the goniometer is aligned with the long axis (midline) of the fibula. The moving arm is aligned with the bottom of the foot (parallel to the fifth metatarsal). Plantarflexion is measured as maximal ROM (the number of degrees) beyond 90° (anatomical position), which is expected to be about 50° beyond anatomical position in the case of normal plantarflexion. Musculoskeletal injuries or neurological disorders can result in ROMs much less than those expected in unaffected persons.

METHODS

Although most authorities would view the Sit-and-Reach (SR) Test as a field test, it has some qualities that meet the criteria for a lab test. The Traditional SR Test requires close interaction between the technician and participant. Additionally, unless there are numerous measuring sticks or sit-and-reach boxes, it does not lend itself to simultaneous testing of many persons, as does a simple bend-over toe-toucher field test.

Six different methods of performing the Sit-and-Reach Test include modifications of the traditional test prescribed by the American Alliance for Health, Physical Education, Recreation and Dance.[2,3,4] The modifications of the Traditional SR Test are the Canadian,[15] YMCA,[18] Wall[22,24,25], V-Sit,[12] and Back-Saver[12] SR tests.

The MacRae and Wright (MW) Test is a criterion measure for lower back flexibility,[40] and the goniometrically measured straight-leg raise is a criterion measure for hamstring flexibility.[16] Other than the subjective aspect of these criteria tests, they meet all of the criteria to qualify as laboratory tests. Comments on the accuracy of the SR Tests and goniometry are presented in Box 22.1.

Equipment

The characteristics of the six SR Tests are presented in Table 22.1. The test apparatus for the Traditional SR Test is a boxlike structure with a measuring scale on its upper surface labeled in 1cm gradations. The 23 cm mark is exactly in line with the vertical plane of the participant's soles and heels, which are underneath the overhang and against the front edge of the box (Figure 22.1). Commercial sit-and-reach flexibility testers are available, one of which is the Acuflex I™ (Novel Products, Inc., Rockton IL). The universal goniometer shown in Figure 22.2 is available from a variety of vendors. There is also a larger metal version.

Procedures for the SR Tests

Certain procedures are the same for all six tests. Because flexion places strain on spinal ligaments, especially when performed ballistically,[1] and raises intradiscal

Table 22.1   Characteristics of Various Sit-and-Reach (SR) Tests

SR Test	Equipment	Position	Index or Heel Line	Time Held (s)	Number of Trials	Trial to Record
Traditional	Sit-and-reach box	Floor or bench	23 cm	1–2 s	4	4th trial
Canadian	Adjustable box, stick	Floor or bench	26 cm	2 s	2	Best trial
YMCA	Measuring stick, tape	Floor	38 cm	2 s	3	Best trial
Wall SR	Sit-and-reach box, stick	Floor or bench	0 cm	≥ 2 s	2	Average
V-Sit	Measuring stick, tape	Floor	23 cm	1–2 s	4	4th trial
Back-Saver	Sit-and-reach box	Floor or bench	23 cm	1–2 s	4 per leg	4th trial

Note: See text for more detailed descriptions of each test.

pressures,[9,41,48] the participant should be "warm and loose" and perform the movement slowly. Although only the Canadian Test prescribes a standard preparatory regimen, it seems that a standard warm-up regimen of slow stretching and walking/jogging in place for 5 minutes would also enhance the reliability and validity of the other tests. It would also validate comparisons among SR Tests.

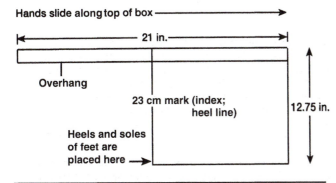

Figure 22.1 The Traditional Sit-and-Reach Test apparatus is boxlike with an overhang.

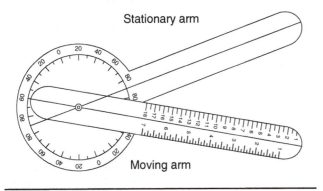

Figure 22.2 Universal goniometer used to measure range of motion (ROM) of various joints.

Participants remove their shoes and fully extend their legs, meaning that the back of the knees are against the floor, table, or bench. The hands are placed with palms down and one palm on top of the back of the other hand. The participant holds the final reach trial for at least a second or two.

The tests are distinct in several ways. The most obvious is the initial body position—distance of the feet spread, a bent leg, hands on floor or on box. They may also vary in their choice of recorded trial—fourth, best, or average. Also, the index line (heel line) may vary—0 cm, 23 cm, 26 cm, and 38 cm. Other distinctions are presented in the specific procedures for each SR Test.

Specific Procedures for the SR Tests

Traditional SR Test

Figure 22.3 illustrates the proper technique to perform the Traditional SR Test. The sit-and-reach box should be braced against an object (e.g., wall) to prevent it from sliding away from the participant. Recognize that the index line (heel line) is at the 23 cm mark. Thus, any participant reaching beyond this line will have a recorded score greater than 23 cm. The procedural steps are as follows:

1. Participant performs a short bout (e.g., 5 min) of prior exercise.
2. Participant removes shoes.
3. Participant sits on the floor, bench, or table with feet against the testing apparatus (index; heel line).
4. Participant fully extends the legs, with the medial sides of the feet about 20 cm (≈ 8 in.) apart.
5. Technician holds one hand lightly against the participant's knees to ensure full leg extension.
6. Participant extends arms forward with the hands placed on top of each other, palms down.

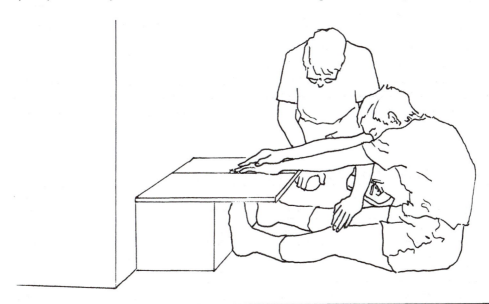

Figure 22.3 A participant performs the Traditional Sit-and-Reach Test while the technician gently holds the knees.

7. Participant slowly bends forward along the measuring scale, not necessarily to the maximal on the first trial.
8. Participant repeats this forward stretch two more times.
9. Participant repeats the same stretch a fourth time, but now holds both hands at the maximal position for at least 1 s, but not necessarily beyond 2 s.
10. Technician observes and records the fourth (final) trial's score to the nearest centimeter onto Form 22.2.
11. Technician interprets the Traditional SR Test value from Table 22.2.

Canadian SR Test[14,15]

Except for the specifically prescribed warm-up regimen, the beginning steps of the Canadian SR Test are similar to those of the Traditional SR Test. The later steps include minor differences related to the height of the meter stick, separation of the participant's feet, the number of trials, and the recorded trial.

1. Participant executes the modified hurdle stretch (bent leg's sole of foot against inside of other leg), holding for 20 s, and repeated twice for each leg.
2. Participant removes shoes, sits on floor, table, or bench, and extends legs.
3. Participant places heels about 5 cm apart.
4. Technician places a meter stick at the participant's toe-level height or uses a height-adjustable box with meter stick attached.
5. The meter stick crosses the heel line (index) at the 26 cm mark.

6. Participant places hands on top of each other and slowly bends forward, running hands along meter stick, keeping head down.
7. Participant holds maximally extended position for 2 s.
8. Technician notes the distance of the reach to the closest centimeter. For example, if the participant reaches exactly to the index line at toe level, the score is recorded as 26 cm.
9. Participant repeats trial.
10. Technician records and interprets the best of the two trials using Form 22.2 and Table 22.3.

YMCA SR Test[18]

Except for the placement of the measuring stick, index line, number of trials, and the recorded trial, most of the Y's procedures are the same as those of the Traditional SR Test.

The technician places a yard/meter stick on the floor, mat, table, or bench so that the zero end is toward the crotch. Because the yardstick is at a lower level than when it is on top of a 12 in. box, the reach scores may be about 1 in. or 2.5 cm lower than the reaches measured on the traditional box.[45] However, this deficit may be partly compensated by the plantar flexion permitted by this nonbox method.

1. Technician intersects the index line with a tape across the yardstick at 15 in. or 38 cm (equivalent to touching toes).
2. After warming up, the participant removes shoes; sits on floor, table, or bench; and extends legs, straddling yard/meter stick or measuring tape.

Table 22.2 Category for Traditional Sit-and-Reach Test Score (cm) by Gender and Age (y)

Category (percentile)	Men			Women		
	18–19 y (N = 209)	20–25 y (N = 171)	20–45 y (N = 52)	18–19 y (N = 506)	20–25 y (N = 221)	20–45 y (N = 52)
Well above ave (> 90th)	> 40	> 40	> 44	> 43	> 42	> 45
Above ave (71st–90th)	34–40	34–40	36–44	39–43	39–42	40–45
Average (31st–70th)	27–33	24–33	24–35	32–38	32–38	32–39
Below ave (10th–30th)	20–26	19–23	16–23	27–31	27–31	26–31
Well below ave (< 10th)	< 20	< 19	< 16	< 27	< 27	< 26
Average	29	28	29	34	34	35

Note: Values for percentiles are estimated for the 20–45 y groups using the reported means and standard deviations assuming the data are normally distributed.
Source: Data for 18–19 y and 20–25 y from Beam (2006)[6]; data for 20–45 y from Jackson & Langford (1989).[31]

Table 22.3 Category for Canadian Sit-and-Reach Test Score (cm) by Gender and Age (y)

Category (percentile)	Men				Women			
	15–19 y	20–29 y	30–39 y	40–49 y	15–19 y	20–29 y	30–39 y	40–49 y
Well above ave (> 90th)	> 40	> 42	> 40	> 37	> 44	> 43	> 42	> 40
Above ave (71st–90th)	37–40	37–42	35–40	31–37	41–44	39–43	38–42	36–40
Average (31st–70th)	27–35	27–36	25–34	21–30	32–40	30–38	29–37	27–35
Below ave (10th–30th)	20–26	19–26	18–24	13–20	26–31	23–29	22–28	20–26
Well below ave (< 10th)	< 20	< 19	< 18	< 13	< 26	< 23	< 22	< 20
Average	31	31	29	25	36	34	33	31

Source: Data adapted from Fitness and Amateur Sport Canada (1987).[14]

3. Participant abducts legs to separate heels by 10–12 in. (25–30 cm) and places heels perpendicular to and at the front edge of the index tape or mark. If the heels slide over the tape, adjust heels accordingly.
4. Participant places hands on top of each other and slowly bends forward with head down, running hands along the top of the yard/meter stick. Technician gently holds participant's knees down.
5. Participant holds the extended position for about 2 s.
6. Technician notes the distance of the reach to the closest 1 cm. For example, if the participant reaches 1 cm past the index line, the score is recorded as 39 cm.
7. Participant performs a second and third trial and can relax and flex legs between trials.
8. Technician records and interprets the best of the three trials using Form 22.2 and Table 22.4, respectively.

Wall SR Test[22,24,25,26]

This test has an added preliminary phase that the other SR Tests do not. This phase is performed against a wall in order to correct for any interindividual differences in appendage proportions, such as leg length versus trunk length.[24,25]

1. Participant executes a short bout ($\approx$ 5 min) of prior exercise.
2. Participant removes shoes.
3. Participant sits on the floor, (or bench or table) with the back, hips, and head against a wall.
4. Participant places soles and heels of feet against the testing apparatus, which can be a commercial box (Acuflex I™) or the traditional box. The apparatus

should be braced against the technician's feet or some object to prevent it from sliding away.
5. Participant fully extends the legs, with the feet about shoulder width (20–30 cm) apart. Technician does not need to hold the participant's knees but legs remain extended.
6. Participant places one hand on top of the other as in the other tests.
7. The **starting (zero) position** is determined by:
   a. **Participant** reaching forward as far as possible along the measuring device without having the head and back leave the wall; however, the shoulders are permitted to hunch forward into a rounded position.
   b. **Technician** records the mark to the closest 1 cm onto Form 22.2; using the Acuflex I™, simply slide the reach indicator to the person's fingertips and observe the score.
8. After the recording or adjustment is made, the participant slowly reaches forward three times during a single maneuver along the device, with the third reach being held for 2 s or more.
9. Technician records the third phase of this reaching maneuver.
10. Technician records the actual back/hamstring flexibility value by subtracting the starting value from the end-reach value.
11. Participant executes another three-phase reach trial.
12. Technician records the second trial, then calculates and records the average flexibility value of the two trials.
13. Technician interprets the flexibility value by referring to Table 22.5.

Table 22.4 Category for YMCA Sit-and-Reach Test Score (cm) by Gender and Age (y)

Category (percentile)	Men				Women			
	18–25 y	26–35 y	36–45 y	46–55 y	18–25 y	26–35 y	36–45 y	46–55 y
Well above ave (> 90th)	> 56	> 53	> 53	> 48	> 61	> 58	> 56	> 53
Above ave (71st–90th)	49–56	44–53	44–53	39–48	54–61	52–58	49–56	47–53
Average (31st–70th)	37–48	34–43	34–43	26–38	44–53	42–51	39–48	37–46
Below ave (10th–30th)	30–36	25–33	20–33	18–25	38–43	36–41	33–38	28–36
Well below ave (< 10th)	< 30	< 25	< 20	< 18	< 38	< 36	< 33	< 28
Average	43	38	38	33	48	48	43	41

Source: Data from Golding (2000).[18]

Table 22.5 Category for Wall Sit-and-Reach Test Score (cm) by Gender and Age (y)

Category (percentile)	Men			Women		
	< 35 y	35–50 y	> 50 y	< 35 y	35–50 y	> 50 y
Well above ave (> 90th)	> 45	> 41	> 38	> 45	> 44	> 38
Above ave (71st–90th)	41–45	36–41	32–38	42–45	40–44	36–38
Average (31st–70th)	34–40	28–35	25–31	36–41	32–39	24–35
Below ave (10th–30th)	24–33	21–27	20–24	26–35	25–31	19–23
Well below ave (< 10th)	< 24	< 21	< 20	< 26	< 25	< 19
Average	37	32	26	38	34	28

Source: Data from Hoeger (1991).[23]

V-Sit SR Test[12]

The V-Sit SR Test is a modification of the Traditional SR Test. The only modifications are the removal of the box and a prescribed 30 cm separation of the heels, hence the V-sit position. All other procedures are the same, such as the following:

1. Participant executes a short bout of prior exercise.
2. Participant removes shoes.
3. Technician places meter stick's 23 cm line between the legs and at the heel line of participant.
4. Participant's legs are fully extended; technician gently holds knees to assure extension.
5. Participant's bottom hand and top hand of outstretched arms are directly aligned.
6. Participant slowly bends forward along the meter stick during three preparatory trials.
7. Participant makes a maximal stretch during the fourth trial.
8. Technician records the fourth trial to the nearest centimeter and interprets according to the same norms as the Traditional SR Test (Table 22.2).

Back-Saver SR Test[12]

Possible excessive posterior disc compression occurs when performing the maneuvers prescribed for the five previously discussed SR tests.[9] The Back-Saver SR Test was devised to reduce this compression when bending forward with *both* legs extended by prescribing forward bending with only *one* leg extended.[12] Unfortunately, some participants feel discomfort at the hip joint of the bent leg during the modified maneuver.[28] The Back-Saver SR Test is identical to the Traditional SR Test (with box) except for the four trials for each leg and the following modified body position:

- Floor-seated participant places the sole of the foot of a fully extended leg against the front and bottom edge of the sit-and-reach box.
- Participant bends the other leg so that the sole of the leg's foot is flat on the floor and about two or three inches ($\approx$ 5–7.5 cm) to the side of the extended knee of the other leg.
- Participant may have to move the bent leg to the side as the body moves forward along the box.

The technician records the fourth trial of the right leg and the left leg. The norms are the same as the Traditional SR Test (Table 22.2).

Procedures for Goniometry

The range of motion (ROM) of any joint may be measured with a plastic or metal goniometer. The two arms of the goniometer are identified as the stationary (or proximal) arm and the moving (or distal) arm. The stationary arm is placed and held by the technician on the proximal limb or portion of the limb or in some cases the torso. The body is provided support by having the participant lying supine or prone or sitting on a padded table. In some cases, the technician also provides manual stabilization to particular body parts. The moving arm of the goniometer is placed and held on the distal portion of the limb. The ROM (in degrees) is determined by the two end points of the joint action. The ROM can be measured passively, where the technician moves the joint through the ROM, or it can be measured with the participant actively contracting the muscles responsible for the joint action. Of all of the joint actions, only six are described here to provide the student with a beginning experience in goniometry. Many good sources exist for providing a more detailed description of measuring all joint actions.[21,37,51]

Measuring Range of Motion

The procedures described are for measuring any ROM. See Table 22.6 and Figure 22.4 for details related to each specific joint action.

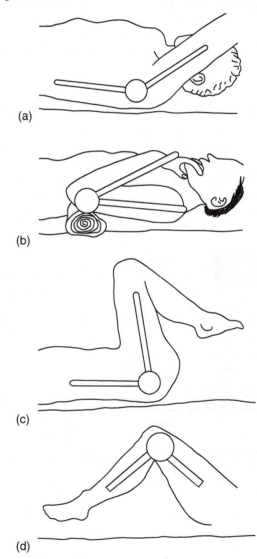

(a)

(b)

(c)

(d)

Figure 22.4 Goniometer placement for measuring range of motion (ROM) of: (a) shoulder flexion, (b) elbow flexion, (c) hip flexion, and (d) knee flexion.

1. Participant lies supine or sits on table determined by joint action being measured.
2. Technician identifies axis of rotation of joint and places the center of the goniometer specifically over this point.
3. Technician places and holds stationary (proximal) arm of goniometer on desired limb or portion of limb or in some cases the torso.
4. Technician places and holds moving (distal) arm on desired limb or portion of limb.
5. Technician instructs participant to move limb to starting point. (For most tests of joint flexion, the starting point is considered 0° of flexion. For measuring ankle ROM, the starting point is 90°, anatomical position.) The starting point is considered the "zero point" and is recorded as 0° in the description of ROM.
6. Participant slowly moves desired limb through full ROM. Technician determines "end point" using the goniometer and records it on Form 22.2.
7. The median of 3 trials is used to describe the ROM for that specific joint action.

Procedures for the Criterion Tests (Optional)

The MacRae and Wright (MW) Test is a criterion measure for lower back flexibility,[40] and the goniometrically measured straight-leg raise is a criterion measure for hamstring flexibility.[16] The MW Test measures the maximal anterior flexion of the lower back and has a high validity coefficient ($r = 0.97$) with radiographically determined vertebral flexion.[52] The criterion test for hamstring flexibility uses a goniometer. The test has a subjective end point whereby the technician and participant both sense tightness during the assisted straight-leg raise. Nevertheless, the reliability of this goniometric test is high.[8] The scores of all performers on the MW and goniometric criterion tests can then be correlated with one or more of the SR tests as a validation check of lower back flexibility and hamstring flexibility, respectively.

Procedures for the MacRae and Wright (MW) Back Criterion Test[40,44]

1. Participant stands erect.
2. Technician locates the sacroiliac joint by palpation and marks it with a pen.
3. Technician measures and marks the points 5 cm below and 10 cm above the lumbosacral joint mark, thus producing a total distance of 15 cm between marks.
4. Participant sits with legs extended on the floor, mat, table, or bench.
5. Technician views the marks on participant's back while placing the tape measure on the low 5 cm mark.
6. As participant bends maximally forward, technician measures the distance from the lowest mark to the highest mark.
7. Technician subtracts the original position's 15 cm from the maximally stretched position's distance.
8. The procedure is repeated three times, with the average being recorded as the flexibility score.

Procedures for the Goniometric Hamstring Criterion Test

The goniometric test received its name because of the goniometer instrument but is often referred to as the straight-leg raise test. The raising of the leg is a passive maneuver on the participant's part because the technician lifts, and gently pushes against, the participant's leg. It may require two technicians—one to lift the participant's leg and another to make the goniometric measurement.

1. Technician aligns the axis of the goniometer with the axis of participant's hip joint.
2. Technician places the stationary arm of the manual goniometer in line with the trunk and the moving arm in line with the femur.
3. Technician holds participant's knee straight while moving that leg toward hip flexion.
4. When technician feels tightness (feedback from participant may help), the leg is held there while a reading to the closest degree is made from the angle produced by the stationary arm and moving arm of the goniometer.
5. The average of three trials is used as the flexibility score.

| Table 22.6 | Procedures for Measuring Range of Motion (ROM) of Selected Joints using Goniometry |

Joint Motion	Body Position	Axis of Rotation	Stationary (Proximal) Arm	Moving (Distal) Arm	Expected ROM	Comment
Shoulder flexion (GH)	Supine	Acromion process	Parallel to thorax (midaxillary line)	Midline of lateral humerus	0–120°	End point is where scapula moves
Elbow flexion	Supine	Epicondyle of humerus	Long axis (midline) of humerus	Long axis (midline) of radius	0–150°	Forearm is fully supinated
Hip flexion	Supine	Greater trochanter	Midline of pelvis	Long axis (midline) of femur	0–120°	Allow knee to flex as hip flexes
Knee flexion	Supine	Epicondyle of femur	Long axis (midline) of femur	Long axis (midline) of fibula	0–140°	Allow hip to flex as knee flexes
Ankle dorsiflxn	Seated with leg hanging	Lateral malleolus	Long axis (midline) of fibula	Parallel to bottom of foot (5th metatarsal)	0–20°	Relative to ankle at 90° (zero point)
Ankle plantarflxn	Seated with leg hanging	Lateral malleolus	Long axis (midline) of fibula	Parallel to bottom of foot (5th metatarsal)	0–50°	Relative to ankle at 90° (zero point)

Source: Compiled from Heyward (2002)[21]; Levangie & Norkin (2001)[37]; Starkey, Brown & Ryan (2010).[51]

RESULTS AND DISCUSSION

The ability to exercise through a full range of motion, thereby demonstrating good flexibility, is desirable. The Traditional Sit-and-Reach (SR) Test provides a reliable and valid method for measuring flexibility. The comparative data for the various SR Tests are seen in Tables 22.2 through 22.5. The percentiles on which the categories are based (e.g., > 90th percentile, 71st–90th percentile, etc.) are somewhat different than those used in previous chapters because they more closely match those used in published studies of SR flexibility. The Traditional SR Test has its limitations, however, in that it is only moderately related (r = 0.70–0.72, p < 0.01) to a direct measure of hamstring extensibility and it correlates relatively poorly (r = 0.29–0.40, p < 0.05) with a direct measure of low back flexibility.[39] It also requires the use of a commercially available or specially constructed box. Alternate tests, including the Canadian SR Test[3,15] and the YMCA SR Test,[18] can be conducted with a measuring stick (a meter stick or yard stick) without the need for the box. Directly comparing scores between two different SR Tests can be difficult. Flexibility scores from floor measuring sticks are lower than scores from boxes.[17,34] A floor score using a measuring stick is typically about 1.75 cm lower than a comparable flexibility measurement taken using a box.[16] And there can also be a difference in the index line or heel line between tests. For example, the index line for the Traditional SR Test is 23 cm, but the index line for the YMCA SR Test is 38 cm, a difference of 15 cm. This is why when you compare the average score of 20–25-year-old men, for example (28 cm) on the Traditional SR Test (Table 22.2), it is 15 cm less than the average of a comparable group of 18–27-year-old men (43 cm) on the YMCA SR Test (Table 22.4).

Other variations of the Traditional SR Test have been created based on anatomical and biomechanical considerations. The Wall SR Test[24,25] attempts to correct for differences in body proportions by measuring inter-individual differences in leg or trunk length. The V-Sit SR Test[12] and the Back-Saver SR[12] Test both utilize body positions different from the Traditional SR Test in an attempt to alleviate back discomfort during the test. Higher scores on any of the SR flexibility tests indicate a higher degree of flexibility. But extremely high flexibility scores are not necessarily considered "excellent." An extreme level of flexibility or hypermobility around a joint can potentially increase the risk of joint injury.

Comparative data for the Traditional SR Test are found in Table 22.2. The data demonstrate a gender difference in flexibility, with women being more flexible than men, indicated by SR scores 5 cm to 6 cm higher in women. The same is observed in the Canadian SR Test (Table 22.3) and the YMCA SR Test (Table 22.4). A study comparing the results of the Traditional SR Test, V-Sit SR Test, and Back-Saver SR Test between men and women showed the mean score of women greater than that of men by 12 cm, 9 cm, and 12 cm, respectively.[28] A study using hip joint angle (HJA) as a measure of sit-and-reach performance reported mean HJAs in women ($M \pm SD$, 92 $\pm$ 10°) on average 12° higher than in men ($M \pm SD$, 80 $\pm$ 9°).[55] Another study comparing older (55 y and above) men and women showed significant (p < 0.05) differences in SR scores between men ($M \pm SD$, 19.3 $\pm$ 9.5 cm) and women ($M \pm SD$, 32.0 $\pm$ 8.2 cm).[38] There is insufficient data to suggest that women are more flexible than men on all tests of flexibility. Interestingly, the gender difference in flexibility is nearly eliminated with the use of the Wall SR Test (Table 22.5). This protocol corrects for proportional differences in leg length versus trunk length.

Flexibility measurements are included in the AAHPERD health-related fitness test for 10- to 18-year-olds.[2] Norms and categories for the fitness test are shown in Table 22.7. Anthropometric factors may cause normal boys and girls between the ages of 10 y and 14 y to be unable to reach the 23 cm index mark (touch their toes) in the Traditional SR Test.[2] This may be due to the preadolescent and adolescent growth spurt, which makes the legs disproportionately longer than the trunk. Except for the Wall SR Test, other tests may favor persons with longer arms and/or a longer trunk and disproportionately shorter legs.[24] However, the criterion MacRae and Wright Test shows that the other SR Tests are just as valid as the Wall SR Test.[28] This might be one of the reasons for higher scores in women than men: lower average leg length compared with their height.[53] Despite the bias attributed to disproportionate lengths, it appears that the "non-Wall" SR Tests would be independent of total height.[49]

In reviewing the data in Table 22.3 through Table 22.5, it can be observed that the flexibility scores of every method are lower in the older age groups compared with the younger age groups. With the Canadian SR Test, the older age groups (40–49 y) average 5 cm to 6 cm lower than the younger age groups (15–19 y). With the YMCA

Table 22.7   Category for Traditional Sit-and-Reach Test Score (cm) for Boys and Girls (10 to 18 y)

Category	Boys					Girls				
	10 y	12 y	14 y	16 y	18 y	10 y	12 y	14 y	16 y	18 y
Optimal/Excellent (≥ 75th %ile)	≥ 29	≥ 31	≥ 32	≥ 36	≥ 37	≥ 34	≥ 36	≥ 40	≥ 41	≥ 41
Acceptable/Good (50th–74th %ile)	27–28	26–30	27–31	31–35	31–36	29–33	32–35	36–39	37–40	37–40
Minimal/Fair (25th–49th %ile)	22–26	20–25	20–26	26–30	26–30	26–28	28–31	31–35	33–36	32–36
Unacceptable/Poor (< 25th %ile)	< 22	< 20	< 20	< 26	< 26	< 26	< 28	< 31	< 33	< 32

Source: Data from AAHPERD (1980).[2]

SR Test, the older groups (46–55 y) average 7 cm to 10 cm lower than the younger groups (18–25 y). And with the Wall SR Test, the older groups (> 50 y) average 10 cm to 11 cm lower than the younger groups (< 35 y). A general decline in joint range of motion and muscle flexibility with age has been reported.[7,33] This decline is possibly due to molecular cross-linking in collagen molecules altering the mechanical structure of collagen[20] and to biological aging of articular structures.[33] But it is also likely due in part to reduced activity levels associated with aging.[33,55]

BOX 22.2 | **Chapter Preview/Review**

What are the characteristics and dimensions of the box used in the Traditional Sit-and-Reach (SR) test?

What are the 6 different tests of SR flexibility described in this chapter?

Which trial is recorded and used to assess flexibility in each of the 6 tests described in this chapter?

How does the Back-Saver SR test differ from the Traditional SR test?

What is the effect of sex/gender on SR flexibility?

What is the effect of aging on SR flexibility?

What is a goniometer? How is it used?

What is the axis of rotation for elbow flexion?

What is the position of the stationary and moving arm during elbow flexion?

What is the expected ROM for ankle dorsiflexion and plantarflexion?

References

1. Adams, M. A., & Hutton, W. C. (1983). The mechanical function of the lumbar apophyseal joints. Spine, 8, 327–330.

2. American Alliance for Health, Physical Education, Recreation and Dance. (1980). *AAHPERD health-related physical fitness test*. Reston, VA: Author.

3. American Alliance for Health, Physical Education, Recreation and Dance. (1985). *Norms for college students—The health-related physical fitness test*. Reston, VA: Author.

4. American Alliance for Health, Physical Education, Recreation and Dance. (1988). *Physical best*. Reston, VA: Author.

5. American College of Sports Medicine. (2000). *ACSM's guidelines for exercise testing and prescription*. Philadelphia: Lippincott Williams & Wilkins.

6. Beam, W. C (2006). Unpublished data.

7. Bell, R. D., & Hoshizaki, T. B. (1981). Relationships of age and sex with range of motion of seventeen joint actions in humans. *Canadian Journal of Applied Sport Science, 6,* 202–206.

8. Boone, D., Azen, S., Lin, G., Spence, C., Baron, C., & Lee, L. (1978). Reliability of goniometric measurements. *Physical Therapy, 58,* 1355–1360.

9. Cailliet, R. (1988). *Low back pain syndrome* (4th ed.). Philadelphia: F. A. Davis.

10. Clark, B., Osness, W., Adrian, M., Hoeger, W. W. K., Raab, D., & Wiswell, R. (1989). Tests for fitness in older adults: AAHPERD Fitness Task Force. *Journal of Physical Education, Recreation and Dance, 60,* 66–71.

11. Clarke, H. H. (1975). Joint and body range of movement. *Physical Fitness Research Digest, 5,* 1–22.

12. Cooper Institute for Aerobics Research. (1992). *The Prudential FITNESSGRAM test administration manual*. Dallas, TX: Author.

13. Corbin, C. B., & Pangrazi, R. P. (1992). Are American children and youth fit? *Research Quarterly for Exercise and Sport, 63,* 96–106.

14. Fitness and Amateur Sport Canada. (1987). *Canadian Standardized Test of Fitness (CSTF) operations manual* (3rd ed.). Ottawa: Canadian Association of Sport Sciences.

15. Fitness and Lifestyle Research Institute. (1983). *Fitness and lifestyle in Canada*. Ottawa: Fitness and Amateur Sport.

16. Goeken, L. N., & Holf, A. L. (1993). Instrumental straight-leg raising: Results in healthy subjects. *Archives of Physical Medicine and Rehabilitation, 74,* 194–203.

17. Golding, L. A. (1997). Flexibility, stretching, and flexibility testing: Recommendations for testing and standards. *ACSM's Health and Fitness Journal, 1,* 17–20, 37–38.

18. Golding, L. A. (Ed.). (2000). *YMCA fitness testing and assessment manual* (4th ed.). Champaign, IL: Human Kinetics.

19. Harris, M. L. (1969). A factor analytic study of flexibility. *Research Quarterly, 40,* 62–70.

20. Hayflick, L. (1998). How and why we age. *Experimental Gerontology, 33,* 639–653.

21. Heyward, V. H. (2002). *Advanced fitness assessment and exercise prescription, 4th ed.* Champaign, IL, Human Kinetics.

22. Hoeger, W. W. K. (1989). *Lifetime physical fitness and wellness*. Englewood, CO: Morton.

23. Hoeger, W. W. K. (1991). *Principles and labs for physical fitness and wellness* (2nd ed.) Englewood, CO: Morton.

24. Hoeger, W. W. K., & Hopkins, D. R. (1992). A comparison of the sit and reach and the modified sit and reach in the measurement of flexibility in women. *Research Quarterly for Exercise and Sport, 63,* 191–195.

25. Hoeger, W. W. K., Hopkins, D. R., Button, S., & Palmer, T. A. (1990). Comparing the sit and reach with the modified sit and reach in measuring flexibility in adolescents. *Pediatric Exercise Science, 2,* 156–162.

26. Hoeger, W. W. K., Hopkins, D. R., & Johnson, L. C. (1993). *The assessment of muscular flexibility*. Rockton, IL: Authors/Novel Products, Inc.

27. Hubley, C. (1982). Testing flexibility. In D. McDougall, H. Wenger, & H. Green (Eds.), *Physiological testing of the elite athlete* (pp. 117–132). Ottawa: Canadian Association of Sport Sciences.

28. Hui, S. C., Yuen, P. Y., Morrow, J. R., & Jackson, A.W. (1999). Comparison of the criterion-related validity of sit-and-reach tests with and without limb length adjustment in Asian adults. *Research Quarterly for Exercise and Sport, 70,* 401–406.

29. Institute for Aerobics Research. (1988). *The FITNESSGRAM.* Dallas, TX: Author.

30. Jackson, A. W., & Baker, A. A. (1986). The relationship of the sit and reach test to criterion measures of hamstring and back flexibility in young females. *Research Quarterly for Exercise and Sport, 57,* 183–186.

31. Jackson, A. W., & Langford, N. J. (1989). The criterion-related validity of the sit and reach test: Replication and extension of previous findings. *Research Quarterly for Exercise and Sport, 60,* 384–387.

32. Jackson, A. W., Morrow, J. R., Brill, P. A., Kohl, H. W., Gordon, N. F., & Blair, S. N. (1998). Relations of sit-up and sit-and-reach test to lower back pain in adults. *Journal of Orthopaedic and Sports Physical Therapy, 27,* 22–26.

33. James, B., & Parker, A.W. (1989). Active and passive mobility of lower limb joints in elderly men and women. *American Journal of Physical Medicine and Rehabilitation, 58,* 162–167.

34. Jones, G. R., Boyce, R. W., Coolidge, W. A., & Hiatt, A. R. (1989). Comparison of two methods of sit and reach trunk flexion assessment. *Medicine and Science in Sports and Exercise, 21* (Suppl.), Abstract #691, S116.

35. Knudson, D. (1999). Stretching during warm-up: Do we have enough evidence? *Journal of Health, Physical Education, Recreation and Dance, 70*(7), 24–27, 51.

36. Kraus, H., & Hirschland, R. P. (1954). Minimum muscular fitness tests in school children. *Research Quarterly, 125,*178–188.

37. Levangie, P. K., & Norkin, C. C. (2001). *Joint structure and function: a comprehensive analysis, 3rd ed.* Philadelphia, F.A. Davis Company.

38. Lemmink, K., Kemper, H., De Greef, M., Rispens, P., & Stevens, M. (2003). The validity of the sit-and-reach test and the modified sit-and-reach test in middle-aged to older men and women. *Research Quarterly for Exercise and Sport, 74,* 331–336.

39. Liemohn, W., Sharpe, G. L., & Wasserman, J. F. (1994). Criterion related validity of the sit-and-reach test. *Journal of Strength and Conditioning Research, 8,* 91–94.

40. MacRae, I. F., & Wright, V. (1969). Measurement of back movement. *Annals of the Rheumatic Diseases, 28,* 584–589.

41. Nachemson, A. (1975). Towards a better understanding of low back pain: A review of the mechanics of the lumbar disc. *Rheumatic Rehabilitation, 14,* 129–143.

42. O'Connor, J. S., Hines, K., & Warner, C. A. (1996). Flexibility and injury incidence. *Medicine and Science in Sports and Exercise, 28*(5), Abstract #376, S63.

43. Osness, W. H., Adrian, M., Clark, B., Hoeger, W., Raab, D., & Wiswell, R. (1990). *Functional fitness assessment for adults over 60 years: A field-bond assessment.* Reston, VA: AAHPERD.

44. Patterson, P., Wiksten, D. L., Ray, L., Flanders, C., & Sanphy, D. (1996). The validity and reliability of the back saver sit-and-reach test in middle school girls and boys. *Research Quarterly for Exercise and Sport, 67,* 448–451.

45. Pope, P. R., Herbert, R. D., Kirwan, J. D., & Graham,B. J. (2000). A randomized trial of preexercise stretching for prevention of lower-limb injury. *Medicine and Science in Sports and Exercise, 32,* 271–277.

46. President's Council on Physical Fitness and Sports. (1990). *PCPFS president's challenge physical fitness program test manual.* Washington, DC: Author.

47. *President's Council on Physical Fitness and Sports.* (2000). Current issues in flexibility fitness. *President's Council on Physical Fitness and Sports Research Digest,* Washington, DC: Author.

48. Schultz, A., Andersson, G., Ortengren, R., Haderspeck, K., & Nachemson, A. (1982). Loads on the lumbar spine: Validation of a biomechanical analysis by measurement of intradiscal pressures and myoelectric signals. *Journal of Bone and Joint Surgery, 64A,* 713–720.

49. Shephard, R. J., Berridge, M., & Montelpare, W. (1990). On the generality of the "sit and reach" test: An analysis of flexibility data for an aging population. *Research Quarterly for Exercise and Sport, 61,* 326–330.

50. Shrier, I. (1999). Stretching before exercise does not reduce the risk of local muscle injury: A critical review of the clinical and basic science literature. *Clinical Journal of Sports Medicine, 9,* 221–227.

51. Starkey, C., Brown, S. D., & Ryan, J. (2010). *Examination of orthopedic and athletic injuries, 3rd ed.* Philadelphia, F.A. Davis Company.

52. Sullivan, M. K., Dejulia, J. J., & Worrell, T. W. (1992). Effect of pelvic position and stretching method on hamstring muscle flexibility. *Medicine and Science in Sports and Exercise, 24,*1383–1389.

53. Wells, C. L. (1985). *Women, sport, and performance: A physiological perspective.* Champaign, IL: Human Kinetics.

54. Worrell, T., Perrin, D., Gansneder, B., & Gieck, J. (1991). Comparison of isokinetic strength and flexibility measures between injured and noninjured athletes. *Journal of Orthopaedic and Sports Physical Therapy, 13,*118–125.

55. Youdas, J. W., Krause, D. A., & Hollman, J. H. (2008). Validity of hamstring muscle length assessment during the sit-and-reach test using an inclinometer to measure hip joint angle. *Journal of Strength and Conditioning Research, 22,* 303–309.

Form 22.1

SIT-AND-REACH AND ROM

Homework

Gender: **M**   Initials: **AA**   Age (y): **22**   Height (cm): **172**   Weight (kg): **84.5**

Sit and Reach

Specific SR Test	Trial 1 (cm)	Trial 2 (cm)	Trial 3 (cm)	Trial 4 (cm)	Score (cm)	Category
Traditional SR	20	23	25	26	(Trial 4)	(Table 22.2)
Canadian SR	28	29	29		( )	( )

Goniometry

Joint Action	Starting point (°)	Ending point (°) Trial 1	Trial 2	Trial 3	Median ROM (°)	Expected ROM (°)
Shoulder flxn (GH)	0	124	120	130	0 -	0 -
Elbow flexion	0	145	150	155	0 -	0 -
Ankle dorsiflxn	0	18	19	20	0 -	0 -

Table 22.6

Comments: _____

_____

_____

Gender: **F**   Initials: **BB**   Age (y): **21**   Height (cm): **158**   Weight (kg): **69.0**

Sit and Reach

Specific SR Test	Trial 1 (cm)	Trial 2 (cm)	Trial 3 (cm)	Trial 4 (cm)	Score (cm)	Category
Back-Saver (R)	30	30	30	30	(Trial 4)	(Table 22.2)
Back-Saver (L)	35	35	35	35	( )	( )

Goniometry

Joint Action	Starting point (°)	Ending point (°) Trial 1	Trial 2	Trial 3	Median ROM (°)	Expected ROM (°)
Hip flexion	0	124	120	130	0 -	0 -
Knee flexion	0	145	150	155	0 -	0 -
Ankle plantarflxn	0	40	46	44	0 -	0 -

Table 22.6

Comments: _____

_____

_____

Form 22.2
SIT-AND-REACH AND ROM

NAME _____ DATE _____ SCORE _____

Lab Results

Gender: _____ Initials: _____ Age (y): _____ Height (cm): _____ Weight (kg): _____

Sit and Reach

Specific SR Test	Trial 1 (cm)	Trial 2 (cm)	Trial 3 (cm)	Trial 4 (cm)	Score (cm)	Category
_____	_____	_____	_____	_____	( )	( )
_____	_____	_____	_____	_____	( )	( )

Goniometry

Joint Action	Starting point (°)	Ending point (°) Trial 1	Trial 2	Trial 3	Median ROM (°)	Expected ROM (°)
_____	0	_____	_____	_____	0 -	0 -
_____	0	_____	_____	_____	0 -	0 -
_____	0	_____	_____	_____	0 -	0 -

Table 22.6

Comments: _____

_____

_____

Gender: _____ Initials: _____ Age (y): _____ Height (cm): _____ Weight (kg): _____

Sit and Reach

Specific SR Test	Trial 1 (cm)	Trial 2 (cm)	Trial 3 (cm)	Trial 4 (cm)	Score (cm)	Category
_____	_____	_____	_____	_____	( )	( )
_____	_____	_____	_____	_____	( )	( )

Goniometry

Joint Action	Starting point (°)	Ending point (°) Trial 1	Trial 2	Trial 3	Median ROM (°)	Expected ROM (°)
_____	0	_____	_____	_____	0 -	0 -
_____	0	_____	_____	_____	0 -	0 -
_____	0	_____	_____	_____	0 -	0 -

Table 22.6

Comments: _____

_____

_____

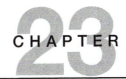
BODY MASS INDEX

The body mass index (BMI), mathematically calculated from a person's height and body mass, is a measure used mostly by epidemiologists to determine the degree to which that person is overweight or obese. BMI became popular in the 1970s through its use by Keys and his colleagues,[9,24] but its origin actually goes back to the 1860s when it was first described by Belgian mathematician Adolphe Quetelet, and was known as the Quetelet Index.[8,11] Of the various stature–weight indices, the BMI has been used the most frequently for categorizing persons with respect to their degree of obesity, health-related fitness, and risk of chronic disease and death. Large epidemiologic studies conducted by the U.S. Surgeon General's office and other public health experts recognize that a high BMI is related to an increased risk of various chronic diseases and conditions, including hypertension, diabetes, metabolic syndrome, and coronary heart disease.[23] The BMI value can be used to classify a person's degree of obesity based on publications by the National Institutes of Health (NIH).[17] A person with a BMI of 18.5–24.9 is classified as normal, whereas a BMI ≥ 25 is considered overweight, and a BMI ≥ 30 is considered obese. Based on these criteria, the prevalence of overweight or obese American men and women has steadily grown over the past 46 years, as seen in Figure 23.1. Further analysis of these data indicates that the prevalence of overweight and obesity is considerably higher in older persons than in younger persons, and that prevalence is also influenced by ethnicity and cultural factors (Table 23.1). Although BMI can be used as a first indicator of the degree to which a person is overweight or obese, it has its limitations. Because it is derived from only height and weight, BMI does not necessarily reflect a person's true body composition. Lean, heavily muscled individuals can have the same BMI as persons of the same height and weight who are obese. For this reason, BMI is used most often to study the relationship between obesity and chronic disease in groups of people, and is not frequently used to assess the specific body composition of one individual. Other tests described in the following chapters (girths, skinfolds, hydrostatic weighing) provide a better indication of a person's actual body composition.

METHOD

Body weight can be assessed from various stature–weight indexes, thus indicating the degree of obesity. Stature–weight indexes for assessing body weight are probably the simplest and least expensive methods of all, requiring only the measurement of body mass and stature (height). See Box 23.1 for a discussion on the accuracy of BMI.

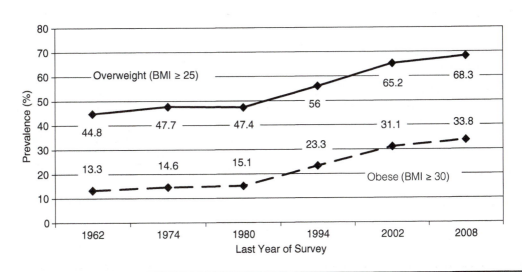

Figure 23.1 Increasing prevalence (%) of American men and women who were overweight (BMI ≥ 25) or obese (BMI ≥ 30) by the year of the survey.
Source: Data from Ogden, Fryar, Carroll, & Flegal (2004)[18] and from Flegal, Carroll, Ogden & Curtin (2010).[6]

Table 23.1	Percentage of Overweight or Obese Adults in U.S.A. by Gender, Age, and Ethnicity	

Overweight (BMI ≥ 25)		
Group	Men	Women
Total	72.3%	64.1%
20–39 y	63.5%	59.5%
40–59 y	77.8%	66.3%
≥ 60 y	78.4%	68.6%
White (Non-Hispanic)	66.7%	61.2%
Black (Non-Hispanic)	73.8%	78.2%
Hispanic	77.9%	76.1%

Obese (BMI ≥ 30)		
Group	Men	Women
Total	32.2%	35.5%
20–39 y	27.5%	34.0%
40–59 y	34.3%	38.2%
≥ 60 y	37.1%	33.6%
White (Non-Hispanic)	31.9%	33.0%
Black (Non-Hispanic)	37.3%	49.6%
Hispanic	34.3%	43.0%

Source: Data from Flegal, Carroll, Ogden & Curtin (2010).[6]

BOX 23.1   Accuracy of BMI

The BMI's formula is accurate; its limitation is the assumption that it estimates body fat in a single individual. BMI has a "somewhat higher" association with body fat than the popular height–weight tables.[14] BMI has moderate correlations *(r)* between 0.70 and 0.80 with the percent fat predicted from hydrostatic weighing[9] and 0.64 to 0.69 for skinfold predictions.[15] These represent a slight improvement of the correlation *(r* = 0.6) between percent fat and body mass alone, hence giving a standard error of predicting percent fat from BMI of 5–6 %.[12,19]

Although the BMI may be acceptable for predicting percent fat in a typical group of persons, and for predicting obesity,[8] it is prone to error in persons exceptionally lean, such as bodybuilders or power athletes,[15] and in older persons,[8] unless the latter group's ages are factored.[2] For example, about 12 % of male athletes were deemed obese (> 27.2 kg·m^{-2}) by BMI; however, only 2 % of the female athletes were falsely positive for obesity.[15] BMI ignores the factor of body-frame size, a factor that may be unnecessary in anthropometry.[21] In summary, BMI plays an important role in epidemiological studies but is lacking accuracy for assessing an individual's body compsition.[12]

Procedures and Calculations

The first two steps in obtaining the BMI are to accurately measure height and weight (body mass). These methods were described in detail in Chapter 3, so only a brief summary of the procedures is included here. The use of a wall-mounted stadiometer and a calibrated electronic scale is preferred for accurately measuring height and weight respectively. The third and final step to obtain BMI is a simple mathematical calculation.

Measuring Height and Weight

1. The participant stands without shoes as tall as possible with the back and heels against the wall and stadiometer. The participant tucks the chin to bring the head into the correct position.
2. The technician places the stadiometer firmly against the participant's head compressing the hair. The technician holds the stadiometer in place as the participant steps out of the way.
3. The technician measures height to the closest 1 cm and records it onto Form 23.2.
4. The participant should remove shoes, socks, jewelry and accessories, empty all pockets, and remove as much clothing as is feasible.
5. The participant steps slowly onto the scale.
6. The technician measures weight to the closest 0.1 kg and records it onto Form 23.2.

Calculation of BMI

BMI is the ratio of the person's body mass (kg) to the height squared (m^2). In other words, BMI (kg·m^{-2}) is the result of dividing a person's mass by the square of that person's height, as seen in Equation 23.1a. For example, if a person weighs 68.0 kg (149.6 lb) and is 1.74 m tall (174 cm; 68.5 in.), the BMI would be calculated as 22.4 kg·m^{-2} (Eq. 23.1b). Although technically the calculated BMI is expressed in kg·m^{-2}, it is common practice to ignore the units and simply refer to the BMI as 22.4.

$$BMI = \text{Body mass (kg)} / \text{Height (m)}^2 \qquad \text{Eq. 23.1a}$$

Assume: Body wt is **68.0** kg (149.6 lb) and Height is **1.74** m (68.5 in)

$$BMI = \textbf{68.0} \text{ kg} / \textbf{1.74} \text{ m}^2 = \textbf{22.4} \text{ kg·m}^{-2} = \textbf{22.4} \quad \text{Eq. 23.1b}$$

RESULTS AND DISCUSSION

Body mass index (BMI) can be used to classify the degree to which a person is underweight, of a normal weight, overweight or obese. Table 23.2 first displays classifications of BMI based on the original guidelines established by the National Heart, Lung, and Blood Institute (NHLBI).[17] A "normal" BMI ranges from 18.5 to 24.9. A BMI below 18.5 is considered "underweight," a BMI of 25.0 or over is considered "overweight," and a BMI of 30.0 or over is classified as "obese." The World Health Organization (WHO) has subsequently provided further classifications of "thinness" and multiple classes of obesity.[25,26,27] The low BMI values are used primarily on populations in countries with limited food supplies where low body weight is associated with specific health problems. High BMI values, used in more affluent, industrialized nations, further classify obesity into class I (mild), class II (moderate), and class III (severe) based on a BMI equal to or greater than 30.0, 35.0, and 40.0, respectively. In combination with waist girth, BMI may also be used to estimate disease risk relative to persons of normal body weight. The risk of disease is greater within the overweight and obese classifications of BMI in males whose waist girth exceeds 102 cm and

in females whose waist girth exceeds 88 cm. Table 23.3 allows the estimation of BMI from height and weight and provides the classification of BMI into underweight, normal, overweight and the three classes of obesity.

Population studies of BMI over a long period of time can indicate trends in overweight and obesity and their correlation to chronic health problems. For example, Figure 23.1 shows the rise in incidence between 1960 and 2008 of those Americans who are classified as overweight (BMI ≥ 25) or obese (BMI ≥ 30) based on data from the National Center for Health Statistics.[18] The prevalence of overweight increased from 44.8 % in 1962 to 68.3 % in 2008, with prevalence of obesity increasing from 13.3 % to 33.8 % over the same period. It is also possible to identify differences in the prevalence of overweight and obesity by gender, age group, and ethnicity, as seen in Table 23.1. The prevalence of overweight is higher in men, but obesity is higher in women. The prevalence of both overweight and obesity is considerably higher in older men and women (45–54 y) when compared to younger men and women (20–34 y). And specific ethnicities, especially when identified by gender, are considerably more likely to be overweight or obese. Categories for BMI can also be created by age group and gender based on mean and percentile data available from the National Center for Health Statistics, as seen in Table 23.3. The mean BMI increases in both men and women across the four decades described. The body mass indexes of a large group (n = 7183) of community-residing older adults (60–94 y) averaged 25.8 and 26.6 in men and women, respectively. Their indexes decreased from the 70–74y age group to the 90–94 y age group in both genders.[20]

Table 23.2 Classifications of Body Mass Index (BMI) and Disease Risk based on Waist Girth (cm)

Classification	BMI	Disease Risk Relative to Normal Weight based on Waist Girth* in Men (M) and Women (W)	
		*M ≤ 102 cm *W ≤ 88 cm	*M > 102 cm *W > 88 cm
Original *NHLBI* Classifications [a]			
Underweight	< 18.5	*See text*	-
Normal	18.5–24.9	Normal	Normal
Overweight	25.0–29.9	Increased	High
Obese	≥ 30.0	High	Very high
Additional *WHO* Cutpoints [b]			
Severe thinness	< 16.0	—	—
Moderate thinness	16.0–16.9	—	—
Mild thinness	17.0–18.4	*See text*	—
Normal	18.5–24.9	Normal	Normal
Pre-obese	25.0–29.9	Increased	High
Obese (I)	30.0–34.9	High	Very high
Obese (II)	35.0–39.9	Very high	Very high
Obese (III)	≥ 40.0	Extreme	Extreme

Note: *See Chapter 24 for description of the measurement of waist girth.
Source: [a]National Heart Lung and Blood Institute (1998).[17] [b]World Health Organization (1995)[25]; WHO (2000)[26]; WHO (2004).[27]

Table 23.3 Estimation of Body Mass Index (BMI) from Height (cm; in.) and Body Weight (kg; lb) and Classification of Degree of Obesity Based on BMI

Body Weight (kg)	(lb)	(cm) (in.)	Height																				
			150 59	153 60	155 61	158 62	160 63	163 64	165 65	168 66	170 67	173 68	175 69	178 70	180 71	183 72	185 73	188 74	190 75	193 76	195 77	198 78
45	99		20	19	19	18	18	17	17	16	16	15	15					Underweight				
50	110	Normal	22	21	21	20	20	19	18	18	17	17	16	16	15	15	15					
55	121		24	24	23	22	21	21	20	20	19	18	18	17	17	17	16	16	15	15	14	14
60	132	Overweight	27	26	25	24	23	23	22	21	21	20	20	19	19	18	18	17	17	16	16	15
65	143		29	28	27	26	25	25	24	23	22	22	21	21	20	20	19	18	18	18	17	17
70	154	Obese (Class I)	31	30	29	28	27	27	26	25	24	24	23	22	22	21	20	20	19	19	18	18
75	165		33	32	31	30	29	28	28	27	26	25	24	24	23	23	22	21	21	20	20	19
80	176	Obese (Class II)	36	34	33	32	31	30	29	29	28	27	26	25	25	24	23	23	22	22	21	21
85	187		38	37	35	34	33	32	31	30	29	29	28	27	26	26	25	24	24	23	22	22
90	198		40	39	37	36	35	34	33	32	31	30	29	29	28	27	26	26	25	24	24	23
95	209		42	41	40	38	37	36	35	34	33	32	31	30	29	29	28	27	26	26	25	24
100	220	Obese (Class III)	44	43	42	40	39	38	37	36	35	34	33	32	31	30	29	28	28	27	26	26
105	231				44	42	41	40	39	37	36	35	34	33	32	32	31	30	29	28	28	27
110	243				46	44	43	42	40	39	38	37	36	35	34	33	32	31	30	30	29	28
115	254					46	45	44	42	41	40	39	38	37	35	35	34	33	32	31	30	29

Note: Based on the equation: Body mass index (BMI) = Body weight (kg) / Height^2 (m). Classifications are based on BMI: underweight (BMI < 18.5), normal (BMI = 18.5–24.9), overweight (BMI = 25.0–29.9), obese class I (BMI = 30.0–34.9), obese class II (BMI = 35.0–39.9), and obese class III (BMI ≥ 40.0).
Source: National Heart, Lung, and Blood Institute (1998).[17]

Table 23.4 Category for BMI by Age Group and Gender

Category (percentile)	20–29 y		30–39 y		40–49 y		50–59 y	
	Men	Women	Men	Women	Men	Women	Men	Women
Well above ave (> 95th)	< 19.4	< 18.4	< 20.5	< 18.7	< 21.2	< 19.2	< 21.4	< 19.9
Above ave (75th–95th)	19.4–21.9	18.4–20.4	20.5–23.4	18.7–21.2	21.2–24.0	19.2–22.3	21.4–24.6	19.9–23.5
Average (25th–74th)	22.0–27.3	20.5–26.2	23.5–28.3	21.3–30.1	24.1–29.5	22.4–30.1	24.7–30.6	23.6–32.0
Below ave (5th–24th)	27.4–33.6	26.3–35.8	28.4–35.5	30.2–39.6	29.6–36.2	30.2–39.9	30.7–35.6	32.1–40.6
Well below ave (< 5th)	> 33.6	> 35.8	> 35.5	> 39.6	> 36.2	> 39.9	> 35.6	> 40.6
Mean	**25.2**	**24.3**	**26.5**	**26.3**	**27.3**	**27.0**	**27.8**	**28.4**

Source: National Center for Health Statistics (2005).[16]

BMI is sometimes used, albeit much less frequently, to evaluate the health risks associated with being underweight (BMI < 18.5). Underweight persons can be found in industrialized nations, but underweight is more of a problem in poor, underdeveloped countries. Being underweight (having a low BMI) increases the risk of developing poor bone health and leads to reduced bone density. Combined with a diet low in folic acid and iron, being underweight increases the risk of developing anemia. Underweight individuals are at increased risk of more severe and frequent infections due to a weakened immune system. Women with a low BMI have a harder time getting pregnant and those who get pregnant are at an increased risk of pregnancy complications and delivering an unhealthy baby.[3] BMI is most frequently used in industrialized countries to indicate the degree of obesity observed in a sample population. High BMI in men is directly related to mortality, indicating a greater risk of death the higher the BMI.[1,4,10,13] For women, BMI values over 29 represent a doubling of mortality risk.[13] The increase in mortality is small for overweight persons (BMI ≥ 25) but is 50–100 % higher in obese persons (BMI ≥ 30) when compared to those persons with a normal BMI of 18.5–24.9.[5] Degree of obesity may also affect motor ability. For an older adult (≥ 60 y), a BMI greater than 25 (overweight) is related to a greater risk of losing functional mobility, such as walking, stair climbing, and standing up from a chair.[7,22] Excess body weight, especially if it consists of excess body fat, is a major public health issue that can be identified in part through the measurement and interpretation of the body mass index.

BOX 23.2 Chapter Preview/Review

How is body mass index (BMI) defined?

How is body mass index calculated?

How is BMI used by epidemiologists?

What is the trend in obesity in the United States?

What is the range of a "normal" BMI?

What values of BMI correspond with the different classifications of body composition?

How is BMI related to mortality?

References

1. American College of Sports Medicine. (2006). *ACSM's guidelines for exercise testing and prescription* (7th ed.). Philadelphia: Lippincott Williams & Wilkins.

2. Deurenberg, P., Weststrate, J. A., & Seidell, J. C. (1991). Body mass index as a measure of body fatness: Age- and sex-specific prediction formulas. *Journal of Nutrition, 65,* 105–114.

3. Dority, J. (2012). *Health risks of a low BMI.* Retrieved August 21, 2012, from http://www.livestrong.com/article/.

4. Dorn, J. P., Trevisan, M., & Winkelstein, W. (1996). The long-term relationship between body mass index, coronary heart disease and all-cause mortality. *Medicine and Science in Sports and Exercise, 28* (Suppl.), Abstract #662, S111.

5. Expert Panel. (1998). Executive summary of the clinical guidelines on the identification, evaluation, and treatment of overweight and obesity in adults. *Archives of Internal Medicine, 158,* 1855–1867.

6. Flegal, K. M., Carroll, M. D., Ogden, C. L., & Curtin, L. R. (2010). Prevalence and trends in obesity among U.S. adults, 1999–2008. *Journal of the American Medical Association, 303,* 235–241.

7. Galanos, A. N., Pieper, C. F., Cornoni-Huntley, J. C., Bales, C. W., & Fillenbaum, G. G. (1994). Nutrition and function: Is there a relationship between body mass index and the functional capabilities of community-dwelling elderly? *Journal of the American Geriatric Society, 42,* 368–373.

8. Garrow, J. S., & Webster, J. (1985). Quetelet's Index (W/H^2) as a measure of fatness. *International Journal of Obesity, 9,* 147–153.

9. Keys, A., Fidanza, F., Karvonen, M. J., Kimura, N., & Taylor, H. L. (1972). Indices of relative weight and obesity. *Journal of Chronic Diseases, 25,* 329–343.

10. Lee, I. M., Manson, J. A., Hennekens, C. H., & Paffenbarger, R. S. (1993). Body weight and mortality: A 27-year follow-up of middle-aged men. *JAMA: The Journal of the American Medical Association, 270,* 2823–2828.

11. Lee, J., Kolonel, L. N., & Hinds, M. W. (1981). Relative merits of the weight-corrected-for-height indices.[1–3] *The American Journal of Clinical Nutrition, 34,* 2521–2529.

12. Lohman, T. G., Houtkooper, L., & Going, S. B. (1997). Body fat measurement goes high-tech. *ACSM's Health and Fitness Journal, 1*(1), 30–35.

13. Manson, J. E., Willett, W. C., Stampfer, M. J., Colditz, G. A., Hunter, D. J., Hankinson, S. E., Hennekens, C. H., & Speizer, F. E. (1995). Body weight and mortality among women. *New England Journal of Medicine, 333,* 677–685.

14. McArdle, W. D., Katch, F. I., & Katch, V. L. (1996). *Exercise physiology: Energy, nutrition, and human performance.* Baltimore: Williams & Wilkins.

15. Mullins, N. M., & Sinning, W. E. (1996). Diagnostic utility of the body mass index as a measure of obesity in athletes and non-athletes. *Medicine and Science in Sports and Exercise, 28,* Abstract #1148, S193.

16. National Center for Health Statistics. (2005). *Anthropometric reference data, United States, 1988–1994.* Hyattsville, MD: Author. Available online at www.cdc.gov/nchs/.

17. National Heart, Lung, and Blood Institute. (1998). *Clinical guidelines on the identification, evaluation, and treatment of overweight and obesity in adults. The evidence report.* (NIH Publication No. 98-4083). Washington DC: U.S. Department of Health and Human Services.

18. Ogden, C. L., Fryar, C. D., Carrol, M. D., & Flegal, K. M. (2004). *Mean body weight, height, and body mass index, United States 1960–2002. Advance data from vital and health statistics.* (Publication No. 347). Hyattsville, MD: National Center for Health Statistics.

19. Pollock, M. (1985). General discussion of sports medicine. In A. F. Roche (Ed.), *Body-composition assessments in youth and adults* (p. 83). Columbus, OH: Ross Laboratories.

20. Rikli, R. E., & Jones, C. J. (1999). Functional fitness normative scores for community-residing older adults, ages 60–94. *Journal of Aging and Physical Activity, 7,* 162–181.

21. Roche, A. F. (1984). Research progress in the field of body composition. *Medicine and Science in Sports and Exercise, 16,* 579–583.

22. Shephard, R. J. (1997). *Aging, physical activity, and health.* Champaign, IL: Human Kinetics.

23. U.S. Surgeon General's Office. (1996). *Physical activity and health: A report of the Surgeon General Executive Summary.* Washington, DC: Author; Government Printing Office.

24. Weigley, E. S. (1989). Adolphe Quetelet (1796–1874): Pioneer anthropometrist. *Nutrition Today, 24,* 12–16.

25. World Health Organization (1995). *Physical status: The use and interpretation of anthropometry. Report of a WHO Expert Committee. WHO Technical Report Series 854.* Geneva: World Health Organization.

26. World Health Organization (2000). *Obesity: Preventing and managing the global epidemic. Report of a WHO Consultation. WHO Technical Report Series 894.* Geneva: World Health Organization.

27. World Health Organization (2004). WHO expert consultation: Appropriate body-mass index for Asian populations and its implications for policy ad intervention strategies. *Lancet, 363,* 157–163.

Form 23.1
BODY MASS INDEX

NAME _____ DATE _____ SCORE _____

Homework

Gender: **M**   Initials: **AA**   Age (y): **22**   Height (cm): **175**   Weight (kg): **96.5**

Height (m) = _____ cm / 100 = _____ m
      Height

Waist girth* (cm) = _____ (optional)   * The measurement of waist girth is described in Chapter 24.

Body mass index (BMI) = _____ kg / (_____ * _____) m^2 = _____ kg·m^{-2}
                  Weight   Ht   Ht

Category for BMI (from Table 23.4)   _____

Classification of BMI (from Table 23.2)   _____

Disease risk from BMI and waist girth (optional)   _____

Evaluation: _____

_____

_____

_____

Gender: **F**   Initials: **BB**   Age (y): **22**   Height (cm): **165**   Weight (kg): **67.3**

Height (m) = _____ cm / 100 = _____ m
      Height

Waist girth* (cm) = _____ (optional)   * The measurement of waist girth is described in Chapter 24.

Body mass index (BMI) = _____ kg / (_____ * _____) m^2 = _____ kg·m^{-2}
                  Weight   Ht   Ht

Category for BMI (from Table 23.4)   _____

Classification of BMI (from Table 23.2)   _____

Disease risk from BMI and waist girth (optional)   _____

Evaluation: _____

_____

_____

_____

Form 23.2
BODY MASS INDEX

Lab Results

Gender: _____ Initials: _____ Age (y): _____ Height (cm): _____ Weight (kg): _____

Height (m) = _____ cm / 100 = _____ m

                  Height

Waist girth* (cm) = _____ (optional) * The measurement of waist girth is described in Chapter 24.

Body mass index (BMI) = _____ kg / (_____ * _____) m^2 = _____ kg·m^{-2}

                           Weight   Ht   Ht

Category for BMI (from Table 23.4) _____

Classification of BMI (from Table 23.2) _____

Disease risk from BMI and waist girth (optional) _____

Evaluation: _____

_____

_____

_____

Gender: _____ Initials: _____ Age (y): _____ Height (cm): _____ Weight (kg): _____

Height (m) = _____ cm / 100 = _____ m

                  Height

Waist girth* (cm) = _____ (optional) * The measurement of waist girth is described in Chapter 24.

Body mass index (BMI) = _____ kg / (_____ * _____) m^2 = _____ kg·m^{-2}

                           Weight   Ht   Ht

Category for BMI (from Table 23.4) _____

Classification of BMI (from Table 23.2) _____

Disease risk from BMI and waist girth (optional) _____

Evaluation: _____

_____

_____

_____

GIRTHS AND RATIOS

A girth measure is simply a circumference measure that results in a linear dimension, such as inches or centimeters. Waist-to-hip and waist-to-height ratios indicating both fat distribution and fat percentage, relate to increased risk of cardiovascular disease.[2,3,13,25,26,38] Persons with a high ratio of waist-to-hip girth are twice as susceptible to heart attack, stroke, hypertension, diabetes, gallbladder disease, and death.[10] This fat patterning is thought to cause a negative effect on liver metabolism due to the release of fat directly into the portal (liver) circulation by the close-proximity abdominal fat cells.[10,11] Waist circumference alone, because it is positively correlated with abdominal fat content, is now being used as a predictor of risk factors and morbidity.[1,14] Men and women increase the relative risk when the waist circumferences are[14,21,32]

- Men: > 102 cm (> 40 in.)
- Women: > 88 cm (> 35 in.)

Various equations, tables, and nomograms are available for predicting percent fat from girth data.[21] Prediction of percent fat can be made from equations derived from a single girth (waist) and body weight of men, or a single girth (hip) and height of women.[40,41] This simple method may be referred to as the **1-Girth Method.** A slightly more complex prediction of percent fat uses height and two or three circumference measures to predict body density in men or women, respectively; then percent fat is calculated from the body density value.[18,19] The more complex methods may be referred to as the **2-Girth Method for Men** and the **3-Girth Method for Women,** or together may be referred to as the Naval Health Research Center (NHRC) method.

PHYSIOLOGICAL RATIONALE

Relationship Between Girth and Percent Fat

Compartmentalization of the body into fat and fat-free divisions may be estimated from such measures as body girths, diameters, skinfolds, and/or hydrostatic weight (hydrodensitometry).[6] Because the hydrodensitometric prediction of percent fat is a valid criterion measure, researchers commonly correlate body density measures from hydrostatic weighing tests with such linear anthropometric measures as skinfolds, diameters, and girths. Regression equations formed from the linear and densitometric relationship are then used to predict the body composition from only the linear measures. Thus, the linear measures can be used to predict the percent fat that would have been determined from hydrodensitometric methods.

In the 1-Girth Method for women, the hip girth at a given height is directly related to percent fat. Thus, higher percent fats occur in women of the same height but with greater hip girths. For men, according to the 1-Girth Method, the lower the midabdominal girth is for any given weight, the lower is the percent fat. Also, the more a man weighs for any given midabdominal girth, the lower is his percent fat. In the 2-Girth and 3-Girth Methods, the neck girth and height favor the lean factor, whereas the hip and abdominal girths favor the fat factor. Thus, the greater the sum of the neck girth and height for a given hip and/or abdominal girth, the lower the percent fat likely will be.

Relationship Between Girth and Fat Distribution

Fat deposits around the upper abdominal area deserve more serious attention with respect to health than fat deposits elsewhere. A greater deposit of fat at this abdominal "waist" area than at the hip area is more common in adult men than adult women; hence, it is often referred to as the android (man) characteristic or the "apple" shape. Women tend to deposit fat in the hip, lower abdominal, gluteal, and appendage areas more than the upper abdominal waist area; hence, this girth is often referred to as the gynoid (woman) characteristic or the "pear" shape.

METHODS FOR GIRTHS AND RATIOS

The equipment for measuring girth is very simple. Ideally, a measuring tape made of reinforced fiberglass or metal should be used. Some anthropometric tapes known as Gulick tapes, have a calibrated spring at the tip. The purported advantage of anthropometric spring tapes is that the proper tape pressure can be applied repeatedly, although not everyone recommends these.[33] The most practical tapes have an inch scale on one side and a metric scale on the other side. The accuracy of girth measurements is presented in Box 24.1.

Because both the 2-Girth and 3-Girth Methods require a height measurement, familiarity with anthropometers or stadiometers is essential. These instruments and the proper procedures for measuring height and body weight are described in Chapter 3.

Procedures for Measuring Girths

1. With the participant standing, the technician measures the body weight and records it to the closest 0.5 kg onto Form 24.2.
2. The technician measures the height of the man or woman and records it to the closest 0.5 cm onto Form 24.2.
3. The technician determines the exact anatomical sites of the girth measurements as shown in Figure 24.1. The measurement sites for the 2-Girth and 3-Girth Methods[18,19] are explained in Table 24.1.
4. The technician measures the girths, careful to avoid any air space between the skin and the tape. On the other hand, the tape should not be pulled so tightly that it indents the skin.[20]
5. The technician holds the tape horizontally, except for neck girth, and reads the tape to the closest 0.5 cm.

BOX 24.1 Accuracy of Girth Measurements

All measures of fat in living bodies are merely estimates. The first anthropometric prediction of body fat was published in 1951.[12] Since then, more than 100 predictive equations have been developed.

Traditionally, hydrostatic weighing has been the criterion by which other predictive methods are evaluated. The standard error of estimate (*SEE*) is about 3.5 % for most linear (not hydrostatic) anthropometric predictive tests.[27,28] For example, if an individual was predicted to be 20 % fat by girth, skinfold, and/or diameter measures, then an assumed error of 3.5 % would mean that there is a 67 % chance that the "true" value as predicted by hydrostatic weighing is between 16.5 and 23.5 % (20 % ± 3.5 %).

The 2-Girth and 3-Girth Methods, which were developed from data on large samples of Navy women and men, have moderate to high correlations (r = 0.85 and 0.90, respectively) and reasonable standard errors (*SEE* = 3.7 % and 2.7 % body fat units, respectively) when compared with hydrostatic weighing. In general, the Naval Health Research equations tend to overpredict body fat in lean persons and underestimate it in fat persons.[18,19]

Investigators evaluating the accuracy of three different military equations (Army, Marine, and Navy) concluded that only the Navy equation was not significantly different from hydrostatic weight for group estimations of percent fat in 50-year-old women, but none were a substitute for underwater weighing for individual estimations for middle-aged women.[37]

Test-retest reliabilities of girth measures are 0.97 or higher.[7]

Determination of Percent Body Fat from Girths

The following methods describe the use of girth measurements to predict percent body fat. Multiple girths are used that reflect body volume and the relationship between differences in regional fat distribution. A 2-Girth method is used for men and a 3-Girth method is used for women.

2-Girth and 3-Girth Method (Naval Health Research)

The 2-Girth and 3-Girth Methods of estimating percent fat were developed at the Naval Health Research Center[18,19] for use by the military. The methods use the height and multiple girths of a participant to estimate body density by way of regression equations. The men's equation (Eq. 24.1a) uses height and two girths, the neck and midabdominal girths, to estimate body density. The women's equation (Eq. 24.1b) uses height and three girths, the neck, upper abdominal, and hip girths, to estimate body density. Percent body fat is then determined from body density by using the Siri[36] equation.

$$D_B \text{ (Men)} = 1.0324 + [0.15456 * Log_{10} (Ht)] - [0.19077 * Log_{10}(CV)] \qquad \text{Eq. 24.1a}$$

Where: Ht = Height (cm); CV (cm) = Midabdominal − Neck grith (cm)

$$D_B \text{ (Women)} = 1.29579 + [0.221 * Log_{10}(Ht)] - [0.35004 * Log_{10}(CV)] \qquad \text{Eq. 24.1b}$$

Where: Ht = Height (cm); CV (cm) = Upper abdominal + Hip − Neck girth (cm)

$$\% \text{ Body Fat} = (495 / D_B) - 450 \quad \textit{Siri equation} \quad \text{Eq. 24.1c}$$

Table 24.1 Measurement Sites for 2-Girth (Men) and 3-Girth (Women) Methods and W:H and W/Ht Ratio

Men: 2-Girth Method[a]	Women: 3-Girth Method[b]
Height (closest 0.5 cm)	Height (closest 0.5 cm)
Neck girth—inferior to the larynx (Adams apple) with tape perpendicular to the axis of the neck	Neck girth—inferior to the larynx (Adams apple) with tape perpendicular to the axis of the neck
Midabdominal girth—at the level of the navel	Upper abdominal girth—at the minimal girth observed between the xiphoid process and the navel
	Hip girth—at the maximal protrusion of the gluteal muscles
Waist-to-Hip Ratio (W:H) for Men and Women[c]	**Waist-to-Height Ratio (W/Ht) for Men and Women[d]**
Upper abdominal girth—at the minimal girth observed between the xiphoid process and the navel	Midabdominal girth—at the level of the navel
Hip girth—at the maximal protrusion of the gluteal muscles	Height (closest 0.5 cm)

Source: [a]Hodgdon & Beckett (1984a)[14]; [b]Hodgdon & Beckett (1984b)[15]; [c]Van Itallie (1988)[38]; [d]Hsieh & Yoshinaga (1995).[22]

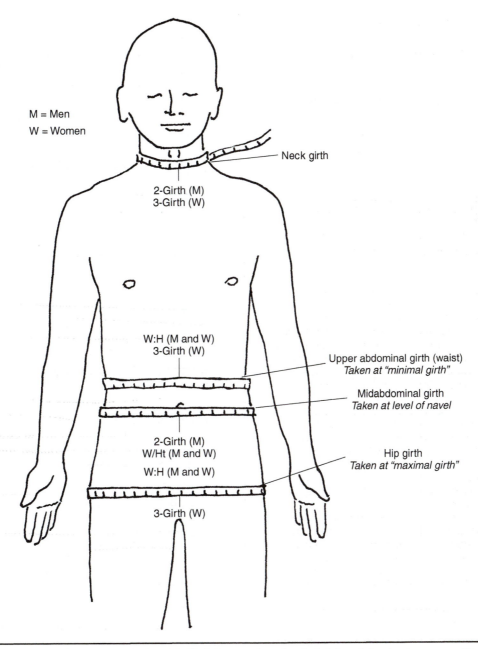

M = Men
W = Women

Neck girth

2-Girth (M)
3-Girth (W)

W:H (M and W)
3-Girth (W)

Upper abdominal girth (waist)
Taken at "minimal girth"

Midabdominal girth
Taken at level of navel

2-Girth (M)
W/Ht (M and W)

W:H (M and W)

Hip girth
Taken at "maximal girth"

3-Girth (W)

Figure 24.1 Girth sites for the 2-Girth (men) and 3-Girth (women) method of determining body composition, and the girth sites for determining waist to hip ratio (W:H) and waist to height ratio (W/Ht) in men and women.

To further describe the determination of body density and percent body fat from multiple girths, sample data and calculations are provided for one man (Eq. 24.2a and 24.2b) and one woman (Eq. 24.2c and 24.2d). The calculation of body density using the regression equations is somewhat difficult due to the use of numerous constants and the $\log_{10}$ function. For this reason, percent body fat may also be estimated by using either Table 24.2 (for men) or Table 24.3 (for women).

Assume: **Male**; Ht = **170** cm; Midabdominal = **88.0** cm, Neck = **40.0** cm

D_B (Men) = 1.0324 + [0.15456 * $\log_{10}$(**170**)] − [0.19077 * $\log_{10}$ (**48.0**)]   Eq. 24.2a

% Fat = (495/**1.056**) − 450 = **19** %   Eq. 24.2b

Assume: **Female**; Ht = **160** cm; Upper ab = **72.0** cm, Hip = **94.0** cm; Neck = **34.0** cm

D_B (Women) = 1.29579 + [0.221] * $\log_{10}$ (**160**)] − [0.35004 * $\log_{10}$ (**132**)]   Eq. 24.2c

% Fat = (495/**1.041**) − 450 = **26** %   Eq. 24.2d

Table 24.2 — Estimation of Percent Body Fat in Men from Height and Circumference Value

Circumference Value (CV) = Midabdominal Girth – Neck Girth

Height (in.)	Height (cm)	32 / 12.6	34 / 13.4	36 / 14.2	38 / 15.0	40 / 15.7	42 / 16.5	44 / 17.3	46 / 18.1	48 / 18.9	50 / 19.7	52 / 20.5	54 / 21.3	56 / 22.0	58 / 22.8	60 / 23.6	62 / 24.4	64 / 25.2
61	155.0	7	9	11	13	15	16	18	20	21	23	24	26	27	28	30	31	32
62	157.5	6	8	10	12	14	16	18	19	21	22	24	25	27	28	29	31	32
63	160.0	6	8	10	12	14	15	17	19	20	22	23	25	26	27	29	30	31
64	162.5	5	8	10	11	13	15	17	18	20	21	23	24	26	27	28	30	31
65	165.0	5	7	9	11	13	15	16	18	19	21	22	24	25	27	28	29	30
66	167.5	5	7	9	11	12	14	16	17	19	21	22	23	25	26	27	29	30
67	170.0		6	8	10	12	14	15	17	19	20	22	23	24	26	27	28	29
68	172.5		6	8	10	12	13	15	17	18	20	21	22	24	25	26	28	29
69	175.0		5	7	9	11	13	15	16	18	19	21	22	23	25	26	27	28
70	177.5		5	7	9	11	12	14	16	17	19	20	22	23	24	26	27	28
71	180.0		5	7	9	10	12	14	15	17	18	20	21	23	24	25	26	28
72	182.5			6	8	10	12	13	15	16	18	19	21	22	23	25	26	27
73	185.0			6	8	10	11	13	15	16	18	19	20	22	23	24	26	27
74	187.5			5	7	9	11	13	14	16	17	19	20	21	23	24	25	26
75	190.0			5	7	9	10	12	14	15	17	18	20	21	22	24	25	26
76	192.5			5	7	8	10	12	13	15	16	18	19	21	22	23	24	26

Circumference Value (CV) = Midabdominal Girth – Neck Girth

Height (in.)	Height (cm)	66 / 26.0	68 / 26.8	70 / 27.6	72 / 28.3	74 / 29.1	76 / 29.9	78 / 30.7	80 / 31.5	82 / 32.3	84 / 33.1	86 / 33.9	88 / 34.6	90 / 35.4	92 / 36.2	94 / 37.0	96 / 37.8	98 / 38.6
61	155.0	33	35	36	37	38	39	40	41	42	43	44	45	45				
62	157.5	33	34	35	36	37	39	40	41	42	43	44	44	45				
63	160.0	32	34	35	36	37	38	39	40	41	42	43	44	45	45			
64	162.5	32	33	34	35	36	38	39	40	41	42	43	43	44	45			
65	165.0	32	33	34	35	36	37	38	39	40	41	42	43	44	45			
66	167.5	31	32	33	34	36	37	38	39	40	41	42	42	43	44	45		
67	170.0	31	32	33	34	35	36	37	38	39	40	41	42	43	44	45		
68	172.5	30	31	32	33	35	36	37	38	39	40	41	41	42	43	44		
69	175.0	30	31	32	33	34	35	36	37	38	39	40	41	42	43	44	45	
70	177.5	29	30	31	33	34	35	36	37	38	39	40	41	41	42	43	44	
71	180.0	29	30	31	32	33	34	35	36	37	38	39	40	41	42	43	44	
72	182.5	28	30	31	32	33	34	35	36	37	38	39	40	41	41	42	43	44
73	185.0	28	29	30	31	32	33	34	35	36	37	38	39	40	41	42	43	44
74	187.5	28	29	30	31	32	33	34	35	36	37	38	39	40	41	41	42	43
75	190.0	27	28	29	30	32	33	34	35	36	36	37	38	39	40	41	42	43
76	192.5	27	28	30	30	31	32	33	34	35	36	37	38	39	40	41	41	42

Note: Based on: $D_B = 1.0324 + [0.15456 * Log_{10} (Ht\ in\ cm)] - [0.19077 * Log_{10} (CV\ in\ cm)]$ and $\%Fat = (495 / D_B) - 450$.

Source: Hodgdon & Beckett (1984).[18]

Table 24.3 **Estimation of Percent Body Fat in Women from Height and Circumference Value**

Circumference Value (CV) = Upper Abdominal Girth + Hip Girth − Neck Girth

Height (in.)	Height (cm)	106 / 41.7	108 / 42.5	110 / 43.3	112 / 44.1	114 / 44.9	116 / 45.7	118 / 46.5	120 / 47.2	122 / 48.0	124 / 48.8	126 / 49.6	128 / 50.4	130 / 51.2	132 / 52.0	134 / 52.8	136 / 53.5	138 / 54.3
59	150.0	14	15	16	17	18	20	21	22	23	24	25	26	27	29	30	31	32
60	152.5	13	14	15	17	18	19	20	21	22	23	25	26	27	28	29	30	31
61	155.0	12	13	15	16	17	18	19	21	22	23	24	25	26	27	28	29	30
62	157.5	12	13	14	15	16	18	19	20	21	22	23	24	25	26	27	28	29
63	160.0	11	12	13	15	16	17	18	19	20	21	22	24	25	26	27	28	29
64	162.5	10	11	13	14	15	16	17	18	20	21	22	23	24	25	26	27	28
65	165.0	10	11	12	13	14	16	17	18	19	20	21	22	23	24	25	26	27
66	167.5		10	11	13	14	15	16	17	18	19	20	22	23	24	25	26	27
67	170.0		10	11	12	13	14	15	17	18	19	20	21	22	23	24	25	26
68	172.5			10	11	13	14	15	16	17	18	19	20	21	22	23	24	25
69	175.0			10	11	12	13	14	15	16	18	19	20	21	22	23	24	25
70	177.5				10	11	13	14	15	16	17	18	19	20	21	22	23	24
71	180.0					11	12	13	14	15	16	17	18	20	21	22	23	24
72	182.5					10	11	12	14	15	16	17	18	19	20	21	22	23
73	185.0						11	12	13	14	15	16	17	18	19	20	21	22
74	187.5						10	11	12	14	15	16	17	18	19	20	21	22

Circumference Value (CV) = Upper Abdominal Girth + Hip Girth − Neck Girth

Height (in.)	Height (cm)	140 / 55.1	142 / 55.9	144 / 56.7	146 / 57.5	148 / 58.3	150 / 59.1	152 / 59.8	154 / 60.6	156 / 61.4	158 / 62.2	160 / 63.0	162 / 63.8	164 / 64.6	166 / 65.4	168 / 66.1	170 / 66.9	172 / 67.7
59	150.0	33	34	35	36	37	38	39	40	41	42	42	43	44	45			
60	152.5	32	33	34	35	36	37	38	39	40	41	42	43	44	44	45		
61	155.0	31	32	33	34	35	36	37	38	39	40	41	42	43	44	45	45	
62	157.5	31	32	33	34	34	35	36	37	38	39	40	41	42	43	44	45	45
63	160.0	30	31	32	33	34	35	36	37	38	39	39	40	41	42	43	44	45
64	162.5	29	30	31	32	33	34	35	36	37	38	39	40	41	41	42	43	44
65	165.0	28	29	30	31	32	33	34	35	36	37	38	39	40	41	42	42	43
66	167.5	28	29	30	31	32	33	34	35	35	36	37	38	39	40	41	42	43
67	170.0	27	28	29	30	31	32	33	34	35	36	37	38	39	39	40	41	42
68	172.5	26	27	28	29	30	31	32	33	34	35	36	37	38	39	40	40	41
69	175.0	26	27	28	29	30	31	32	33	33	34	35	36	37	38	39	40	41
70	177.5	25	26	27	28	29	30	31	32	33	34	35	36	37	37	38	39	40
71	180.0	25	26	27	28	28	29	30	31	32	33	34	35	36	37	38	38	39
72	182.5	24	25	26	27	28	29	30	31	32	32	33	34	35	36	37	38	39
73	185.0	23	24	25	26	27	28	29	30	31	32	33	34	35	35	36	37	38
74	187.5	23	24	25	26	27	28	29	29	30	31	32	33	34	35	36	37	37

Note: Based on: D_B = 1.29579 + [0.221 * Log_{10} (Ht in cm)] − [0.35004 * Log_{10} (CV in cm)] and % Fat = (495 / D_B) − 450.
Source: Hodgdon & Beckett (1984).[19]

Determination of Waist-to-Hip Ratio (W:H)

Although a nomogram is available for determining waist-to-hip (W:H) ratio, it is actually less convenient than calculating the ratio by hand with a calculator. The girth sites (Figure 24.1) and the calculation of the W:H ratio are the same for men and women. The ratio is found simply by dividing the upper abdominal (waist) girth by the hip girth (Eq. 24.3a). The sample girth data provided below are in metric units (cm), but because the calculation is of a ratio, the girth values could also be measured in inches. The resultant W:H ratio of 0.88 (Eq. 24.3b) can be used to estimate risk of coronary heart disease and other chronic diseases and conditions.

Waist-to-hip ratio (W:H) = Upper abdominal (waist)
girth / Hip (gluteal) girth   Eq. 24.3a

Assume: Upper abdominal girth = **80** cm;
Hip girth = **91** cm

W:H ratio = **80** cm / **91** cm = **0.88**   Eq. 24.3b

Determination of Waist-to-Height Ratio (W/Ht)

Another ratio which is sometimes used to relate central fat distribution to metabolic risk is the waist-to-height (W/Ht) ratio. The girth sites (Figure 24.1) and the calculation of the W/Ht ratio are also the same for men and women. The ratio is calculated by dividing the midabdominal girth (measured at the level of the navel) by the height (Eq. 24.4a). The sample data provided result in a W/Ht ratio of 0.50 (Eq. 24.4b) which can be used to estimate risk of coronary heart disease and other chronic metabolic diseases and conditions.

Waist-to-height ratio (W/Ht) = Midabdominal
girth / Height   Eq. 24.4a

Assume: Midabdominal girth = **80** cm; Height = **160** cm

W:H ratio = **80** cm / **160** cm = **0.50**   Eq. 24.4b

RESULTS AND DISCUSSION

Methods are described in this chapter for using circumferences to assess percent body fat and risk of chronic disease based on fat distribution as measured by the waist-to-hip ratio. Circumference measurements around the waist and hips reflect body volume and can be used in conjunction with height and weight to estimate percent body fat. The addition of neck girth further allows for some differentiation of lean weight. The waist girth and the ratio of the waist-to-hip girths also help identify those individuals with more visceral fat who may be at increased risk of developing type II diabetes and coronary heart disease.

Percent Body Fat Interpretation

The use of girth measurements is one of the simplest and least expensive methods for the evaluation of body composition. It requires far less practice and expertise than many other methods, in particular methods using the measurement of skinfold thicknesses or hydrostatic weighing, both of which are described in subsequent chapters. And percent body fat determined by circumferences has been shown to relate closely ($r = 0.95$ in young men and $r = 0.90$ in middle-aged men) to percent body fat derived by the skinfold method.[17] As noted earlier, the 2-Girth and 3-Girth Methods for determining body composition in this chapter were developed for use by the U.S. Navy.[18,19] Other branches of the U.S. Armed Forces use the same methods or similar methods also based on circumference measures to assess body composition. The preference for circumference measurements appears to be based not only on the simplicity and inexpensiveness of the method, but on other factors as well.[16] Changes with training are not represented well by changes in body weight alone, due to the fact that the body weights of many military personnel do not change with training as a result of the fat loss being counteracted by an increase in muscle mass. Adding the measurement of circumferences to the measurement of body weight alone increases the ability to detect fat loss. In men, a reduced mid-abdominal girth represents a loss of fat, in particular a loss of visceral fat.[15] Measuring skinfold thicknesses may not adequately detect this loss because it does not measure visceral fat. Accurately detecting fat loss in women presents a bigger problem because women lose fat in the thighs, hips, abdomen, and upper arms, while men lose fat predominantly in the abdomen. In women, there is no single site of fat deposition and therefore no single girth measurement that accurately reflects fat loss.[39] For this reason, two girths are used in women, the upper abdominal girth and the hip girth, to increase the likelihood of detecting fat loss and more accurately estimating body composition.

Since the 1980s, it has been military policy to assess the body weight and body composition of military personnel annually.[16] Individuals who exceed a weight-for-height limit subsequently go through a girth assessment of percent body fat. Men with percent body fat values of less than 20 % and women less than 30 % are considered "within standards." Percent body fat values for men of 20–26 % and women of 30–36 % are considered "cautionary," and acceptance of their body fat content depends on their performance on a physical fitness test. Several different criteria for the evaluation of percent body fat are presented in Table 24.4. Essential body fat in men (5 %) and women (8 %) is considered the minimal fat necessary to sustain normal physiological function.[34] The average percent body fat for a young, college-aged population is 12–16 % for men and 22–26 % for women.[37] Body fat standards for fitness generally run a little lower than standards for health. Percent body fats over 20 % in men and 30 % in women are typically classified as overweight or overfat.[30] And obesity is typically classified as a percent body fat over 25 % in men and a value over 30–35 % for women.[34,37] These criteria are all fairly general. More

Table 24.4 Health and Fitness Standards for Percent Body Fat

Classification/Category	Percent Fat (%) Men	Percent Fat (%) Women
Essential fat[34]	5	8
Fitness standard (< 40 y)[34]	5–15	16–28
Optimal fitness[34]	12–18	16–25
Average[37]	12–16	22–26
Health standard (< 40 y)[34]	8–22	20–35
Optimal health[34]	10–25	18–30
Overfat[30]	> 20	> 30
Obese[34]	> 25	> 30
Obese[37]	> 25	> 35

Sources: McArdle, Katch, & Katch (1991);[30] Roundtable (1986);[34] U.S. Department of the Navy (1986).[37]

specific comparative data are presented in subsequent chapters involving the measurement of body fat by skinfold thicknesses and hydrostatic weighing.

Waist-to-Hip Ratio Interpretation

Girth measurements, in addition to being used to estimate percent body fat, are also used to directly reflect regional fat distribution and risk of chronic disease. Greater neck girths and greater waist girths have both been studied as simple indicators of increased adiposity. Neck girth can be used as an indicator of upper body fat distribution.[8] Men with a neck girth ≥ 37 cm and women with a neck girth of ≥ 34 cm are recommended to have additional evaluation of their overweight and obesity status. Furthermore, neck girth as an index of upper body obesity is correlated with factors indicative of metabolic syndrome and therefore likely increases the risk of cardiovascular disease.[9] Comparative data for waist girth as an indicator of abdominal adiposity are presented in Table 24.5. The average waist girth in this large sample of adults is 87.6 cm and 80.5 cm in 20–29-year-old men and women, respectively, with an increase in waist girth of about 4 cm observed per decade.[31] According to standards published by the National Heart, Lung, and Blood Institute (NHLBI), a waist girth over 102 cm (40 in.) in men and over 88 cm (35 in.) in women identify increased obesity-associated risk factors.[32] Alternative waist girth measurements specific to BMI category have also been described. The waist girth used to identify those at increased risk of disease in four BMI categories (normal weight, overweight, class I obesity, and class II obesity) is 90, 100, 110, and 125 cm in men and 80, 90, 105, and 115 cm in women.[4,5] A higher waist-to-hip ratio is also related to increased risk of chronic disease, with comparative data provided in Table 24.6. The average W:H ratio for young males (20–29 y) according to one reference is 0.90 and for females is 0.82. Other references identify elevated health risk with W:H ratios exceeding 0.94–1.00 for men[3,10,24] and 0.80–0.86 for women.[2,10,24]

Waist-to-Height Ratio Interpretation

Another simple, less frequently used measure for assessing central fat distribution and metabolic risk in men and women is the waist-to-height ratio (W/Ht). Many believe the degree of central fat distribution is more closely tied to metabolic risks than waist-to-hip ratio, BMI or skinfolds. Studies of the W/Ht ratio have been published since the mid-1990s,[22] but there has been a recent resurgence in interest in this index.[29] A person with a waist girth of 90 cm who is 180 cm tall would have a W/Ht of 0.50. Nearly all overweight persons (BMI ≥ 25) in a recent study had a W/Ht ratio ≥ 0.5 (98.5 % of men and 97.5 % of women), while none (literally 0 %) of the underweight persons had a W/Ht ratio ≥ 0.5. Waist-to-height ratio can be used to identify higher metabolic risk equally well in people of normal weight as those who are overweight. The prevalence of metabolic risks has been shown to be significantly higher among both men and women when W/Ht ratio ≥ 0.5 compared to those with W/Ht < 0.5.[23] W/Ht has also been reported to be useful in screening for cardiovascular risk factors in children.[35] Waist-to-height ratio may offer several advantages over other measures of central adiposity. It does not differ greatly between men and women, it provides more accurate tracking of fat distribution and accumulation by age, it is more closely related with death due to coronary risk factors, it better

Table 24.5 Category for Waist Girth (cm) by Gender and Age Group

Category (percentile)	20–29 y Men	20–29 y Women	30–39 y Men	30–39 y Women	40–49 y Men	40–49 y Women
Well above ave (> 95th)	< 72.3	< 65.6	< 76.4	< 67.1	< 79.1	< 69.6
Above ave (75th–95th)	72.3–79.1	65.6–70.9	76.4–85.7	67.1–74.8	79.1–89.5	69.6–78.2
Average (25th–74th)	79.2–94.0	71.0–87.1	85.8–100.0	74.9–94.6	89.6–104.2	78.3–98.8
Below ave (5th–24th)	94.1–111.5	87.2–107.0	100.1–115.1	94.7–116.3	104.3–121.1	98.9–116.7
Well below ave (< 5th)	≥ 111.6	≥ 107.1	≥ 115.2	≥ 116.4	≥ 121.2	≥ 116.8
Mean	87.6	80.5	93.6	86.4	97.7	89.7

Source: National Center for Health Statistics (2005).[31]

Table 24.6   Category for Waist-to-Hip Ratio (W:H) by Gender and Age Group

Category (percentile)	20–29 y		30–39 y		40–49 y	
	Men	Women	Men	Women	Men	Women
Well above ave (> *95th*)	< 0.85	< 0.78	< 0.87	< 0.78	< 0.91	< 0.79
Above ave (*75th–95th*)	0.85–0.87	0.78–0.79	0.87–0.92	0.78–0.80	0.91–0.95	0.79–0.82
Average (*25th–74th*)	0.88–0.92	0.80–0.84	0.93–0.96	0.81–0.87	0.96–0.99	0.83–0.90
Below ave (*5th–24th*)	0.93–0.98	0.85–0.89	0.97–0.99	0.88–0.91	1.00–1.03	0.91–0.92
Well below ave (< *5th*)	≥ 0.99	≥ 0.90	≥ 1.00	≥ 0.92	≥ 1.04	≥ 0.93
Mean	0.90	0.82	0.94	0.84	0.97	0.86

Source: National Center for Health Statistics (2005).[31]

BOX 24.2   Chapter Preview/Review

What is the rationale for using girths to estimate body composition?

Which girth measurements are used in assessing body composition in men and women?

What is the *SEE* for most girth methods?

How is the upper abdominal (waist) girth identified?

What percent body fat range defines the "optimal fitness" category in men and in women?

What waist girth in men and women is related to an increased obesity-associated risk of disease?

What are the average waist-to-hip ratios in young (20–29-year-old) men and women?

What is the value of waist-to-height ratio used to distinguish between higher and lower risk of disease?

---

identifies risk in normal weight and overweight persons, and it is extremely simple.[23] There is one single rule with W/Ht ratio—keep your waist girth below half your height (W/Ht < 0.50) to minimize your risk of chronic disease and to increase your life expectancy.

References

1. American College of Sports Medicine. (1995). *ACSM's guidelines for exercise testing and prescription.* Philadelphia: Williams & Wilkins.

2. American College of Sports Medicine. (2000). *ACSM's guidelines for exercise testing and prescription.* Philadelphia: Lippincott Williams & Wilkins.

3. American Heart Association. (1991). *1992 heart and stroke facts.* Dallas, TX: Author.

4. Ardern, C. I., Janssen, I., Ross, R., & Katzmarzyk, P. T. (2004). Development of health-related waist circumference threshold within BMI categories. *Obesity Research, 12,* 1094–1103.

5. Ardern, C. I., Katzmarzyk, P. T., Janssen, I., & Ross, R. (2003). Discrimination of health risk by combined body mass index and waist circumference. *Obesity Research, 11,* 13–142.

6. Behnke, A. R., & Wilmore, J. H. (1974). *Evaluation and regulation of body build and composition.* Englewood Cliffs, NJ: Prentice-Hall.

7. Bemben, M. G., Massey, B. H., Bemben, D. A., Boileau, R. A., & Misner, J. E. (1995). Age-related patterns in body composition for men aged 20–79 y. *Medicine and Science in Sports and Exercise, 27,* 264–269.

8. Ben-Noun, L., & Laor, A. (2001). Neck girth as a simple screening measure for identifying overweight and obese patients. *Obesity Research, 9,* 470–477.

9. Ben-Noun, L., & Laor, A. (2003). Relationship of neckcircumference to cardiovascular risk factors. *Obesity Research, 11,* 226–231.

10. Bray, G. A., & Gray, D. S. (1988). Obesity, Part 1—Pathogenesis. *Western Journal of Medicine, 149,* 429–441.

11. Brooks, G. A., Fahey, T. D., White, T. P., & Baldwin, K. M. (2000). *Exercise physiology: Human bioenergetics and its application* (p. 582). Mountain View, CA: Mayfield.

12. Brozek, J., & Keys, A. (1951). The evaluation of leanness-fatness in man: Norms and intercorrelations. *British Journal of Nutrition, 5,* 194–205.

13. Despres, J.-P., Moorjani, S., Lupien, P. J., Tremblay, A., Nadeau, A., & Bouchard, C. (1990). Regional distribution of body fat, plasma lipoproteins, and cardiovascular disease. *Arteriosclerosis, 10,* 497–511.

14. Expert Panel. (1998). Executive summary of the clinical guidelines on the identification, evaluation, and treatment of overweight and obesity in adults. *Archives of Internal Medicine, 158,* 1855–1867.

15. Friedl, K., Moore, R., Martinez-Lopez, L., Vogel, J., Askew, E., Marchitelli, L., Hoyt, R., & Gordon, C. (1994). Lower limit of body fat in healthy active men. *Journal of Applied Physiology, 77,* 933–940.

16. Friedl, K., Wesphal, K., Marchitelli, L., Patton, J., Chumlea, C., & Guo, S. (2001). Evaluation of anthropometric equations to assess body composition changes in young women. *American Journal of Clinical Nutrition, 73,* 268–275.

17. Hedge, S., & Aluja, S. (1996). Assessment of percent body fat content in young and middle aged men: Skinfold method versus girth method. *Journal of Postgraduate Medicine, 42,* 97–100.

18. Hodgdon, J. A., & Beckett, M. B. (1984a). *Prediction of percent body fat for U.S. Navy men from body circumferences and height.* Report No. 84-11. San Diego, CA: Naval Health Research Center.

19. Hodgdon, J. A., & Beckett, M. B. (1984b). *Prediction of percent body fat for U.S. Navy women from body circumferences and height.* Report No. 84-29. San Diego, CA: Naval Health Research Center.

20. Hodgdon, J. A., & Beckett, M. B. (1984c). *Technique for measuring body circumferences and skinfold thicknesses.* Report No. 84-39. San Diego, CA: Naval Health Research Center.

21. Howley, E. T. (2000). You asked for it. *ACSM's Health & Fitness Journal, 4*(6), 6, 26.

22. Hsieh, S. D., & Yoshinaga, H. (1995). Abdominal fat distribution and coronary heart disease risk factors in men—waist/height ratio as a simple and useful predictor. *International Journal of Obesity and Related Metabolic Disorders, 19,* 585–589.

23. Hsieh, S. D., Yoshinaga, H., & Muto, T. (2003). Waist-to-height ratio, a simple and practical index for assessing central fat distribution and metabolic risk in Japanese men and women. *International Journal of Obesity, 27,* 610–616.

24. Johnson, P. B., Updyke, W. F., Schaefer, M., & Stolberg, D. C. (1975). *Sport, exercise, and you.* San Francisco: Holt, Rinehart & Winston.

25. Joint Dietary Guidelines Advisory Committee of the United States Departments of Agriculture, and Health and Human Services. (1990). U.S. Dept of Agriculture.

26. Larsson, B., Svardsudd, K., Welin, L., Wilhelmsen, L., Bjorntorp, P., & Tibblin, G. (1984). Abdominal adipose tissue distribution, obesity, and risk of cardiovascular disease and death: 13-year follow-up of participants in the study of men born in 1913. *British Medical Journal, 288,* 1401–1404.

27. Lohman, T. G. (1981). Skinfolds and body density and their relation to body fatness: A review. *Human Biology, 53,* 181–225.

28. Lohman, T. G. (1986). Body composition—A round-table. *The Physician and Sportsmedicine, 14,* 157–162.

29. Mann, D. (2012). *An easier way to assess body fat and health risks. Waist-to-height ratio may predict health risks more accurately than BMI.* Retrieved August 28, 2012, from http://www.webmd.com/diet/news/20120511/better-way-assess-body-fat-health-risk

30. McArdle, W. D., Katch, F. I., & Katch, V. L. (1996). *Exercise physiology: Energy, nutrition, and human performance.* Baltimore: Williams & Wilkins.

31. National Center for Health Statistics. (2005). *Anthropometric reference data, United States, 1988–1994.* Hyattsville, MD: Author. Available online at www.cdc.gov/nchs/.

32. National Heart, Lung, and Blood Institute. (1998). *Clinical guidelines on the identification, evaluation, and treatment of overweight and obesity in adults.* Washington, DC: U.S. Government Printing Office.

33. Ross, W. D., & Marfell-Jones, M. J. (1991). Kinanthopometry. In J. D. MacDougall, H. A. Wenger, & H. J. Green (Eds.), *Physiological testing of the high performance athlete* (pp. 223–308). Champaign, IL: Human Kinetics.

34. Roundtable. (1986). Body composition methodology in sportsmedicine. *The Physician and Sportsmedicine,* 46–58.

35. Savva, S. C., Tornaritis, M., Savva, M. E., Kourides, Y., Panagi, A., Silikiotou, N., Georgiou, C., & Kafatos, A. (2000). Waist circumference and waist-to-height ratio are better predictors of cardiovascular disease risk factors in children than body mass index. *International Journal of Obesity and Related Metabolic Disorders, 24,* 1453–1458.

36. Siri, W. E. (1961). *Body composition from fluid spaces and density: Analysis of methods in techniques for measuring body composition.* Washington, DC: National Academy of Science, National Research Council.

37. U.S. Department of the Navy, Navy Military Personnel Command, Code 6H. (1986, August). Office of the Chief of Naval Operations Instruction 6110.1C. Physical Readiness Program.

38. Van Itallie, T. B. (1988). Topography of body fat: Relationship to risk of cardiovascular and other diseases. In T. G. Lohman, A. F. Roche, & R.Martorell (Eds.), *Anthropometric standardization reference manual* (pp. 143–149). Champaign, IL: Human Kinetics.

39. Vogel, J., & Friedl, K. (1992). Body fat assessment in women—special considerations. *Sports Medicine, 13,* 245–269.

40. Wilmore, J. H. (1986). *Sensible fitness.* Champaign, IL: Human Kinetics.

41. Wilmore, J. H., & Behnke, A. R. (1969). An anthropometric estimation of body density and lean body weight in young men. *Journal of Applied Physiology, 27,* 25–31.

Form 24.1
GIRTHS

NAME _____ DATE _____ SCORE _____

Homework

Gender: **M**   Initials: **AA**   Age (y): **22**   Height (cm): **170**   Weight (kg): **70.5**

Midabdominal girth *(closest 0.5 cm)* T_1 **88.5** T_2 **89.0** T_3 **89.5**   Median _____ cm

Neck girth T_1 **37.5** T_2 **37.0** T_3 **37.0**   Median _____ cm

Upper abdom girth* *(for W:H ratio)* T_1 **82.5** T_2 **83.0** T_3 **83.5**   Median _____ cm

Hip girth* *(for W:H ratio)* T_1 **92.0** T_2 **92.0** T_3 **91.0**   Median _____ cm

2-Girth Body Comp   Circumference value (CV) = _____ – _____ = _____ cm

                                                        Midabdom   Neck

D_B = 1.0324 + [0.15456 * _____] – [0.19077 * _____] = _____ $g \cdot ml^{-1}$

                          Log$_{10}$ (Ht)   Log$_{10}$ (CV)

% Fat = (495 / D_B _____) – 450 = _____ %   % Fat = _____   *(from Table 24.2)*

Category _____   *(Table 24.4)*

Waist-to-Hip Ratio (W:H)   _____ cm / _____ cm = _____

                              Upper abdom   Hip   W:H Ratio

Category for waist _____   *(Table 24.5)*   Category for W:H _____   *(Table 24.6)*

Waist-to-Height Ratio (W/Ht)   _____ cm / _____ cm = _____

                                Midabdom   Height   W/Ht Ratio

Evaluation of W/Ht ratio: [ ] < 0.50 Lower risk   [ ] ≥ 0.50 Higher risk of disease

---

Gender: **F**   Initials: **BB**   Age (y): **22**   Height (cm): **165**   Weight (kg): **64.8**

Upper abdom girth *(closest 0.5 cm)* T_1 **76.0** T_2 **77.0** T_3 **77.5**   Median _____ cm

Hip girth T_1 **94.5** T_2 **95.0** T_3 **94.0**   Median _____ cm

Neck girth T_1 **34.0** T_2 **33.0** T_3 **33.5**   Median _____ cm

Midabdominal girth* *(for W/Ht)* T_1 **81.0** T_2 **80.5** T_3 **81.5**   Median _____ cm

3-Girth Body Comp   Circumference value (CV) = _____ + _____ – _____ = _____ cm

                                                        Upper abd   Hip   Neck

D_B = 1.29579 + [0.221 * _____] – [0.35004 * _____] = _____ $g \cdot ml^{-1}$

                         Log$_{10}$ (Ht)   Log$_{10}$ (CV)

% Fat = (495 / D_B _____) – 450 = _____ %   % Fat = _____   *(from Table 24.3)*

Category _____   *(Table 24.4)*

Waist-to-Hip Ratio (W:H)   _____ cm / _____ cm = _____

                              Upper abdom   Hip   W:H Ratio

Category for waist _____   *(Table 24.5)*   Category for W:H _____   *(Table 24.6)*

Waist-to-Height Ratio (W/Ht)   _____ cm / _____ cm = _____

                                Midabdom   Height   W/Ht Ratio

Evaluation of W/Ht ratio: [ ] < 0.50 Lower risk   [ ] ≥ 0.50 Higher risk of disease

Form 24.2
GIRTHS

NAME _____ DATE _____ SCORE _____

Lab Results

Gender: **M**   Initials: _____   Age (y): _____   Height (cm): _____   Weight (kg): _____

Midabdominal girth (closest 0.5 cm)	T_1 _____	T_2 _____	T_3 _____	Median _____	cm
Neck girth	T_1 _____	T_2 _____	T_3 _____	Median _____	cm
Upper abdom girth* (for W:H ratio)	T_1 _____	T_2 _____	T_3 _____	Median _____	cm
Hip girth* (for W:H ratio)	T_1 _____	T_2 _____	T_3 _____	Median _____	cm

2-Girth Body Comp   Circumference value (CV) = _____ – _____ = _____ cm

            Midabdom   Neck

$D_B = 1.0324 + [0.15456 * \underline{\hspace{2cm}}] - [0.19077 * \underline{\hspace{2cm}}] = \underline{\hspace{2cm}}$ g·ml^{-1}

          Log_{10} (Ht) Log_{10} (CV)

% Fat = (495 / D_B _____) – 450 = _____ %   % Fat = _____   (from Table 24.2)

Category _____ (Table 24.4)

Waist-to-Hip Ratio (W:H)   _____ cm / _____ cm = _____

         Upper abdom   Hip   W:H Ratio

Category for waist _____ (Table 24.5)   Category for W:H _____ (Table 24.6)

Waist-to-Height Ratio (W/Ht)   _____ cm / _____ cm = _____

         Midabdom   Height   W/Ht Ratio

Evaluation of W/Ht ratio: ☐ < 0.50 Lower risk   ☐ ≥ 0.50 Higher risk of disease

Gender: **F**   Initials: _____   Age (y): _____   Height (cm): _____   Weight (kg): _____

Upper abdom girth (closest 0.5 cm)	T_1 _____	T_2 _____	T_3 _____	Median _____	cm
Hip girth	T_1 _____	T_2 _____	T_3 _____	Median _____	cm
Neck girth	T_1 _____	T_2 _____	T_3 _____	Median _____	cm
Midabdominal girth* (for W/Ht)	T_1 _____	T_2 _____	T_3 _____	Median _____	cm

3-Girth Body Comp   Circumference value (CV) = _____ + _____ – _____ = _____ cm

            Upper abd   Hip   Neck

$D_B = 1.29579 + [0.221 * \underline{\hspace{2cm}}] - [0.35004 * \underline{\hspace{2cm}}] = \underline{\hspace{2cm}}$ g·ml^{-1}

          Log_{10} (Ht) Log_{10} (CV)

% Fat = (495 / D_B _____) – 450 = _____ %   % Fat = _____   (from Table 24.3)

Category _____ (Table 24.4)

Waist-to-Hip Ratio (W:H)   _____ cm / _____ cm = _____

         Upper abdom   Hip   W:H Ratio

Category for waist _____ (Table 24.5)   Category for W:H _____ (Table 24.6)

Waist-to-Height Ratio (W/Ht)   _____ cm / _____ cm = _____

         Midabdom   Height   W/Ht Ratio

Evaluation of W/Ht ratio: ☐ < 0.50 Lower risk   ☐ ≥ 0.50 Higher risk of disease

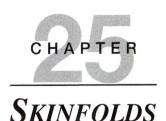

CHAPTER

SKINFOLDS

The use of calipers to measure subcutaneous skinfolds for predicting percent body fat is popular not only in laboratories and health clinics but also in commercial fitness centers. Although traditionally the skinfold caliper has been thought of as a laboratory instrument, its portability and recent modification to an inexpensive plastic version would qualify it also as a field instrument. In addition, the recommendation of AAHPERD to incorporate skinfold measures in physical education classes,[2,3] characterizes skinfold testing as a field test. Because the location of fat (regional distribution) may be as important clinically and aesthetically as the total amount of fat, skinfolds have an advantage over some other body composition measures.

PHYSIOLOGICAL RATIONALE

Fat is not bad. In fact, it is a very economical way to store energy. For instance, one gram of fat contains slightly more than twice the amount of kilocalories (or kilojoules) as do either carbohydrates or proteins. In addition to its economical storage of fuel, fat also provides a storage place for vitamins. Also, fat is important because it serves as an insulator. Because of these important roles, fat is often subdivided into two compartments—essential fat and storage fat.

The **essential fat** necessary to sustain life in the theoretical reference male (ht = 174 cm or 68.5 in.; 70 kg or 154 lb) represents about 2 % to 5 % of total body mass[29] and that of the reference female (ht = 163.8 cm or 64.5 in.; 57 kg or 125 lb) up to 12 % of total body mass (Table 25.1).[6,29] Essential fat may be stored in the bone marrow, heart, intestines, kidneys, liver, spleen, central nervous system (myelination), muscles, and other organs and tissues. In women, an additional, gender-related site for essential fat is the breast area and possibly the pelvis, buttocks, and thighs.[29]

Storage fat is stored subcutaneously between the skin and muscles; it is also stored between muscles (intermuscularly) and surrounding various organs. The subcutaneous fat represents about half of the fat in the body of a young adult,[34] whereas the other half is internalized. In older adults the visceral (internal) fat becomes proportionally greater.[29]

Regression equations for predicting percent body fat and/or body density are based upon correlations between

Table 25.1	Body Composition of the Reference Man and Woman, 20–30 y of Age					
	Reference Man			Reference Woman		
	kg	lb	%*	kg	lb	%*
Total fat mass	11	23	15 %	16	35	27 %
Essential fat	2	5	3 %	7	15	12 %
Storage fat	9	19	12 %	9	20	15 %
Total lean mass	59	131	85 %	41	91	73 %
Muscle	31	69	45 %	20	45	36 %
Bone	10	23	15 %	7	15	12 %
Remainder	18	39	25 %	14	31	25 %
Total body mass	70	154	100 %	57	126	100 %

Note: *Percent (%) of total body mass.
Source: Behnke & Wilmore (1974).[6]

anthropometric measures (e.g., skinfolds) and hydrostatic measures of body density. Numerous skinfold sites may be measured originally, with the combination of sites best predicting body density and/or body fat being chosen for the regression equation. In some cases, the regression equation is transformed into a table or nomogram based upon two or more skinfolds (or their sum), which is then used to find the corresponding percent body fat.

METHODS

A detailed description of skinfold techniques is found in Chapter 5 of the *Anthropometric Standardization Reference Manual.*[18] The technique of measuring skinfolds accurately requires practice—the technician must learn to sense (feel) the participant's subcutaneous fold. This feel, however, is not consistent in participants or from one site to another in the same participant. Thus, the ease with which the skinfold, or fatfold, can be separated from the underlying muscle varies between persons and at different sites within the same person. There are also variations in the compressibility of the skin or adipose tissue, which may affect the feel and the measurement. For example, the skinfold is more likely to change its dimension while being grasped in younger persons due to their greater tissue hydration.[18] A description of the accuracy of predicting percent body fat from skinfold dimensions is presented in Box 25.1.

BOX 25.1   Accuracy of the Skinfold-Prediction of Body Fat

Of the more than 100 equations for the prediction of body density from anthropometric data (with subsequent conversion to percent body fat), the ones from skinfold measurements are considered the most accurate.[30] The relationship between body density and skinfold fat is nonlinear. Thus, when using a linear equation, accurate predictions would be made for those in the middle values but not at the extremes, where the obese person would be underestimated and the lean person overestimated. On the other hand, quadratic equations eliminate this bias.[21]

Reliability

The reliability of skinfold measurements is high with test-retest reliabilities of 0.94–0.98.[8,24] As with girth estimations, skinfold predictions of body fat are not without controversy. One investigator said that using skinfolds to predict body fat mass "is like trying to find the weight of the peel of an orange by measuring the thickness of the peel, but ignoring the size of the orange."[13] Nevertheless, for the determination of desirable weights, it is logical to conclude that skinfolds are superior to the height-weight-age tables, girths, and diameters.

Validity

Correlation coefficients between skinfolds and hydrostatically determined body fatness have consistently ranged from 0.70 to 0.90.[1,4] In general, the inclusion of three skinfold sites in the regression equation produces a better prediction (lower standard error of estimate; *SEE*) of body density than fewer sites. However, neither the feasibility nor accuracy is improved by using more than three sites.[33] The standard error of the estimate for skinfold prediction of hydrodensitometrically determined body fat is about 3.5 % body fat units with the acceptable *SEE* of 1 %–1.5 %—probably impossible to attain via skinfold methods.[7,14,22,35,39] For example, using the sum of three skinfolds, described as the J-P Method in this chapter, resulted in an *SEE* of 2.7 % fat in young adult men.[38] The skinfold *SEE* should be added to the error of hydrodensitometry, making the error of determining true body fat from skinfolds about 4.6 %.[12] The sum of the skinfolds itself may be a more valid indicator of adiposity and better for progressive monitoring of fatness than the prediction of percent fat derived from the skinfolds. The J-P researchers used Lange™ calipers, which reportedly overestimate measures from Harpenden™ calipers.[17,26] This leads to an underestimation of 1–2 % body fat relative to J-P estimations.[17] Consequently, one group of reviewers recommends that the sum of Harpenden™ skinfolds be adjusted upward by multiplying them by 1.10 to account for the 10 % difference.[32]

Equipment

The caliper is the basic instrument for skinfold measurements. It simplifies and improves the crude use of a ruler to measure the pinch of skinfold held by the technician's fingers. Thus, calipers apply a standard pinch pressure and provide an easily readable measure of the width (mm) of the pinch. High-quality calipers, such as the Harpenden™ Lafayette™, and Lange™, have scales that can be read within a range of 0.2 mm and 1.0 mm. Descriptions of several calipers are in various sources.[11,30] Comments on the calibration of calipers are in Box 25.2.

A tape measure is used to locate the precise site of some skinfolds (e.g., triceps). It is best to use a metric tape because the midpoint of any measure is often simpler to find using a metric dimension than an inches dimension (e.g., the halfway point of 13.75 in. vs. 34.2 cm). A felt marker (or body marker) or ballpoint pen is used to mark the site of the skinfolds on the participant.

Participant Preparation

Participants should wear loose-fitting shirts and shorts. Males are encouraged to go shirtless, while females are encouraged to wear a bathing-suit top. The participant should not be overheated while being measured, due to the increased fluid volume in the skinfold from cutaneous capillary blood flow. On the other hand, the skinfold will be reduced up to 15 % if the participant is hypohydrated.[9]

General Procedures for Measuring Skinfolds

Position of Participant

The participant stands while all skinfold sites are measured. Although some authorities state that there is little practical difference as to which side of the body to use for girth measures,[28] it appears that most skinfold equations, including those in this manual, are based on right-side measurements. The description of the skinfold sites corresponds mainly with those methods described by Jackson and Pollock (J-P),[20,23] and the *Anthropometric Standardization Reference Manual*.[18,27]

Skinfold Technique

The caliper should be handled very carefully. While holding it in the right hand, the technician uses the thumb and index finger of the left hand to pinch the skinfold at a distance of about 1 cm above the skinfold site (or mark). This fold represents two layers of skin and fat. The long axis of the fold is a natural, smooth, and untwisted fold. This may be referred to as the natural cleavage of the skin. The axis direction of the cleavage may be different in obese persons than in those of normal weight.

The points of the caliper should be placed perpendicular across the long axis of the skinfold at the designated skinfold site (mark). The 1 cm separation between the technician's fingers and the caliper should prevent the skinfold dimension from being affected by the pressure of the fingers. The depth of caliper placement is about half the

The scale of a caliper is in units of millimeters (mm). Two of the main characteristics to consider when judging the accuracy of a skinfold caliper are (1) the precision of the tension spring on the jaws of the caliper and (2) the precision of the scale reflecting the width of the caliper opening. Other important characteristics that may affect both of these are the mechanical condition of the caliper pivot, the mechanical resistance of the indicator gauge, and the caliper jaw alignment.[10] The closing jaw tension of earlier calipers ranged from 9 g/mm^2 to 20 g/mm^2 for any given type of caliper; most calipers were about 10 g/mm^2 ± 2.0 throughout the range of the caliper opening. The closing jaw pressure (tension) of 7.82 g/mm^2 reported by one group of researchers[16] testing Harpenden calipers is less than most other newer calipers. The 9.36 g/mm^2 reported by another group of researchers, however, is virtually the same as the Lange caliper.[17] The jaw pressure of a caliper is inversely related to the size of the skinfold.[16] Thus, lower skinfolds reported by some researchers[17] using Harpenden calipers can not be attributed to pressure differences. It is apparent that, for greater accuracy in predicting percent fat, the technician should use the same caliper that was used by the researcher(s) who developed the prediction equation.[17]

One group of investigators recommends the following:[16]

- Service the caliper pivot, indicator gauge, and jaw alignment about every 12 mo, never exceeding 24 mo.
- Wipe the caliper springs with a lightly oiled rag periodically.

Harpenden calipers usually include a stublike piece of metal that has a precise diameter (15.9 mm). The calipers can be checked for accuracy at this dimension. The technician should recognize that this does not assure that the calipers are accurate at other jaw gap dimensions.

---

distance between the base of the normal skin perimeter and the crest (top) of the skinfold.

Because of the compressibility of the skinfold,[5] the jaws of the caliper should not press longer than 4 s at the skinfold site so they do not force fluid from the tissues and reduce the measurement.[25,34] However, the technician should wait 1–2 s before reading the gauge.[4] Technicians should be consistent in the timing of the reading, not relying on the end of the rapid decrease in the measurement.[18] For example, all technicians should agree that they will record the reading observed at the third or fourth second. While still holding the skinfold, the technician reads the gauge (dial) of the skinfold caliper to the closest 0.5 mm or 1 mm (e.g., Lange caliper) to 0.1 mm or 0.2 mm (e.g., Harpenden caliper), depending on what type of caliper is used.

Number of Measurements

Although many technicians take two or three measurements at one site before moving on to another skinfold site, some make a complete circuit of the measurement sites, then repeat the circuit. The measurements should be repeated three times (three circuits) or more if the skinfold thicknesses differ by more than 10 %[42] or 2 mm.[4] If making consecutive measurements at the same site, the technician should give enough time to allow the skin to return to normal texture and thickness.[4] Either the median (middle) or mean value of the two or three trials is used for evaluation, depending on the instructions for the different skinfold equations. There is no need for a third measurement if the first two are the same for equations using median values.

Summary of General Procedures

1. The technician marks the sites to be measured on the right side of the participant's body.

2. The technician pinches the skinfold, at about 1 cm proximal to the marked site, using the thumb and index finger.
3. The jaw points of the caliper are placed on the marked site at a depth of about half the distance between the base of the normal skin perimeter and the crest of the fold.
4. The technician maintains a firm grip on the skinfold while reading the gauge of the skinfold caliper within 4 s to the closest 0.5–1 mm (e.g., Lange) or closest 0.1–0.2 mm (e.g., Harpenden).
5. The technician makes three circuits of skinfold measurements and records for each site during each circuit.
6. The technician uses the median value for analytical purposes.

Specific Procedures for Identifying and Marking Skinfold Sites

Each of the seven skinfold sites used in the Jackson and Pollock method should be identified and marked with a nontoxic marker prior to measuring skinfold thickness. A "cross" should be made at each site, with the long part of the cross identifying the axis of the skinfold. If the seven-site method is used, all seven sites including triceps, subscapula, chest, axilla, suprailium, abdomen, and thigh are marked and used. If the three-site method is used, for men the chest, abdomen, and thigh skinfold sites are used, and for women the triceps, suprailium, and thigh skinfold sites are used. A measuring tape should be used to identify the triceps and thigh skinfold sites. The description of the following skinfold sites corresponds closely with the methods described by Jackson and Pollock[20,23] and the *Anthropometric Standardization Reference Manual*.[18,27]

Triceps Skinfold (Figure 25.1a)

The participant bends the right arm at a right angle, keeping the elbow close to the side to mark the skinfold site. The

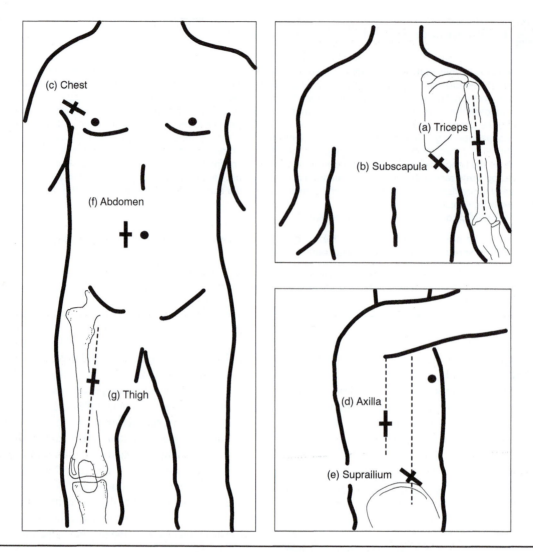

Figure 25.1 Locations for marking and measuring the seven skinfold sites for use with the Jackson and Pollock method for determining percent body fat. Skinfold sites include (a) triceps, (b) subscapula, (c) chest, (d) axilla, (e) suprailium, (f) abdomen, and (g) thigh.

tester identifies the posterior midline of the upper arm, the acromion process of the scapula, and the olecranon process of the ulna (elbow) of the participant. The **triceps skinfold** is a vertical skinfold taken in the posterior midline of the right upper arm, midway (as measured with a tape measure) between the acromion and olecranon processes. The arm should be straight, relaxed, and hanging at the participant's side during the measurement of the skinfold.

Subscapula Skinfold (Figure 25.1b)

The participant looks straight ahead with both shoulders relaxed. The tester identifies the inferior angle of the right scapula of the participant. The identification of the scapula may be accentuated by having the participant place the right hand in the middle of the back. Once the scapula is identified, the arm should be returned to the side. The **subscapula skinfold** is a diagonal skinfold running downward and laterally away from the inferiormost point of the right scapula.

Chest Skinfold (Figure 25.1c)

The tester identifies the axillary fold at the front of the right axilla (armpit) and the nipple of the right breast of the participant. The **chest skinfold** is a diagonal skinfold taken in a line one-half the distance in men and one-third the distance in women from the front of the axilla (axillary fold) to the nipple.

Axilla Skinfold (Figure 25.1d)

The participant places the right arm on the shoulder of the tester. The tester identifies the xiphoid process of the sternum and the midaxillary line below the right axilla. The **axilla skinfold** is a vertical skinfold in the midaxillary line at a point horizontal to the xiphoid process.

Suprailium Skinfold (Figure 25.1e)

The participant places the right arm on the shoulder of the tester. The tester identifies the ridge of fat that naturally runs along the suprailiac crest of the right side of the pelvis and the anterior axillary line (a line running vertically down from the front of the axilla). The **suprailium skinfold** is a diagonal skinfold taken along the natural ridge of fat over the iliac crest at the crossing of the anterior axillary line.

Abdomen Skinfold (Figure 25.1f)

The tester identifies the navel (umbilicus) of the participant. The **abdomen skinfold** is a vertical skinfold taken about 2 cm (1 in.) to the right of the navel.

Thigh Skinfold (Figure 25.1g)

The tester identifies the anterior midline of the right thigh, the inguinal fold (made by raising the right leg parallel to the floor), and the patella (knee cap) of the participant. The **thigh skinfold** is a vertical skinfold taken in the anterior midline of the right thigh midway (as measured with a tape measure) between the inguinal fold and the top of the patella.

Determining Percent Fat from Three Skinfold Sites by the Jackson and Pollock Method

The Jackson and Pollock methods of determining percent body fat actually provide numerous regression equations based on varying numbers of skinfold sites and circumference measures.[20,23] The equations shown below are those for estimating percent body fat based on gender, age, and the sum of three skinfold sites for men (Eq. 25.1a) and women (Eq. 25.1b).

$$D_B \text{ (Men)}^{20} = 1.10938 - (0.0008267 * SSF) + (0.0000016 * SSF^2) - (0.0002574 * Age) \quad \text{Eq. 25.1a}$$

Where: SSF (Men) = Sum (mm) of chest, abdomen, and thigh skinfolds

$$D_B \text{ (Women)}^{23} = 1.0994921 - (0.0009929 * SSF) + (0.0000023 * SSF^2) - (0.0001392 * Age) \quad \text{Eq. 25.1b}$$

Where: SSF (Women) = Sum (mm) of triceps, suprailium, and thigh skinfolds

$$\% \text{ Body Fat} = (495 / D_B) - 450 \quad \textit{Siri equation}^{36} \quad \text{Eq. 25.1c}$$

By way of example, the following data are provided for two participants. A 27-year-old man whose chest, abdomen, and thigh skinfolds total 82 mm, would have a body density of 1.045 g·ml^{-1} corresponding to a percent body fat of 24 % (Eq. 25.2a and 25.2b). A 32-year-old woman whose triceps, suprailium, and thigh skinfolds total 92 mm, would have a body density of 1.023 g·ml^{-1} corresponding to a percent body fat of 34 % (Eq. 25.2c and 25.2d). Percent body fat can also be determined knowing only the gender, age, and sum of three skinfold sites for the participant using Table 25.2.

Assume: **Man**, SSF = **82** mm, Age = **27** y

$$D_B \text{ (Men)} = 1.10938 - (0.0008267 * \mathbf{82}) + (0.0000016 * \mathbf{82}^2) - (0.0002574 * \mathbf{27}) = 1.045 \quad \text{Eq. 25.2a}$$

$$\% \text{ Fat (Men)} = (495 / \mathbf{1.045}) - 450 = \mathbf{24} \% \quad \text{Eq. 25.2b}$$

Assume: **Woman**, SSF = **92** mm, Age = **32** y

$$D_B \text{ (Women)} = 1.0994921 - (0.0009929 * \mathbf{92}) + (0.0000023 * \mathbf{92}^2) - (0.0001392 * \mathbf{32}) = 1.023 \quad \text{Eq. 25.2c}$$

$$\% \text{ Fat (Women)} = (495 / \mathbf{1.023}) - 450 = \mathbf{34} \% \quad \text{Eq. 25.2d}$$

Determining Percent Fat from Seven Skinfold Sites by the Jackson and Pollock Method

The equations below (Eq. 25.3a and 25.3b) provide a means of estimating body fat from the combination of all seven sites described in the Jackson and Pollock method. The calculations for the seven-site method are virtually the same as the three-site method, so no particular example is provided. Percent body fat can also be determined using the gender, age, and sum of seven skinfold sites for the participant using Table 25.3.

$$D_B \text{ (Men)}^{20} = 1.112 - (0.00043499 * SSF) + (0.00000055 * SSF^2) - (0.00028826 * Age) \quad \text{Eq. 25.3a}$$

$$D_B \text{ (Women)}^{23} = 1.097 - (0.00046971 * SSF) + (0.00000056 * SSF^2) - (0.00012828 * Age) \quad \text{Eq. 25.3b}$$

Where: SSF = Sum of triceps, subscapular, chest, axilla, suprailium, abdomen, and thigh

RESULTS AND DISCUSSION

The Jackson and Pollock method of determining percent body fat is only one of many methods based on the measurement of skinfold thickness and other anthropometric measures (i.e., circumferences, bone breadths). It was chosen for inclusion in this lab manual as the primary method of determining body fat from skinfolds for three main reasons. First, the authors of the method, Jackson and Pollock, have the well-deserved reputation of being an outstanding statistician and exercise physiologist, respectively. Second, the relationship between skinfold thickness and percent body fat was observed to be curvilinear, and as a result, the regression equations used to estimate percent fat were based on quadratic equations including the square of the sums of three or seven skinfold sites. Third, the samples used in deriving the methods were large (308 men and 249 women) and covered a wide range of ages (18–61 y in men and 18–55 y in women).

Table 25.4 can be used to evaluate percent body fat derived from either the three-site or seven-site Jackson and Pollock skinfold method. The male sample (*N* = 308), with a mean age of 32.6 y and mean body weight of 74.8 kg, averaged 59.4 mm for the sum of three skinfolds and

Table 25.2   Estimation of Percent Body Fat in Men and Women from Age and Sum of Three Skinfolds

Sum of 3 Skinfolds (mm)	Men (Chest, Abdomen, Thigh) Age (y)						Women (Triceps, Suprailium, Thigh) Age (y)					
	18–19	20–24	25–29	30–34	35–39	40–44	18–19	20–24	25–29	30–34	35–39	40–44
15–19	4	4	5	5	6	6	8	8	9	9	9	9
20–24	5	6	6	7	7	8	10	10	10	11	11	11
25–29	7	7	8	8	9	9	12	12	12	13	13	13
30–34	8	9	9	10	10	11	14	14	14	15	15	15
35–39	10	10	11	11	12	13	16	16	16	16	17	17
40–44	11	12	12	13	14	14	17	18	18	18	18	19
45–49	13	13	14	14	15	16	19	19	20	20	20	21
50–54	14	15	15	16	16	17	21	21	21	22	22	22
55–59	16	16	17	17	18	18	22	23	23	23	24	24
60–64	17	18	18	19	19	20	24	24	25	25	25	26
65–69	19	19	20	20	21	21	26	26	26	26	27	27
70–74	20	20	21	21	22	23	27	27	28	28	28	29
75–79	21	22	22	23	23	24	29	29	29	30	30	30
80–84	23	23	24	24	25	25	30	30	31	31	31	32
85–89	24	24	25	25	26	27	32	32	32	32	33	33
90–94	25	25	26	27	27	28	33	33	33	34	34	34
95–99	26	27	27	28	28	29	34	34	35	35	35	36
100–104	27	28	28	29	30	30	35	36	36	36	37	37
105–109	29	29	30	30	31	31	37	37	37	38	38	38
110–114	30	30	31	31	32	32	38	38	38	39	39	39
115–119	31	31	32	32	33	34	39	39	40	40	40	41
120–124	32	32	33	33	34	35	40	40	41	41	41	42
125–129	33	33	34	34	35	36	41	41	42	42	42	43
130–134	34	34	35	35	36	37	42	42	43	43	43	44
135–139	35	35	36	36	37	38	43	43	44	44	44	45
140–144	36	36	37	37	38	38	44	44	44	45	45	45
145–149	36	37	37	38	39	39	45	45	45	46	46	46
150–154	37	38	38	39	40	40	45	46	46	46	47	47
155–159	38	38	39	40	40	41	46	46	47	47	47	48
≥ 160	39	39	40	40	41	42	47	47	47	48	48	48

Sources: Values based on regression equations from Jackson & Pollock (1978) for men[20] and Jackson, Pollock, & Ward (1980) for women.[23]

122.8 mm for the sum of seven skinfolds, corresponding to a mean percent body fat of 17.7 %. The female sample ($N = 249$), with a mean age of 31.4 y and mean body weight of 57.2 kg, averaged 60.3 mm for the sum of three skinfolds and 122.7 mm for the sum of seven skinfolds, corresponding to a mean percent body fat of 24.1 %. Although the mean values for skinfold thickness are similar between men and women, women at the same skinfold thickness as men have about 7–10 % more body fat, which is necessary for childbirth and nursing.[29] It can also be noted from Table 25.2 and Table 25.3 that older persons (40–44 y) with the same skinfold sum as younger persons (18–19 y), have 2–3 % more body fat. This is because older adults store a greater proportion of body fat internally, especially in the visceral area.[29] This violates the assumption of the skinfold method that half the body fat is stored internally and half is stored subcutaneously. Older adults also demonstrate a decrease in skin thickness, an increase in skinfold compressibility, and a loss of bone density.[40] So,

the percent body fat of older adults is corrected statistically and their values are higher than younger adults at the same skinfold sum.

In fact, it is important to realize that any skinfold method should only be used on participants who are similar in age and gender to the sample on which that method was derived. That is to say, young adults (typically 18–55 y) should be assessed with a method derived on young adults, children or youth (under age 18 y) should be assessed with a method derived on children, and methods derived on older adults (typically over 55 or 65 y) should be used when testing older adults. Equations for estimating body fat from skinfolds in children and equations for older adults are found in Box 25.3. The older adult equations are derived from a three-component model (fat, water, and bone) that enhances their validity ($SEE = 2.9$ % and 3.8 % for men and women, respectively) compared with the Jackson and Pollock two—component models (fat and fat-free weight).[41] Other investigators have determined body fat

Table 25.3 Estimation of Percent Body Fat in Men and Women from Age and Sum of Seven Skinfolds (Chest, Axilla, Triceps, Subscapula, Abdomen, Suprailium, Thigh)

Sum of 7 Skinfolds (mm)	Men Age (y)						Women Age (y)					
	18–19	20–24	25–29	30–34	35–39	40–44	18–19	20–24	25–29	30–34	35–39	40–44
40–49	5	5	6	7	7	8	11	11	11	11	12	12
50–59	6	7	8	8	9	9	12	13	13	13	13	14
60–69	8	8	9	10	10	11	14	14	15	15	15	15
70–79	10	10	11	11	12	12	16	16	16	17	17	17
80–89	11	11	12	13	13	14	18	18	18	18	19	19
90–99	12	13	14	14	15	15	19	19	20	20	20	21
100–109	14	14	15	16	16	17	21	21	21	22	22	22
110–119	15	16	16	17	18	18	22	23	23	23	23	24
120–129	17	17	18	18	19	20	24	24	24	25	25	25
130–139	18	18	19	20	20	21	25	26	26	26	26	27
140–149	19	20	20	21	22	22	27	27	27	28	28	28
150–159	20	21	21	22	23	23	28	28	29	29	29	30
160–169	21	22	23	23	24	25	29	30	30	30	31	31
170–179	23	23	24	24	25	26	31	31	31	32	32	32
180–189	24	24	25	25	26	27	32	32	33	33	33	33
190–199	25	25	26	26	27	28	33	33	34	34	34	35
200–209	26	26	27	27	28	29	34	35	35	35	36	36
210–219	27	27	28	28	29	30	36	36	36	36	37	37
220–229	28	28	29	29	30	31	37	37	37	37	38	38
230–239	28	29	29	30	31	31	38	38	38	38	39	39
240–254	29	30	30	31	32	32	39	39	39	40	40	40
255–269	30	31	32	32	33	34	40	40	41	41	41	42
270–284	31	32	32	33	34	35	41	42	42	42	42	43
285–299	32	33	33	34	35	35	42	43	43	43	44	44
300–314	33	33	34	35	35	36	43	44	44	44	45	45
315–334	34	34	35	36	36	37	44	45	45	45	46	46
335–354	34	35	35	36	37	38	45	46	46	46	47	47
355–374	35	35	36	37	37	38	46	46	47	47	47	48
375–394	35	35	36	37	37	38	47	47	47	47	48	48
≥ 395	35	35	36	37	38	38	47	47	47	48	48	48

Sources: Values based on regression equations from Jackson & Pollock (1978)[20] for men and Jackson, Pollock, & Ward (1980)[23] for women.

Table 25.4 Category (Descriptor) for Sum of 3 and 7 Skinfold Thicknesses and Percent Body Fat (% Fat)

Category	Descriptor	Men (N = 308)			Women (N = 249)		
		Sum of 3	Sum of 7	% Fat	Sum of 3	Sum of 7	% Fat
Well above ave (> 95th %ile)	"Very lean"	< 19	< 37	< 4.5	< 30	< 56	< 12.2
Above ave (75th–95th %ile)	"Lean"	19–43	37–87	4.5–12.3	30–48	56–76	12.2–19.2
Average (25th–74th %ile)	"Average"	44–76	88–158	12.4–23.1	49–73	77–169	19.3–29.0
Below ave (5th–24th %ile)	"Overfat"	77–99	159–208	23.2–30.9	74–91	170–190	29.1–36.0
Well below ave (< 5th %ile)	"Obese"	> 99	> 208	> 30.9	> 91	> 190	> 36.0
Mean		59.4	122.6	17.7	60.3	122.7	24.1

Source: Data from Jackson & Pollock (1978)[20] and Jackson, Pollock & Ward (1980).[23] Values for percentiles are estimated using the reported means and standard deviations from the studies, assuming the data for all variables are normally distributed.

using a four component model (fat, water, bone, and residual).[15,31,40] These recently described methods should be considered along with the previously described methods when choosing an appropriate skinfold or anthropometric methodology. Still other studies have looked at the benefit of combining skinfolds with other additional anthropometric measures. Equations for estimating body density from skinfolds and circumferences[20,23] and for estimating body fat mass from skinfolds, circumferences, and bone breadths[14] are also included in Box 25.3.

BOX 25.3 Equations for Assessing Body Composition from Skinfolds and Anthropometry

Equations for Children (8 to 18 y)[37]

% Fat (Boys) = 1.0 + (0.735 ∗ SSF)
% Fat (Girls) = 5.1 + (0.610 ∗ SSF)
    Where: SSF = Sum of triceps and calf skinfolds (mm)
See Ref # 37 for specific details on measuring skinfolds.

Equations for Older Adults (34 to 84 y)[41]

% Fat (Men) = $(0.486 * SSF) - (0.0015 * SSF^2) + (0.067 * Age) - 3.83$
    Where: SSF = Sum (mm) of chest, subscapula, axilla and thigh skinfolds
% Fat (Women) = $(0.573 * SSF) - (0.0022 * SSF^2) + (0.107 * Age) - 9.35$
    Where: SSF = Sum of triceps, subscapula, abdomen and calf skinfolds (mm)
See Ref # 41 for specific details on measuring skinfolds.

Equations using Skinfolds and Circumferences[20,23]

D_B (Men) = $1.101 - (.0004115 * SSF) + (.00000069 * SSF^2) - (.00022631 * Age) - (.0059239 * C_w) + (.0190632 * C_F)$
    Where: SSF = Sum of triceps, subscapula, chest, axilla, suprailium, abdomen and thigh skinfolds (mm)
        C_w = Waist circumference (cm); C_F = Forearm circumference (cm)

D_B (Women) = $1.147 - (.00042359 * SSF) + (.00000061 * SSF^2) - (.000652 * C_H)$
    Where: SSF = Sum of triceps, subscapula, chest, axilla, suprailium, abdomen and thigh skinfolds (mm)
        C_H = Hip circumference (cm)
See Ref # 20 and # 23 for specific details on measuring skinfolds and circumferences.

Equations using Skinfolds, Circumferences, and Bone Breadths[14]

BFM (Men) = $-40.75 + (0.397 * C_W) + [6.568 * ((Log (SF_{TRI}) + Log (SF_{SUB}) + Log (SF_{ABD}))]$
    Where: BFM = Body fat mass (kg); C_W = Waist circumference (cm); Triceps, subscapula and abdomen SF (mm)
BFM (Women) = $-75.231 + (0.512 * C_H) + [8.889 * (Log (SF_{CHI}) + Log (SF_{TRI}) + Log (SF_{SUB})] + (1.905 * B_K)$
    Where: BFM = Body fat mass (kg); C_H = Hip circumference (cm); Chin, triceps, and subscapula skinfolds (mm)
        B_K = Knee breadth (cm)
See Ref # 14 for specific details on measuring skinfolds, circumferences and bone breadths.

BOX 25.4 Chapter Preview/Review

What is the rationale for using skinfold thickness to estimate percent body fat?

What is essential fat and stored fat?

How well do percent body fats estimated by skinfolds correlate with those measured hydrostatically?

What are the skinfold sites used in the three- and seven-site Jackson and Pollock methods?

How is a triceps skinfold specifically identified?

What is the average percent body fat of adult (18–55-year-old) men and women?

How is skinfold thickness affected by aging?

References

1. American Alliance for Health, Physical Education, Recreation and Dance (AAHPERD). (1980). *AAHPERD health-related physical fitness test.* Reston, VA: Author.

2. American Alliance for Health, Physical Education, Recreation and Dance (AAHPERD). (1985). *Norms for college students.* Reston, VA: Author.

3. American Alliance for Health, Physical Education, Recreation and Dance (AAHPERD). (1988). *Physical best.* Reston, VA: Author.

4. American College of Sports Medicine. (2000). *ACSM's guidelines for exercise testing and prescription* (pp. 60–66). Philadelphia: Lippincott Williams & Wilkins.

5. Becque, B. D., Katch, V. L., & Moffatt, K. J. (1986). Time course of skin-plus-fat compression in males and females. *Human Biology, 58,* 33–42.

6. Behnke, A. R., & Wilmore, J. H. (1974). *Evaluation and regulation of body build and composition.* Englewood Cliffs, NJ: Prentice-Hall.

7. Bouchard, C. (1985). General discussion of sports medicine. In A. F. Roche (Ed.), *Body-composition assessments in youth and adults* (p. 95). Columbus, OH: Ross Laboratories.

8. Bouchard, C. (1985). Reproducibility of body-composition and adipose-tissue measurements in

humans. In A. F. Roche (Ed.), *Body-composition assessments in youth and adults* (pp. 9–13). Columbus, OH: Ross Laboratories.

9. Brooks, G. A., Fahey, T. D., & White, T. P. (1996). *Exercise physiology: Human bioenergetics and its application.* Mountain View, CA: Mayfield.

10. Carlyon, R., Bryant, R., Gore, C., & Walker, R. (1998). Apparatus for precision calibration of skinfold calipers. *American Journal of Human Biology, 10,* 689–697.

11. Cataldo, D., & Heyward, V. H. (2000). Pinch an inch: A comparison of several high-quality and plastic skinfold calipers. *ACSM's Health and Fitness Journal, 4*(3), 12–16.

12. Cureton, K. J. (1984). A reaction to the manuscript of Jackson. *Medicine and Science in Sports and Exercise, 16,* 621–622.

13. Dugdale, A. E., & Griffiths, M. (1979). Estimating fat body mass from anthropometric data. *American Journal of Clinical Nutrition, 32,* 2400–2403.

14. Garcia, A., Wagner, K., Hothorn, T., Koebnick, C., Zunft, H., & Trippo, U. (2005). Improved prediction of body fat by measuring skinfold thickness, circumferences, and bone breadths. *Obesity Research, 13,* 626–634.

15. Goran, M., Toth, M., & Poehlman, E. (1997). Cross-validation of anthropometric and bioelectrical resistance prediction equations for body composition in older people using the 4-compartment model as a criterion method. *Journal of the American Geriatric Society, 45,* 837–843.

16. Gore, C. J., Carlyon, R. G., Franks, S. W., & Woolford, S. M. (2000). Skinfold thickness varies directly with spring coefficient and inversely with jaw pressure. *Medicine and Science in Sports and Exercise, 32,* 540–546.

17. Gruber, J. J., Pollock, M. L., Graves, J. E., Colvin, A. B., & Braith, R. W. (1990). Comparison of Harpenden and Lange calipers in predicting body composition. *Research Quarterly for Exercise and Sport, 61,* 184–190.

18. Harrison, G. G., Buskirk, E. R., Carter, J. E. L., Johnston, F. E., Lohman, T. G., Pollock, M. L., Roche, A. F., & Wilmore, J. H. (1988). Skinfold thicknesses and measurement technique. In T. G. Lohman, A. F. Roche, & R. Martorell (Eds.), *Anthropometric standardization reference manual* (pp. 55–70). Champaign, IL: Human Kinetics.

19. Israel, R. G., Houmard, J. A., O'Brien, K. F., McCammon, M. R., Zamora, B. S., & Eaton, A. W. (1989). Validity of a near-infrared spectrophotometry device for estimating human body composition. *Research Quarterly for Exercise and Sport, 60,* 379–383.

20. Jackson, A. S., & Pollock, M. L. (1978). Generalized equations for predicting body density of men. *British Journal of Nutrition, 40,* 497–504.

21. Jackson, A. S., & Pollock, M. L. (1985). Practical assessment of body composition. *The Physician and Sportsmedicine, 13*(5), 76–80, 82–90.

22. Jackson, A. S., Pollock, M. L., Graves, J. E., & Mahar, M. T. (1988). Reliability and validity of bioelectrical impedance in determining body composition. *Journal of Applied Physiology, 64,* 529–534.

23. Jackson, A. S., Pollock, M. L., & Ward, A. (1980). Generalized equations for predicting body density of women. *Medicine and Science in Sports and Exercise, 12,* 175–182.

24. Kolkhorst, F. W., & Dolgener, F. A. (1994). Nonexercise model fails to predict aerobic capacity in college students with high $\dot{V}O_2$ peak. *Research Quarterly for Exercise and Sport, 65,* 78–83.

25. Lohman, T. G. (1987). *Measuring body fat using skinfolds* [Video]. Champaign, IL: Human Kinetics.

26. Lohman, T. G., Pollock, M. L., Slaughter, M. H., Brandon, L. J., & Boileau, R. A. (1984). Methodological factors and the predicting of body fat in female athletes. *Medicine and Science in Sports and Exercise, 16,* 92–96.

27. Lohman, T. G., Roche, A. F., & Martorell, R. (Eds.). (1988). *Anthropometric standardization reference manual.* Champaign, IL: Human Kinetics.

28. Martorell, R., Mendoza, F., Mueller, W. H., & Pawson, I. G. (1988). Which side to measure: Right or left? In A. F. Roche (Ed.), *Body-composition assessments in youth and adults* (pp. 73–78). Columbus, OH: Ross Laboratories.

29. McArdle, W. D., Katch, F. I., & Katch, V. L. (1996). *Exercise physiology: Energy, nutrition, and human performance* (4th ed.). Baltimore: Williams & Wilkins.

30. Nieman, D. C. (1999). *Exercise testing and prescription: A health-related approach.* Mountain View, CA: Mayfield.

31. Peterson, M., Czerwinski, S., & Siervogel, R. (2003). Development and validation of skinfold-thickness prediction equations with a 4-compartment model. *Clinical Nutrition, 77,* 1186–1191.

32. Pollock, M. L., Garzarella, L., & Graves, J. E. (1995). The measurement of body composition. In P. J. Maud & Carl Foster (Eds.), *Physiological assessment of human fitness* (pp. 167–204). Champaign, IL: Human Kinetics.

33. Pollock, M. L., & Jackson, A. S. (1984). Research progress in validation of clinical methods of assessing body composition. *Medicine and Science in Sports and Exercise, 16,* 606–613.

34. Pollock, M. L., Schmidt, D. H., & Jackson, A. S. (1980). Measurement of cardiorespiratory fitness and body composition in the clinical setting. *Comprehensive Therapy, 6,* 12–27.

35. Sinning, W. E., Dolny, D. G., Little, K. D., Cunningham, L. N., Racaniello, A., Siconolfi, S. F., & Sholes, J. L. (1985). Validity of "generalized"

equations for body composition in male athletes. *Medicine and Science in Sports and Exercise, 17,* 124–130.

36. Siri, W. E. (1961). *Body composition from fluid spaces and density: Analysis of methods in techniques for measuring body composition.* Washington, DC: National Academy of Science, National Research Council.

37. Slaughter, M. H., Lohman, T. G., Boileau, R. A., Horswill, C. A., Stillman, R. J., Van Loan, M. D., & Bemben, D. A. (1988). Skinfold equations for estimation of body fatness in children and youth. *Human Biology, 60,* 709–723.

38. Stout, J. R., Eckerson, J. M., Housh, T. J., Johnson, G.O., & Betts, N. M. (1994). Validity of percent body fat estimations in males. *Medicine and Science in Sports and Exercise, 26,* 632–636.

39. Thorland, W. G., Johnson, G. O., & Tharp, G. D. (1984). Validity of anthropometric equations for the estimation of body density in adolescent athletes. *Medicine and Science in Sports and Exercise, 16,* 77–81.

40. van der Ploeg, G., Gunn, S., Withers, R., & Modra, A. (2003). Use of anthropometric variables to predict relative body fat determined by a four-compartment body composition model. *European Journal of Clinical Nutrition, 57,* 1009–1016.

41. Williams, D. P., Going, S. B., Lohman, T. G., Hewitt, M. J., & Haber, A. E. (1992). Estimation of body fat from skinfold thickness in middle-aged and older men and women: A multiple component approach. *American Journal of Human Biology, 4,* 595–605.

42. Williams, D. P., Going, S. B., Milliken, L. A., Hall, M.C., & Lohman, T. G. (1995). Practical techniques for assessing body composition in middle-aged and older adults. *Medicine and Science in Sports and Exercise, 27,* 776–783.

Form 25.1
SKINFOLDS

Homework

Gender: **M** Initials: **AA** Age (y): **30** Height (cm): **163** Weight (kg): **89.0**

	T_1	T_2	T_3	Median	
Triceps *(closest 0.5 mm)*	18.0	18.5	18.0	_____ mm	
Subscapular skinfold	27.0	26.0	25.0	_____ mm	_____ mm
Chest skinfold *	17.0	16.0	17.0	_____ mm	* Sum of 3 skinfolds
Axilla skinfold	30.0	30.0	28.5	_____ mm	
Suprailium skinfold	21.5	21.0	20.5	_____ mm	_____ mm
Abdomen skinfold *	34.0	35.5	34.0	_____ mm	Sum of 7 skinfolds
Thigh skinfold *	27.0	26.0	25.0	_____ mm	

3-Site $D_B = 1.10938 - [0.0008267 * \underline{\quad}_{\text{SF sum}}] + [0.0000016 * \underline{\quad}^2_{\text{SF sum}}] - [0.0002574 * \underline{\quad}_{\text{Age}}]$

% Fat = (495 / _____) − 450 = _____ %   *Table 25.2* : _____ %   Category: _____   *Table 25.4*
(under: D_B)

7-Site $D_B = 1.112 - [0.00043499 * \underline{\quad}_{\text{SF sum}}] + [0.00000055 * \underline{\quad}^2_{\text{SF sum}}] - [0.00028826 * \underline{\quad}_{\text{Age}}]$

% Fat = (495 / _____) − 450 = _____ %   *Table 25.3* : _____ %   Category: _____   *Table 25.4*
(under: D_B)

Evaluation _____

_____

Gender: **F** Initials: **BB** Age (y): **23** Height (cm): **158** Weight (kg): **73.6**

	T_1	T_2	T_3	Median	
Triceps * *(closest 0.5 mm)*	30.0	30.0	30.0	_____ mm	
Subscapular skinfold	22.0	21.0	21.0	_____ mm	_____ mm
Chest skinfold	18.5	18.0	18.0	_____ mm	* Sum of 3 skinfolds
Axilla skinfold	16.0	17.0	16.5	_____ mm	
Suprailium skinfold *	15.5	15.5	14.5	_____ mm	_____ mm
Abdomen skinfold	28.0	29.0	29.0	_____ mm	Sum of 7 skinfolds
Thigh skinfold *	32.0	31.5	33.0	_____ mm	

3-Site $D_B = 1.0994921 - [0.0009929 * \underline{\quad}_{\text{SF sum}}] + [0.0000023 * \underline{\quad}^2_{\text{SF sum}}] - [0.0001392 * \underline{\quad}_{\text{Age}}]$

% Fat = (495 / _____) − 450 = _____ %   *Table 25.2* : _____ %   Category: _____   *Table 25.4*
(under: D_B)

7-Site $D_B = 1.097 - [0.00046971 * \underline{\quad}_{\text{SF sum}}] + [0.00000056 * \underline{\quad}^2_{\text{SF sum}}] - [0.00012828 * \underline{\quad}_{\text{Age}}]$

% Fat = (495 / _____) − 450 = _____ %   *Table 25.3* : _____ %   Category: _____   *Table 25.4*
(under: D_B)

Evaluation _____

_____

Form 25.2

SKINFOLDS

NAME _____ DATE _____ SCORE _____

Lab Results

Gender: **M**   Initials: _____   Age (y): _____   Height (cm): _____   Weight (kg): _____

	T_1	T_2	T_3	Median	
Triceps *(closest 0.5 mm)*	____	____	____	____	mm
Subscapular skinfold	____	____	____	____	mm
Chest skinfold *	____	____	____	____	mm
Axilla skinfold	____	____	____	____	mm
Suprailium skinfold	____	____	____	____	mm
Abdomen skinfold *	____	____	____	____	mm
Thigh skinfold *	____	____	____	____	mm

_____ mm   * Sum of 3 skinfolds

_____ mm   Sum of 7 skinfolds

3-Site $D_B = 1.10938 - [\,0.0008267 * \underline{\quad}_{\text{SF sum}}\,] + [\,0.0000016 * \underline{\quad}_{\text{SF sum}}{}^2\,] - [\,0.0002574 * \underline{\quad}_{\text{Age}}\,]$

% Fat = (495 / _____$_{D_B}$) − 450 = _____ %   *Table 25.2 :* _____ %   Category: _____   *Table 25.4*

7-Site $D_B = 1.112 - [\,0.00043499 * \underline{\quad}_{\text{SF sum}}\,] + [\,0.00000055 * \underline{\quad}_{\text{SF sum}}{}^2\,] - [\,0.00028826 * \underline{\quad}_{\text{Age}}\,]$

% Fat = (495 / _____$_{D_B}$) − 450 = _____ %   *Table 25.3 :* _____ %   Category: _____   *Table 25.4*

Evaluation _____

_____

Gender: **F**   Initials: _____   Age (y): _____   Height (cm): _____   Weight (kg): _____

	T_1	T_2	T_3	Median	
Triceps * *(closest 0.5 mm)*	____	____	____	____	mm
Subscapular skinfold	____	____	____	____	mm
Chest skinfold	____	____	____	____	mm
Axilla skinfold	____	____	____	____	mm
Suprailium skinfold *	____	____	____	____	mm
Abdomen skinfold	____	____	____	____	mm
Thigh skinfold *	____	____	____	____	mm

_____ mm   * Sum of 3 skinfolds

_____ mm   Sum of 7 skinfolds

3-Site $D_B = 1.0994921 - [\,0.0009929 * \underline{\quad}_{\text{SF sum}}\,] + [\,0.0000023 * \underline{\quad}_{\text{SF sum}}{}^2\,] - [\,0.0001392 * \underline{\quad}_{\text{Age}}\,]$

% Fat = (495 / _____$_{D_B}$) − 450 = _____ %   *Table 25.2 :* _____ %   Category: _____   *Table 25.4*

7-Site $D_B = 1.097 - [\,0.00046971 * \underline{\quad}_{\text{SF sum}}\,] + [\,0.00000056 * \underline{\quad}_{\text{SF sum}}{}^2\,] - [\,0.00012828 * \underline{\quad}_{\text{Age}}\,]$

% Fat = (495 / _____$_{D_B}$) − 450 = _____ %   *Table 25.3 :* _____ %   Category: _____   *Table 25.4*

Evaluation _____

_____

CHAPTER

HYDROSTATIC WEIGHING

Hydrostatic weighing is often referred to as underwater weighing because the participant's weight is measured while being submerged in water. Researchers also refer to it as hydrodensitometry because its unit of measure is body density in units of grams per milliliter (g·ml^{-1}). A multicomponent model utilizing the combination of dual-energy X-ray absorptiometry (DXA), isotope dilution, and hydrodensitometry "is now widely recognized as the 'gold standard' in body composition assessment,"[57] meaning that it is the criterion by which other methods are compared. Despite hydrostatic weighing's prominent position among tests of body composition, it can qualify as a simple field test under certain conditions. For example, hydrostatic weighings can be performed in any body of water, such as jacuzzis, swimming pools, or lakes. By indirectly predicting residual volume, rather than measuring it, the hydrostatic technique is greatly simplified. However, when residual volume is measured directly and the underwater weight is measured under controlled conditions, it truly is a laboratory test, not a field test.

PHYSICAL AND ANATOMICAL RATIONALES

The rationales for hydrostatic weighing are based on the interaction between physical and anatomical factors. For example, the buoyancy of the human body during hydrostatic weighing is affected by its anatomical compartments, some being more buoyant or less dense than others.

Fat can be disadvantageous, both mechanically and aesthetically, because its density—that is, weight (mass) for any given volume—is lower than lean tissue. Thus, 1 kg of fat occupies more volume than 1 kg of muscle (Figure 26.1).

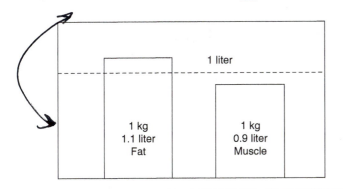

Figure 26.1 Because the density of fat is less than that of muscle, 1 kg of fat occupies a greater volume than 1 kg of muscle.

This means that different gains in circumference occur even if identical weight gains are from fat storage or from muscle growth (e.g., muscle hypertrophy). Thus, if two people of identical stature and body mass were of different body compositions, the leaner person would occupy less space than the fatter person.

Physical Rationale

Hydrostatic weighing, or densitometry, is a method for determining the density of the human body. Once the density of the body is known, equations can be used to convert it to percent body fat. The density (D) of any object is a function of its mass (M) per unit volume (V) and may be calculated as seen in Equation 26.1a. Therefore, density of the body is equal to body mass divided by body volume (Eq. 26.1b).

Density (g·ml^{-1}) = Mass (g) / Volume (ml)   Eq. 26.1a

Body density (D$_B$) = Body mass (BM)
    / Body volume (BV)   Eq. 26.1b

Thus the density (g·ml^{-1}) of the body can be determined by knowing the mass (or weight) of the body in grams and the volume of the body in milliliters.[6] The normal mass of the body weighed on a scale is referred to as body mass in air (Body mass$_{AIR}$). When weighed totally immersed underwater, the mass of the body is referred to as body mass in water (Body mass$_{WATER}$). From Archimedes' principle we know that "a body immersed in water is buoyed up with a force equal to the weight of the water displaced."[7,10] In other words, the apparent loss in mass between the body mass-in-air and the body mass-in-water is equal to the mass (or weight) of the water displaced (Eq. 26.2a). Once the mass of the water displaced is known, the volume of the water can be determined by dividing the mass of the water by the density of the water (Eq. 26.2b). This volume of water is assumed to be equal to body volume.

Mass of water displaced = (Body mass$_{AIR}$
    − Body mass$_{WATER}$)   Eq. 26.2a

Volume of water = (Body mass$_{AIR}$ − Body mass$_{WATER}$)
    / Density$_{WATER}$ Eq. 26.2b

An example of water displacement would be when a person enters a spa or Jacuzzi filled completely to the top. If all of the water that spills over the brim is collected as the person completely submerges under the water, then the mass of that collected water is equal to the mass lost by the person due to submersion. The mass of the displaced water can therefore either be measured directly by displacement (volumetric method) or measured indirectly by use of Archimedes' principle (underwater weighing method). Typically, most laboratories measure the mass of the submerged body rather than the volume of the displaced water.

Anatomical Rationale

The rationale for hydrostatic weighing is based on dividing the total body mass into two compartments, or components. This method is described as a two-compartment or two-component model. Most studies use the term *compartment*, but some investigators use the term *component* instead. The two compartments into which the total body mass is separated are the fat mass and the fat-free mass, as seen in Equation 26.3a. From this compartmentalization, the percent body fat can then be determined by dividing the fat mass by the total body mass (Eq. 26.3b).

Total body mass (TBM) = Fat mass (FM)
  + Fat-free mass (FFM)   Eq. 26.3a

% Fat = (Fat mass / Total body mass) * 100   Eq. 26.3b

The fat mass is stored mainly in fat cells or adipocytes. However, not even this fat is all fat—fat cells are about 62 % pure fat, 31 % water, and 7 % protein.[49] The fat-free mass is composed mainly of muscle and bone tissue, and secondarily of skin, blood, brain, and organs.[3] The primary constituents of fat-free mass are water, mineral, protein, and glycogen.[4] Although the terms fat-free mass (FFM) and lean body mass (LBM) are often used interchangeably, the LBM is actually a slightly greater mass than the FFM because the LBM includes some essential fat found inside internal organs, bone marrow, and the central nervous system.

Interaction of Physical and Anatomical Rationales

Because fat is less dense than lean body mass, fat weighs less than fat-free tissue when both are placed in water. Thus, greater differences between the person's mass on land (in air) versus the mass in water mean lower densities and, consequently, higher fat percentages.

When the body density is known, that number is inserted into another equation that relates it to the density of lean and fat tissue. Figure 26.1 depicts the fact that a less dense tissue, such as fat, occupies more space (volume) than that of a more dense tissue, such as muscle, at any given mass.[9] This concept can be stated another way: The mass of a less dense tissue is less than the mass of a more dense tissue for any given volume. Bone has a density of 1.280 $g \cdot ml^{-1}$, lean tissue a density of 1.100, and fat a density of 0.9001, all compared to 1.000 $g \cdot ml^{-1}$, the density of water.[3] As a result, bone and lean tissue both have a tendency to sink in water due to their greater density, whereas fat floats because it is less dense than water.

METHODS OF HYDROSTATIC WEIGHING

There are at least two methods to determine body density from the submersion of a human in water. One of these methods, the volumetric method, uses a narrow, cylindrical chamber (a volumeter or a spill-over burette) that facilitates the measurement of the displaced water from the submerged human. The conversion of this volume change to a density measure was first proposed in 1942.[7] The hydrostatic weighing method derives body volume by determining body density from the mass of the body when completely submerged in water. Body density is the technique that is the focus of this manual. Box 26.1 contains a discussion of the accuracy of hydrostatic weighing.

Equipment

Scale

For nearly 50 years, most laboratories used the spring-loaded Chatillon autopsy scale to weigh a person underwater. It resembles a supermarket's produce scale and usually has a maximum range of 9 kg to 15 kg (Figure 26.2). In the 9 kg autopsy scale, there are 1 kg, 2 kg, and 3 kg (1000 g, 2000 g, and 3000 g) markers on the main face of the dial; another gauge is on the cycle bar extending from the bottom of the scale, which represents the number of cycles made by the main dial's pointer. For example, if the

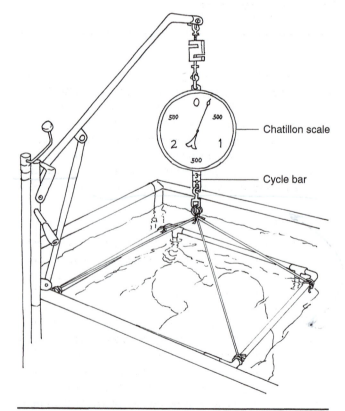

Figure 26.2 A participant's body mass is measured underwater to determine body density.

BOX 26.1 Accuracy of Hydrostatic Weighing

Although hydrostatic weighing is often considered a gold standard of body composition methods, it does receive some criticism.

Reliability

The reliability of body densitometry is high ($r \geq 0.95$).[15,58] This obviously can vary with the experience of the investigators, the accuracy of the equipment, and the experience and control of the participant. Correlative statistics, however, are not always the best reflector of the repeatability of a test. Statistics may produce high correlations on a heterogeneous group (e.g., widely varied in fat content). Thus, both the correlation values and the standard error values should be used to interpret the accuracy of a test.

Validity

Its validity has been questioned mainly because of the limitations of the cadaver studies that have provided the typical tissue densities. For example, a classic equation for predicting body fat from body density is based upon a sample of only six cadavers.[12] In a study of 12 cadavers, investigators revealed a much larger variability in muscle and body density than originally supposed.[36] The 1.100 g·ml^{-1} density value for lean tissue used in the equation to predict body fat now is recognized as a varying value in various population subgroups. For example, the densities of children (1.085), blacks (1.113), and the elderly, especially the lower values in postmenopausal women,[24] differ significantly. The greater skeletal densities of black males[2,55] contribute to their greater lean tissue density. Children have lower densities than adults due to their greater water concentration and lower bone mineral levels in their lean tissue component.[14] Older adults also have a less dense skeleton than younger adults. Thus, unless specific population equations[1,26,46,47] are used, the fat percentage will be underestimated or overestimated when using such popular equations as the Brozek and the Siri equations.

The variability of the volume component of the density value is a major problem with hydrostatic weighing; consequently, this problem transfers to all of the other anthropometric methods, such as girths and skinfolds, that predict the hydrostatically determined body density. The problem is not with the density of fat but with that of the highly variable density of the fat-free mass.[40] The standard error of the estimate by hydrostatic weighing is about 2.5 % body fat,[47] with most of this error attributed to biological variability, not measurement error.[49,50] Ideally, to reduce inherent errors in the two-compartment models or equations (Brozek and Siri), laboratory procedures should measure not only body density but also total body water and bone mineral density. Although equations using the combination of three or four components were once rare,[27] such equations are now available.[1,26]

Errors in body density up to 10 % may result from estimating residual volume.[32] An average error of 0.7 % body fat units occurs for each error of 100 ml in lung volume; the error may accumulate to 3.6 % body fat units.[60] Indirectly measuring residual volume by using the standard 24 % and 28 % vital capacity values for men and women, respectively, may overestimate the residual volume of persons with large vital capacities. Hence, the accuracy of densitometry is improved by directly measuring the residual lung volume (RV) rather than by predicting it from regression equations or from a certain percentage of the vital capacity.[39]

---

large-faced dial is at 1500 g (1.5 kg), and the protruding bar is between the 2 and 3, then the actual underwater body mass is 7.5 kg or 7500 g [(2 cycles × 3000 g) + 1500].

Presently, the choice of scale is the strain-gauge, load-cell, or force-transducer scale, which is more precise, is more accurate, and can be interfaced with a recorder and/or a computer.[1,37,43] A regular platform scale may be used to measure the participant's body mass in air (BM$_a$).

Water Tank

Water tanks vary in style and weight (e.g., redwood, cedar, plexiglass, stainless steel, fiberglass, tile, etc.), but are usually similar in size—just large enough to allow the participant to sit (usually) totally submerged in the water without touching the bottom or sides of the tank. The water tanks include a water filter and heater. The mass of a body immersed in a fluid varies according to the temperature of the fluid. The temperature of the water can be monitored with a water thermometer, such as a basic pool thermometer. The water density may be monitored with a hydrometer or be derived from an appropriate table for water temperature versus density (Table 26.1). People are more buoyant in cool water than in warm water.

Table 26.1 Relationship Between Water Temperature (*T*w) and Water Density (Dw)

*T*w °C	*T*w °F	Dw g·ml^{-1}		*T*w °C	*T*w °F	Dw g·ml^{-1}
0	32	0.999		32	90	0.9950
4	39	1.000	Comfort	33	91	0.9947
24	75	0.9973		34	93	0.9944
25	77	0.9971		35	95	0.9941
26	79	0.9968		36	97	0.9937
27	81	0.9965	Range	37	99	0.9934
28	82	0.9963		38	100	0.9930
29	84	0.9960		39	102	0.9926
30	86	0.9957		40	104	0.9922
31	88	0.9954				

Lung Volume Equipment

The direct measurement of residual volume (RV) is preferred when underwater weighing is performed. RV can be measured by helium dilution, in which case a helium analyzer is required, or by nitrogen washout, requiring a nitrogen analyzer. Another simplified method, described in Chapter 20, is known as the oxygen dilution method and can be done with an oxygen analyzer and a carbon dioxide analyzer.[63] This method is convenient because many exercise laboratories already possess these analyzers for metabolic measurement. Additional equipment (mouthpieces, valves, breathing bags, etc.) is needed for these methods, as is a supply of the required gas (helium or oxygen). To avoid the difficulty and expense of directly measuring RV, some laboratories choose to estimate RV from some other measure of lung function, usually from a measured vital capacity (VC). VC is measured with a spirometer or pneumotachometer, after which various methods can be used to estimate RV.

Participant Preparation

It is best to have participants somewhat fasted (3–4 h) prior to completing the underwater weighing so that the last meal has had a chance to move through the gastrointestinal (GI) tract. Instruct participants not to eat 3–4 h prior to the underwater weighing, and to attempt to rid the body of all fluids, solids, and gas by urinating and defecating before arriving in the laboratory. They should further avoid eating gas-producing foods 12 h prior to the test. This is all to help get as true a body weight as possible on land, and to help the participant sink and weigh as much as possible underwater. Even with proper preparation, gas can be trapped in the GI tract, which can reduce the underwater weight. For this reason, many laboratories add 100 ml to the residual lung volume to help account for trapped GI gas. Proper hydration is also important. Participants should not be hypohydrated, nor should they be hyperhydrated. Some investigators advise against testing females who are retaining water due to their menstrual cycle,[13,30] while others find the fluid retention during normal menstruation is not enough to affect the body density.[16] In any case, it should be recognized that a hydration change equivalent to about 1 kg to 2 kg of body weight may affect the percent body fat estimation by hydrostatic weighing.[25]

Participants should wear a swimsuit to avoid trapping air in the clothing when submerged under the water. A small nylon swimsuit is preferred over other possible clothing. Loose fitting or baggy shorts and shirts should not be worn. If skinfold measurements are to be taken at the same time, a two-piece swimsuit is preferred for women so that it does not interfere with the marking and measurement of the skinfolds. All jewelry should be removed, if possible, including necklaces, bracelets, watches, earrings, and other body jewelry. Gold jewelry can add to the participant's underwater weight because it has a density of 19.3 $g \cdot ml^{-1}$, about 18 times heavier than an equivalent volume of muscle. To help keep the tank clean, participants are strongly encouraged to shower just before the test to remove body oils and lotions. The participant should also be instructed to bring a towel and a change of clothing.

Technician Preparation

The technician ensures that the water in the tank is clean, chlorinated appropriately, and at a comfortable temperature. Water temperature should range between 32 and 36 °C. The water temperature should be recorded during the test so that the density of the water can be determined (Table 26.1). Water that is cooler and harder (due to increased mineral content) is denser and will therefore increase the buoyancy of the participant. The technician should determine the tare weight of the hydrostatic weighing apparatus (i.e., the chair, supporting cables, other supporting materials, and possibly a weight belt) at the water level likely to be encountered during the underwater weighing. This tare weight typically ranges from 3 to 6 kg[41] and needs to be taken into account in the calculation of body density. If an electronic load-scale cell is being used, instead of a Chatillon scale or its equivalent, the tare weight can be removed electronically such that the weight displayed is already the net underwater weight, and no adjustment for tare weight is necessary. A swimmer's noseclip should be available if the participant requests one to assist in exhaling as much air from the lungs as possible. All preparations associated with the measurement of RV or VC should also be completed before the test. Lastly, because of the possible risk associated with water immersion and maximal lung exhalation, it is good practice to have participants complete an informed consent process so that they are fully informed of any risks involved (drowning, water aspiration, dizziness, etc.) prior to the test.

Procedures

Besides comforting and positioning the participant, three other concerns in the hydrostatic weighing procedures are to account for essential air, to eliminate excess air, and to read the underwater weight accurately.

Nonessential and Essential Air

In addition to fat, only two other parts of the body float: (1) the nonessential air trapped in hair, and (2) the essential air compartments in the lungs and the gastrointestinal (GI) tract.

Nonessential Air

The first thing the participant should do upon entering the water is to dunk under the water and then press the hands against the suit and body hairs in order to push the pockets of nonessential air from these sources. Nylon bathing suits trap air to a lesser extent than most conventional suits.

Essential GI Air

The GI air is a constant value of 100 ml assumed for all persons. But gas-producing foods and GI disturbances can increase this value to several hundred milliliters.[49]

Essential Lung Air

The lung volume can be any known volume, such as total lung capacity (TLC), functional residual capacity (FRC), or residual volume (RV). The person does not have to expel air during submersion if using the TLC, FRC, or partial expiration methods. These methods are more comfortable than the RV method but less common.[38] The FRC,[53] TLC,[17,54,59] and partial expiration[33] methods appear to be as accurate as the RV method. The TLC or partial exhalation methods may be especially convenient for testing the older adult.[34,52]

The **RV method** of underwater weighing calls for the person to rid the body of all lung air except the residual air by exhaling maximally. Usually, the person is in the seated position and moves the head toward the knees during the effort to expel the air. The technician can observe the formed bubbles of air as they escape from the participant's mouth to the surface of the water. As long as there are noticeable bubbles, the participant still is not down to residual volume. The amount of time that participants can remain underwater while exhaling to residual volume is quite variable. Typically, it is 5–10 s, but some persons remain totally submerged for 15 s or more.[54]

Although a true research laboratory test of hydrostatic weighing would include the direct measurement of RV, it is possible to modify the hydrostatic test so that the RV is predicted by equations from either the prior measurement of vital capacity for men (Eq. 26.4a) or women (Eq. 26.4b).[62] Sometimes the vital capacity is measured with the person submerged to the neck.[52]

Men: $RV \ (L) = 24 \% \ (or \ 0.24) * VC_{BTPS}$ Eq. 26.4a

Women: $RV \ (L) = 28 \% \ (or \ 0.28) * VC_{BTPS}$ Eq. 26.4b

Reading the Scale for Underwater Weight

The technician does not have much time to read the oscillating pointer or digital display of the autopsy scale or force transducer, respectively. The time may depend upon the participant's breath-holding ability and the degree of oscillation of the scale. Force transducers reduce fluctuations, compared with spring autopsy scales, but do not eliminate them.[43] The oscillations may depend upon the size of the tank, larger tanks requiring greater time. The oscillations should be small enough to be read to the nearest 20 g[29] or 25 g. However, it is not unusual to be able to read it to only the nearest 50 g. The technician reads the midpoint of the oscillations or the consistently highest value. The oscillations can be dampened if the technician loosely grasps the chair with the fingers while the participant submerges. Before reading the scale, the technician should check to be sure that all parts of the person's body are submerged and that no air bubbles are visible. When the technician is satisfied with the reading, a prearranged signal (e.g., knocking on the tank) may be given to let the participant know it is time to surface. However, all participants should feel free to ascend according to their own comfort.

The number of trials may vary according to the experience of the participants. Usually, submerged persons will reach their consistently highest expiratory capacities (hence, heaviest weights), within 5 to 12 trials. Some technicians repeat the procedure until 3 trials are within 100 g of each other.[62] Others may exclude the heaviest underwater body mass and use only the mean of the next two highest masses for the body density equations.[31] Other researchers use either the average of the last 2 or 3 trials or the average of the two heaviest weighings. Ideally, none of the readings used to calculate the average should differ by more than 100 g.[8,45]

Summary of Procedures

1. The technician records the participant's age, height, and body weight. If other anthropometric measurements are to be made (e.g., skinfolds, circumferences, bone diameters), they are also made and recorded at this time.
2. The technician measures and records either the participant's residual volume or vital capacity prior to the underwater weighing. (Ideally, the volume of air in the participant's lungs at the actual time of the underwater weighing would be measured, but this presents numerous logistical challenges and is infrequently done.)
3. The participant carefully enters the tank dressed only in a swimsuit, briefly submerges to wet the hair and suit, and makes an attempt to further remove all trapped air from the hair and suit.
4. The participant, before getting into the chair, submerges to chin level so that the technician can record the tare weight, or set the electronic scale to zero so that net underwater weight can be directly recorded. The technician also records the water temperature at this time.
5. The participant then gets into the chair. The participant may strap on a weighted belt at this point, if part of the protocol. The participant may also affix a swimmer's noseclip to the nose, if so desired and available. It is also a good idea for any participant with long hair to have a hair tie to keep the hair out of the face upon surfacing.
6. The technician directs the participant on how to sit properly in the chair, how to submerge fully under the water by pulling the head down to the knees (if seated), and how to exhale forcefully and maximally as much air from the lungs as possible (assuming the goal is to reach RV).
7. The participant begins to exhale and slowly bends forward to submerge the head and shoulders under the water until the entire body is fully submerged. The technician at this point dampens the oscillations of the scale by lightly holding onto the chair and watches for no more bubbles to appear. The participant continues to exhale toward RV.

8. Once it appears that all bubbles have stopped and the participant is at RV, usually near the 10th second, the technician lets go of the chair, reads and records the underwater weight (or mass) to the nearest 0.02–0.05kg (20–50 g), and knocks on the tank to signal the participant to surface.

9. The procedure is repeated 5–12 times, depending on the consistency of the values. The average of either the last two (or three) trials or the average of the two highest overall values is designated as the underwater weight (or mass).

10. The participant carefully exits the tank and dries off, which completes the test. The technician performs the required calculations, prepares the test results, and explains the results to the participant.

Many modifications of the hydrostatic method have focused on ways to make the participant more comfortable in the water without losing any of the accuracy from the traditional technique. The FRC and TLC methods are two examples. Another example is one that permits the person's head to remain above the water during the procedure.[20] Another modification eliminates the weight scale by having the participant grasp a 5.5 L plastic bottle to achieve neutral buoyancy in the measurement of body volume.[19] In general, it appears that modifications of the hydrodensitometry technique will continue to occur.

Calculations

The density of the body was shown to be a function of body mass per unit of body volume in Equation 26.1b. Body mass is determined simply by weighing the participant on land using an accurate scale. Body volume is more difficult to determine, but can be estimated through the use of Archimedes' principle by observing the difference between the body mass-in-air (BM_A) and the body mass-in-water (BM_W). This difference in mass, representing the mass of the water displaced, is divided by the density of the water (D_W) to determine the volume of the water displaced and thereby the body volume. The essential air (lung air and gastrointestinal gas) is then subtracted to yield the actual body volume, as seen in Equation 26.5a. The next step is to determine body density (D_B) by dividing the body mass by the terms representing the body volume, as seen in Equation 26.5b. The final step is to estimate the percent body fat using, in this case, the Siri equation (Eq. 26.5c).

$$\text{Body volume} = ((BM_A - BM_W) / D_W) - (RV_{BTPS} + V_{GI}) \quad \text{Eq. 26.5a}$$

$$D_B (g \cdot ml^{-1}) = BM_A / [((BM_A - BM_W) / D_W) - (RV_{BTPS} + V_{GI})] \quad \text{Eq. 26.5b}$$

Where: BM_A = Body mass$_{AIR}$ (g)
Where: BM_W = Body mass$_{WATER}$ (g)

Where: D_W = Water density (g·ml^{-1})

Where: RV_{BTPS} = Residual volume (ml)

Where: V_{GI} = Volume of gastrointestinal air (ml), *assumed to be 100 ml*

$$\text{\% Body fat} = (495 / D_B) - 450 \quad \text{Siri equation}[50] \quad \text{Eq. 26.5c}$$

To demonstrate these calculations, the following example is provided. A 30-year-old man with a body weight (BM_A) of 70 kg (70,000 g) has an immersed weight (BM_W) of 2.5 kg (2500 g) and a residual volume (RV_{BTPS}) of 1.15 liters (or 1150 ml). Body density is calculated in Equation 26.6a as 1.051 g·ml^{-1}, which translates into a percent body fat of about 21 % (Eq. 26.6b).

Assume: BM_A = **70,000** g; BM_W = **2500** g; D_W = **0.9950** g·ml^{-1}; RV_{BTPS} ml = **1150** ml

$$D_B = 70,000 / [((70,000 - 2500) / 0.9950) - (1150 + 100)] = 1.051 \text{ g·ml}^{-1} \quad \text{Eq. 26.6a}$$

$$\text{\% Body fat} = (495 / 1.051) - 450 = 20.9 \% \approx 21 \% \quad \text{Eq. 26.6b}$$

Combined with body weight, the percent body fat can be used to calculate the actual fat weight of the participant, which can then be used to determine the lean weight (Eq. 26.7a and 26.7b). In the example, fat weight is calculated as 21 % of the body weight (70.0 kg), which is 14.7 kg of fat (Eq. 26.7c). Removing 14.7 kg of fat from a body weight of 70.0 kg leaves 55.3 kg of lean weight (Eq. 26.7d).

$$\text{Fat weight} = \text{Body weight} * (\% \text{ Fat} / 100) \quad \text{Eq. 26.7a}$$

$$\text{Lean weight} = \text{Body weight} - \text{Fat weight} \quad \text{Eq. 26.7b}$$

Assume: Body wt (kg) = **70.0** kg; % Fat = **21%**

$$\text{Fat weight} = 70.0 \text{ kg} * (21\% / 100) = 70.0 * 0.21 = 14.7 \text{ kg} \quad \text{Eq. 26.7c}$$

$$\text{Lean weight} = 70.0 \text{ kg} - 14.7 \text{ kg} = 55.3 \text{ kg} \quad \text{Eq. 26.7d}$$

The values for percent body fat, fat weight, and lean weight can be evaluated based on data provided in Tables 26.2 and 26.3. A percent body fat of 21 % for a 30-year-old male is somewhat higher than the average adult male (17.7 %). If the man in our example was interested in losing weight and had a goal of reaching 17 % fat, to be slightly leaner than average, a body weight could be estimated that would make him 17 % fat. Theoretically, if lean weight is known, then fat weight can be added to yield an estimated total body weight at any particular percent body fat. This estimated body weight is determined by dividing the lean weight of the participant by (1.00 − (E % 100)), where E% is the desired percent body fat at which the body weight is being estimated (Eq. 26.8a). For the man in our example to reduce his percent body fat from 21 % to 17 %, he would need to slowly lose 3.4 kg of weight (assumed

Table 26.2 Mean Values for Body Composition Variables by Gender and Age

MALES Category	Method	M	Age (y) (Range)	Height (cm)	% Fat M ± SD	Body wt (kg)	Fat wt (kg)	Lean wt (kg)
Young boys (N = 58)[51]	Hydrostatic	15.8		172.2	14.7 ± 6.4	64.0	9.4	54.6
Young boys (N = 57)[21]	3 Compartment	16.7	(15–18)	174.2	15.6 ± 7.7	70.3	11.0	59.3
College athletes (N = 265)[23]	Hydrostatic	20.3		178.5	9.2 ± 4.4	75.7	7.0	68.7
College students (N = 312)[5]	Skinfolds	19.7	(18–25)	175.1	15.5 ± 6.0	75.9	11.8	64.1
Adult men (N = 308)[28]	Skinfolds	32.6	(18–61)	179.0	17.7 ± 8.0	74.8	13.2	61.6
Older men (N = 91)[61]	Hydrostatic	59.9	(34–84)	175.8	22.9 ± 6.5	77.8	17.8	60.0
Very old men (N = 35)[4]	Hydrostatic	74.1	(65–94)	171.0	25.0 ± 5.6	71.3	17.8	53.4

FEMALES Category	Method	M	Age (y) (Range)	Height (cm)	% Fat M ± SD	Body wt (kg)	Fat wt (kg)	Lean wt (kg)
Young girls (N = 59)[51]	Hydrostatic	15.3		167.7	25.4 ± 5.8	56.6	14.4	42.2
Young girls (N = 90)[22]	3 Compartment	15.6	(15–18)	162.7	30.4 ± 7.1	60.7	18.5	42.2
College athletes (N = 132)[48]	3 Compartment	20.4		166.4	20.4 ± 3.1	63.1	12.9	50.2
College students (N = 601)[5]	Skinfolds	19.4	(18–25)	162.7	24.5 ± 5.7	61.1	15.0	46.1
Adult women (N = 249)[30]	Skinfolds	31.4	(18–55)	165.0	24.1 ± 7.2	57.2	13.8	43.4
Older women (N = 116)[61]	Hydrostatic	58.0	(34–84)	162.2	32.3 ± 7.5	63.8	20.6	43.2
Very old women (N = 63)[4]	Hydrostatic	74.7	(65–94)	158.2	33.2 ± 7.4	59.1	19.6	39.5

Sources: Data from Baumgartner, et al. (1991)[4]; Beam (2005)[5]; Ellis (1997)[21]; Ellis, Abrams, & Wong (1997)[22]; Fornetti, Pivarnik, Foley, & Fiechtner (1999)[23]; Jackson & Pollock (1978)[28]; Jackson, Pollock, & Ward (1980)[30]; Sinning, et al.(1985)[48]; Slaughter, et al. (1988)[51]; Williams, et al.(1992).[61]

Table 26.3 Categories for Percent Body Fat Based on College Sport Participation, Gender and Age

Category	(Percentile)	Men					Women				
		College athletes	College[a] men	Adult[b] men	Older[c] men	Very old[d] men	College athletes	College[a] women	Adult[b] women	Older[c] women	Very old[d] women
"Very lean"	(> 95th %ile)	< 3	< 6	< 5	< 12	< 16	< 15	< 15	< 12	< 20	< 21
"Lean"	(75th–95th %ile)	3–6	6–11	5–12	12–18	17–21	16–18	16–21	13–19	21–27	22–28
"Average"	(25th–75th %ile)	7–12	12–20	13–23	19–27	22–29	19–23	22–28	20–29	28–37	29–38
"Overfat"	(5th–25th %ile)	13–16	21–25	24–31	28–34	30–34	24–26	29–34	30–36	39–45	39–45
"Obese"	(< 5th %ile)	> 16	> 25	> 31	> 34	> 34	> 26	> 34	> 36	> 45	> 45
Mean		9.2	15.5	17.7	22.9	25.0	20.4	24.5	24.1	32.3	33.2

Note: Values for percentiles are estimated using the reported means and standard deviations from the studies, assuming the data for all variables are normally distributed. Approximate ages, [a]18–24 y, [b]25–54 y, [c]55–74 y, [d]75 y.
Source: Data from Baumgartner, et al. (1991)[4]; Beam (2005)[5]; Fornetti, et al. (1999)[23]; Jackson & Pollock (1978)[28]; Jackson, Pollock & Ward (1980)[30]; Sinning, et al. (1985)[48]; Slaughter, et al. (1988)[51]; Williams, et al. (1992).[61]

to be fat weight if lost appropriately) and reduce his body weight from 70.0 kg to 66.6 kg (Eq. 26.8b). This method of estimating body weights at lower percent body fats is only valid if lean weight stays the same and any weight loss is due to a loss of fat. In many cases, however, lean weight is not held constant; it either decreases because of caloric restriction, or it increases as a result of resistance training, which invalidates the estimated weights. For this reason, if any significant weight loss is achieved, it is always better to remeasure the percent body fat following the weight loss to evaluate the composition of the weight loss.

Estimated body weight at E % fat = Lean weight
/ (1.00 − (E % / 100))   Eq. 26.8a

Estimated body weight at 17 % = 55.3 kg
/ (1.00 − 0.17) = 66.6 kg   Eq. 26.8b

RESULTS AND DISCUSSION

The hydrostatic weighing method is used to assess the body volume and subsequently the body density of a human. Once body density is determined, it is used to estimate percent body fat. Within the limitations of the method, hydrostatic weighing is considered to yield a more accurate estimate of percent body fat than anthropometric measures, including the measurement of girths and skinfold thicknesses. The mean values for numerous body composition variables are given in Table 26.2. Many of these studies assessed body fat by hydrostatic weighing, as indicated in the table. Hydrostatic weighing is based on the two-compartment model, where total body mass is divided into fat mass and fat-free mass. Other results in Table 26.2 are from studies that used a three-compartment model (a methodology that will be discussed in more detail shortly) or from studies that used skinfold thickness to assess body fat.

One trend observed in Table 26.2 is the effect of age on body composition. The percent body fat of males appears to stay relatively constant at about 15 % from adolescence (15–18 y) through young adulthood (25–30 y).[5,21,51] Over this same time, body weight increased by about 10 kg due to a nearly 10 kg increase in lean weight with little change in fat weight. A sample of male college athletes averaged 9.2 % body fat.[23] The mean percent body fat observed in a sample of older men (34–84 y)[61] increased to 22.9 % and in a sample of very old men (65–94 y),[4] to 25.0 %. Further comparison shows the very old men had the same amount of fat weight (17.8 kg) but had 6.6 kg less lean weight. In summary, it appears that body weight in men peaks in middle adulthood, then begins to decrease in late adulthood; fat weight peaks in middle adulthood and remains unchanged through later adulthood; and lean weight peaks in young adulthood, decreases slowly through middle adulthood, then decreases more rapidly in later adulthood. Remember, however, that these data are cross-sectional, and data collected longitudinally may not show the same trends. In general, many of these same trends are observed in women. Young women through early adulthood (35 y) average about 25 % body fat.[5,30,51] A study of female college athletes[48] reported a mean percent body fat of 20.4 %. The mean percent body fat observed in a sample of older women (34–84 y)[61] increased to 32.3 % and in a sample of very old women (65–94 y),[4] to 33.2 %.

Fat weight was similar between the two age groups, but the very old women possessed nearly 4 kg less lean weight.

Another consideration when comparing body composition results between different studies is the methodology used. Hydrostatic weighing was described earlier as a two-compartment (2C) method, where total body mass is divided into fat mass and fat-free mass, with assumed densities of 0.9007 $g \cdot ml^{-1}$ for fat tissue and 1.099–1.1000 $g \cdot ml^{-1}$ for fat-free tissue.[4,56] The two-compartment model also assumes that body hydration and bone mineral content are both stable. There is considerable debate, however, over the validity of these assumptions due to significant observed variations in densities of fat-free tissues, body hydration levels, and bone mineral content between genders, ages, and races.[4,21,22,46,61] The three-compartment model (3C) begins with total body densitometry (2C model) but then additionally measures total-body bone mineral (TBBM) content measured by dual-energy X-ray absorbtiometry (DXA). The four-compartment model (4C) further adds the measurement of total body water (TBW) by deuterium oxide dilution. The four compartments or components, then, of the 4C method are fat, mineral, water, and residual.

Several studies have used the 3C and 4C methods to create more valid equations for predicting percent body fat from body density and from anthropometric variables in persons differing by gender, age, and race.[4,21,22,46,61] Table 26.4 shows estimated percent body fat derived from the Siri[50] and Brozek[11] equations (generally used for all persons regardless of gender, age, or race), and percent

Table 26.4 Estimation of Percent Body Fat from Body Density by Different Equations

Source: Race: Gender: Equation:	Siri[50] General Both $495/D_B - 450$	Brozek[12] General Both $457/D_B - 414$	Lohman[35] General Young Women $509/D_B - 465$	Schutte[46] Afr-Amer Both $437/D_B - 393$	Ortiz[44] Afr- Amer Women $483/D_B - 437$	Range in % Fat Between Equations	Maximum Difference Between Equations
D_B (g·ml⁻¹)	% Fat	% Fat	% Fat	% Fat	% Fat	(%)	(%)
1.085	6	7	4	10	8	4–10	6
1.080	8	9	6	12	10	6–12	6
1.075	10	11	8	14	12	8–14	6
1.070	13	13	11	15	14	11–15	4
1.065	15	15	13	17	17	13–17	4
1.060	17	17	15	19	19	15–19	4
1.055	19	19	17	21	21	17–21	4
1.050	21	21	20	23	23	20–23	3
1.045	24	23	22	25	25	22–25	3
1.040	26	25	24	27	27	24–27	3
1.035	28	28	27	29	30	27–30	3
1.030	31	30	29	31	32	29–32	3
1.025	33	32	32	33	34	32–34	2
1.020	35	34	34	35	37	34–37	3
1.015	38	36	36	38	39	36–39	3
1.010	40	38	39	40	41	38–41	3
1.005	43	41	41	42	44	41–44	3
1.000	45	43	44	44	46	43–46	3

Sources: Equations from Siri (1961)[50]; Brozek et al. (1963)[12]; Lohman et al. (1984)[35]; Schutte et al. (1984)[46]; and Ortiz et al. (1992).[44]

What is the rationale for using hydrostatic weighing to determine body density and percent body fat?

Which weighs more, a kilogram of fat or a kilogram of muscle? Which occupies a greater volume?

What is Archimedes' principle and how does it relate to determining body density?

What is the effect of temperature on water density?

What is meant by essential GI and essential lung air?

What is meant by a two-, three-, and/or four-compartment model for predicting percent body fat?

What is the average percent fat in young (18–24 y) men and women? Does it differ in athletes?

What is the effect of aging on percent fat in men and women?

How is the estimation of percent body fat from body density affected by gender and race?

body fat derived for the same body density by three other equations assuming differences in the density of the fat-free tissues.[35,44,46] Differences in estimated percent body fats of up to 6 % are observed at the same body density. Aging results in losses of bone mineral, total body water, and total body protein, all resulting in a lower and more variable fat-free tissue density in elderly people.[4,61] In the case of differences in percent body fat observed in specific racial or ethnic groups, it is suspected that differences in bone mineral content and density,[18,21,22,46] muscle density,[46] and the density and mass of other lean tissues[21,22,42] explain most of the variability. It should be noted, however, that resistance-trained athletes in general, regardless of race, likely possess higher fat-free densities than untrained subjects.[42] For this reason, equations estimating percent body fat from body density should be corrected for those persons with denser fat-free tissues whether due to race or training status.

References

1. American College of Sports Medicine. (2000). *ACSM's guidelines for exercise testing and prescription* (p. 62). Philadelphia: Lippincott Williams & Wilkins.

2. Baker, P. T., & Angel, J. L. (1965). Old age changes in body density: Sex and race factors in the United States. *Human Biology, 37,* 104–119.

3. Bakker, H. K., & Struikenkamp, R. S. (1977). Biological variability and lean body mass estimates. *Human Biology, 49,* 187–202.

4. Baumgartner, R. N., Heymsfield, S. B., Lichtman, S., Wang, J., & Pierson, R. N. (1991). Body composition in elderly people: Effect of criterion estimates on predictive equations. *American Journal of Clinical Nutrition, 53,* 1345–1353.

5. Beam, W. (2005). Unpublished data.

6. Behnke, A. R., Feen, B. G., & Welham, A. C. (1942). The specific gravity of healthy men: Body weight divided by volume as an index of obesity. *JAMA: The Journal of the American Medical Association, 118,* 495–498.

7. Behnke, A. R., & Wilmore, J. H. (1974). *Evaluation and regulation of body build and composition.* Englewood Cliffs, NJ: Prentice-Hall.

8. Bonge, D., & Donnelly, J. E. (1989). Trials to criteria for hydrostatic weighing at residual volume. *Research Quarterly for Exercise and Sport, 60,* 176–179.

9. Brobek, J. R. (1968). Energy balance and food intake. In V. B. Mountcastle (Ed.), *Medical physiology* (pp. 498–519). St. Louis, MO: C. V. Mosby.

10. Brooks, G. A., Fahey, T. D., & White, T. P. (1996). *Exercise physiology: Human bioenergetics and its application.* Mountain View, CA: Mayfield.

11. Brozek, J., Grande, F., Anderson, J., & Keys, A. (1963). Densitometric analysis of body composition: Revision of some quantitative assumptions. *Annals of New York Academy of Science, 110,* 113–140.

12. Brozek, J., & Keys, A. (1951). The evaluation of leanness-fatness in man: Norms and intercorrelations. *British Journal of Nutrition, 5,* 194–205.

13. Bunt, J. C., Lohman, T. G., & Boileau, R. A. (1989). Impact of total body water fluctuations on estimation of body fat from body density. *Medicine and Science in Sports and Exercise, 21,* 96–100.

14. Bunt, J. C., Lohman, T. G., Slaughter, M. H., Boileau, R. A., Lussier, L., & Van Loan, M. (1983). Bone mineral content as a source of variation in body density in children and youth. *Medicine and Science in Sports and Exercise, 15* (Abstract), 172.

15. Buskirk, E., & Taylor, H. L. (1957). Maximal oxygen intake and its relation to body composition with special reference to chronic physical activity and obesity. *Journal of Applied Physiology, 11,* 72–78.

16. Byrd, P. J., & Thomas, T. R. (1983). Hydrostatic weighing during different stages of the menstrual cycle. *Research Quarterly for Exercise and Sport, 54,* 296–298.

17. Coffman, J. L., Timson, B. F., Beneke, W. M., & Paulsen, B. K. (1983). Measurement of body composition by hydrostatic weighing at residual volume and total lung capacity. *Medicine and Science in Sports and Exercise, 15* (Abstract), 172–173.

18. Cote, K. D., & Adams, W. C. (1993). Effect of bone density on body composition estimates in young adult black and white women. *Medicine and Science in Sports and Exercise, 25,* 290–296.

19. Denahan, T., Hortobagyl, T., & Katch, F. I. (1988). Validation of a new method of hydrostatic weighing. *Medicine and Science in Sports and Exercise, 20* (2 Suppl.), Abstract #44, S8.

20. Donnelly, J. E., Brown, T. E., Israel, R. G., Smith-Sintek, S., O'Brien, K. F., & Caslavka, B. (1988).

Hydrostatic weighing without head submersion: Description of a method. *Medicine and Science in Sports and Exercise, 20,* 66–69.

21. Ellis, K. J. (1997). Body composition of a young, multiethnic male population. *American Journal of Clinical Nutrition, 66,* 1323–1331.

22. Ellis, K. J., Abrams, S. A., & Wong, W. W. (1997). Body composition of a young, multiethnic female population. *American Journal of Clinical Nutrition, 65,* 724–731.

23. Fornetti, W. C., Pivarnik, J. M., Foley, J. M., & Fiechtner, J. J. (1999). Reliability and validity of body composition measures in female athletes. *Journal of Applied Physiology, 87,* 1114–1122.

24. Freund, B. J., Wilmore, J. H., Boyden, T. W., Stimi, W. A., & Harrington, R. J. (1984). Relationships of aerobic fitness and body composition measurements to bone density in post-menopausal women. *International Journal of Sports Medicine, 5,* 159.

25. Girandola, R. N., Wiswell, R. A., & Romero, G. T. (1977). Body composition changes resulting from fluid ingestion and dehydration. *Research Quarterly for Exercise and Sport, 48,* 299–303.

26. Heyward, V. H., & Stolarczyk, L. M. (1996). *Applied body composition assessment.* Champaign, IL: Human Kinetics.

27. Houtkooper, L. B., & Going, S. B. (1994). Body composition: How should it be measured? Does it affect sport performance? *Sports Science Exchange, 7*(5), 1–9.

28. Jackson, A. S., & Pollock, M. L. (1978). Generalized equations for predicting body density of men. *British Journal of Nutrition, 40,* 497–504.

29. Jackson, A. S., & Pollock, M. L. (1985). Practical assessment of body composition. *The Physician and Sportsmedicine, 15*(5), 76–80, 82–90.

30. Jackson, A. S., Pollock, M. L., & Ward, A. (1980). Generalized equations for predicting body density of women. *Medicine and Science in Sports and Exercise, 12,* 175–182.

31. Johansson, A. G., Forslund, A., Sjödin, A., Mallmin, H., Hambraeus, L., & Ljunghall, S. (1993). Determination of body composition of dual-energy X-ray absorptiometry and hydrodensitometry. *American Journal of Clinical Nutrition, 57,* 323–326.

32. Katch, F. I., & Katch, V. L. (1980). Measurement and prediction errors in body composition assessment and the search for the perfect equation. *Research Quarterly for Exercise and Sport, 51,* 249–260.

33. Kohrt, W. M., Malley, M. T., Dalsky, G. P., & Holloszy, J. O. (1992). Body composition of healthy sedentary and trained young and older men and women. *Medicine and Science in Sports and Exercise, 24,* 832–837.

34. Latin, R. W., & Ruhling, R. O. (1986). Total lung capacity, residual volume and predicted residual volume in a densitometric study of older men. *British Journal of Sports Medicine, 20* (2), 66–68.

35. Lohman, T. G., Slaughter, M. H., Boileau, R. A., Bunt, J., & Lussier, L. (1984). Bone mineral measurements and their relation to body density in children, youth, and adults. *Human Biology, 56,* 667.

36. Martin, A. D., Drinkwater, D. T., Clarys, J. P., & Ross, W. D. (1981). Estimation of body fat: A new look at some old assumptions. *The Physician and Sportsmedicine, 9,* 21–22.

37. McClenaghan, B. A., & Rocchis, L. (1986). Design and validation of an automated hydrostatic weighing system. *Medicine and Science in Sports and Exercise, 18,* 479–484.

38. McGarty, J. M., Butts, N. K., Hall, L. K., & Fletcher, R. A. (1983). Comparison of three hydrostatic weighing methods. *Medicine and Science in Sports and Exercise, 15,* (Abstract), 181.

39. Morrow, J. R., Jackson, A. S., Bradley, P. W., & Hartung, G. H. (1986). Accuracy of measured and predicted residual lung volume on body density measurement. *Medicine and Science in Sports and Exercise, 18,* 647–652.

40. Nash, H. L. (1985). Body fat measurement: Weighing the pros and cons of electrical impedance. *The Physician and Sportsmedicine, 13*(11), 124–128.

41. Nieman, D. C. (1995). *Fitness and sports medicine: A health-related approach.* Palo Alto, CA: Bull.

42. Nindl, B. C., Kraemer, W. J., Emmert, W. H., Mazzetti, S. A., Gotshalk, L. A., Putukian, M., Sebastianelli, W. J., & Patton, J. F. (1998). Comparison of body composition assessment among lean black and white male collegiate athletes. *Medicine and Science in Sports and Exercise, 30,* 769–776.

43. Organ, L. W., Eklund, A. D., & Ledbetter, J. D. (1994). An automated real time underwater weighing system. *Medicine and Science in Sports and Exercise, 26,* 383–391.

44. Ortiz, O., Russel, M., Daley, T. L., Baumgartner, R.N., Waki, M., Lichtman, S., Wang, J., Pierson, R.N., & Heymsfield, S. B. (1992). Differences in skeletal muscle and bone mineral mass between black and white females and their relevance to estimates of body composition. *American Journal of Clinical Nutrition, 55,* 8–13.

45. Quatrochi, J. A., Hicks, V. L., Heyward, V. H., Colville, B. C., Cook, K. L., Jenkins, K. A., & Wilson, W. L. (1992). Relationship of optical density and skinfold measurements: Effects of age and level of body fatness. *Research Quarterly for Exercise and Sport, 63,* 402–409.

46. Schutte, J., Townsend, E., Hugg, J., Shoup, R., Malina, R., & Blomqvist, G. (1984). Density of lean body mass is greater in Blacks than in Whites. *Journal of Applied Physiology, 56,* 1647–1649.

47. Schutte, J. E., Longhurst, J. C., Gaffney, F. A., Bastian, B. C., & Blomqvist, C. G. (1981). Total plasma

creatinine: An accurate measure of total striated muscle mass. *Journal of Applied Physiology, 51,* 762–766.

48. Sinning, W. E., Dolny, D. G., Little, K. D., Cunningham, L. N., Racaniello, A., Siconolfi, S. F., & Sholes, J. L. (1985). Validity of "generalized" equations for body composition in male athletes. *Medicine and Science in Sports and Exercise, 17,* 124–130.

49. Siri, W. E. (1956). The gross composition of the body. *Advances in Biological Medical Physiology, 4,* 239–280.

50. Siri, W. E. (1961). *Body composition from fluid spaces and density: Analysis of methods in techniques for measuring body composition* (pp. 223–244). Washington, DC: National Academy of Science, National Research Council.

51. Slaughter, M. H., Lohman, T. G., Boileau, R. A., Horswill, C. A., Stillman, R. J., Van Loan, M. D., & Bemben, D. A. (1988). Skinfold equations for estimation of body fatness in children and youth. *Human Biology, 60,* 709–723.

52. Snead, D. B., Birge, S. J., & Kohrt, W. M. (1993). Age-related differences in body composition by hydrodensitometry and dual-energy X-ray absorptiometry. *Journal of Applied Physiology, 74,* 770–775.

53. Thomas, T. R., & Etheridge, G. L. (1980). Hydrostatic weighing at residual volume and functional residual capacity. *Journal of Applied Physiology: Respiratory, Environmental and Exercise Physiology, 49,* 157–159.

54. Timson, B. F., & Coffman, J. L. (1984). Body composition by hydrostatic weighing at total lung capacity and residual volume. *Medicine and Science in Sports and Exercise, 16,* 411–414.

55. Trotter, M., Broman, G. E., & Peterson, R. R. (1959). Density of cervical vertebrae and comparison with densities of other bones. *American Journal of Physical Anthropology, 17,* 19–25.

56. van der Ploeg, G., Gunn, S., Wither, R., & Modra, A. (2003). Use of anthropometric variables to predict relative body fat determined by a four-compartment body composition model. *European Journal of Clinical Nutrition, 57,* 1009–1016.

57. Wagner, D. R., & Heyward, V. H. (1999). Techniques of body composition assessment: A review of laboratory and field methods. *Research Quarterly for Exercise and Sport, 70,* 135–149.

58. Ward, A., Pollock, M. L., Jackson, A. S., Ayres, J. J., & Pape, G. (1978). A comparison of body fat determined by underwater weighing and volume displacement. *American Journal of Physiology, 234,* E94–E96.

59. Weltman, A., & Katch, V. (1981). Comparison of hydrostatic weighing at residual volume and total lung capacity. *Medicine and Science in Sports and Exercise, 13,* 210–213.

60. Williams, L., & Davis, J. A. (1987). Influence of functional residual capacity methodology on body fat determined by hydrostatic weighing. *International Journal of Sports Medicine, 8* (Abstract), 243.

61. Williams, D., Going, S., Lohman, T., Hewitt, M., & Haber, A. (1992). Estimation of body fat from skinfold thicknesses in middle-aged and older men and women: A multiple component approach. *American Journal of Human Biology, 4,* 595–605.

62. Wilmore, J. H. (1969). The use of actual, predicted, and constant residual volumes in the assessment of body composition by underwater weighing. *Medicine and Science in Sports and Exercise, 1,* 87–90.

63. Wilmore, J. H. (1980). A simplified method for determination of residual volume. *Journal of Applied Physiology, 27,* 96–100.

Form 26.1

NAME _____ **DATE** _____ **SCORE** _____

HYDROSTATIC WEIGHING

Homework

Gender: **M**   Initials: **AA**   Age (y): **24**   Height (cm): **178**   Weight (kg): **90.6**

BM_A = _____ kg * 1000 = _____ g VC_{BTPS} = **4750** ml or RV_{BTPS} = _____ ml
       Body wt   Measured

BM_W = **4.150** kg * 1000 = _____ g RV_{BTPS} = _____ * 0.24 = _____ ml
                                           VC_{BTPS} Estimated

T_W = **32** °C D_W = _____ g·ml^{-1} Gastrointestinal (GI) air = **100** ml

D_{Body} = [_____ g] / [((_____ g − _____ g) / _____ g·ml^{-1}) − (_____ ml + 100 ml)]
          BM_A BM_A BM_W D_W RV_{BTPS}

D_{Body} = _____ g·ml^{-1} % Fat (Siri) = (495 / _____) − 450 = _____ %
                                                  D_{Body}

Fat wt (kg) = _____ kg * _____ /100 = _____ kg   Lean wt (kg) = _____ − _____ = _____ kg
          Body wt   % Fat   Body wt   Fat wt

Athlete (Y/N): **N**   Comparison: **College men**   Category (*Table 26.3*) _____

Preferred % fat = **11** %   Est'd wt at _____ % fat = _____ kg / (1 − (_____ / 100)) = _____ kg
                                           Lean wt   Pref % fat

Evaluation _____

Gender: **F**   Initials: **BB**   Age (y): **22**   Height (cm): **166**   Weight (kg): **64.9**

BM_A = _____ kg * 1000 = _____ g VC_{BTPS} = **3300** ml or RV_{BTPS} = _____ ml
       Body wt   Measured

BM_W = **1.750** kg * 1000 = _____ g RV_{BTPS} = _____ * 0.28 = _____ ml
                                           VC_{BTPS} Estimated

T_W = **32** °C D_W = _____ g·ml^{-1} Gastrointestinal (GI) air = **100** ml

D_{Body} = [_____ g] / [((_____ g − _____ g) / _____ g·ml^{-1}) − (_____ ml + 100 ml)]
          BM_A BM_A BM_W D_W RV_{BTPS}

D_{Body} = _____ g·ml^{-1} % Fat (Lohman) = (509 / _____) − 465 = _____ %
                                                  D_{Body}

Fat wt (kg) = _____ kg * _____ /100 = _____ kg   Lean wt (kg) = _____ − _____ = _____ kg
          Body wt   % Fat   Body wt   Fat wt

Athlete (Y/N): **N**   Comparison: **College women**   Category (*Table 26.3*) _____

Preferred % fat = **21** %   Est'd wt at _____ % fat = _____ kg / (1 − (_____ / 100)) = _____ kg
                                           Lean wt   Pref % fat

Evaluation _____

Form 26.2

HYDROSTATIC WEIGHING

Lab Results

Gender: **M**   Initials: _____   Age (y): _____   Height (cm): _____   Weight (kg): _____

BM_A = _____ kg * 1000 = _____ g VC_{BTPS} = _____ ml or RV_{BTPS} = _____ ml
<u>Body wt</u>   Measured

BM_W = _____ kg * 1000 = _____ g RV_{BTPS} = _____ * 0.24 = _____ ml
<u>VC_{BTPS}</u>   Estimated

T_W = _____ °C D_W = _____ g·ml^{-1} Gastrointestinal (GI) air = **100** ml

D_{Body} = [_____ g] / [((_____ g – _____ g) / _____ g·ml^{-1}) – (_____ ml + 100 ml)]
<u>BM_A</u>   <u>BM_A</u>   <u>BM_W</u>   <u>D_W</u>   <u>RV_{BTPS}</u>

D_{Body} = _____ g·ml^{-1} % Fat (Siri) = (495 / _____) – 450 = _____ %
<u>D_{Body}</u>

Fat wt (kg) = _____ kg * _____ /100 = _____ kg   Lean wt (kg) = _____ – _____ = _____ kg
<u>Body wt</u>   <u>% Fat</u>   <u>Body wt</u>   <u>Fat wt</u>

Athlete (Y/N): _____   Comparison: _____   Category *(Table 26.3)* _____

Preferred % fat = _____ %   Est'd wt at _____ % fat = _____ kg / (1 – (_____ / 100)) = _____ kg
<u>Lean wt</u>   <u>Pref % fat</u>

Evaluation _____

_____

Gender: **F**   Initials: _____   Age (y): _____   Height (cm): _____   Weight (kg): _____

BM_A = _____ kg * 1000 = _____ g VC_{BTPS} = _____ ml or RV_{BTPS} = _____ ml
<u>Body wt</u>   Measured

BM_W = _____ kg * 1000 = _____ g RV_{BTPS} = _____ * 0.28 = _____ ml
<u>VC_{BTPS}</u>   Estimated

T_W = _____ °C D_W = _____ g·ml^{-1} Gastrointestinal (GI) air = **100** ml

D_{Body} = [_____ g] / [((_____ g – _____ g) / _____ g·ml^{-1}) – (_____ ml + 100 ml)]
<u>BM_A</u>   <u>BM_A</u>   <u>BM_W</u>   <u>D_W</u>   <u>RV_{BTPS}</u>

D_{Body} = _____ g·ml^{-1} % Fat (Lohman) = (509 / _____) – 465 = _____ %
<u>D_{Body}</u>

Fat wt (kg) = _____ kg * _____ /100 = _____ kg   Lean wt (kg) = _____ – _____ = _____ kg
<u>Body wt</u>   <u>% Fat</u>   <u>Body wt</u>   <u>Fat wt</u>

Athlete (Y/N): _____   Comparison: _____   Category *(Table 26.3)* _____

Preferred % fat = _____ %   Est'd wt at _____ % fat = _____ kg / (1 – (_____ / 100)) = _____ kg
<u>Lean wt</u>   <u>Pref % fat</u>

Evaluation _____

_____

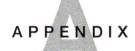

APPENDIX A

EXERCISE RISK ASSESSMENT

Name _____ Gender _____ Age _____

Email address _____

Phone _____

Please provide the following information as accurately and completely as possible so that it can be used to assess your cardiovascular exercise risk.

KNOWN CARDIOVASCULAR, PULMONARY, OR METABOLIC DISEASE

Have you been diagnosed with any of the following diseases/disorders/conditions or undergone any of the following procedures?

☐ Yes ☐ No   Myocardial infarction ("heart attack") _____

☐ Yes ☐ No   Stroke or ischemic attack ("mini-stroke") _____

☐ Yes ☐ No   Heart bypass surgery or other heart surgery _____

☐ Yes ☐ No   Coronary catheterization and/or angioplasty _____

☐ Yes ☐ No   Abnormal ECG (tachycardia, heart block, etc.) _____

☐ Yes ☐ No   Other cardiovascular disease/disorder (aneurysm, etc.) _____

☐ Yes ☐ No   Chronic obstructive lung disease (asthma, COPD, etc.) _____

☐ Yes ☐ No   Diabetes (insulin dependent, non-insulin dependent) _____

☐ Yes ☐ No   Hyperlipidemia (high LDL, low HDL, etc.) _____

Comment: _____

_____

_____

SIGNS OR SYMPTOMS SUGGESTIVE OF CARDIOVASCULAR AND PULMONARY DISEASE

Have you experienced any of the following?

☐ Yes ☐ No   Pain/discomfort in your chest, jaw, or arms _____

☐ Yes ☐ No   Shortness of breath at rest or mild exertion _____

☐ Yes ☐ No   Dizziness or fainting spells _____

☐ Yes ☐ No   Difficulty breathing while lying down _____

☐ Yes ☐ No   Swelling of your ankles _____

☐ Yes ☐ No   Skipped heartbeats or a racing heartbeat _____

☐ Yes ☐ No   Occasional leg pain, especially while walking _____

☐ Yes ☐ No   Heart murmur _____

☐ Yes ☐ No   Fatigue or shortness of breath with usual activities _____

Comment: _____

_____

_____

RISK FACTORS OF CARDIOVASCULAR DISEASE

Do you have a personal history of any of the following?

☐ Yes ☐ No   Cigarette smoking: packs/day _____, years smoked _____

☐ Yes ☐ No   Obese or highly overweight: body weight _____

☐ Yes ☐ No   Physical inactivity: _____

☐ Yes ☐ No   High blood pressure (SBP > 140, DBP > 90), BP _____ mm Hg

☐ Yes ☐ No   High cholesterol (total > 200, LDL > 130): total _____ , LDL _____ mg/dl

☐ Yes ☐ No   Diabetes or high blood glucose (> 110): blood glucose _____ mg/dl

☐ Yes ☐ No   Family history of heart attack/stroke at young age: _____

Comment: _____

_____

_____

DRUGS/MEDICATIONS

Please list any prescription or over-the-counter drugs/medications you are currently taking.

Drug/medication   **Purpose/reason for taking**

_____   _____

_____   _____

_____   _____

CLASSIFICATION OF EXERCISE RISK (*ACSM GUIDELINES*)

☐ **Low Risk:** Free of cardiovascular, pulmonary, and metabolic disease; and free of any signs or symptoms of cardiovascular disease; and possess no more than 1 major risk factor of cardiovascular disease; and male ≤ 45 y, female ≤ 55 y

☐ **Moderate Risk (age):** Free of cardiovascular, pulmonary, and metabolic disease; and free of any signs or symptoms of cardiovascular disease; and possess no more than 1 major risk factor of cardiovascular disease; and male > 45 y, female > 55 y

☐ **Moderate Risk (risk factors):** Free of cardiovascular, pulmonary, and metabolic disease; free of any signs or symptoms of cardiovascular disease; regardless of age; possess 2 or more major risk factors of cardiovascular disease

☐ **High Risk:** Regardless of age; diagnosed with cardiovascular, pulmonary, or metabolic disease; or possess any one or more signs or symptoms of cardiovascular disease

Participants in the *low risk* category can participate in maximal intensity exercise with little risk of cardiovascular problems (e.g., arrhythmia, etc.). It is not necessary that they get medical clearance before participating in exercise or any lab test.

Participants in the *moderate risk* category have a somewhat higher risk of experiencing cardiovascular problems with vigorous (60 % $\dot{V}O_2max$) to maximal exercise intensity. ACSM recommends anyone in the moderate risk category get medical clearance before vigorous exercise. Lower intensity exercise (< 60 % $\dot{V}O_2max$) poses less cardiovascular risk and can be done without prior medical clearance.

ACSM recommends that participants in the *high risk* category get medical clearance before participating in any type of exercise test or exercise program.

Reference: American College of Sports Medicine. (2010). *ACSM's guidelines for exercise testing and prescription* (8th ed.). Philadelphia: Lippincott Williams & Wilkins.

IN CASE OF EMERGENCY

Name _____   Phone _____

PAR-Q & YOU

(A Questionnaire for People Aged 15 to 69)

Regular physical activity is fun and healthy, and increasingly more people are starting to become more active every day. Being more active is very safe for most people. However, some people should check with their doctor before they start becoming much more physically active.

If you are planning to become much more physically active than you are now, start by answering the seven questions in the box below. If you are between the ages of 15 and 69, the PAR-Q will tell you if you should check with your doctor before you start. If you are over 69 years of age, and you are not used to being very active, check with your doctor.

Common sense is your best guide when you answer these questions. Please read the questions carefully and answer each one honestly: check YES or NO.

YES	NO	
☐	☐	**1. Has your doctor ever said that you have a heart condition <u>and</u> that you should only do physical activity recommended by a doctor?**
☐	☐	**2. Do you feel pain in your chest when you do physical activity?**
☐	☐	**3. In the past month, have you had chest pain when you were not doing physical activity?**
☐	☐	**4. Do you lose your balance because of dizziness or do you ever lose consciousness?**
☐	☐	**5. Do you have a bone or joint problem (for example, back, knee or hip) that could be made worse by a change in your physical activity?**
☐	☐	**6. Is your doctor currently prescribing drugs (for example, water pills) for your blood pressure or heart condition?**
☐	☐	**7. Do you know of <u>any other reason</u> why you should not do physical activity?**

If you answered

YES to one or more questions

Talk with your doctor by phone or in person BEFORE you start becoming much more physically active or BEFORE you have a fitness appraisal. Tell your doctor about the PAR-Q and which questions you answered YES.

- You may be able to do any activity you want — as long as you start slowly and build up gradually. Or, you may need to restrict your activities to those which are safe for you. Talk with your doctor about the kinds of activities you wish to participate in and follow his/her advice.
- Find out which community programs are safe and helpful for you.

NO to all questions

If you answered NO honestly to <u>all</u> PAR-Q questions, you can be reasonably sure that you can:
- start becoming much more physically active — begin slowly and build up gradually. This is the safest and easiest way to go.
- take part in a fitness appraisal — this is an excellent way to determine your basic fitness so that you can plan the best way for you to live actively. It is also highly recommended that you have your blood pressure evaluated. If your reading is over 144/94, talk with your doctor before you start becoming much more physically active.

DELAY BECOMING MUCH MORE ACTIVE:
- if you are not feeling well because of a temporary illness such as a cold or a fever — wait until you feel better; or
- if you are or may be pregnant — talk to your doctor before you start becoming more active.

PLEASE NOTE: If your health changes so that you then answer YES to any of the above questions, tell your fitness or health professional. Ask whether you should change your physical activity plan.

<u>Informed Use of the PAR-Q</u>: The Canadian Society for Exercise Physiology, Health Canada, and their agents assume no liability for persons who undertake physical activity, and if in doubt after completing this questionnaire, consult your doctor prior to physical activity.

No changes permitted. You are encouraged to photocopy the PAR-Q but only if you use the entire form.

NOTE: If the PAR-Q is being given to a person before he or she participates in a physical activity program or a fitness appraisal, this section may be used for legal or administrative purposes.

"I have read, understood and completed this questionnaire. Any questions I had were answered to my full satisfaction."

NAME _____

SIGNATURE _____ DATE_____

SIGNATURE OF PARENT _____ WITNESS _____
or GUARDIAN (for participants under the age of majority)

Note: This physical activity clearance is valid for a maximum of 12 months from the date it is completed and becomes invalid if your condition changes so that you would answer YES to any of the seven questions.

 © Canadian Society for Exercise Physiology   Supported by: Health   Santé
                                                                                          Canada Canada   continued on other side...

Source: Physical Activity Readiness Questionnaire (PAR-Q) © 2002. Reprinted with permission from the Canadian Society for Exercise Physiology. http://www.csep.ca.

PAR-Q & YOU

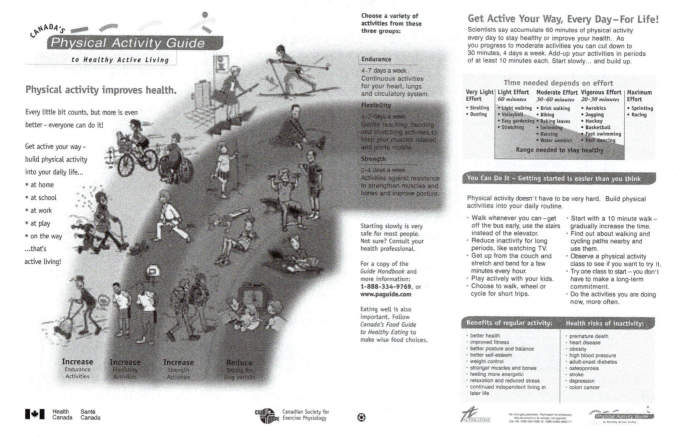

Source: Canada's Physical Activity Guide to Healthy Active Living, Health Canada, 1998 http://www.hc-sc.gc.ca/hppb/paguide/pdf/guideEng.pdf.
© Reproduced with permission from the Minister of Public Works and Government Services Canada, 2002.

FITNESS AND HEALTH PROFESSIONALS MAY BE INTERESTED IN THE INFORMATION BELOW:

The following companion forms are available for doctors' use by contacting the Canadian Society for Exercise Physiology (address below):

The **Physical Activity Readiness Medical Examination (PARmed-X)** – to be used by doctors with people who answer YES to one or more questions on the PAR-Q.

The **Physical Activity Readiness Medical Examination for Pregnancy (PARmed-X for Pregnancy)** – to be used by doctors with pregnant patients who wish to become more active.

References:
Arraix, G.A., Wigle, D.T., Mao, Y. (1992). Risk Assessment of Physical Activity and Physical Fitness in the Canada Health Survey
    Follow-Up Study. **J. Clin. Epidemiol.** 45:4 419-428.
Mottola, M., Wolfe, L.A. (1994). Active Living and Pregnancy, In: A. Quinney, L. Gauvin, T. Wall (eds.), **Toward Active Living: Proceedings of the International
    Conference on Physical Activity, Fitness and Health**. Champaign, IL: Human Kinetics.
PAR-Q Validation Report, British Columbia Ministry of Health, 1978.
Thomas, S., Reading, J., Shephard, R.J. (1992). Revision of the Physical Activity Readiness Questionnaire (PAR-Q). **Can. J. Spt. Sci.** 17:4 338-345.

For more information, please contact the:

Canadian Society for Exercise Physiology
202-185 Somerset Street West
Ottawa, ON K2P 0J2
Tel. 1-877-651-3755 • FAX (613) 234-3565
Online: www.csep.ca

The original PAR-Q was developed by the British Columbia Ministry of Health. It has been revised by an Expert Advisory Committee of the Canadian Society for Exercise Physiology chaired by Dr. N. Gledhill (2002).

Disponible en français sous le titre «Questionnaire sur l'aptitude à l'activité physique - Q-AAP (revisé 2002)».

 © Canadian Society for Exercise Physiology

Supported by: Health Santé
Canada Canada

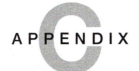

INFORMED CONSENT FOR PARTICIPATING IN EXERCISE PHYSIOLOGY LABORATORY

EXPLANATION OF THE GRADED (PROGRESSIVE) EXERCISE TEST

You will perform a graded exercise test on a cycle ergometer and/or treadmill. The exercise intensity will increase each 2 to 4 minutes. Depending on your heart rate or other symptoms and variables, you may continue to work harder or the test will end. We may stop the test at any time because of signs of fatigue or discomfort. Also, you may stop the test for any reason at any time.

EXPLANATION OF OTHER TESTS

You will also perform several other tests, including evaluations of your muscular strength, anaerobic power, body composition, pulmonary function, blood pressure, and flexibility.

RISKS AND DISCOMFORTS

The possibility does exist that certain changes will occur during the graded exercise test. They include abnormal blood pressure, fainting, disorders of heartbeat, and, in very rare instances, heart attack or death. Every effort will be made to minimize the risk of these changes through preliminary screening and by observation during the testing. Emergency procedures and trained laboratory personnel are available to deal with any unusual situations that may arise. All of the other tests involve minimal risk but could result in muscle strains, respiratory difficulties, and light-headedness. Psychological distress is possible when performing these tests in front of your student peers and the instructor. Although informed consents contain statements indicating the confidentiality of test results, this Informed Consent for Participating in Exercise Physiology Laboratory states that not only is it difficult in an instructional setting to keep test data confidential, but confidentiality may minimize learning. Discussing freely the individual and group data enhances the visualization, personalization, and retention of information. Therefore, confidentiality cannot be guaranteed in most instances.

Please inform the instructor of your present health status, medications, or former symptoms of concern associated with the tests mentioned within this Informed Consent, Course Syllabus (Outline), or *Exercise Physiology Laboratory Manual*. Symptoms of special importance are those related to your heart, such as pain in the chest, neck, jaw, back, and arms, or shortness of breath. Report symptoms immediately upon their occurrence during the test. The Physical Activity Readiness Questionnaire (PAR-Q) form is a popular questionnaire that can guide you and the laboratory personnel toward a safe test.

BENEFITS TO BE EXPECTED

The results obtained from the graded exercise test and related tests will assist in the assessment of your current level of physical fitness. You will learn how it feels to perform these tests and how to administer them, in addition to learning how to interpret them.

INQUIRIES

Any questions about the procedures used in the exercise tests are encouraged. If you have any doubts or questions, please ask for further explanations.

FREEDOM OF CONSENT

Your permission to perform the tests is voluntary. We will work together toward making an effort to find a substitute assignment for any of the tests you do not feel comfortable in performing.

"I have read this form and I understand the test procedures that I will perform. I freely consent to participate voluntarily in all of the described laboratory tests."

_____   _____

(Signature of Participant)   (Date)

_____   _____

(Witness)   (Date)

INDEX

Note: Page numbers with *f* indicate figures, page numbers with *t* indicate tables, page numbers with *b* indicate boxes, page numbers with *n* indicate notes.

hydrostatic weighing, 310,
    312–313, 312*t*
isotonic strength tests, 40–41
Maximal Oxygen Consumption
    (Vo$_2$ max) Test, 170–175, 171*f*,
    172*t*, 173*t*, 175*t*
resting lung volume tests, 237–240,
    238*t*
skinfold measurements, 300*b*
waist-to-height ratio, 286
waist-to-hip ratio, 286
calibration
    calipers, 295*b*
    cycle ergometers, 146*b*
    electrocardiograph, 214*b*
    handgrip dynamometers, 49*b*
    isokinetic dynamometers, 58*b*
    isotonic strength test equipment, 36
    metabolic measurement
        equipment, 166*b*
    metronomes, 137*b*
    platform scales, 23*b*
    sphygmomanometers, 186*b*,
        187, 187*f*
    spirometers, 235*b*
calibration syringe, 166, 166*f*
calipers, 293, 294, 294*b*, 295*b*
caloric expenditure, 12, 174, 175*t*
calorimetry, 4, 12
Canadian SR Test, 262, 263, 264,
    264*t*, 268
Canadian Standardization Test, 7
carbon dioxide analyzers
    exercise ventilation tests, 252, 252*b*
    hydrostatic weighing, 308
    maximal oxygen consumption
        (Vo$_2$ max), 165*f*, 166, 166*b*
carbon dioxide (F$_E$CO$_2$), 165–167,
    165*f*, 171*f*, 172–174
cardiac output (Q), 197–198,
    198*f*, 198*t*
cardiorespiratory endurance, 2
cardiorespiratory system, 163
cardiovascular disease (CVD)
    blood pressure, 183
    exercise electrocardiogram (ECG)
        tests, 215, 219–220, 220*b*, 221,
        226, 227
    Exercise Risk Assessment form,
        317–318
    fat distribution and percentage, 281
    girth measurements, 286, 287–288
    resting blood pressure
        measurement, 190
    systolic blood pressure, 197
    total peripheral resistance and, 198

cardiovascular fitness. *See* aerobic
    fitness
categorization scores, 7, 7*t*
Caucasians. *See* whites
Celsius, Anders, 5
celsius scale, 5, 13, 13*f*
centimeters (cm), 11
CF (correction factor), 172, 172*t*,
    239–240, 239*t*
Chatillon scales, 306–307, 306*f*, 308
CHD (coronary heart disease). *See*
    cardiovascular disease
chest leads, 211, 211*f*, 212*f*
chest skinfold measurements, 296,
    296*f*, 298*t*, 299*t*
Chester Step Test, 141
children
    flexibility, 261
    girth measurements, 287
    hydrostatic weighing, 307*b*
    one repetition maximum, 33
    sit-and-reach (SR) tests, 268, 268*t*
    skinfold measurements, 298, 300*b*
chondromalacia patellae, 60, 61*f*
chronic disease, 273, 275, 286, 287
chronic obstructive pulmonary disease
    (COPD), 243
circumference measurements. *See*
    girth measurements
CKCE (closed kinetic chain
    exercise), 56
clinical populations
    12-lead electrocardiograph, 211
    aerobic cycling tests, 154
    aerobic step tests, 141
    exercise electrocardiogram (ECG)
        tests, 219
    rate-pressure product, 202, 203*t*
closed kinetic chain exercise
    (CKCE), 56
CMJ (counter movement jump),
    83–84, 84*b*
coasting, 74
college-age persons
    absolute and relative strength of,
        41, 41*t*, 42*t*
    aerobic run/jog/walk tests, 129*t*
    anaerobic step tests, 112, 113*t*
    anaerobic treadmill tests, 120, 120*t*
    fat percentage, 311*t*, 312
    George Jog Test, 125
    knee extension and flexion, 62
    sprint tests, 76–77, 76*t*, 77*t*
Collins 9 L Vitalometer, 234
comparative scores, 7
construct validity, 7

content validity, 7
cool-down
    aerobic cycling tests, 152
    aerobic step tests, 138
    anaerobic treadmill tests, 118, 118*t*
    sprint tests, 75
    Wingate Anaerobic Test, 98, 98*t*, 99
Cooper, Kenneth, 125
Cooper Run Test, 125–134
    accuracy of, 126*b*
    forms, 130–131
    methods and procedures, 126–128,
        127*f*, 127*t*, 128*t*
    rationale for, 125
    results and discussion, 130
COPD (chronic obstructive pulmonary
    disease), 243
coronary heart disease. *See*
    cardiovascular disease
correction factor (CF), 172, 172*t*,
    239–240, 239*t*
correlation, 5, 6
correlation coefficient, 5, 6
counter movement jump (CMJ),
    83–84, 84*b*
CP (creatine phosphate), 47, 73, 74
creatine phosphate (CP), 47, 73,
    74, 96
criterion validity, 6–7
cross-sectional data, 24–25
cuff manometry
    accuracy of, 199*b*
    exercise blood pressure
        measurement, 199
    resting blood pressure measurement,
        186–190, 186*b*, 186*f*, 187*f*,
        188*f*, 188*t*
CUNY (City University of New
    York), 135
customary (American) units of mea-
    sure, 10, 16
CVD. *See* cardiovascular disease
Cybex II, 57*b*, 58–59, 58*b*, 60*f*
cycle ergometers
    accuracy of, 96*b*, 146*b*
    aerobic cycling tests, 146*b*,
        147–148, 147*f*
    anaerobic cycling tests, 96*b*, 97, 97*f*
    calibration of, 146*b*
    electromagnetically braked, 148
    exercise blood pressure
        measurement, 197, 199–201, 200*f*,
        200*t*, 202
    exercise electrocardiogram (ECG)
        tests, 224, 225*t*
    exercise ventilation tests, 253*t*

mechanical rationale, 56, 56f
mechanically braked cycle ergometers, 147–148, 147f
mercury (mm Hg), 13, 184, 185
MET (metabolic equivalent), 201, 225–226, 226t
metabolic diseases, 317
metabolic equivalent (MET), 201, 225–226, 226t
metabolic measurement equipment, 165–167, 165f, 166b
metabolic syndrome, 287
metabolism, aerobic, 2, 163
meteorological balloons, 252b
meteorological conditions. See environmental conditions
meteorological units of measure, 12–13, 13f
meter (m), 11, 14t
meter-second, 14t
metric conversion, 14–16, 14t
metric units, 10–19
  decimal expression, 11, 11t
  measurement error, 15–16, 15f
  meteorological, 12–13
  for variables, 11–12
metronomes, 136, 137b, 148
Mexican-Americans. See Hispanics
midabdominal girth, 282–283, 282t, 284t, 286
mixing chambers, 165f, 167
Moderate Test (treadmill), 117, 118t
modified Bruce protocol, 224
moment of force, 12
Monark cycle ergometer, 97, 97f, 99–100, 99f, 147–148
mouthpiece, rubber, 166, 251
muscle, density of, 306
muscle fibers. See also fast-twitch (FT) fibers
  characteristics of, 55–56
  slow-twitch (ST) fibers, 55–56, 59, 96
  type distribution of, 59, 63, 63t, 64
muscle strains, 55
muscular endurance, 1, 2
muscular strength. See also absolute strength
  definition of, 1
  isokinetic, 55, 60–61
  isotonic, 33
  relative, 41, 41t, 42t, 49, 50t, 61, 62t, 63t
muscular strength tests, 1, 33
muscular strength tests, isokinetic, 55–72

accuracy of, 57b
forms, 69–72
methods and procedures, 57–60, 57f, 58b, 60f, 61f
rationale for, 56–57, 56f
results and discussion, 60–64, 62t, 63t
muscular strength tests, isometric
  accuracy of, 48b
  forms, 53–54
  methods and procedures, 47–49, 48f, 49f
  rationale for, 47
  results and discussion, 49–51, 50f, 50t
muscular strength tests, isotonic, 33–46
  calculations, 40–41
  directly measured 1 RM, 33, 37
  forms, 45–46
  indirectly measured 1 RM, 37–39, 38t, 39t
  methods and procedures, 34–41, 36f, 38t
  rationale for, 33–34
  results and discussion, 40t, 41–42, 41t, 42t
  work and mean power in, 39–41
MVV (maximal voluntary ventilation), 251–254, 252b, 252f, 255t, 256t
MW (MacRae and Wright) Test, 262, 267, 268
myocardial ischemia, 210f, 214, 221, 222, 223f, 227. See also cardiovascular disease
myosin-actin interactions, 74, 125
Myotest system, 84b

name (basic data collection), 20
National Center for Health Statistics, 275
National Heart, Lung, and Blood Institute (NHLBI), 191, 274, 275t, 287
National High Blood Pressure Education Program, 190, 191
National Institute of Standards and Technology, 10
National Institutes of Health (NIH), 273
National Strength and Conditioning Association, 33
Naughton protocol (treadmill), 224
Naval Health Research Center (NHRC), 281, 282b, 286
neck girth, 282–283, 282t, 284t, 285t, 286, 287
negative work, 40

newton meter (N-m), 12, 14t, 56
NFL-225 Test, 41–42
NHLBI (National Heart, Lung, and Blood Institute), 191, 274, 275t, 287
NHRC (Naval Health Research Center), 281, 282b, 286
NIH (National Institutes of Health), 273
nitrogen washout method, 237
nomogram, 7
nonessential air, 308
norms
  aerobic cycling tests, 154–155, 155t
  anaerobic treadmill tests, 119–120, 120t
  definition of, 7, 7t
  Maximal Oxygen Consumption (V_{O_2} max) Test, 165
  resting lung volume tests, 240
numbers, rounding off, 21

obesity
  BMI, 273, 274–276, 275t
  fat percentage, 286
  prevalence of, 273, 273f, 274t, 275
  waist-to-hip ratio, 287
objectivity, 5, 6f, 7
obstructive lung diseases, 234, 243, 243t
OKCE (open kinetic chain exercise), 56
older adults
  BMI, 273
  body composition, 300b, 313
  hydrostatic weighing, 307b, 312
  isokinetic strength tests, 55
  one repetition maximum and, 33
  Rockport Walk Test, 125
  self-reported height and weight, 21b
  skinfold measurements, 298, 300b
one repetition maximum (1 RM)
  accuracy of, 35b
  directly measured, 33, 37
  forms, 45–46
  indirectly measured, 33–34, 37–39, 38t, 39t
  rationale for, 33–34
  repetitions to fatigue and, 33–34, 34f, 41–42
  results and discussion, 40t, 41–42, 41t, 42t
1-Girth Method, 281
open kinetic chain exercise (OKCE), 56
Optojump system, 84–85, 84b
Ortiz equation, 312t